Organ System Crosstalk in Critical Illness

Denise Battaglini • Silvia De Rosa
Daniel Agustin Godoy
Editors

Organ System Crosstalk in Critical Illness

From Basic Pathophysiology to Clinical Management

Springer

Editors
Denise Battaglini
Department of Surgical Sciences
and Integrated Diagnostics
University of Genoa
Genoa, Italy

Silvia De Rosa
Centre for Medical Sciences-CISMed
University of Trento
Trento, Italy

Daniel Agustin Godoy
Unidad de Cuidados Neurointensivos,
Sanatorio Pasteur
Human Resources and Planning
(Government of Catamarca)
Catamarca, Argentina

ISBN 978-3-032-01023-0 ISBN 978-3-032-01024-7 (eBook)
https://doi.org/10.1007/978-3-032-01024-7

This Springer imprint is published by the registered company Springer Nature Switzerland AG
The registered company address is: Gewerbestrasse 11, 6330 Cham, Switzerland

Contents

Part I

General Aspects

Organ System Crosstalk in Critical Illness

1

Silvia De Rosa, Daniel Agustin Godoy,
and Denise Battaglini

1.1 Introduction

The human body operates as a finely tuned, interconnected system where constant communication between organs is crucial for maintaining physiological stability. This ongoing dialogue—referred to as *organ system crosstalk*—relies on a complex network of neuroendocrine, immune, metabolic, and vascular signals that help coordinate responses to both routine and extreme physiological demands [1] (Table 1.1).

In critical illness, this balance is often severely disrupted. When one organ begins to fail, it rarely does so in isolation. Instead, dysfunction can rapidly propagate across systems, creating a cascade that culminates in multi-organ failure [2]. Conditions like sepsis, acute respiratory distress syndrome (ARDS), acute kidney injury (AKI), and acute brain injury (ABI) highlight the systemic interdependence at play: what begins as a localized insult can quickly become a full-body crisis [2].

This concept is not just theoretical—it has direct implications for how we monitor, manage, and treat critically ill patients. Understanding how one organ's distress impacts others allows clinicians to recognize early warning signs and intervene before deterioration becomes irreversible. This chapter explores the physiological

S. De Rosa (✉)
Centre for Medical Sciences-CISMed, University of Trento, Trento, Italy

D. A. Godoy
Unidad de Cuidados Neurointensivos, Sanatorio Pasteur, Human Resources and Planning (Government of Catamarca), Catamarca, Argentina

D. Battaglini
Department of Surgical Sciences and Integrated Diagnostics, University of Genoa, Genoa, Italy

D. Battaglini et al. (eds.), *Organ System Crosstalk in Critical Illness*,
https://doi.org/10.1007/978-3-032-01024-7_1

Table 1.1 Key inter-organ crosstalk mechanisms in critical illness

Primary organ involved	Connected organs	Crosstalk mechanisms	Clinical consequences
Brain (ABI)	Gut, lungs, heart, kidneys, liver	Neuroinflammation, BBB dysfunction, dysbiosis, sympathetic overactivity	Gut paralysis, neurogenic pulmonary edema, AKI, liver dysfunction, worsened neurological status
Lungs (ARDS)	Heart, kidneys, liver, brain	Systemic hypoxia, cytokine release, endothelial dysfunction	Multiorgan failure, pulmonary hypertension, AKI, encephalopathy
Kidneys (AKI/CKD)	Heart, brain, liver, gut	Uremia, systemic inflammation, oxidative stress, intestinal barrier disruption	Cardiorenal syndrome, uremic encephalopathy, hepatic injury, dysbiosis
Liver (acute/chronic)	Heart, brain, kidneys, muscle, gut	Toxin accumulation, metabolic derangement, immune dysregulation	Hepatic encephalopathy, hepatorenal syndrome, sarcopenia, metabolic syndrome
Heart (MI, HF)	Kidneys, liver, muscle, spleen, adipose, gut	RAAS activation, cytokines, hypoperfusion, sympathetic drive	Cardiorenal syndrome, liver congestion, muscle wasting, systemic inflammation
Gut	Brain, liver, kidneys, lungs	Dysbiosis, increased permeability, endotoxemia	Sepsis, systemic inflammation, multiorgan dysfunction

Note. *ABI* acute brain injury, *ARDS* acute respiratory distress syndrome, *AKI* acute kidney Injury, *CKD* chronic kidney disease, *MI* myocardial infarction, *HF* heart failure, *RAAS* renin–angiotensin–aldosterone system, *BBB* blood–brain barrier.

and molecular foundations of organ crosstalk, emphasizing real-world clinical consequences and therapeutic considerations in the intensive care setting.

1.2 Mechanisms of Organ Crosstalk

1.2.1 Inflammation, Immunity, and Coagulation

Critical illness is frequently accompanied by a powerful and widespread inflammatory response. Central to this process is the release of key cytokines, including TNF-α, IL-1, IL-6, and IL-8, which act as primary drivers of systemic inflammation [3]. These mediators not only influence immune activity but also activate the endothelium and disrupt microvascular integrity. The resulting imbalance in vascular function and perfusion lays the groundwork for organ injury. Organs with high metabolic demand and delicate microcirculation—such as the kidneys, lungs, and liver—are particularly susceptible, often leading to clinical manifestations like AKI, ARDS, and hepatic dysfunction [4].

As the inflammatory response progresses, a paradoxical phase of immune suppression often follows. This secondary immunosuppression increases susceptibility to opportunistic and nosocomial infections and is a common challenge in prolonged critical illness. The shift reflects a complex interplay between organs—particularly the gut, lungs, and cardiovascular system—as frequently observed in septic shock. Dysbiosis, altered barrier function, and neurohumoral signaling all contribute to this immunological imbalance [5].

Inflammation also interfaces closely with coagulation. In conditions like sepsis and major trauma, systemic inflammatory signals trigger the coagulation cascade, resulting in widespread formation of microthrombi. These clots impair tissue perfusion, driving further organ dysfunction. At the same time, platelet activation and endothelial injury perpetuate a vicious cycle, reinforcing both inflammation and microvascular damage [6].

1.2.2 Neuroendocrine and Metabolic Crosstalk

The neuroendocrine system plays a central regulatory role in the body's response to critical illness. One of the key responses is activation of the hypothalamic–pituitary–adrenal (HPA) axis, which leads to the release of glucocorticoids [7]. These hormones help modulate the inflammatory response and maintain metabolic stability. At the same time, elevated levels of catecholamines—though vital for preserving blood pressure—often lead to excessive vasoconstriction, reducing perfusion to vulnerable organs like the kidneys and gastrointestinal tract. Activation of the renin–angiotensin–aldosterone system (RAAS) further complicates this picture by promoting sodium and water retention, contributing to volume overload and congestion, particularly affecting the heart and lungs [8].

In parallel, critical illness disrupts normal metabolic homeostasis. Stress-induced hyperglycemia and insulin resistance are common and can impair immune responses while promoting endothelial dysfunction [9]. The systemic stress response also accelerates muscle catabolism and alters nutrient utilization, leading to sarcopenia and diminished respiratory muscle strength—factors that can significantly delay recovery and complicate ventilator weaning and rehabilitation [10].

1.2.3 Oxygen Transport and Hypoxic Injury

Hypoxia is a common and often critical factor in the pathophysiology of severe illness, particularly in patients with ARDS or impaired systemic perfusion. Its effects are far-reaching and systemic. At the cellular level, oxygen is indispensable for mitochondrial oxidative phosphorylation—the primary pathway for adenosine triphosphate (ATP) production [11]. When oxygen delivery is compromised, mitochondrial efficiency declines, leading to reduced ATP generation. This cellular energy shortfall disrupts essential functions across organ systems, contributing to cellular dysfunction, injury, and eventually apoptosis [11].

In response, anaerobic metabolism becomes more prominent, resulting in the accumulation of lactic acid and the onset of metabolic acidosis. This acidotic state further hampers enzymatic processes, intensifies systemic inflammation, and impairs oxygen unloading from hemoglobin due to a leftward shift in the oxygen–hemoglobin dissociation curve, compounding tissue hypoxia.

The organs most vulnerable to systemic hypoxia include the heart, liver, and skeletal muscles. In the heart, reduced oxygen availability impairs myocardial contractility and promotes arrhythmias, undermining cardiac output and further compromising perfusion [12]. The liver, with its high metabolic demand, exhibits decreased detoxification capacity, impaired protein synthesis, and altered glucose regulation under hypoxic stress. In skeletal muscle, oxygen deprivation accelerates muscle wasting and weakness—frequently delaying weaning from mechanical ventilation and prolonging ICU recovery [13].

Beyond metabolic dysfunction, hypoxia exerts significant effects on immune regulation. Hypoxia-inducible factors (HIFs), activated under low-oxygen conditions, play a dual role by modifying cytokine expression, vascular permeability, and leukocyte behavior. This ties tissue hypoxia directly to immune dysregulation and endothelial dysfunction, further impairing microcirculatory flow and amplifying systemic inflammation [14].

Together, these processes—hypoxia, metabolic disruption, immune activation, and neuroendocrine stress—form a self-reinforcing cycle of inter-organ dysfunction. If not promptly interrupted, this cascade can progress to full-blown multi-organ failure. Early recognition and correction of hypoxia through strategies such as lung-protective ventilation, optimized oxygen delivery, and management of acidosis are therefore essential components of critical care, aimed at preventing irreversible organ damage and improving survival outcomes.

1.3 Crosstalk Between Brain and Other Organs

The brain is deeply interconnected with peripheral organs through a complex network of neural, hormonal, immune, and metabolic pathways. This bidirectional communication is fundamental to maintaining systemic homeostasis [15]. However, when the brain is injured—as in acute brain injury (ABI)—these same connections can drive widespread physiological disruption. The consequences are often systemic, with neuroinflammation, autonomic instability, and blood–brain barrier (BBB) dysfunction triggering a cascade of events that affect nearly every major organ [15].

One of the most prominent examples of this is the gut–brain axis. Following ABI, gastrointestinal motility slows, and intestinal permeability increases, promoting microbial dysbiosis [16]. This altered microbial environment perpetuates systemic inflammation and can even worsen neuronal injury. The production of short-chain fatty acids—key metabolites for gut integrity and immune modulation—is often impaired, weakening the mucosal barrier and blunting local immune defenses [17]. Clinical studies have shown a rapid decline in gut microbial diversity after ABI, with certain microbial profiles associated with poorer neurological outcomes [18].

The brain also communicates closely with the liver, primarily via autonomic and inflammatory pathways. In the aftermath of ABI, the liver plays a role in systemic immune regulation by producing acute-phase proteins such as serum amyloid A1, which can modulate microglial activity and influence the neuroimmune response [19]. However, this protective mechanism can be disrupted by metabolic stressors—for example, diets high in fructose may exacerbate hepatic inflammation, ultimately hindering cerebral recovery.

Kidney dysfunction is another common complication post-ABI. AKI may be driven by systemic inflammation, hormonal dysregulation, and BBB disruption. On the flip side, renal impairment can worsen neurological status through the buildup of uremic toxins and increased sympathetic activity—a phenomenon referred to as the *reno-cerebral reflex*. This feedback loop underscores how kidney-brain interactions can amplify injury in both systems [20].

The brain–lung axis is equally critical. Patients with ABI often experience impaired airway protection, leading to aspiration and complications like neurogenic pulmonary edema. Mechanical ventilation, while essential for respiratory support, must be carefully managed to avoid unintended effects on both cerebral dynamics and the composition of the lung and gut microbiome [21].

Cardiac function, too, is tightly linked to brain injury. Surges in catecholamines following ABI can result in arrhythmias, myocardial stunning, or even stress-induced cardiomyopathy (Takotsubo syndrome). Genetic variations in β-adrenergic receptors may modulate this susceptibility. Importantly, this heart–brain crosstalk can lead to reduced cerebral perfusion and elevated intracranial pressure (ICP), setting up a harmful feedback cycle [22].

Altogether, the intricate communication between the brain and other organs in the context of injury illustrates the need for a systems-based approach in neurocritical care. Recognizing and understanding these connections is vital—not only to prevent the progression to multi-organ failure but also to guide therapeutic strategies that support both neurological recovery and systemic stability [23].

1.4 Crosstalk Between Kidneys and Other Organs

The kidneys are traditionally viewed as regulators of fluid balance, electrolytes, and waste excretion—but their role extends far beyond. In both acute and chronic kidney disease, the kidneys become active participants in systemic pathophysiology through the accumulation of uremic toxins, persistent inflammation, and oxidative stress [24]. These disturbances contribute to secondary injury in distant organs such as the heart, lungs, brain, liver, gastrointestinal tract, and vasculature. Importantly, this crosstalk is bidirectional: the kidneys may be the source of dysfunction, but they can also be downstream victims of pathology originating elsewhere [25].

A well-recognized example is the cardio–renal axis. Chronic kidney disease (CKD) significantly increases the risk of cardiovascular events, while heart failure—both acute and chronic—can precipitate acute kidney injury (AKI). This mutual relationship is mediated by shared mechanisms, including hemodynamic compromise, activation of the renin–angiotensin–aldosterone system (RAAS), sympathetic overactivity, and cytokine-driven inflammation. Emerging biomarkers such as interferon-γ and stem cell growth factor-β are showing promise in detecting early kidney stress, particularly in high-risk scenarios like post-cardiac surgery [26].

The gut–kidney axis also illustrates the far-reaching impact of renal disease. In CKD, alterations in the gut microbiota and increased intestinal permeability drive low-grade systemic inflammation [27, 28]. Intestinal dysbiosis not only worsens renal outcomes but also amplifies cardiovascular and metabolic complications. Experimental therapies, including targeted probiotics and herbal compounds such as *Astragalus mongholicus* and *Panax notoginseng*, have demonstrated protective effects on both gut and kidney tissues by modulating macrophage-mediated inflammation through the Mincle/NF-κB pathway [29, 30].

The brain is another vulnerable target. AKI has been associated with long-term neurological sequelae, including increased risk of stroke and cognitive impairment [31]. Experimental studies have shown that uremic toxins can directly affect the integrity of the blood–brain barrier (BBB), altering transporter function and tight junction proteins—evidence of a direct kidney-to-brain signaling axis [32].

Liver injury, too, may result from renal dysfunction, particularly in the context of ischemic AKI, where oxidative stress and immune cell infiltration contribute to hepatic damage. In patients with advanced kidney disease or on dialysis, systemic complications such as thrombocytopenia and valvular dysfunction—particularly tricuspid regurgitation—are frequently observed, reflecting the broad vascular and hematologic effects of renal failure [33].

These interconnected relationships highlight that kidney disease is not confined to the renal system alone—it is a systemic disorder. Management strategies should therefore move beyond organ-specific treatment and adopt an integrative, cross-disciplinary approach [34]. A deeper understanding of the molecular and physiological pathways involved in kidney-organ crosstalk will be key to developing targeted interventions aimed at mitigating multi-organ complications and improving long-term outcomes in patients with renal dysfunction [35].

1.5 Crosstalk Between Liver and Other Organs

The liver, as a central metabolic organ, does not function in isolation but continuously communicates with other organs through a complex network of biochemical, hormonal, and neural signals [36]. This dialogue, known as inter-organ crosstalk, is essential for maintaining systemic homeostasis and regulating vital functions such as energy metabolism, immune response, and fluid-electrolyte balance. The liver interacts closely with the heart, brain, skeletal muscle, adipose tissue, and kidneys, influencing their physiology reciprocally [36].

The liver-heart communication is particularly evident in conditions of advanced heart failure, where hepatic venous congestion impairs hepatocellular function, contributing to the development of the hepato-cardiac-renal syndrome [37]. In this condition, liver dysfunction leads to cardiac and renal impairment through inflammatory, neuroendocrine, and perfusion-related mechanisms. Recent studies have highlighted the role of IL-22, an interleukin involved in immune response, in cardiac protection following myocardial infarction (MI). Its activity is regulated through a liver–heart axis, suggesting that the liver can modulate cardiac recovery via immunometabolic pathways [38]. Regarding liver–brain crosstalk, the liver plays a crucial role in cognitive function and neuroinflammatory regulation, as seen in patients with hepatic encephalopathy, where toxin accumulation due to liver dysfunction impairs neuronal function. Additionally, the liver influences the hypothalamic–pituitary–adrenal axis, affecting metabolism and stress responses [39].

The liver–skeletal muscle interaction is another key element in metabolic regulation. The liver supplies glucose to muscles during physical activity, while muscle-derived signals, such as myokines, can modulate liver function. For example, the liver secretes hepatokines such as fetuin-A and fetuin-B, which influence insulin sensitivity in muscles and adipose tissue, contributing to the development or prevention of insulin resistance [40]. The liver–kidney crosstalk is evident in conditions of advanced liver failure, where liver dysfunction negatively impacts renal perfusion, contributing to the hepatorenal syndrome. Inflammatory mechanisms and portal hypertension alterations play a key role in this pathological connection, suggesting that therapeutic strategies aimed at improving liver function could also benefit renal function [41]. Finally, the liver–adipose tissue interaction regulates lipid and glucose metabolism. The liver processes free fatty acids released from adipose tissue, determining their conversion into energy or storage. However, in pathological conditions such as non-alcoholic fatty liver disease (NAFLD), this interaction becomes dysfunctional, promoting systemic inflammation and increasing the risk of metabolic and cardiovascular diseases [42].

Understanding these intricate liver–organ communication mechanisms is essential for developing innovative therapeutic strategies for metabolic, cardiovascular, and neurological diseases, focusing not only on a single affected organ but on the entire physiological network that connects the liver to other vital organs.

1.6 Crosstalk Between Heart and Other Organs

The heart, while often viewed primarily as a mechanical pump, is also an active endocrine and immunomodulatory organ. Through a network of hormonal, neural, and inflammatory signals, it maintains dynamic communication with peripheral systems. This inter-organ crosstalk becomes particularly relevant in the setting of cardiovascular disease—especially myocardial infarction (MI) and heart failure (HF)—where cardiac injury sets off a cascade of systemic effects [43].

Following cardiac injury, the heart releases a variety of bioactive molecules, collectively known as cardiokines, including IL-1β, IL-18, TNF-α, and atrial natriuretic peptide (ANP) [44]. These mediators do not act locally alone—they exert influence over distant organs such as the kidneys, liver, spleen, adipose tissue, skeletal muscle, and bone marrow. In heart failure, activation of the myocardial NLRP3 inflammasome is a key driver of systemic inflammation. The resulting cytokine surge contributes to adverse cardiac remodeling, but also initiates damage in other organs [44].

One of the clearest examples of this systemic interplay is the cardiorenal syndrome [45]. Here, a failing heart compromises renal perfusion and function, while renal dysfunction feeds back through neurohormonal and inflammatory pathways to worsen cardiac output. Mechanisms like RAAS activation, sympathetic overactivity, and oxidative stress are shared across both organs, creating a self-perpetuating cycle of dysfunction [45].

The spleen is also involved in this multi-organ dialogue. In the so-called cardio–splenic axis, monocytes and dendritic cells from the spleen are mobilized in response to myocardial injury. While this response can be initially adaptive, chronic activation promotes persistent inflammation and fibrosis within the heart [46]. Similarly, adipose tissue—particularly in the context of obesity—secretes pro-inflammatory adipokines such as IL-6 and MCP-1, while levels of protective molecules like adiponectin are reduced. These altered adipokine profiles further exacerbate myocardial injury and remodeling. Of note, epicardial fat, located in direct contact with the myocardium, exerts potent paracrine effects that influence post-MI recovery [47].

Skeletal muscle is not immune to these systemic effects. Muscle wasting and weakness are common in chronic heart failure, driven in part by inflammatory cytokines such as TNF-α and IL-1β, which activate catabolic pathways like NF-κB and accelerate protein breakdown. Angiotensin II, a hormone elevated in heart failure, also contributes to muscle atrophy [48]. Meanwhile, the bone marrow responds to cardiac stress by producing pro-inflammatory myeloid cells, which can migrate to the heart, intensifying local inflammation. In some cases, this chronic inflammatory signaling may even promote clonal hematopoiesis—a risk factor for cardiovascular events in itself [49].

Altogether, these pathways reflect the deeply systemic nature of cardiac disease. When the heart suffers, other organs follow. This recognition is fueling the development of targeted therapies aimed at disrupting this harmful inter-organ communication [50]. Treatments such as IL-1β inhibitors, PCSK9 inhibitors, sodium-glucose co-transporter 2 (SGLT2) inhibitors, and even emerging cell-based therapies like CAR-T are being explored not just for their cardiac benefits, but for their potential to prevent or limit multi-organ dysfunction [51].

1.7 Crosstalk Between Lungs and Other Organs

Respiratory diseases, particularly those involving acute inflammation, have far-reaching effects beyond the lungs themselves [52]. One of the most striking examples is ARDS, a life-threatening condition often triggered by pneumonia, sepsis, or major trauma [53]. Characterized by diffuse alveolar damage and increased permeability of the alveolar-capillary barrier, ARDS results in pulmonary edema, impaired gas exchange, and severe hypoxemia [53]. However, ARDS is not solely a pulmonary issue—it quickly becomes a systemic one. The interaction between the lungs and the cardiovascular system plays a central role in its progression. Inflammatory mediators released from injured lung tissue can spill into the circulation, leading to endothelial dysfunction, vasoconstriction, and increased pulmonary vascular resistance [54]. This, in turn, can strain the right ventricle, contribute to pulmonary hypertension, and further compromise oxygen delivery in a vicious cycle that accelerates respiratory and cardiac failure [55].

Beyond the heart, this inflammatory burden also affects other organs. The kidneys and liver are particularly susceptible, with systemic inflammation and hypoxia contributing to acute kidney injury and hepatic dysfunction [56]. In many cases, these secondary injuries are not just byproducts but active components of the multi-organ response to lung injury. Hypoperfusion, oxidative stress, and dysregulated immune responses amplify the damage, creating a complex, interdependent pathophysiological state [57]. Even after the acute phase, the consequences of lung-organ crosstalk can persist. Survivors of ARDS often face long-term respiratory impairment, reduced exercise tolerance, and diminished quality of life [57]. These chronic effects are not limited to the lungs—muscle wasting, cognitive dysfunction, and psychological distress are also common. Effective recovery, therefore, requires a multidisciplinary approach that addresses not just pulmonary rehabilitation but also systemic recovery, nutrition, mobility, and mental health. Recognizing the lungs as both an origin and a target of systemic inflammation is essential in managing critically ill patients. Interventions aimed at protecting lung integrity—such as lung-protective ventilation, fluid management, and early identification of extrapulmonary complications—can have cascading benefits across organ systems [58–60].

1.8 Multi-organ Failure

Multi-organ failure (MOF) represents one of the most severe manifestations of critical illness, defined by the simultaneous dysfunction of two or more organ systems [61]. It is not a single disease entity but rather the result of a complex, self-perpetuating process that often begins with an insult to a single organ—most commonly the lungs or cardiovascular system, which are especially vulnerable to initial stress [61]. Once one organ begins to fail, its dysfunction can set off a cascade of adverse effects on others. For instance, respiratory failure leads to systemic hypoxia, which compromises renal perfusion and oxygen delivery, setting the stage for acute kidney injury. Meanwhile, hepatic function may deteriorate as the liver struggles to clear circulating toxins and inflammatory mediators, further exacerbating systemic instability. This dynamic illustrates the intricate web of organ interdependence that defines MOF.

Understanding the mechanisms of organ crosstalk is vital in recognizing how these failures evolve and how they might be interrupted. Early intervention in one system can often prevent deterioration in others. For example, timely correction of hypoxia may protect the kidneys, or managing fluid balance in heart failure may reduce the risk of pulmonary edema and respiratory compromise [62]. Supportive strategies may include mechanical ventilation for respiratory failure, renal replacement therapy for kidney dysfunction, and vasopressors or inotropes to stabilize cardiovascular function. Hemodynamic monitoring, lactate clearance, and dynamic perfusion markers guide ongoing resuscitation and therapeutic decisions [62, 63].

Table 1.2 Early indicators, biomarkers, and management strategies in organ crosstalk

Organ dysfunction	Early warning signs	Key biomarkers	Initial management priorities
Brain (ABI)	Altered mental status, autonomic instability, GCS drop	NSE, S100B, IL-6, ICP trends	Prevent secondary injury, optimize CPP, manage systemic inflammation
Lungs (ARDS)	Tachypnea, desaturation, high ventilatory pressures	PaO_2/FiO_2 ratio, IL-8, SP-D, lactate	Lung-protective ventilation, fluid management, prone positioning
Kidneys (AKI)	Oliguria, rising creatinine, fluid overload	NGAL, cystatin C, creatinine, KIM-1	Avoid nephrotoxins, optimize perfusion, consider early RRT
Liver	Elevated LFTs, jaundice, coagulopathy	Bilirubin, AST/ALT, INR, ammonia	Treat underlying cause, support metabolism, monitor coagulation
Heart	Hypotension, arrhythmia, elevated JVP	Troponin, BNP/NT-proBNP, lactate	Hemodynamic support, manage preload/afterload, treat ischemia
Gut	Abdominal distension, high gastric residuals	I-FABP, citrulline, calprotectin	Early enteral nutrition, prevent dysbiosis, maintain perfusion

Note. *ABI* acute brain injury, *ARDS* acute respiratory distress syndrome, *AKI* acute kidney injury, *LFTs* liver function tests, *GCS* Glasgow Coma Scale, *NSE* neuron-specific enolase, *ICP* intracranial pressure, *CPP* cerebral perfusion pressure, *PaO2/FiO2* arterial oxygen partial pressure to fractional inspired oxygen ratio, *SP-D* surfactant protein D, *NGAL* neutrophil gelatinase-associated lipocalin, *KIM-1* kidney injury molecule-1, *AST* aspartate aminotransferase, *ALT* alanine aminotransferase, *INR* international normalized ratio, *BNP* B-type natriuretic peptide, *NT-proBNP* N-terminal pro B-type natriuretic peptide, *I-FABP* intestinal fatty acid–binding protein, *RRT* renal replacement therapy

Ultimately, preventing progression to multi-organ failure hinges on early recognition, a systems-based approach to care, and a nuanced understanding of how organ systems interact in both health and disease [63, 64].

To support clinical recognition and timely management of early organ dysfunction, the following Table 1.2 summarizes key warning signs, relevant biomarkers, and initial therapeutic strategies associated with inter-organ crosstalk in critical illness.

1.9 Conclusions

The human body operates as an integrated system, and critical illness unravels this integration in ways that are both complex and consequential. As this chapter has outlined, no organ system functions in isolation—particularly in the context of life-threatening conditions such as sepsis, acute brain injury, ARDS, or multi-organ failure. The concept of organ crosstalk is not just a theoretical framework but a daily reality in intensive care units, where dysfunction in one organ frequently influences the trajectory of others. From the gut–brain axis following ABI to the cardiorenal and hepato-skeletal muscle networks, the pathways of communication are diverse—mediated by neural, endocrine, immune, and metabolic signals. These interconnections can be protective in homeostasis but become maladaptive under physiological stress [61, 63]. The inflammatory response, oxidative stress, and neurohumoral activation serve as common denominators that link organ systems in a web of mutual vulnerability. Recognizing these connections is critical for early diagnosis, timely intervention, and personalized treatment. A systems-level approach—one that anticipates the downstream effects of single-organ dysfunction—can make the difference between recovery and progression to multi-organ failure. Advances in biomarkers, immunomodulatory therapies, and metabolic interventions are beginning to provide tools for clinicians to not only support failing organs but to break the cycles of inter-organ injury [15].

Ultimately, improving outcomes in critical illness demands a shift in perspective: from viewing organs as separate targets of therapy to understanding the body as an interconnected whole. Continued research into the mechanisms of organ crosstalk will be key to developing smarter, more integrated strategies for the prevention, diagnosis, and treatment of critical illness—bringing us closer to precision critical care.

References

1. Mrozek S, Gobin J, Constantin JM, Fourcade O, Geeraerts T. Crosstalk between brain, lung and heart in critical care. Anaesth Crit Care Pain Med. 2020;39(4):519–30.
2. Singer M, De Santis V, Vitale D, Jeffcoate W. Multiorgan failure is an adaptive, endocrine-mediated, metabolic response to overwhelming systemic inflammation. Lancet. 2004;364(9433):545–8.
3. Riyaz Tramboo S, Elkhalifa AME, Quibtiya S, Ali SI, Nazir Shah N, Taifa S, et al. The critical impacts of cytokine storms in respiratory disorders. Heliyon. 2024;10(9):e29769.
4. Rengarajan A, Goldblatt HE, Beebe DJ, Virumbrales-Muñoz M, Boeldt DS. Immune cells and inflammatory mediators cause endothelial dysfunction in a vascular microphysiological system. Lab Chip. 2024;24(6):1808–20.
5. Delano MJ, Ward PA. The immune system's role in sepsis progression, resolution, and long-term outcome. Immunol Rev. 2016;274(1):330–53.
6. Tsantes AG, Parastatidou S, Tsantes EA, Bonova E, Tsante KA, Mantzios PG, et al. Sepsis-induced coagulopathy: an update on pathophysiology, biomarkers, and current guidelines. Life. 2023;13(2):350.
7. Gulyaeva NV. Neuroendocrine control of Hyperglutamatergic states in brain pathologies: the effects of glucocorticoids. J Evol Biochem Physiol. 2022;58(5):1425–38.
8. Singh A, Singh K. Pathology of the renin-angiotensin-aldosterone system. In: Renin-angiotensin-aldosterone system – latest trends [Working title]. IntechOpen; 2024.
9. Guo S. Insulin signaling, resistance, and the metabolic syndrome: insights from mouse models into disease mechanisms. J Endocrinol. 2014;220(2):T1–T23.
10. Larsson L, Degens H, Li M, Salviati L, Lee Y il, Thompson W, et al. Sarcopenia: aging-related loss of muscle mass and function. Physiol Rev. 2019;99(1):427–511.
11. Samaja M, Ottolenghi S. The oxygen Cascade from atmosphere to mitochondria as a tool to understand the (Mal)adaptation to hypoxia. Int J Mol Sci. 2023;24(4)
12. Dijkman M, Heslinga J, Sipkema P, Westerhof N. Perfusion-induced changes in cardiac contractility and oxygen consumption are not endothelium-dependent. Cardiovasc Res. 1997;33(3):593–600.
13. Kumar R, Prakash SS, Priyadarshi RN, Anand U. Sarcopenia in chronic liver disease: a metabolic perspective. J Clin Transl Hepatol. 2022;
14. Liu Y, Xiang D, Zhang H, Yao H, Wang Y. Hypoxia-inducible Factor-1: a potential target to treat acute lung injury. Barreto E, editor. Oxidative Med Cell Longev. 2020;2020:1–13.
15. Battaglini D, De Rosa S, Godoy DA. Crosstalk between the nervous system and systemic organs in acute brain injury. Neurocrit Care. 2024;40(1):337–48.

16. Battaglini D, Robba C, Fedele A, Trancă S, Sukkar SG, Di Pilato V, et al. The role of dysbiosis in critically ill patients with COVID-19 and acute respiratory distress syndrome. Front Med (Lausanne). 2021;8
17. Ney LM, Wipplinger M, Grossmann M, Engert N, Wegner VD, Mosig AS. Short chain fatty acids: key regulators of the local and systemic immune response in inflammatory diseases and infections. Open Biol. 2023;13(3):230014.
18. Taraskina A, Ignatyeva O, Lisovaya D, Ivanov M, Ivanova L, Golovicheva V, et al. Effects of traumatic brain injury on the gut microbiota composition and serum amino acid profile in rats. Cells. 2022;11(9):1409.
19. Zou J, Li J, Wang X, Tang D, Chen R. Neuroimmune modulation in liver pathophysiology. J Neuroinflammation. 2024;21(1):188.
20. De Rosa S, Battaglini D, Robba C. Kidney dysfunction after acute brain injury. Nephrol Dial Transplant. 2024;39(2):170–3.
21. Frisvold S, Coppola S, Ehrmann S, Chiumello D, Guérin C. Respiratory challenges and ventilatory management in different types of acute brain-injured patients. Crit Care. 2023;27(1):247.
22. Chen Z, Venkat P, Seyfried D, Chopp M, Yan T, Chen J. Brain–heart interaction. Circ Res. 2017;121(4):451–68.
23. Fan TH, Rosenthal ES. Physiological monitoring in patients with acute brain injury. Crit Care Clin. 2023;39(1):221–33.
24. Basile DP, Anderson MD, Sutton TA. Pathophysiology of acute kidney injury. In: Comprehensive physiology. Wiley; 2012. p. 1303–53.
25. López-Andrés N, Jaisser F, Barrera-Chimal J. Editorial: kidney and distant organ crosstalk in health and disease. Front Physiol. 2021;12:712535.
26. Abassi Z, Hamo-Giladi DB, Kinaneh S, Heyman SN. The endocrine basis of the cardio-renal axis: new perspectives regarding corin. Physiol Rep. 2024;12(13)
27. Rangaswami J, Bhalla V, Blair JEA, Chang TI, Costa S, Lentine KL, et al. Cardiorenal syndrome: classification, pathophysiology, diagnosis, and treatment strategies: a scientific statement from the American Heart Association. Circulation. 2019;139(16)
28. Mafra D, Kemp JA, Borges NA, Wong M, Stenvinkel P. Gut microbiota interventions to retain residual kidney function. Toxins (Basel). 2023;15(8):499.
29. Tsuji K, Uchida N, Nakanoh H, Fukushima K, Haraguchi S, Kitamura S, et al. The gut–kidney axis in chronic kidney diseases. Diagnostics. 2024;15(1):21.
30. Zheng L, Luo M, Zhou H, Chen J. Natural products from plants and microorganisms: novel therapeutics for chronic kidney disease via gut microbiota regulation. Front Pharmacol. 2022;13:1068613.
31. Wang J, Xu X, Wang C, Ye D, Chen R, Peng P, et al. Association of acute kidney injury with the risk of cognitive impairment or dementia: a systematic review and meta-analysis. Ren Fail. 2023;45(2):2279647.
32. Faucher Q, van der Made TK, De Lange E, Masereeuw R. Blood-brain barrier perturbations by uremic toxins: key contributors in chronic kidney disease-induced neurological disorders? Eur J Pharm Sci. 2023;187:106462.
33. Lee HT, Park SW, Kim M, D'Agati VD. Acute kidney injury after hepatic ischemia and reperfusion injury in mice. Lab Investig. 2009;89(2):196–208.
34. Chawla LS, Eggers PW, Star RA, Kimmel PL. Acute kidney injury and chronic kidney disease as interconnected syndromes. N Engl J Med. 2014;371(1):58–66.
35. Wang X, Zhou XJ, Qiao X, Falchi M, Liu J, Zhang H. The evolving understanding of systemic mechanisms in organ-specific IgA nephropathy: a focus on gut-kidney crosstalk. Theranostics. 2025;15(2):656–81.
36. Wang F, So KF, Xiao J, Wang H. Organ-organ communication: the liver's perspective. Theranostics. 2021;11(7):3317–30.
37. El Hadi H, Di Vincenzo A, Vettor R, Rossato M. Relationship between heart disease and liver disease: a two-way street. Cells. 2020;9(3):567.
38. Tang TT, Li YY, Li JJ, Wang K, Han Y, Dong WY, et al. Liver-heart crosstalk controls IL-22 activity in cardiac protection after myocardial infarction. Theranostics. 2018;8(16):4552–62.

39. Butterworth RF. The liver–brain axis in liver failure: neuroinflammation and encephalopathy. Nat Rev Gastroenterol Hepatol. 2013;10(9):522–8.
40. Chen C, Xie L, Zhang M, Shama CKKY, Jia W. The interplay between the muscle and liver in the regulation of glucolipid metabolism. J Mol Cell Biol. 2024;15(12)
41. Nassar M, Nso N, Medina L, Ghernautan V, Novikov A, El-Ijla A, et al. Liver kidney crosstalk: Hepatorenal syndrome. World J Hepatol. 2021;13(9):1058–68.
42. Azzu V, Vacca M, Virtue S, Allison M, Vidal-Puig A. Adipose tissue-liver cross talk in the control of whole-body metabolism: implications in nonalcoholic fatty liver disease. Gastroenterology. 2020;158(7):1899–912.
43. Jahng JWS, Song E, Sweeney G. Crosstalk between the heart and peripheral organs in heart failure. Exp Mol Med. 2016;48(3):e217.
44. Wu YS, Zhu B, Luo AL, Yang L, Yang C. The role of Cardiokines in heart diseases: beneficial or detrimental? Biomed Res Int. 2018;2018:1–14.
45. Meche V, Kundnani NR, Sharma A, Căpăstraru FM, Nistor D, Sarau CA, et al. Cardio-renal syndrome: latest developments in device-based therapy. J Clin Med. 2024;13(24)
46. Hiraiwa H, Okumura T, Murohara T. The cardiosplenic axis: the prognostic role of the spleen in heart failure. Heart Fail Rev. 2022;27(6):2005–15.
47. Feijóo-Bandín S, Aragón-Herrera A, Moraña-Fernández S, Anido-Varela L, Tarazón E, Roselló-Lletí E, et al. Adipokines and inflammation: focus on cardiovascular diseases. Int J Mol Sci. 2020;21(20)
48. Londhe P, Guttridge DC. Inflammation induced loss of skeletal muscle. Bone. 2015;80:131–42.
49. Mitroulis I, Hajishengallis G, Chavakis T. Bone marrow inflammatory memory in cardiometabolic disease and inflammatory comorbidities. Cardiovasc Res. 2024;119(18):2801–12.
50. Pearce L, Galán-Arriola C, Bell RM, Carr RD, Cunningham J, Davidson SM, et al. Inter-organ communication: pathways and targets to cardioprotection and neuro-protection. A report from the 12th Hatter Cardiovascular Institute workshop. Basic Res Cardiol. 2024;
51. Simela C, Walker JM, Ghosh AK, Chen DH. SGLT2 inhibitors for prevention and management of cancer treatment-related cardiovascular toxicity: a review of potential mechanisms and clinical insights. Cardio-Oncology. 2025;11(1):15.
52. Bezerra FS, Lanzetti M, Nesi RT, Nagato AC, Silva CPE, Kennedy-Feitosa E, et al. Oxidative stress and inflammation in acute and chronic lung injuries. Antioxidants (Basel). 2023;12(3)
53. Swenson KE, Swenson ER. Pathophysiology of acute respiratory distress syndrome and COVID-19 lung injury. Crit Care Clin. 2021;37(4):749–76.
54. Han S, Mallampalli RK. The acute respiratory distress syndrome: from mechanism to translation. J Immunol. 2015;194(3):855–60.
55. Westerhof BE, Saouti N, van der Laarse WJ, Westerhof N, Vonk NA. Treatment strategies for the right heart in pulmonary hypertension. Cardiovasc Res. 2017;113(12):1465–73.
56. Wang B, Li ZL, Zhang YL, Wen Y, Gao YM, Liu BC. Hypoxia and chronic kidney disease. EBioMedicine. 2022;77:103942.
57. Ziaka M, Exadaktylos A. Pathophysiology of acute lung injury in patients with acute brain injury: the triple-hit hypothesis. Crit Care. 2024;28(1):71.
58. Maciolek LM, Harmon TS, He J, Sadruddin S, Nguyen QD. Pseudoangiomatous stromal hyperplasia of the breast: a rare finding in a male patient. Cureus. 2019;
59. Palakshappa JA, Krall JTW, Belfield LT, Files DC. Long-term outcomes in acute respiratory distress syndrome. Crit Care Clin. 2021;37(4):895–911.
60. Ziaka M, Exadaktylos A. Exploring the lung-gut direction of the gut-lung axis in patients with ARDS. Crit Care. 2024;28(1):179.
61. Asim M, Amin F, El-Menyar A. Multiple organ dysfunction syndrome: contemporary insights on the clinicopathological spectrum. Qatar Med J. 2020;2020(1):22.
62. Lee SA, Cozzi M, Bush EL, Rabb H. Distant organ dysfunction in acute kidney injury: a review. Am J Kidney Dis. 2018;72(6):846–56.
63. Ronco C, Ricci Z, Husain-Syed F. From multiple organ support therapy to extracorporeal organ support in critically ill patients. Blood Purif. 2019;48(2):99–105.
64. Sakr Y, Lobo SM, Moreno RP, Gerlach H, Ranieri VM, Michalopoulos A, et al. Patterns and early evolution of organ failure in the intensive care unit and their relation to outcome. Crit Care. 2012;16(6):R222.

Endocrine Emergencies

2

Barbara Altieri, Antea Ciafardini, Giuseppina De Filpo, Roberto Novizio, Chiara Sabbadin, Irene Samperi, Marianna Torchio, and Walter Vena

2.1 Introduction

Endocrine emergencies are uncommon but potentially life-threatening conditions arising from either the excess or deficiency of critical hormones. Their clinical manifestations are often nonspecific and mimic other acute illnesses, posing significant diagnostic challenges. As the burden of endocrine disorders continues to grow globally, clinicians are increasingly likely to encounter acute presentations that demand urgent recognition and specialized treatment. This chapter provides a comprehensive overview of key endocrine emergencies—including thyroid storm,

B. Altieri (✉)
Department of Medicine and Surgery, Division of Endocrinology and Metabolic Diseases, University of Parma, Parma, Italy

Division of Endocrinology and Diabetes, Department of Internal Medicine I, University Hospital, University of Würzburg, Würzburg, Germany
e-mail: barbara.altieri@unipr.it

A. Ciafardini · W. Vena
Department of Biomedical Sciences, Humanitas University, Pieve Emanuele (MI), Rozzano, Italy

Endocrinology and Diabetology Center, Humanitas Gavazzeni Institute, Bergamo, Italy
e-mail: anteaciafardini@gmail.com; walter.vena@gmail.com

G. De Filpo
Unit of Internal Medicine and Oncological Endocrinology, University Hospital of Parma, Parma, Italy
e-mail: gdefilpo@ao.pr.it

R. Novizio
Unit of Endocrinology and Diabetology, Catholic University of The Sacred Heart, Policlinico Universitario "A. Gemelli" IRCCS, Rome, Italy
e-mail: robertonovizio@gmail.com

D. Battaglini et al. (eds.), *Organ System Crosstalk in Critical Illness*,
https://doi.org/10.1007/978-3-032-01024-7_2

hypertensive crisis due to catecholamine excess, adrenal crisis, diabetic ketoacidosis, and hypoglycemia. Each section covers the underlying pathophysiological mechanisms, identifiable triggers, hallmark clinical features, and standardized treatment protocols. The goal is to equip frontline healthcare providers with the knowledge to swiftly identify and manage these emergencies, improve patient outcomes, and implement effective strategies for recurrence prevention.

2.2 Thyroid Storm: A Life-Threatening Exacerbation of Thyrotoxicosis

2.2.1 Definition and Clinical Relevance

Thyroid storm (TS) is a rare but life-threatening endocrine emergency that represents an extreme manifestation of thyrotoxicosis.

In clinical endocrinology, it is essential to distinguish between the terms "thyrotoxicosis" and "hyperthyroidism," which are often mistakenly interchangeably used. Thyrotoxicosis refers to elevated levels of circulating thyroid hormones, regardless of their source. This condition may result from overproduction of hormones by the thyroid gland itself or from other causes such as thyroiditis or the exogenous intake of thyroid hormones. In contrast, hyperthyroidism is a specific subset of thyrotoxicosis, defined by the autonomous overactivity of the thyroid gland leading to increased hormone synthesis and secretion.

Although thyrotoxicosis encompasses all conditions leading to elevated thyroid hormones, TS is distinguished by systemic decompensation involving multiple organ systems (Fig. 2.1).

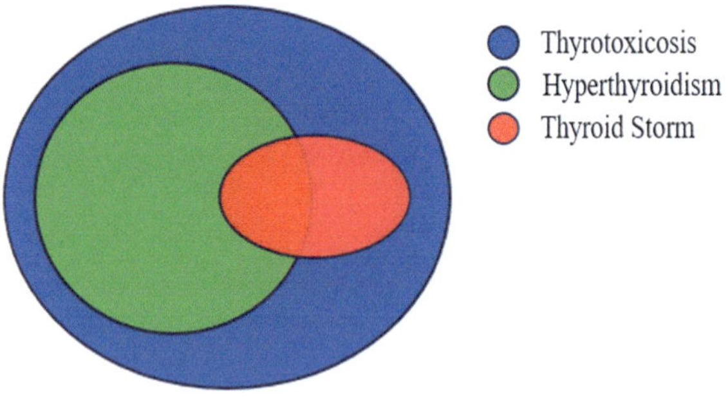

Fig. 2.1 Correlation of thyroid storm with hyperthyroidism and thyrotoxicosis

C. Sabbadin · M. Torchio
Department of Medicine DIMED, Endocrine Unit, Padua, Italy

Endocrine Unit, University-Hospital of Padova, Padua, Italy
e-mail: chiara.sabbadin@unipd.it; mariannatorchio@gmail.com

I. Samperi
SSD of Diabetology and Metabolic Diseases – Azienda Sanitaria Locale Novara, Borgomanero, Italy
e-mail: irene.samperi89@gmail.com

It is characterized by heightened thermogenesis, profound metabolic derangements, and neuro-cardiovascular dysfunction.

While thyrotoxicosis is relatively common, TS accounts for only 0.5–0.8 cases per 100,000 population per year, and 5–15% of hospital admissions for thyrotoxicosis. Despite its rarity, TS carries a disproportionately high in-hospital mortality rate (3.6% vs. 0.3%) and significantly higher healthcare costs compared to uncomplicated thyrotoxicosis [1].

2.2.2 Pathophysiology

The pathophysiological basis of TS remains not completely understood but involves several synergistic mechanisms [2].

One key factor is an acute increase in the availability of unbound (free) thyroid hormones in circulation. Severe illness often reduces levels of thyroid hormone binding, thereby elevating the fraction of free T_3 and T_4 and increasing their bioactivity. Moreover, peripheral tissues become more sensitive to thyroid hormones under conditions of stress (such as infection, hypoxia, diabetic ketoacidosis, or lactic acidosis).

Furthermore, TS usually exhibits features of profound sympathetic overactivity despite normal circulating catecholamine levels. The striking clinical improvement observed with β-adrenergic blockade suggests that thyroid hormone excess confers a permissive effect on catecholamines, for example, by upregulating β-adrenergic receptors and enhancing post-receptor signaling. So, even ordinary catecholamine concentrations drive an exaggerated adrenergic response.

2.2.3 Etiology and Triggers

TS typically arises on a background of unrecognized, untreated, or inadequately managed hyperthyroidism. Among these, Graves' disease is the most common underlying cause of this crisis, but toxic multinodular goiter, thyroiditis, and exogenous thyroid hormone intake can also be implicated.

In most cases, poorly controlled hyperthyroidism alone does not escalate into a TS unless provoked by an acute precipitating event. Common triggers include infection, trauma, surgery (thyroid and non-thyroid), childbirth, and abrupt discontinuation of antithyroid drugs. A variety of less common triggers for TS have been documented, encompassing treatment with amiodarone, checkpoint inhibitors, molar pregnancy, or even vigorous palpation of the thyroid gland [3].

2.2.4 Clinical Presentation

TS presents as an extreme exacerbation of thyrotoxicosis, characterized by an abrupt onset of severe hypermetabolic and multisystemic manifestations.

One of the hallmark signs is high-grade fever, with body temperatures often exceeding 39–41 °C, accompanied by profuse sweating and heat intolerance.

The cardiovascular system is particularly vulnerable, with patients typically developing severe tachycardia (>140 bpm). This hyperdynamic circulatory state may precipitate atrial fibrillation and progress to high-output heart failure, especially in individuals with pre-existing cardiac disease. In more advanced cases, hypotension and cardiovascular collapse may ensue.

Neurological manifestations are also prominent and reflect the central effects of excess thyroid hormone. Patients may present with agitation, anxiety, confusion, and delirium, which can rapidly deteriorate into seizures or coma if left untreated. The gastrointestinal and hepatic systems are commonly affected as well: nausea, vomiting, diarrhea, and abdominal pain are frequent complaints, often contributing to significant dehydration and electrolyte imbalance.

In some cases, jaundice and elevated liver enzymes indicate hepatic dysfunction, likely due to a combination of increased metabolic demand, systemic congestion, and direct hepatocellular injury.

Importantly, not all patients display the classic hypermetabolic profile. In the elderly or debilitated, "apathetic" presentations may occur, characterized by lethargy, weakness, and minimal sympathetic activation, potentially leading to misdiagnosis or delayed recognition.

2.2.5 Diagnosis

Due to the lack of universally accepted diagnostic criteria, TS remains a clinical diagnosis. The Burch-Wartofsky Point Scale is commonly used to assess the likelihood of TS, considering thermoregulatory, cardiovascular, central nervous system, and gastrointestinal parameters, along with precipitating history (Table 2.1). A score >45 is suggestive of TS, while <25 makes it unlikely. Still, these tools are meant to support, not replace, bedside clinical judgment [4].

2.2.6 Treatment

The management of TS must be prompt, intensive, and multidisciplinary. Treatment begins with the inhibition of thyroid hormone synthesis, typically using high-dose propylthiouracil (PTU) or methimazole (MMI). PTU is often preferred initially due to its additional effect in blocking peripheral T4-to-T3 conversion. After thionamides are initiated, iodine (e.g., Lugol's solution or potassium iodide) is administered at least 1 hour later to inhibit the release of preformed hormone through the acute Wolff–Chaikoff effect. In patients with iodine intolerance, lithium represents a valid alternative for suppressing hormone release.

Beta-blockers such as propranolol (or esmolol in unstable patients) are critical to counteract the adrenergic manifestations of the storm, while glucocorticoids (e.g., hydrocortisone) are used both to support adrenal function and to reduce peripheral hormone activation. Supportive care plays a central role and includes fever control

Table 2.1 Wartoffky Scale to assess the likelihood of thyroid storm

	Thyroid storm >45	Points
Temperature	99–99.9	5
	100–100.9	10
	101–101.9	15
	102–102.9	20
	103–103.9	25
	≥104	30
Central nervous system	Absent	0
	Mild agitation	10
	Delirium, psychosis, lethargy	20
	Seizure or coma	30
GI dysfunction	Absent	0
	Diarrhea, N&V, pain	10
	Unexplained jaundice	20
Tachycardia	90–109	5
	110–119	10
	120–129	15
	130–139	20
	≥140	25
CHF	Absent	0
	Mild (edema)	5
	Moderate (bibasilar rales)	10
	Severe (pulmonary edema)	15
AF	Absent/present	0 / 10
History of precipitating event	Absent/present	0 / 10

with acetaminophen, aggressive fluid resuscitation, oxygen therapy, and targeted treatment of precipitating factors such as infections or cardiac events.

Adjunctive therapies can enhance hormone elimination. Bile acid sequestrants, such as cholestyramine, reduce enterohepatic recirculation of thyroid hormones. In rare and refractory cases, especially when standard therapy is contraindicated or ineffective, extracorporeal therapies like plasmapheresis or hemodialysis may be considered to rapidly reduce circulating hormone levels.

Once the acute phase is controlled, definitive treatment of the underlying hyperthyroidism—via radioiodine therapy or thyroidectomy—is essential to prevent recurrence. The choice depends on patient-specific factors and the timing relative to iodine exposure. Early planning for definitive therapy is a key component of long-term management.

In patients stabilized after the acute phase, definitive therapy (radioiodine or thyroidectomy) should be considered to prevent recurrence.

2.2.7 Prognosis and Follow-Up

With prompt recognition and appropriate treatment, patients typically show clinical improvement within 12–24 hours. Anti-thyroid drugs are continued post-crisis to maintain euthyroidism until definitive therapy is performed.

Long-term outcomes are generally favorable, but early mortality remains a risk in the presence of multiorgan failure, delayed treatment, or inadequate supportive care.

2.3 Hypertensive Crisis

2.3.1 Definition

Hypertensive crisis is defined as the presence of severe hypertension (HT), usually reported as the occurrence of systolic blood pressure (SBP) ≥ 180 mmHg and/or diastolic blood pressure (DBP) ≥ 110–120 mmHg, depending on the source [5, 6].

The hypertensive crisis includes hypertensive urgency, without or with minimal symptoms and no acute target organ damage, and hypertensive emergency, characterized by organ damage and related symptoms [7].

A recent Task Force of the European Society of Cardiology (ESC) proposed to quit using the term hypertensive crisis and urgency because physicians should be focused on recognizing hypertensive emergency, which present hypertension-mediated organ damage (HMOD) and require an immediate reduction of blood pressure levels to limit vital organ impairment [8]. Nevertheless, the terms hypertensive crisis and urgency are still frequently used at present.

Specifically, the hypertensive emergency occurs in 1/200 patients presenting to the Emergency Department, and the most frequent HMOD reported are ischemic stroke (28.1%), pulmonary edema, and heart failure (24.1%) [9].

2.3.2 Hypertensive Crisis Due to Pheochromocytoma and Paraganglioma

One of the most dangerous causes of endocrine hypertensive crisis is catecholamine (CA) excess due to chromaffin tumors, which is related to a very high risk of life-threatening cardiovascular complications. Pheochromocytoma (PCC, or intra-adrenal paraganglioma) and paraganglioma (PGL, together PPGL) are rare tumors arising from the neural crest, occurring in about 0.6–0.8 cases per 100.000 persons/year. PCCs derive from the chromaffin cells of the adrenal medulla and PGLs of those of the extra-adrenal paraganglia. Sympathetic PGLs, which include PGLs originating from thorax, abdomen, pelvis, and PCCs, largely produce and release CA. On the contrary, tumors located in the parasympathetic ganglia of the head and neck region, named head and neck paragangliomas (HNPGLs), are usually unable to produce and release CA and provoke HC less frequently than sympathetic PGLs [10].

Hypertension in PPGL occurs in up to 95% of cases (sustained HT 50%, paroxysmal HT 45%), and it is caused by CA action on the adreno-receptors (AR) located in target organs. Noradrenaline (NA) and adrenaline (A) show a different affinity for AR, leading to distinct clinical manifestations. Noradrenergic tumors are usually associated with sustained HT (α1-AR mediated), due to the continuous NA release, and less noticeable tachycardia (β1-AR mediated). Adrenergic tumors generally present an episodic CA release with a paroxysmal HT and tachycardia [11].

Several factors can induce a massive release of CA leading to HC. First of all, a wide variety of drugs used to treat several medical conditions, acting on mechanisms involved in CA release and metabolism, may precipitate hypertensive crises in patients with PPGL [12] (Table 2.2). For instance, non-selective β-AR antagonists should be administered only after a previous α-AR antagonism to prevent the rise of blood pressure levels due to the inhibition of vascular β2AR-mediated vasodilation. Another critical issue in patients affected by PPGL is surgery, both performed in patients with diagnosed PPGL (surgery for primary tumor or metastatic disease) and in those with undiagnosed PPGL (surgery for other causes). Indeed, during surgical procedures, the intubation or, for example, the manipulation of the tumor and drugs administered during the anesthesia can provoke a huge release of CA worsening patients' prognosis. With the aim to limit peri-surgical complications, a multidisciplinary management is essential. Moreover, PPGL guidelines suggest the use of α-AR antagonists before surgery (at least 2 weeks prior to the procedure) to achive an adeguate blood pressure control.

Table 2.2 Main classes of drugs and surgical procedures associated with an increased risk of hypertensive crises in patients with in pheochromocytoma/paraganglioma

Drugs/procedures	Details
β-Adrenergic receptor antagonists (β-blockers)	Used in hypertension, heart failure, migraine, tachycardia, and cardiac dysrhythmias
Dopamine D2 receptor antagonists	Control of nausea, vomiting
Tricyclic antidepressants	Treatment of insomnia, neuropathic pain, headache
Monoamine oxidase inhibitors	Rarely used as antidepressants
Peptide and corticosteroid hormones	Used in diagnostic tests
Sympathomimetics	Control of blood pressure during surgery
Opioid analgesics	Used in surgical anesthesia
Neuromuscular blocking agents	Used in surgical anesthesia
Vagolytic agents	Control of heart rate (raise)
Surgical procedures	Intubation; insufflation of peritoneum; manipulation of tumors

Adapted from Eisenhofer et al. [12]

2.3.3 Treatment

It is worth remembering that the therapeutic approach is chosen according to physicians' experience and agent availability. Considering pathophysiological aspects, the use of α-AR antagonists provides the most rational treatment of hypertensive crisis caused by PPGL (Table 2.3). Phentolamine is a competitive (reversible) non-selective α1- and α2-AR antagonist with an immediate onset (1–2 minutes), but it is unavailable in some countries [11]. A suitable alternative is urapidil, a competitive selective α1-AR antagonist and serotonin agonist, which has been shown to be effective in controlling blood pressure during surgery [13]. It is worth mentioning to avoid using labetalol, an α and β-antagonist, as a first-line agent because its activity is unbalanced in favor of β-antagonism (ratio α:β antagonistic activity 1:7). Tachyarrhythmias can be managed with cardio-selective β-AR antagonists (e.g., esmolol, metoprolol). Additionally, also calcium channel blocking agents may be helpful in dealing with tachyarrhythmias, and verapamil is preferred for its strong antihypertensive effect. Nitrites are recommended for patients with heart failure; nitroprusside is the most used in PPGL. In specific conditions, such as pregnancy and in a pediatric setting, magnesium sulfate can be administered. Fenoldopam, a selective dopamine-1-receptor agonist, is rarely used given the lack of experience in

Table 2.3 Main classes and surgical procedures associated with an increased risk of hypertensive crises in patients with pheochromocytoma / paraganglioma

Class of drugs	Agents	Mechanism of action	Clinical aspects
α-Adrenoreceptor blocking agents	IV Phentolamine	Competitive (reversible) non-selective α1- and α2-adrenoceptor antagonist	AEs: reflex tachycardia; abdominal cramps, diarrhea, vomiting
	IV Urapidil	Competitive selective α1-adrenoreceptor antagonist and serotonin agonist	Contraindications: cardiac or cerebrovascular ischemia and cardiac arrhythmias
β-adrenoreceptor blocking agents	IV Esmolol, Metoprolol	β1-selective adrenoceptor antagonists	Only after adequate α-adrenoceptor blockade: at high doses, β-blockers inhibit β2-adrenoceptor activity AEs: bradycardia, asystole, heart block (especially combined with verapamil) Contraindications: overt heart failure and severe obstructive lung disease

(continued)

Table 2.3 (continued)

Class of drugs	Agents	Mechanism of action	Clinical aspects
Calcium channel blocking agents	IV Nicardipine (vascular action); Diltiazem, Verapamil (cardiac action)	Inhibit vascular and cardiac L-type calcium channels	AEs: intracranial hemorrhage; bradycardia, atrioventricular nodal block Contraindications: advanced aortic stenosis; decompensated heart failure
Nitrates	IV Nitroprusside	Nitric oxide-mediated vasodilator. Action on arterioles (reducing afterload) and venules (reducing preload)	AEs: may increase intracranial pressure Contraindications: myocardial infarction and concomitant use of phosphodiesterase inhibitors
	IV Nitroglycerine	Preferential vasodilator at lower doses (reducing preload, preserving afterload)	AEs: reflex tachycardia Contraindications: preload-dependent states (e.g., right ventricular myocardial infarction)
Other agents	IV Magnesium sulfate	Acts contrasting calcium-mediated catecholamine release, vasoconstriction, and arrythmias	Preferred agent in children and pregnant patients AEs and contraindications: toxicity in patients with renal insufficiency
	IV Fenoldopam	Dopamine-1-receptor agonist	AEs: reflex tachycardia Contraindications: glaucoma and sulfite allergy

Adapted from Nazari et al. [11]
Abbreviation: *IV* intravenous, *AEs* adverse events

the treatment of CA-induced HC. On the other hand, diuretics should be avoided for the risk of hypovolemia, because of the prolonged vasoconstriction consequent to CA excess, inducing relative hypovolemia. In addition, up to 30% of patients experience hypotension during the treatment. In this case, intravenous (IV) fluids (approximately 1 L of crystalloids) are recommended, and vasopressors can be used and are more effective than sympathomimetic agents, because of the α1AR down-regulation caused by the continuous and persistent CA release and action [11].

2.4 Adrenal Crisis

2.4.1 Definition, Epidemiology, and Mortality

Adrenal crisis (AC) is a severe, life-threatening condition that requires prompt recognition and immediate intervention due to its high mortality rate (0.5 per 100 patient-years) [14–21]. It occurs when cortisol levels fail to adequately meet an increased demand, either due to internal or external factors.

AC may be the first manifestation of adrenal insufficiency (AI) or it may develop in individuals with known chronic AI. In the latter case, AC occurs approximately in 6–8% of AI patients annually, more frequently in those with primary AI (PAI) than in those with secondary AI (SAI), presumably because of the lack of aldosterone and more severe hypocortisolism [14–21].

There is no consensus on the definition of AC, but it can be defined as an acute deterioration in health status associated with several signs and symptoms, such as hypotension, abdominal symptoms, and laboratory abnormalities, that improve after parenteral glucocorticoid administration.

2.4.2 Pathophysiology

Absolute or relative deficiency of cortisol is the defining characteristic of the AC. This deficiency results in increased inflammatory cytokine activity due to the loss of cortisol's normal suppressive effects, leading to symptoms such as fever, gastrointestinal disorders, and severe fatigue [22–24]. Cortisol deficiency also contributes to vasodilation and hypotension by disrupting its synergistic interaction with catecholamines on vascular reactivity and impacts on hepatic metabolism, reducing gluconeogenesis and glycogenolysis leading to hypoglycemia. Furthermore, in PAI, the concurrent mineralocorticoid deficiency exacerbates AC by worsening water loss and electrolyte imbalances [22–24].

2.4.3 Precipitating Events and Risk Factors

Infections, especially gastroenteritis, are the most common precipitating events of AC (Table 2.4). Bacterial infections are more common in adults, whereas viral infections predominate among children. Other stressful events, such as trauma, surgery, major psychological distress, or inadequate intake of replacement therapy, can act as triggers for AC [15–18, 22–26].

Table 2.4 Precipitating events of adrenal crisis

Major events that precipitate adrenal crisis
Infections especially gastrointestinal and flu-like illnesses
Trauma or surgery
Significant emotional distress or strenuous physical activity
Nonadherence to glucocorticoid replacement therapy or abrupt cessation of chronic glucocorticoid therapy
Thyrotoxicosis, or levothyroxine therapy initiation in an undiagnosed adrenal insufficiency
Anti-adrenal medications (e.g., mitotane, metyrapone, ketoconazole)
Anticancer medications (e.g., immunotherapy with checkpoint inhibitors and tyrosine kinase inhibitors)
No identifiable cause (10% of cases of adrenal crisis)

Several drugs can interfere with cortisol metabolism by increasing its clearance or altering its activity. These include levothyroxine and medications that induce the CYP3A4 enzyme (e.g., antiepileptics such as carbamazepine, mitotane, rifampicin, and phenytoin). Conversely, CYP3A4 inhibitors (e.g., antibiotics like clarithromycin and telithromycin, or antivirals such as ritonavir and telaprevir) can elevate cortisol levels, potentially increasing the risk of AC once these drugs are discontinued [15–18, 22–26]. Certain immunotherapies or chemotherapies may precipitate AC by inducing hypophysitis or adrenalitis. Finally, some conditions, such as adrenal or pituitary gland infarction, hemorrhage, trauma, apoplexy, or Sheehan's syndrome, can lead directly to an AC [15–18, 22–26].

Among patients with chronic AI, the susceptibility to AC varies. Factors that may exacerbate the risk of AC are older age, a history of prior AC, autoimmune polyglandular syndromes, PAI, type 1 diabetes mellitus, diabetes insipidus, and the presence of comorbidities [15–18, 22–26]. The underlying mechanism of action of these factors in AC is still unknown and may be specific to coexisting conditions.

2.4.4 Physical and Biochemical Features of Adrenal Crisis

Proper and timely recognition of AC can be challenging due to its nonspecific presentation, often leading to delays in treatment initiation. The predominant clinical features include hypotension and hypovolemia, though patients may also present with symptoms such as fatigue, nausea, vomiting, abdominal pain, and altered consciousness [15–17, 22, 23].

Biochemically, in addition to key alterations in cortisol, renin, ACTH, and aldosterone levels, common findings include hyponatremia and hyperkalemia (particularly in PAI due to mineralocorticoid deficiency), hypoglycemia (especially in children, which may result in seizures), hypercalcemia, elevated creatinine levels (attributable to dehydration), anemia, lymphocytosis, and eosinophilia. Moreover, patients may exhibit symptoms related to the underlying trigger that precipitated the crisis (e.g., infections) [15–17, 22, 23].

2.4.5 Treatment

The treatment of an AC is highly effective if administered promptly and should not be delayed by performing diagnostic tests or waiting for their results.

Glucocorticoid Therapy [15–17, 22, 23, 25]
Hypertensive crisis is the first-choice steroid for the treatment of AC due to its physiological glucocorticoid and mineralocorticoid effects, as well as its favorable pharmacokinetics and pharmacodynamics. In contrast, mineralocorticoid therapy (fludrocortisone), when indicated, is usually resumed once the AC has resolved and oral therapy is initiated.

- *Adults:*

Treatment begins with an initial 100 mg dose of HC administered via intravenous or intramuscular (IV/IM) bolus injection. This is followed by an additional 200 mg of HC over the next 24 hours (IV/IM), given either as 50 mg every 6 hours or as a continuous infusion. Subsequent steroid doses should be tailored to the patient's clinical response. If HC is unavailable, other parenteral glucocorticoid may be used (e.g., prednisolone 25 mg as initial dose, followed by two additional 25 mg doses, and then 50 mg in 24 hours). Once parenteral steroid therapy is successful, oral glucocorticoid treatment doses should be tapered in 2–3 days to the patient's usual maintenance dose.

Meanwhile, adequate rehydration with crystalloid fluids (e.g., 0.9% isotonic sodium chloride) is crucial, especially during the first hours. Circulatory status, electrolyte balance, and glycemic levels should be monitored frequently, with careful management of maintenance fluids, especially in the presence of any relevant coexisting conditions.

- *Children:*

Treatment involves a parenteral bolus of HC at 50 mg/m^2 of body surface area, followed by 50–100 mg/m^2 of body surface area every 24 hours (administered IM/IV, either divided into equal doses every 6 hours or as a continuous infusion).

Regarding fluid resuscitation in children, the recommended treatment regimen involves administering a normal saline bolus of 20 mL/kg of body weight, with

Table 2.5 Strategies for adrenal crisis prevention

"Sick day rules": strategies for adrenal crisis prevention	
Stressors	Dosage adjustments
Infection with fever >38 °C	Patients should double/triple the dose of oral glucocorticoids until recovery and then gradually decrease it to the baseline dose in 2 days
Severe infections requiring admission to the intensive care unit	Patients should receive parenteral hydrocortisone administered at 50–100 mg every 6 to 12 hours until recovery
Major surgery	Patients should receive parental hydrocortisone administered at 100 mg during the induction of anesthesia, followed by 50–100 mg every 6 to 12 hours until recovery
Minor surgery or major dental surgery	Patients should receive 50–100 mg of hydrocortisone during the induction of anesthesia, followed by a double oral dose for 24 hours, and then gradually return to the baseline dose
During labor	Patients should receive 100 mg of hydrocortisone at the onset of labor, followed by an additional 25–50 mg every 6 hours, and then gradually reduce the dose over the next 3 days
Significant emotional stress	Patients should receive additional 10–20 mg of hydrocortisone to their baseline dose
Prolonged intensive strenuous exercise	Patients should receive additional 10 mg of hydrocortisone 30–60 minutes before exercise
Dental procedure	Patients should take an additional dose of hydrocortisone 1 hour before the procedure, followed by a double dose for the next 24 hours. Subsequently, they can return to their regular dosage

From Hanner et al. *J Clin Endocrinol Metab.* 2015 [26]

repeated doses up to 60 mL/kg within the first hour. If hypoglycemia is present, additional dextrose should be considered at a dose of 0.5 to 1 g/kg.

Addressing the Precipitating Cause [15–17, 22, 23, 25]

Treatment for the precipitating cause of the AC should be initiated, and specific treatment (e.g., antibiotic therapy) should be started promptly.

2.4.6 Prevention Strategies

Patient education plays a crucial role in preventing AC [15–17, 22, 23, 25]. Patients and their families must be well-informed about "sick day rules" (Table 2.2) to adjust their medication in response to stressful events, even without the presence of their treating physician. This includes injectable intramuscular HC at home, as part of an emergency injection kit that every patient should have. All patients should carry a steroid emergency card and present it to any healthcare professional they consult, to ensure proper and prompt treatment in case of AC or to prevent it [15–17, 22, 23, 25].

A history of a previous AC is one of the most significant risk factors for future crises. Therefore, it is essential to review the appropriate actions to avoid AC and re-educate patients and families at each endocrinology appointment (Table 2.5) [15–17, 22, 23, 25].

2.5 Diabetic Ketoacidosis

2.5.1 Definition and Mortality

Diabetic ketoacidosis (DKA) is a critical and potentially fatal complication of diabetes mellitus (DM) that often necessitates intensive care admission characterized by the presence of: (1) hyperglycemia, (2) ketonemia, and (3) metabolic acidosis with an elevated anion gap [27, 28]. Although DKA is more frequently observed in younger patients with type 1 diabetes (T1D), it can also develop in individuals with type 2 diabetes (T2D) [29]. Early detection in emergency settings is essential, as appropriate and timely treatment can be life-saving. Despite significant progress in both diagnostic methods and therapeutic strategies, DKA continues to be a major cause of complications and mortality in diabetic patients. DKA contributes to approximately 1% of emergency department visits among adults with diabetes and is responsible for nearly 25% of hospital admissions associated with T2D [30]. Encouragingly, mortality associated with DKA has steadily declined over the last decades dropping from 1.1% to 0.4%, with an average annual reduction of 6.8%. However, the highest mortality rates continue to be recorded among patients aged 75 and older [31].

2.5.2 Pathophysiology and Clinical Presentation

The primary determinant of DKA is either a complete or relative deficiency of insulin, along with significant activation of counter-regulatory mechanisms that lead to an increase in glucagon, catecholamines, cortisol, and growth hormone levels [28] ultimately leading to increased hepatic glycogenolysis, free fatty acids breakdown, and beta-oxidation and accumulation of ketone bodies. The primary ketones that accumulate are acetoacetic acid and β-hydroxybutyrate, both of which are strongly acidic and release significant amounts of hydrogen ions ($H+$), which are initially neutralized by bicarbonate. However, the excessive production of $H+$ quickly overwhelms the buffering capacity, resulting in the onset of anion gap metabolic acidosis [32]. The hallmark features of DKA are the triad of hyperglycemia, ketonemia, and acidosis. Nevertheless, certain exceptions, like euglycemic diabetic ketoacidosis (eDKA), can occur, which presents with anion gap metabolic acidosis, the presence of ketones in the blood or urine, and blood glucose levels that remain within the normal range or are mildly elevated (<250 mg/dL) [33]. Individuals with DKA frequently seek medical attention in the emergency department with symptoms such as profound fatigue, nausea, vomiting, abdominal discomfort, excessive urination (polyuria), increased thirst (polydipsia), heightened appetite (polyphagia), and unintended weight loss [34]. DKA can be confirmed when the following conditions are

Table 2.6 Diagnostic criteria for DKA

Diagnostic criteria for DKA				
		Mild	Moderate	Severe
D: blood glucose concentration	Glucose ≥11.0 mmol/L (200 mg/dL) or known to have DM	≥11.1 mmol/l (200 mg/dL)	≥11.1 mmol/l (200 mg/dL)	≥11.1 mmol/l (200 mg/dL)
K: ketones	β-Hydroxybutyrate blood concentration ≥3.0 mmol/L or ketonuria (urine ketone strip 2+ or more)	β-Hydroxybutyrate 3.0–6.0 mmol/l	β-Hydroxybutyrate 3.0–6.0 mmol/l	β-Hydroxybutyrate >6.0 mmol/l
A: acidosis	pH <7.3 and/or serum bicarbonate concentration < 18 mmol/L	pH >7.25 to <7.30 or bicarbonate 15–18 mmol/l	pH 7.0–7.25 or bicarbonate 10 to <15 mmol/l	pH <7.0 or bicarbonate <10 mmol/l
Mental status	–	Alert	Alert/drowsy	Stupor/coma

Adapted from Umpierrez et al. [9]

met: a blood glucose level of ≥200 mg/dL (11.0 mmol/L) or a documented history of DM, a venous or capillary β-hydroxybutyrate concentration of ≥3.0 mmol/L or the presence of significant ketonuria (≥ 2+ on standard urine dipsticks), and a pH < 7.3 and/or a bicarbonate concentration below 18.0 mmol/L [35]. DKA severity is categorized as mild, moderate, or severe based on the degree of acidosis (Table 2.6) [35].

2.5.3 Treatment

The initial and most essential step in the management of DKA is appropriate fluid resuscitation, which serves to restore intravascular volume, enhance renal perfusion, promote urinary excretion of glucose and ketone bodies, and mitigate insulin resistance by reducing circulating counter-regulatory hormone levels. The estimated water deficit is approximately 100 ml/kg, which should be corrected within 24 to 48 hours following diagnosis [36]. Isotonic saline (0.9% NaCl) is generally the preferred initial fluid replacement with well-documented efficacy in restoring circulatory volume [37]. In patients without cardiac or renal impairment, 0.9% NaCl is recommended at an infusion rate of 500–1000 ml/h during the first 2–4 hours [35]. The cornerstone of DKA management is insulin therapy, which reduces blood glucose levels by suppressing hepatic glucose production and enhancing peripheral glucose uptake. Continuous intravenous (IV) infusion of short-acting insulin remains the preferred approach. The choice between a fixed-rate IV insulin infusion, typically initiated at 0.1 U/kg/h, or a nurse-driven protocol with variable insulin infusion rates depends on the available resources and the severity of the patient's clinical condition [27–29]. Once blood glucose falls below 250 mg/dL (14 mmol/L), a 5–10% dextrose infusion should be introduced alongside 0.9% saline, and the IV insulin infusion rate can be reduced to 0.05 U/kg/h to minimize the risk of hypoglycemia and hypokalemia [35]. Insulin and fluid adjustments should be made to maintain blood glucose at approximately 200 mg/dL (11.1 mmol/L) until DKA resolves [28, 30]. To prevent recurrence of hyperglycemia or ketosis during the transition to subcutaneous insulin, IV insulin should be continued for 1 to 2 hours after subcutaneous insulin is initiated. Patients previously on insulin therapy should resume their regular regimen with appropriate dose modifications. Insulin-naive individuals should receive long-acting insulin analogs subcutaneously at an initial dose of 0.15–0.3 U/kg, administered either as a single daily dose or divided into two equal doses given twice daily. DKA is frequently linked to a range of electrolyte imbalances, especially disturbances in sodium and potassium levels, primarily driven by insulin deficiency and the increased extracellular osmolarity associated with hyperglycemia. It is essential to recognize that sodium and potassium levels measured in blood tests may be falsely normal. Therefore, it is crucial to calculate the corrected sodium concentration based on blood glucose levels and to consider that once insulin therapy is initiated, potassium will shift back into the cells, potentially resulting in hypokalemia. The guidelines recommend initiating potassium supplementation once levels fall below 5 mmol/L to prevent hypokalemia and maintain a steady potassium level of 4–5 mmol/L [29, 37]. Instead, routine administration of bicarbonate is not recommended, as proper fluid and insulin therapy typically resolves acidosis in DKA, especially when the arterial pH is above 7.0 [38].

Therefore, bicarbonate therapy should be reserved for patients with a pH below 7.0 and those with heart failure. The resolution of DKA is defined by biochemical markers, which include: (a) plasma ketone levels <0.6 mmol/L; (b) serum bicarbonate levels ≥18 mmol/L; (c) venous pH ≥ 7.3; and (d) ideally, blood glucose levels <200 mg/dL (11.2 mmol/L) [35].

2.6 Hypoglycemia

2.6.1 Definition and Risk Factors

Hypoglycemia (HG) can be defined biochemically as a blood glucose below 3.9 mmol/l. HG is the most frequent emergency in diabetes individuals and is associated with significant morbidity and mortality and is frequently associated with inappropriate use of insulin treatment and/or other hypoglycemic medications (e.g., sulfonylureas). Multiple factors contribute to an individual's susceptibility to hypoglycemic episodes, including discrepancies in the timing, dosage, or formulation of insulin administration, as well as inadequate caloric intake due to missed meals, reduced portion sizes, or irregular eating patterns. Additional predisposing conditions include alcohol consumption, obesity, advanced age, hepatic dysfunction, renal impairment, adrenal insufficiency (resulting from glucocorticoid or catecholamine deficits), and pituitary insufficiency which may increase the likelihood of hypoglycemia [39].

2.6.2 Clinical Presentation

While mild hypoglycemia (blood glucose 3.9–3.0 mmol/L) can present with sympathetic nervous system activation symptoms, including hunger, sweating, tachycardia, palpitations, and tremors, moderate hypoglycemia (blood glucose 3.0–2.2 mmol/L) can be supported by confusion, drowsiness, and irritability as a result of impaired function of the central nervous system. In presence of severe HG (blood glucose <2.2 mmol/L), the symptoms can escalate to seizures, stupor, and loss of consciousness with the need for immediate medical support. In the diabetic population, most episodes of hypoglycemia are indeed iatrogenic, either due to an excessive administration of insulin or skipping of a meal or a deficient education on how to schedule physical activity and its impact on glycemia.

2.6.3 Treatment

The management of HG largely depends on the mental status of the patient. Indeed, for alert patients, fast-acting carbohydrates and dietary sugars (e.g., sucrose, fructose, glucose tablets) can be sufficient to effectively restore blood serum glucose levels [40]. Due to its strong association with short- and long-term mortality, in hospitalized subjects, hypoglycemia should be promptly managed [41].

Severe hypoglycemic episodes among patients either not awake or unable to ingest oral nutrition require the administration of intravenous solutions that contain dextrose 10% (10% dextrose solution seems to be better for reducing the risk of rebound hyperglycemia) [42]. Usually, a starting bolus dose of 12.5–15 g of intravenous (IV) dextrose is recommended and can be administered by slow IV push over 3–5 minutes. Whenever IV access is not already available, then IM or subcutaneous administration of glucagon is recommended, with a single dose of glucagon 1 mg. Alternatively, if available, intranasal glucagon 3 mg can be safely administered, and it was found to be non-inferior to intramuscular (IM) glucagon for either adult or pediatric subjects (above age of 4 years old) [43]. Independent of the treatment choice, monitoring of serum blood glucose after treatment initiation should be performed within 15 minutes, and treatment should be repeated if blood glucose is still below 3.9 mmol/L, until the patient is no longer in hypoglycemic state. Once the patient is in stable conditions, the cause of hypoglycemia should be determined and appropriate adjustments to the ongoing anti-hyperglycemic therapy regimen should be considered [44].

Acknowledgments *Antonio Bossi*, Department of Biomedical Sciences, Humanitas University, Pieve Emanuele (MI), Rozzano, Italy, and Endocrinology and Diabetology Center, Humanitas Gavazzeni Institute, Bergamo, Italy.

Andrea Dall'Oca, Department of Biomedical Sciences, Humanitas University, Pieve Emanuele (MI), Rozzano, Italy, and Endocrinology and Diabetology Center, Humanitas Gavazzeni Institute, Bergamo, Italy.

Q&A Section

1. What are the three primary therapeutic targets in the acute management of thyroid storm, and which interventions address each?
2. Why β-AR antagonists should be administered only after α-AR blockade in patients affected by PHEO/PGL?
3. Which signs suggest the occurrence of an adrenal crisis?
4. What is the cornerstone of initial management in a patient presenting with diabetic ketoacidosis (DKA)?
5. What are the first-line treatment options for a conscious patient experiencing mild-to-moderate hypoglycemia?

References

1. Galindo RJ, Hurtado CR, Pasquel FJ, Garcia Tome R, Peng L, Umpierrez GE. National trends in incidence, mortality, and clinical outcomes of patients hospitalized for thyrotoxicosis with and without thyroid storm in the United States, 2004-2013. Thyroid. 2019;29(1):36–43. https://doi.org/10.1089/thy.2018.0275.

2. Bahn Chair RS, Burch HB, Cooper DS, Garber JR, Greenlee MC, Klein I, Laurberg P, McDougall IR, Montori VM, Rivkees SA, Ross DS, Sosa JA, Stan MN, American Thyroid, A., American Association of Clinical, E. Hyperthyroidism and other causes of thyrotoxicosis: management guidelines of the American Thyroid Association and American Association of Clinical Endocrinologists. Thyroid. 2011;21(6):593–646. https://doi.org/10.1089/thy.2010.0417.
3. Warnock AL, Cooper DS, Burch HB. Thyroid storm and adverse effects of antithyroid drugs. In: Matfin G, editor. Endocrine and metabolic medical emergencies: a clinician's guide. John Wiley & Sons Ltd; 2018. p. 262–83.
4. Burch HB, Wartofsky L. Life-threatening thyrotoxicosis. Thyroid storm. Endocrinol Metab Clin N Am. 1993;22(2):263–77.
5. Mancia G, Kreutz R, Brunstrom M, Burnier M, Grassi G, Januszewicz A, Muiesan ML, Tsioufis K, Agabiti-Rosei E, Algharably EAE, Azizi M, Benetos A, Borghi C, Hitij JB, Cifkova R, Coca A, Cornelissen V, Cruickshank JK, Cunha PG, Danser AHJ, Pinho RM, Delles C, Dominiczak AF, Dorobantu M, Doumas M, Fernandez-Alfonso MS, Halimi JM, Jarai Z, Jelakovic B, Jordan J, Kuznetsova T, Laurent S, Lovic D, Lurbe E, Mahfoud F, Manolis A, Miglinas M, Narkiewicz K, Niiranen T, Palatini P, Parati G, Pathak A, Persu A, Polonia J, Redon J, Sarafidis P, Schmieder R, Spronck B, Stabouli S, Stergiou G, Taddei S, Thomopoulos C, Tomaszewski M, Van de Borne P, Wanner C, Weber T, Williams B, Zhang ZY, Kjeldsen SE. 2023 ESH guidelines for the management of arterial hypertension the task force for the management of arterial hypertension of the European Society of Hypertension: endorsed by the International Society of Hypertension (ISH) and the European Renal Association (ERA). J Hypertens. 2023;41(12):1874–2071. https://doi.org/10.1097/HJH.0000000000003480.
6. Whelton PK, Carey RM, Aronow WS, Casey DE Jr, Collins KJ, Dennison Himmelfarb C, DePalma SM, Gidding S, Jamerson KA, Jones DW, MacLaughlin EJ, Muntner P, Ovbiagele B, Smith SC Jr, Spencer CC, Stafford RS, Taler SJ, Thomas RJ, Williams KA Sr, Williamson JD, Wright JT Jr. 2017 ACC/AHA/AAPA/ABC/ACPM/AGS/APhA/ASH/ASPC/NMA/PCNA guideline for the prevention, detection, evaluation, and management of high blood pressure in adults: a report of the American College of Cardiology/American Heart Association Task Force on Clinical Practice Guidelines. Hypertension. 2018;71(6):e13–e115. https://doi.org/10.1161/HYP.0000000000000065.
7. Muiesan ML, Salvetti M, Amadoro V, di Somma S, Perlini S, Semplicini A, Borghi C, Volpe M, Saba PS, Cameli M, Ciccone MM, Maiello M, Modesti PA, Novo S, Palmiero P, Scicchitano P, Rosei EA, Pedrinelli R, Working Group on Hypertension, P.R.o.t.I.S.o.C.t.S.I.d.I.A. An update on hypertensive emergencies and urgencies. J Cardiovasc Med (Hagerstown). 2015;16(5):372–82. https://doi.org/10.2459/JCM.0000000000000223.
8. van den Born BH, Lip GYH, Brguljan-Hitij J, Cremer A, Segura J, Morales E, Mahfoud F, Amraoui F, Persu A, Kahan T, Agabiti Rosei E, de Simone G, Gosse P, Williams B. ESC Council on hypertension position document on the management of hypertensive emergencies. Eur Heart J Cardiovasc Pharmacother. 2019;5(1):37–46. https://doi.org/10.1093/ehjcvp/pvy032.
9. Siddiqi TJ, Usman MS, Rashid AM, Javaid SS, Ahmed A, Clark D 3rd, Flack JM, Shimbo D, Choi E, Jones DW, Hall ME. Clinical outcomes in hypertensive emergency: a systematic review and meta-analysis. J Am Heart Assoc. 2023;12(14):e029355. https://doi.org/10.1161/JAHA.122.029355.
10. Lenders JW, Duh QY, Eisenhofer G, Gimenez-Roqueplo AP, Grebe SK, Murad MH, Naruse M, Pacak K, Young WF Jr, Endocrine S. Pheochromocytoma and paraganglioma: an endocrine society clinical practice guideline. J Clin Endocrinol Metab. 2014;99(6):1915–42. https://doi.org/10.1210/jc.2014-1498.
11. Nazari MA, Hasan R, Haigney M, Maghsoudi A, Lenders JWM, Carey RM, Pacak K. Catecholamine-induced hypertensive crises: current insights and management. Lancet Diabetes Endocrinol. 2023;11(12):942–54. https://doi.org/10.1016/S2213-8587(23)00256-5.

12. Eisenhofer G, Rivers G, Rosas AL, Quezado Z, Manger WM, Pacak K. Adverse drug reactions in patients with phaeochromocytoma: incidence, prevention and management. Drug Saf. 2007;30(11):1031–62. https://doi.org/10.2165/00002018-200730110-00004.
13. Rossi GP, Rossitto G, Maifredini C, Barchitta A, Bettella A, Cerruti L, Latella R, Ruzza L, Sabini B, Vigolo S, Seccia TM. Modern management of hypertensive emergencies. High Blood Press Cardiovasc Prev. 2022;29(1):33–40. https://doi.org/10.1007/s40292-021-00487-1.
14. Hahner S, Loeffler M, Bleicken B, Drechsler C, Milovanovic D, Fassnacht M, Ventz M, Quinkler M, Allolio B. Epidemiology of adrenal crisis in chronic adrenal insufficiency: the need for new prevention strategies. Eur J Endocrinol. 2010;162(3):597–602. https://doi.org/10.1530/EJE-09-0884.
15. Allolio B. Extensive expertise in endocrinology. Adrenal crisis. Eur J Endocrinol. 2015;172(3):R115–24. https://doi.org/10.1530/EJE-14-0824.
16. Rushworth RL, Torpy DJ, Stratakis CA, Falhammar H. Adrenal crises in children: perspectives and research directions. Horm Res Paediatr. 2018;89(5):341–51. https://doi.org/10.1159/000481660.
17. Bornstein SR, Allolio B, Arlt W, Barthel A, Don-Wauchope A, Hammer GD, Husebye ES, Merke DP, Murad MH, Stratakis CA, Torpy DJ. Diagnosis and treatment of primary adrenal insufficiency: an Endocrine Society Clinical Practice Guideline. J Clin Endocrinol Metab. 2016;101(2):364–89. https://doi.org/10.1210/jc.2015-1710.
18. Simpson H, Tomlinson J, Wass J, Dean J, Arlt W. Guidance for the prevention and emergency management of adult patients with adrenal insufficiency. Clin Med (Lond). 2020;20(4):371–8. https://doi.org/10.7861/clinmed.2019-0324.
19. Puar TH, Stikkelbroeck NM, Smans LC, Zelissen PM, Hermus AR. Adrenal crisis: still a deadly event in the 21st century. Am J Med. 2016;129(3):339 e331–9. https://doi.org/10.1016/j.amjmed.2015.08.021.
20. Smans LC, Van der Valk ES, Hermus AR, Zelissen PM. Incidence of adrenal crisis in patients with adrenal insufficiency. Clin Endocrinol. 2016;84(1):17–22. https://doi.org/10.1111/cen.12865.
21. Rushworth RL, Torpy DJ, Falhammar H. Adrenal crises: perspectives and research directions. Endocrine. 2017;55(2):336–45. https://doi.org/10.1007/s12020-016-1204-2.
22. Dineen R, Thompson CJ, Sherlock M. Adrenal crisis: prevention and management in adult patients. Ther Adv Endocrinol Metab. 2019;10:2042018819848218. https://doi.org/10.1177/2042018819848218.
23. Rushworth RL, Torpy DJ, Falhammar H. Adrenal crisis. N Engl J Med. 2019;381(9):852–61. https://doi.org/10.1056/NEJMra1807486.
24. Elshimy G, Chippa V, Kaur J, Jeong JM. Adrenal crisis. In: StatPearls. Treasure Island (FL) ineligible companies. Disclosure: Venu Chippa declares no relevant financial relationships with ineligible companies. Disclosure: Jasleen Kaur declares no relevant financial relationships with ineligible companies. Disclosure: Jordan Jeong declares no relevant financial relationships with ineligible companies; 2025.
25. Husebye ES, Allolio B, Arlt W, Badenhoop K, Bensing S, Betterle C, Falorni A, Gan EH, Hulting AL, Kasperlik-Zaluska A, Kampe O, Lovas K, Meyer G, Pearce SH. Consensus statement on the diagnosis, treatment and follow-up of patients with primary adrenal insufficiency. J Intern Med. 2014;275(2):104–15. https://doi.org/10.1111/joim.12162.
26. Hahner S, Spinnler C, Fassnacht M, Burger-Stritt S, Lang K, Milovanovic D, Beuschlein F, Willenberg HS, Quinkler M, Allolio B. High incidence of adrenal crisis in educated patients with chronic adrenal insufficiency: a prospective study. J Clin Endocrinol Metab. 2015;100(2):407–16. https://doi.org/10.1210/jc.2014-3191.
27. Umpierrez G, Korytkowski M. Diabetic emergencies – ketoacidosis, hyperglycaemic hyperosmolar state and hypoglycaemia. Nat Rev Endocrinol. 2016;12(4):222–32. https://doi.org/10.1038/nrendo.2016.15.
28. Dhatariya KK, Glaser NS, Codner E, Umpierrez GE. Diabetic ketoacidosis. Nat Rev Dis Primers. 2020;6(1):40. https://doi.org/10.1038/s41572-020-0165-1.

29. Dhatariya KK, Joint British Diabetes Societies for Inpatient, C. The management of diabetic ketoacidosis in adults-an updated guideline from the Joint British Diabetes Society for Inpatient Care. Diabet Med. 2022;39(6):e14788. https://doi.org/10.1111/dme.14788.
30. Calimag APP, Chlebek S, Lerma EV, Chaiban JT. Diabetic ketoacidosis. Dis Mon. 2023;69(3):101418. https://doi.org/10.1016/j.disamonth.2022.101418.
31. Benoit SR, Zhang Y, Geiss LS, Gregg EW, Albright A. Trends in diabetic ketoacidosis hospitalizations and in-hospital mortality – United States, 2000-2014. MMWR Morb Mortal Wkly Rep. 2018;67(12):362–5. https://doi.org/10.15585/mmwr.mm6712a3.
32. Besen B, Ranzani OT, Singer M. Management of diabetic ketoacidosis. Intensive Care Med. 2023;49(1):95–8. https://doi.org/10.1007/s00134-022-06894-9.
33. Diaz-Ramos A, Eilbert W, Marquez D. Euglycemic diabetic ketoacidosis associated with sodium-glucose cotransporter-2 inhibitor use: a case report and review of the literature. Int J Emerg Med. 2019;12(1):27. https://doi.org/10.1186/s12245-019-0240-0.
34. Umpierrez G, Freire AX. Abdominal pain in patients with hyperglycemic crises. J Crit Care. 2002;17(1):63–7. https://doi.org/10.1053/jcrc.2002.33030.
35. Umpierrez GE, Davis GM, ElSayed NA, Fadini GP, Galindo RJ, Hirsch IB, Klonoff DC, McCoy RG, Misra S, Gabbay RA, Bannuru RR, Dhatariya KK. Hyperglycaemic crises in adults with diabetes: a consensus report. Diabetologia. 2024;67(8):1455–79. https://doi.org/10.1007/s00125-024-06183-8.
36. Mustafa OG, Haq M, Dashora U, Castro E, Dhatariya KK, Joint British Diabetes Societies for Inpatient Care, G. Management of Hyperosmolar Hyperglycaemic State (HHS) in adults: an updated guideline from the Joint British Diabetes Societies (JBDS) for Inpatient Care Group. Diabet Med. 2023;40(3):e15005. https://doi.org/10.1111/dme.15005.
37. Kitabchi AE, Umpierrez GE, Miles JM, Fisher JN. Hyperglycemic crises in adult patients with diabetes. Diabetes Care. 2009;32(7):1335–43. https://doi.org/10.2337/dc09-9032.
38. Chua HR, Schneider A, Bellomo R. Bicarbonate in diabetic ketoacidosis – a systematic review. Ann Intensive Care. 2011;1(1):23. https://doi.org/10.1186/2110-5820-1-23.
39. McCall AL, Lieb DC, Gianchandani R, MacMaster H, Maynard GA, Murad MH, Seaquist E, Wolfsdorf JI, Wright RF, Wiercioch W. Management of individuals with diabetes at high risk for hypoglycemia: an Endocrine Society Clinical Practice Guideline. J Clin Endocrinol Metab. 2023;108(3):529–62. https://doi.org/10.1210/clinem/dgac596.
40. Carlson JN, Schunder-Tatzber S, Neilson CJ, Hood N. Dietary sugars versus glucose tablets for first-aid treatment of symptomatic hypoglycaemia in awake patients with diabetes: a systematic review and meta-analysis. Emerg Med J. 2017;34(2):100–6. https://doi.org/10.1136/emermed-2015-205637.
41. Akirov A, Grossman A, Shochat T, Shimon I. Mortality among hospitalized patients with hypoglycemia: insulin related and noninsulin related. J Clin Endocrinol Metab. 2017;102(2):416–24. https://doi.org/10.1210/jc.2016-2653.
42. Moore C, Woollard M. Dextrose 10% or 50% in the treatment of hypoglycaemia out of hospital? A randomised controlled trial. Emerg Med J. 2005;22(7):512–5. https://doi.org/10.1136/emj.2004.020693.
43. Sherr JL, Ruedy KJ, Foster NC, Piche CA, Dulude H, Rickels MR, Tamborlane WV, Bethin KE, DiMeglio LA, Fox LA, Wadwa RP, Schatz DA, Nathan BM, Marcovina SM, Rampakakis E, Meng L, Beck RW, Investigators, T.D.E.I.G. Glucagon nasal powder: a promising alternative to intramuscular glucagon in youth with type 1 diabetes. Diabetes Care. 2016;39(4):555–62. https://doi.org/10.2337/dc15-1606.
44. Lowe RN, Williams B, Claus LW. Diabetes: how to manage patients experiencing hypoglycaemia. Drugs Context. 2022:11. https://doi.org/10.7573/dic.2021-9-11.

3 Immune-Inflammatory Mechanisms in Organ Crosstalk: Rheumatic Conditions in Intensive Care Unit

María C. Cuéllar-Gutiérrez, Alí Duarte-García, Francesco Muratore, and Alvise Berti

3.1 Introduction

Despite their relatively low prevalence in the general population, 10–25% of patients presenting to the emergency room with autoimmune and autoinflammatory diseases require hospitalization, with 30% requiring intensive care unit (ICU) admission [1]. Mortality ranges between 20% and 54%, being, in general, higher for those admitted for infections as compared to those admitted for disease flare, and it is associated with high scores of Acute Physiology and Chronic Health Evaluation (APACHE)-II or Sequential Organ Failure Assessment (SOFA), need of vasopressors, and prolonged hospital stay [2, 3].

The conditions more frequently admitted in the ICU are rheumatoid arthritis, systemic vasculitis (particularly antineutrophilic cytoplasmic antibody

M. C. Cuéllar-Gutiérrez
Division of Rheumatology, Department of Medicine, Mayo Clinic, Rochester, MN, USA

Division of Rheumatology, Hospital del Salvador, Universidad de Chile, Santiago, Chile

A. Duarte-García
Division of Rheumatology, Department of Medicine, Mayo Clinic, Rochester, MN, USA

F. Muratore
Department of Surgery, Medicine, Dentistry and Morphological Sciences with interest in Transplant, Oncology and Regenerative Medicine, University of Modena and Reggio Emilia, Modena, Italy

Rheumatology Unit, Azienda USL – IRCCS di Reggio Emilia, Reggio Emilia, Italy

A. Berti (✉)
Center for Medical Sciences (CISMed) and Department of Cellular, Computational and Integrative Biology (CIBIO), University of Trento, Trento, Italy

Rheumatology Unit, Santa Chiara Regional Hospital, APSS, Trento, Italy
e-mail: alvise.berti@unitn.it

D. Battaglini et al. (eds.), *Organ System Crosstalk in Critical Illness*,
https://doi.org/10.1007/978-3-032-01024-7_3

(ANCA)-associated vasculitis (AAV)), systemic lupus erythematosus (SLE), catastrophic antiphospholipid syndrome (CAPS), systemic sclerosis, and myositis.

These patients can be admitted to the ICU for several reasons: over 50% of hospitalizations are due to infections because of concomitant immunosuppression (with respiratory tract being the most frequently involved), between 25% and 35% result from exacerbation of the underlying rheumatic condition (with a new diagnosis made in ICU in 20% of these cases), and the remaining 15–25% are due to other life-threatening complications of the rheumatologic disease (e.g., macrophage activation syndrome, MAS) [4]. Only a minority is due to the toxicity of the drugs or acute serious illnesses unrelated to the rheumatic disease. In most cases, the biggest challenge in these patients is establishing the diagnosis between infection and disease flare, which requires significantly different treatments.

The crosstalk between the immune system and the different organs affected is the key to understanding the pathophysiology of these immune-inflammatory conditions. Some rheumatic conditions should always be considered as a possible diagnosis, especially in the context of a multisystem disease, when the diagnosis is not immediately evident. For instance, the combination of respiratory and renal failure could be a new diagnosis of AAV, presenting with pulmonary-renal syndrome. Therefore, a prompt assessment should be undertaken (i.e., thoracic CT scan, urinalysis, bronchoscopy, etc.) [5]. Another example is that the combination of digital ischemia, ulceration, and superficial gangrene of the lower extremities with multiorgan failure, livedo reticularis, and splinter hemorrhages should suggest CAPS syndrome [6]. In all these cases, it is essential to involve rheumatologists early in the management of the patients, even if the condition is only suspected.

Here, we summarized the most frequent severe manifestations and complications of rheumatic diseases that could be seen by physicians working in the ICU, providing some basic concepts and practical guidance on the clinical presentation, diagnosis, and management of these conditions.

3.2 Vasculitides

3.2.1 Diffuse Alveolar Hemorrhage

Diffuse alveolar hemorrhage (DAH) is a clinical syndrome caused by nonimmune-mediated and immune-mediated etiologies, including but not limited to AAV, as summarized in Fig. 3.1. DAH is a life-threatening manifestation of AAV, presenting in both granulomatosis with polyangiitis and microscopic polyangiitis, occurring in up to 25% of patients in total, counting both severe and non-severe forms [7]. One-year survival ranges between 63.7% and 88.0%, being worse in the elderly, those who have severe renal disease (serum creatinine >500 micromol/L), a ratio of partial pressure of arterial O_2 to fraction of inspired O_2 (PaO_2/FiO_2) <300 mmHg, and involved lung area at CT scan ≥50% at presentation [7, 8].

Typical symptoms are dyspnea, cough, and hemoptysis, with symptoms developing rapidly in hours or days. The DAH triad includes lung opacities, hemoptysis,

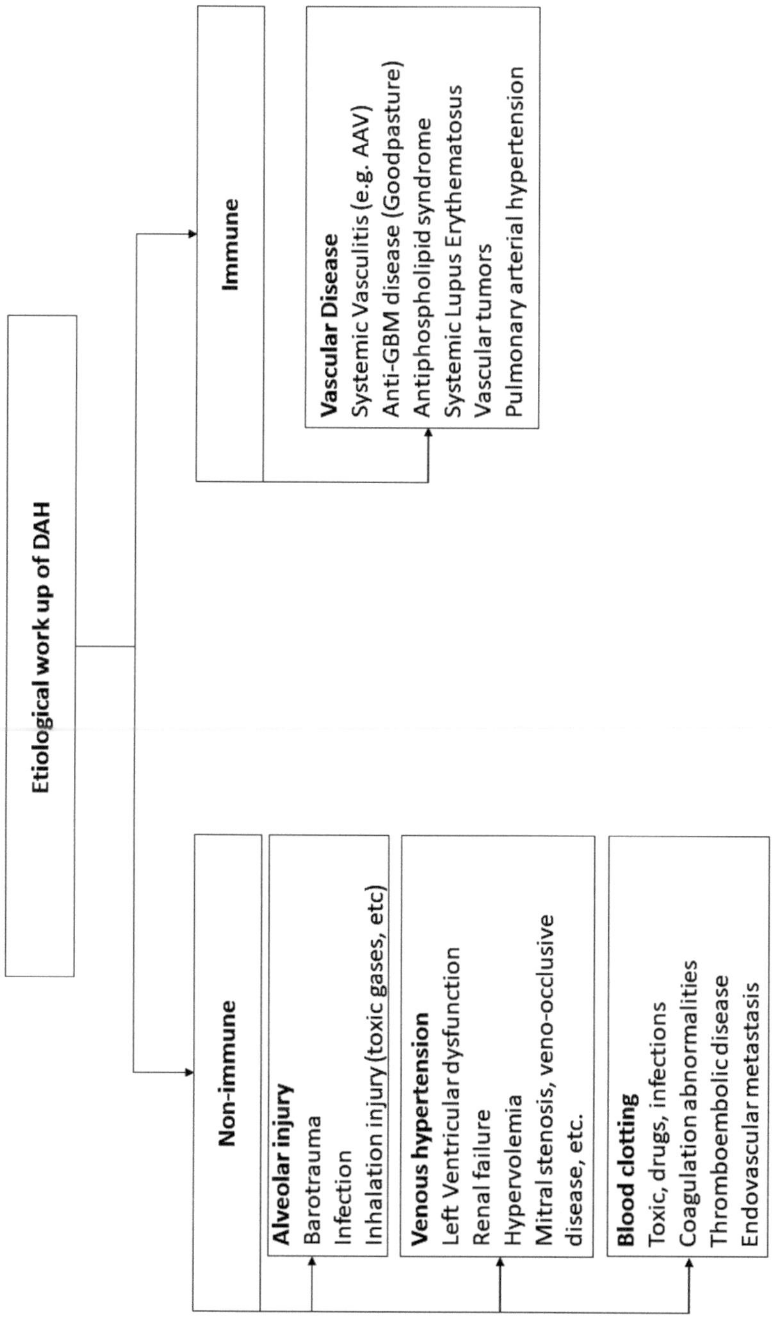

Fig. 3.1 The spectrum of nonimmune-mediated and immune-mediated etiologies of DAH. (DAH diffuse alveolar hemorrhage, GBM glomerular basement membrane, AAV ANCA-associated vasculitis)

and anemia, but they are not always present simultaneously in all patients. Severe DAH is defined by oxygen saturation of ≤85% in room air or the need for mechanical ventilation.

The diagnosis of AAV is often suggested by the presence of a concomitant rapidly progressive glomerulonephritis (i.e., with elevated plasma creatinine and an abnormal urinalysis, suggesting a pulmonary-renal syndrome [9]) and/or of a multisystemic involvement (skin purpura, scleritis, mononeuritis multiplex, bloody enterocolitis, bloody nasal discharge/nasal crusting, arthralgia, fever, and systemic inflammation) [10]. Testing for ANCA and anti-glomerular basement membrane (GBM) antibodies is essential in these cases. CT scan of the thorax shows a diffuse infiltrative opacification pattern; the bronchoscopy with bronchoalveolar lavage demonstrates the presence of alveolar hemorrhage (that should not be confused with bronchial hemorrhage with alveolar flooding) in the most acute forms and siderophages in the subacute ones. It is important to rule out other DAH differential diagnoses such as anticoagulation excess, infections, and other conditions such as heart failure.

There is low-quality evidence for the best treatment of idiopathic DAH or AAV-related DAH. Intravenous methylprednisolone 0.5–1 g/day for up to 3 days, followed by oral prednisone 1 mg/kg/day, should be immediately started in all patients to control the symptoms. Cyclophosphamide and Rituximab, alone or in combination, are added to induce remission. The use of plasmapheresis did not add a clear benefit in any outcomes; in achieving complete remission, in reducing mortality, or in reducing hypoxemia/need for mechanical ventilantion [8, 11].

3.2.2 Rapidly Progressive Glomerulonephritis

Rapidly progressive glomerulonephritis (RPGN) is a type of nephritic syndrome leading to the inflammation of the glomeruli. This inflammation ultimately causes a proliferation of epithelial cells in the Bowman's capsule, forming "crescents" -moon-shaped cell proliferation - that lead to hematuria and glomerular damage, decreasing glomerular filtration, and causing rapidly progressive glomerulonephritis to renal failure (days to weeks). Most often, this condition affects adults between 50 and 60, with a poor prognosis if not treated early. If the renal failure becomes irreversible (i.e., crescents from cellular become fibrous), patients may require long-term renal replacement therapy or kidney transplantation [12].

The development of crescents in Bowman's space could be the consequence of different underlying mechanisms that correspond to different pathological pictures and diagnoses, summarized in Fig. 3.2. Briefly, there are three main immune-mediated mechanisms leading to RPGN, which are: (1) immune-complex mediated, meaning that the process is caused by the deposition in the glomeruli of immune complexes, composed of antigens and circulating antibodies, leading to cell-mediated inflammation and/or complement activation; (2) anti-GBM antibody-mediated, meaning that circulating autoantibodies directed against type IV collagen (alfa-3 chain) bind their target which is expressed in the kidney and alveolar membranes;

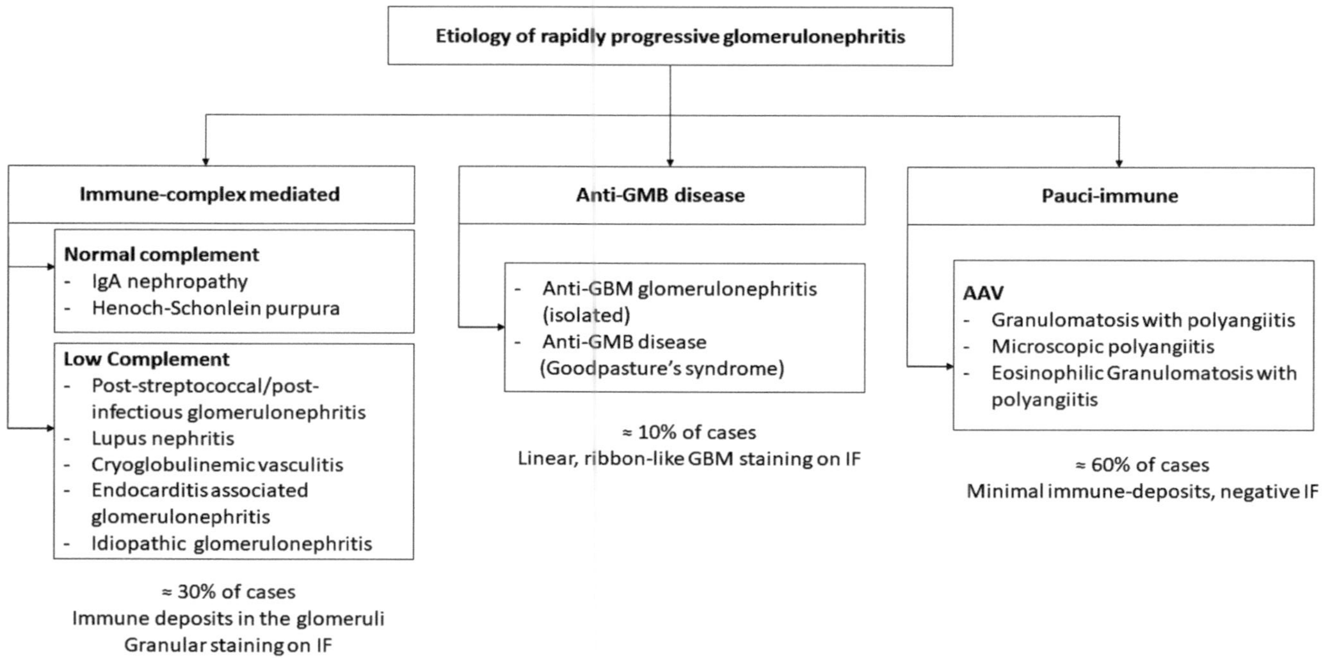

Fig. 3.2 The spectrum of rapidly progressive glomerulonephritis etiologies. (IF immunofluorescence, IgA Immunoglobulin A, GBM glomerular basement membrane, AAV ANCA-associated vasculitis)

(3) pauci-immune, typically resulting from activation of neutrophils by circulating ANCA, which induces inflammation at the small vessel interface (i.e. in the glomeruli) [13–19].

The typical clinical presentation is nephritic syndrome, with glomerular inflammation leading to active urinary sediment (microscopic hematuria and red blood casts in the urine; proteinuria is usually present and below 3.5 g/day), increasing creatinine and blood urea nitrogen, and, in more severe cases, oligo-anuria, blood hypertension, and anemia [16]. As previously mentioned, the concomitant presence of DAH should promptly suggest a pulmonary-renal syndrome (e.g., anti-GBM disease or AAV) [9], and multisystemic manifestations should suggest vasculitis (AAV, cryoglobulinemic, IgA, or immune-complex vasculitis). Histological confirmation is needed when technically possible, but this should not delay the treatment with systemic glucocorticoids, which should be started as soon as possible at 0.5–1 g/day for up to 3 days, followed by oral glucocorticoids in more severe cases or by oral prednisone 1 mg/kg/day. Oral or intravenous cyclophosphamide, rituximab, or mycophenolate mofetil (MMF) should be added after renal biopsy when performed to induce remission. According to the specific type of disease and severity, different treatments could be preferred, while plasmapheresis may be considered in more severe cases (serum creatinine >300 micromol/L) and is usually added in anti-GMB disease. In acute renal failure due to glomerulonephritis, dialysis may be required [16–19].

3.2.3 Large Vessel Vasculitis with Ischemic Symptoms

Giant cell arteritis (GCA) and Takayasu arteritis (TAK) are granulomatous large-vessel vasculitides (LVV) affecting the aorta and/or its major branches that share many clinical and radiographic features [20]. In both diseases, inflammation of the vessel wall triggers a remodeling process of the artery that has two major outcomes: lumen-occluding intimal hyperplasia and aneurysm formation.

GCA (also known as Horton disease and temporal arteritis) is the most common vasculitis in Western countries in individuals older than 50 years [21]. The greatest risk factor for GCA is age. It is a disease of the elderly, occurring between the ages of 60 and 80, while it never occurs under the age of 50.

Headache, systemic symptoms (such as fever, fatigue, and weight loss), polymyalgia rheumatica, jaw claudication, and visual disturbance are the common manifestations of this disease. The laboratory features of GCA reflect the systemic inflammatory response. Erythrocyte sedimentation rate (ESR) and C-reactive protein (CRP) are (often extremely) elevated, but they are not per se specific to GCA. The onset of symptoms tends to be subacute, and its manifestations rarely prompt admission to the ICU. However, abrupt presentations over a few days can occur.

Visual loss and cerebrovascular events are the ischemic manifestations of the disease [22]. These clinical manifestations are typically an early event in the disease course and occur in up to 20% and 7.5% of patients, respectively, usually before glucocorticoid (GC) therapy is started. Visual loss is painless and sudden in onset, generally resulting from arteritic anterior ischemic optic neuropathy (AION). Amaurosis fugax may precede permanent visual loss. Cerebrovascular events are rarer and result from the stenosis or occlusion of the extradural carotid or, more commonly, vertebral arteries. Intracranial involvement is extremely rare [23]. A suspected diagnosis of GCA should be confirmed by temporal artery imaging (ultrasound or MRI) or biopsy or by extracranial large vessel imaging (MRA, CTA, or PET-CT) [24]. Patients with GCA have an increased risk of developing aneurysm and/or dissection of the thoracic aorta, especially of the ascending aorta. These are generally late complications of the disease, occurring 3–5 years after GCA diagnosis, but early evidence of aortic dilation is increasingly reported in patients with GCA [25, 26].

High-dose GCs are the mainstay of treatment for GCA and are effective in controlling symptoms and preventing the ischemic manifestations of the disease. Intravenous methylprednisolone 0.5–1 g/day for up to 3 days, followed by oral prednisone 1 mg/kg/day, should be immediately started in all patients presenting with ischemic manifestations secondary to GCA.

TAK is an uncommon vasculitis affecting individuals younger than 50 years. Women are affected in 80–90% of cases, with an age of onset between 10 and 40 years [25]. The onset of symptoms tends to be subacute. Nonspecific constitutional inflammatory symptoms are frequently the early manifestations of the disease, leading to a delay in diagnosis, and the consequences of the arterial disease are often the first sign at presentation. Arterial inflammation, stenosis, occlusion, and aneurysms lead to various symptoms and signs according to the involved arteries (carotidynia, chest pain, back pain, limb claudication, bruits, absent or diminished pulses). Laboratory abnormalities in patients with TAK are nonspecific and generally reflect an inflammatory process. ESR and CRP may be elevated; however, these tests do not reliably reflect disease activity and can be normal in patients with active disease. TAK generally follows an insidious course at onset, but ischemic manifestations may require admission to the ICU during the disease course [27]. Hypertension develops in more than 50% of patients due to stenosis of one or both renal arteries, and malignant hypertension may occur. Invasive blood pressure monitoring may be required in cases with bilateral subclavian occlusion. Cardiac involvement is common [28, 29]. Moderate to severe aortic regurgitation is the most common manifestation. Angina pectoris may occur in the case of coronary artery ostial narrowing from aortitis, while coronary arteritis is rarer. Pulmonary hypertension secondary to pulmonary arterial involvement may occur, and it is associated with increased mortality. Vertebral and carotid involvement is often asymptomatic, but transient ischemic attacks, stroke, dizziness, or syncope may occur. Although mesenteric involvement is frequent, ischemic abdominal pain is rare. Like GCA, patients with TAK are at increased risk of aortic aneurysm and/or dissection [26, 28]. The diagnosis of TAK should be suspected in young women presenting with constitutional symptoms, hypertension, diminished or absent pulses, and/or arterial bruits and should be confirmed by non-invasive angiography (CTA or MRA) of the entire aorta and its major branches [24]. High-dose GC therapy (40–60 mg/day prednisone-equivalent) in combination with conventional (methotrexate, azathioprine, or mycophenolate mofetil) or biological immunosuppressants (TNF-inhibitors or tocilizumab) should be initiated early in patients with active TAK. Vascular intervention may be necessary for the treatment of stenosed or occluded arteries leading to organ ischemia or hypertension and for the management of aneurysmal disease. Except for emergency indications, procedures should preferably be performed during the remission phase of the disease.

3.2.4 Polyarteritis Nodosa

Polyarteritis nodosa (PAN) is a rare systemic necrotizing vasculitis predominantly affecting medium-sized arteries with variable presenting features [20]. Constitutional symptoms, cutaneous findings (purpura, livedo, nodules, and ulcers), and peripheral nerve involvement (mononeuritis multiplex) are common.

Among the most serious complications of PAN is digital infarction, which may result in gangrene. Severe renovascular hypertension can result from renal artery stenosis and renal infarcts from occlusion of intrarenal arteries or rupture of microaneurysms. Mesenteric arteritis can result in ischemic bowel perforation and rupture of a visceral artery aneurysm. Coronary arteritis resulting in angina and myocardial infarctions is rarer [30].

There are no specific laboratory markers for PAN. Laboratory abnormalities reflect an inflammatory process, and autoantibodies are absent. The diagnosis of PAN requires evidence of the typical angiographic features (saccular or fusiform microaneurysms alternating with stenotic lesions) or a biopsy of an affected organ showing necrotizing inflammation of medium-sized arteries [31].

Patients with mild disease may be treated with GC monotherapy, while those with cardiac, renal, gastrointestinal, and central nervous system involvement have a poorer prognosis and require more aggressive treatment with high-dose GCs (1 mg/kg/day of prednisone-equivalent) in combination with oral or intravenous cyclophosphamide [32]. Emergency endovascular (or surgical) stenting of the aneurysms could be required.

3.2.5 CNS Vasculitis

Central nervous system (CNS) vasculitis refers to a broad spectrum of diseases that result in inflammation and destruction of the blood vessels of the brain, spinal cord, and meninges. CNS vasculitis is considered secondary when it occurs in the context of a systemic inflammatory disease, while primary CNS vasculitis (PCNSV) denotes a vasculitis that is limited to the CNS. PCNSV is a rare disease, and it represents the most frequent vasculitis involving the CNS [33]. The onset of disease can be acute or insidious, with variable and non-specific clinical manifestations, including headache, cognitive impairment, transient ischemic attack, and stroke. Strokes are usually multiple and involve different anatomic territories. Less common symptoms include ataxia, seizure, coma, intracerebral hemorrhage, and myelopathy. Rapidly progressive PCNSV represents the most severe subset of this vasculitis [34]. Typically, bilateral large cerebral vessel lesions with several bilateral cerebral infarctions are present. Constitutional symptoms such as fever are uncommon in PCNSV, and inflammatory markers and autoantibodies are usually normal. CSF analysis shows mildly increased leucocyte count and total protein concentration in 80–90% of patients.

MRI has a high sensitivity for PCNSV, and the diagnosis is unlikely if the MRI is normal. However, abnormal MRI findings are non-specific and include infarction, parenchymal and leptomeningeal enhancement, intracranial hemorrhage, and tumor-like mass lesions [35]. A biopsy of CNS tissue showing vasculitis is the only definitive test. Cerebral angiography may support the diagnosis of PCNSV in the context of a strongly suggestive presentation when a biopsy is not performed, or it is negative. Typical findings are segments of stenotic or occluded artery alternating with normal or dilated segments. The limit of angiography is its low specificity, and findings compatible with vasculitis might be present in cerebral angiography of patients with different non-vasculitic disorders. MRA is less invasive but also less sensitive than angiography, especially for the cerebellar district. Early recognition is important because treatment with GCs and cytotoxic drugs may prevent serious outcomes [33]. For treatment of PCNSV, see Fig. 3.3.

The variable manifestations of PCNSV and the non-specificity of laboratory and imaging findings pose a challenge to accurate diagnosis. The differential diagnosis is broad and includes reversible cerebral vasoconstriction syndromes, infections, malignancy, and secondary cerebral vasculitis (Table 3.1).

Different forms of systemic vasculitides and other rheumatic diseases can involve the CNS (Table 3.2). Systemic disease is generally an established diagnosis before the CNS is involved, and patients usually have evidence of active disease elsewhere.

3.2.6 Behçet's Disease (BD)

Behçet's disease (BD) is a systemic inflammatory disease characterized by oral and genital ulcers, ocular manifestations, and systemic involvement. Vascular and neurological involvement are the major causes of mortality and morbidity of BD and may require the admission of the patient to the ICU. Vascular involvement is observed in up to 40% of the patients with BD, especially in young males [37, 38].

Venous disease is more common than arterial disease. Deep vein thrombosis of lower extremities is the most common manifestation, observed in approximately 70% of patients with vascular Behçet, followed by thrombosis of superior and inferior vena cava (10% of patients). Budd-Chiari syndrome is a rare manifestation of BD (<5%). Pulmonary arterial involvement is the most frequent arterial disease observed in BD, affecting around 5% of patients with vascular Behçet. It can manifest as aneurysm formation, thrombosis, or both and is associated with a high mortality rate [39]. Hemoptysis (sometimes massive) is the most frequent symptom of pulmonary arterial aneurysm. Peripheral arterial involvement is a rare and generally

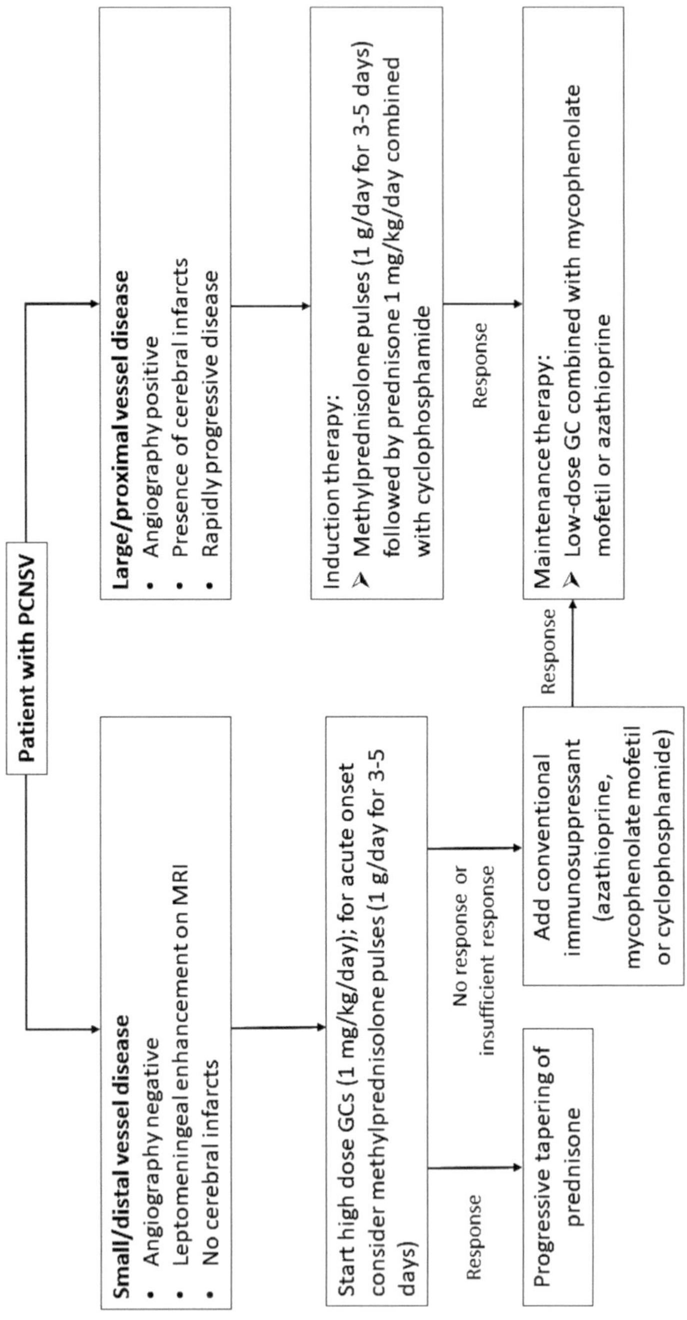

Fig. 3.3 Treatment algorithm for PCNSV. (Adapted from [36])

Table 3.1 Causes of secondary CNS vasculitis

Viral infections
Varicella zoster virus, HIV, hepatitis C virus, cytomegalovirus, parvovirus B19
Bacterial infections
Treponema pallidum, *Borrelia burgdorferi*, *Mycobacterium tuberculosis*, *Mycoplasma pneumoniae*, *Bartonella henselae*, *Rickettsia* spp.
Fungal infections
Aspergillosis, mucormycosis, coccidioidomycosis, candidosis
Parasitic infections
Cysticercosis
Systemic vasculitides
Granulomatosis with polyangiitis, eosinophilic granulomatosis with polyangiitis, Behçet's disease, polyarteritis nodosa, IgA vasculitis, Kawasaki disease, giant cell arteritis, Takayasu's arteritis
Connective Tissue Diseases and other Systemic Autoimmune Conditions
Systemic lupus erythematosus, rheumatoid arthritis, Sjogren's syndrome, dermatomyositis, mixed connective tissue disease
Miscellaneous
Antiphospholipid antibodies syndrome, Hodgkin's and non-Hodgkin lymphomas, neurosarcoidosis, inflammatory bowel disease, graft-versus-host disease, bacterial endocarditis, acute bacterial meningitis, drug-induced CNS vasculitis (cocaine, amphetamine, ephedrine, phenylpropanolamine)

Adapted from [33]

Table 3.2 Neurological syndromes in the ICU secondary to rheumatic disease

Neurological syndromes	Conditions
Acute stroke	CNS vasculitis, Takayasu arteritis, giant cell arteritis, antiphospholipid syndrome, systemic lupus erythematosus, Behçet's disease, DADA2
Status epilepticus	Central nervous system vasculitis, systemic lupus erythematosus, Behçet's disease, sarcoidosis
Meningoencephalitis	Systemic lupus erythematosus, CNS vasculitis, systemic vasculitis, Behçet's disease, rheumatoid arthritis, sarcoidosis
Pachymeningitis	IgG4-related disease, granulomatosis with polyangiitis, sarcoidosis, rheumatoid arthritis
Demyelinating syndrome	Systemic lupus erythematosus, antiphospholipid syndrome, CNS vasculitis, Behçet's disease
Myelopathy	Antiphospholipid syndrome, systemic lupus erythematosus, CNS vasculitis, sarcoidosis, Behçet disease, ankylosing spondylitis
Cerebral venous sinus thrombosis	Behçet's disease, antiphospholipid syndrome
Peripheral or cranial neuropathy	ANCA-associated vasculitis, polyarteritis nodosa, sarcoidosis, systemic lupus erythematosus, Sjogren syndrome, rheumatoid arthritis

late manifestation of the disease (<5% of patients with vascular Behçet). The primary pathology leading to thrombosis in BD is the inflammation of the vessel wall, and high-dose GCs in combination with conventional (azathioprine, cyclosporine-A, or cyclophosphamide) or biological immunosuppressants (TNF-inhibitors) are used to reduce this inflammation. The role of anticoagulation in the treatment of venous vascular Behçet remains unclear [40].

Neurologic involvement occurs in around 10% of patients with BD [41]. Cerebral sinus thrombosis consists of approximately one-third of neurologic involvement of BD. It is mainly seen in males, and it is strongly associated with peripheral venous involvement [42]. The most common neurologic manifestation of BD is parenchymal disease, with meningoencephalitis predominantly affecting the brainstem, generally occurring as a late manifestation of the disease. High-dose GCs in combination with conventional immunosuppressants (azathioprine or cyclophosphamide) are recommended in patients with active neurological Behçet. TNF inhibitors are reserved for patients with chronic progressive course or recurrences [40].

3.2.7 Monogenic Autoinflammatory Syndromes in Adults

Autoinflammatory diseases are rare conditions that have episodic features of inflammation with little or no evidence of systemic autoantibodies or autoreactive T lymphocytes.

Deficiency of adenosine deaminase 2 (DADA2) is a rare, autoinflammatory disease characterized by systemic inflammation, vasculitis, early-onset stroke, cytopenias, and immunodeficiency [43]. It is caused by an autosomal recessive mutation in the Adenosine Deaminase 2 gene (ADA2, formerly known as CECR1) on chromosome 22q11.

Early diagnosis is important because the use of TNF inhibitors is associated with a significantly lower risk for additional strokes [44]. The diagnosis of DADA2 should be suspected in children and young adults who present with PAN-like vasculitis and ischemic or hemorrhagic stroke, especially in the presence of livedo, systemic inflammation, cytopenias, and hypogammaglobulinemia.

VEXAS (Vacuoles, E1 enzyme, X-linked, autoinflammatory, somatic) syndrome is a systemic autoinflammatory disease caused by somatic mutations in the UBA1 gene and presents with adult-onset long-term refractory inflammatory symptoms associated with macrocytic anemia that may progress to pancytopenia, progressive bone marrow failure, as well as myelodysplastic syndrome, and plasma cell neoplasm [45]. VEXAS syndrome should be suspected in male patients older than 50 years with clinical features that bridge hematologic and rheumatologic conditions: cytopenia and inflammatory symptoms, such as fever, skin eruption, chondritis, lung infiltrates, and venous thromboembolism. Vacuolization of myeloid and erythrocytic precursors constitutes a ubiquitous, although not specific, feature of the disease. Patients with VEXAS syndrome may present with organ failure requiring hospitalization in the ICU. Multidisciplinary team involvement is recommended for patient management.

Since VEXAS syndrome remains a rare and novel pathologic entity, clinical evidence stems mainly from observational studies, including case reports and series. High-dose GCs are effective in controlling symptoms in most patients, but steroid dependency is common. Therapies targeting the inflammatory response (anti-IL6 and Janus kinase inhibitors) may have a role in patients with predominant inflammatory manifestations, while therapies targeting the clone (azacytidine) should be considered in patients with myelodysplastic syndrome. Allogeneic stem cell transplantation represents a curative therapeutic approach but has a high risk for adverse events, and careful selection of patients is required [46].

3.3 Connective Tissue Diseases and other Systemic Autoimmune Conditions

3.3.1 Diffuse Alveolar Hemorrhage in Systemic Lupus Erythematosus (SLE)

In SLE, the incidence of DAH ranges from 0.6% to 5.4%, with a reported mortality rate as high as 50% [47]. All the three mechanisms characterizing DAH (capillaritis, bland hemorrhage, and diffuse alveolar damage) are present in SLE [47], and could be further complicated by microvascular thrombosis if APS is present (approximately in 10% of patients with SLE) [48]. High SLE disease activity, positive antiphospholipid antibodies (aPL), thrombocytopenia, or lupus nephritis is associated with an increased risk of DAH [49].

Clinical picture is characterize by dyspnea, cough, and hemoptysis, with symptoms developing rapidly in hours or days. A combination of physical examination, imaging, laboratory results, and BAL analysis provides evidence for diagnosis (Fig. 3.1) [47]. As with DAH due to AAV (see above), patients should be assessed for excessive anticoagulation, infections, concomitant renal disease, and heart failure [49].

Patients with DAH have decreased hemoglobin levels and increased diffusing capacity for carbon monoxide (DLCO) [9]. Elevated plasma creatinine and an abnormal urinalysis suggest a pulmonary-renal syndrome [9]. Initial testing for SLE as an underlying cause of DAH includes antinuclear antibodies, C3, C4, anti-DNA antibodies, and extractable nuclear antigen antibodies. We recommend obtaining microbiologic studies, testing for aPL, antineutrophil cytoplasmic antibodies (ANCA), anti-glomerular basement membrane antibodies (anti-GBM), and a drug screen (if cocaine abuse is suspected).

The imaging findings of DAH on chest X-ray include airspace opacities with central and basilar predominance. Computerized tomography (CT) findings include ground glass opacities that are usually diffuse and bilateral. If the DAH is subacute, these opacities are accompanied by septal thickening [47].

There is a paucity of evidence regarding the treatment of DAH in SLE. Multiple combinations of immunosuppression have been reported, including pulses of methylprednisolone and cyclophosphamide. Plasmapheresis and intravenous immunoglobulins have been used for patients with inadequate response [49].

3.3.2 Severe Lupus Nephritis (LN)

The kidney is affected in 40–60% of SLE patients, and the impairment of renal function results from glomerular, tubule-interstitial, and vascular lesions. Glomerular involvement is produced by the deposition of immunocomplexes (IC), leading to complement leukocyte activation. The spectrum of clinical presentation ranges from silent urinary abnormalities, nephritic and nephrotic syndromes, and rapidly progressive renal insufficiency [50].

In SLE patients, an erythrocyte sedimentation rate (ESR)/ C-reactive protein (CRP) ratio > 15 indicates a probable flare, while <2 indicates more likely an infection. However, in case of a disease flare with serositis (as pericarditis or pleuritis), the CRP is usually elevated. Similarly, new circulating biomarkers such as neutrophil CD64 expression, 2′5′-oligoadenylate synthetase (OAS), and soluble triggering receptor expressed on myeloid cell type 1 (sTREM1) can be helpful in differentiating infection from flares SLE patients with systemic inflammatory response (SIRS) [1, 51].

Clinical manifestations of lupus nephritis (LN) include proteinuria, hypertension, edema, abnormal urinalysis, or renal impairment. A renal biopsy is necessary for the diagnosis of LN. Specific microscopic lesions and the distribution of IC define six histological classes.

Treatment choice depends on the histological class and activity, and chronicity indexes. Classes I and II usually do not need specific immunosuppressive therapy. For classes III and IV, treatment included pulses of methylprednisolone (250–500 mg/day for 3 days), then prednisone 0.6–1 mg/kg/day p.o., with MMF 2–3 g per day p.o. (or mycophenolic acid at equivalent dose) or low cyclophosphamide doses (Eurolupus regimen) 500 mg iv every 2 weeks for six doses. A complete renal response is defined, according to the 2019 update of EULAR/ERA-EDTA recommendations for LN, by a urine protein creatinine ratio (UPCR) <500–700 mg/g (<50–70 mg/mmol) by 12 months with normal or near-normal GFR [17]. In case of no response, reasonable alternatives include MMF combined with a calcineurin inhibitor (voclosporine or tacrolimus), belimumab, or cyclophosphamide combined with belimumab. For Class V LN, immunosuppressive treatment is indicated in patients with nephrotic syndrome and those with proteinuria >1 g/day despite renin-angiotensin-aldosterone system therapy [52]. Both hydroxychloroquine and kidney protective measures should be given in all classes [17].

3.3.3 Thrombotic Microangiopathy in SLE

Thrombotic microangiopathy (TMA) is a life-threatening condition characterized by thrombocytopenia, microangiopathic hemolytic anemia, and platelet microthrombi in small-sized blood vessels [53].

Presence of anemia with hemolysis elements, such as increased reticulocyte count, high LDH, increased indirect bilirubin, and decreased haptoglobin.

Microangiopathic elements such as schistocytes can be found in the blood smear. As it is not an immune process, direct Coombs is negative.

The causes of TMA in SLE are listed in Table 3.3.

The etiology of a TMA in a patient with SLE includes complement-mediated TMA, also called atypical hemolytic uremic syndrome (atypical HUS). In this regard, several studies suggest that the dysregulation of the alternative complement pathway may play a role in SLE patients [53]. Other causes are TTP, APS, especially in the form of Catastrophic APS (CAPS), and drug-mediated TMA. Often, the cause is multifactorial [53].

Thrombocytopenic thrombotic purpura (TTP), caused by ADAMTS 13 deficiency, may present with the pentad of microangiopathic hemolytic anemia, thrombocytopenia, fever, kidney involvement, and/or neurological symptoms. This is an acute condition with a well characterized pathogenesis.

It is recommended to take the following laboratory tests in an SLE patient with TMA (See Fig. 3.4).

Treatment depends on the cause of TMA. If proven to be TTP, the patient should receive therapeutic plasma exchange (TPE) and, in refractory cases, Rituximab [54]. Eculizumab, an anti-complement agent, is currently the first-line therapy in the presence of a clear diagnosis of complement-mediated TMA [54]. The treatment of CAPS is discussed in section "Catastrophic Antiphospholipid Syndrome (CAPS)".

Table 3.3 Differential diagnosis of thrombotic microangiopathies in SLE

Etiology	Supported features
Thrombotic thrombocytopenic purpura (TTP)	ADAMTS 13 deficiency (<10% activity is diagnostic) It could be hereditary or acquired Obtain ADAMTS13 activity, inhibitor screen, and mutational analysis
Complement-mediated TMA (atypical HUS)	Most common cause is abnormalities of complement regulation with uncontrolled complement activation It could be hereditary or acquired Obtain panel: CH50 (functional assay), AH50 (functional assay), C3, C4, C4d, sC5b-9, CFB, CFBb, and CFH
Shiga toxin-Hemolytic Uremic Syndrome (ST-HUS)	Bacteria produce Shiga toxin: *Shigella dysenteriae* type 1, *Escherichia coli* O157:H7, *E coli* O104:H4 Diarrhea prodrome (+) Ask for Shiga toxin stool PCR
Other causes	
Drugs	Calcineurin inhibitors
Infection	HIV, Streptococcus pneumoniae
Antiphospholipid antibodies	Antiphospholipid syndrome Catastrophic antiphospholipid syndrome (CAPS)
Miscellaneous	Coagulopathy, pregnancy, malignancy, malignant hypertension

ADAMTS13 = a disintegrin and metalloprotease with a thrombospondin type 1 motif, member 13; CH50 = total hemolytic complement assay; AH50 = complement alternate pathway assay; *CFB* complement factor B, *CFBb* complement factor Bb, *CFH* complement factor H

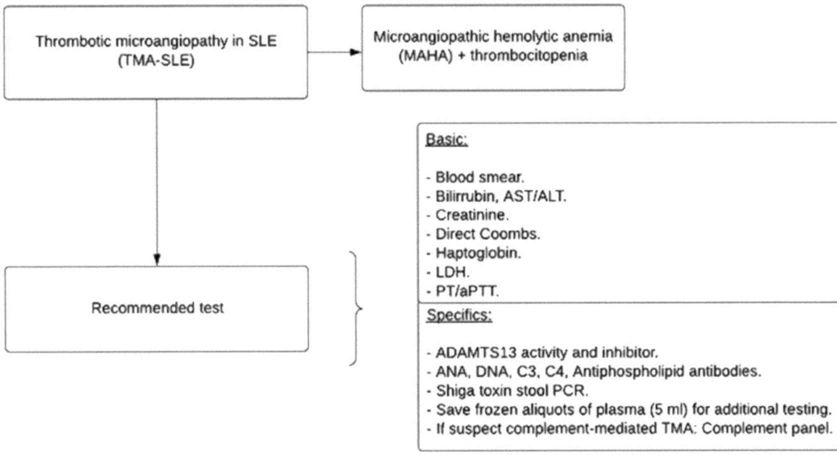

Fig. 3.4 Recommended laboratory workup in thrombotic microangiopathy in SLE

3.3.4 Severe Neuropsychiatric SLE

Neuropsychiatric manifestations in SLE (NPSLE) may involve the central and peripheral nervous systems. While multiple neuropsychiatric syndromes have been described, most of the neuropsychiatric manifestations in SLE are due to non-lupus causes, such as infections, medications (i.e., glucocorticoids), and metabolic disturbances.

The manifestations can be divided pathophysiologically into inflammatory, thrombotic, or a combination thereof [55]. Inflammatory syndromes include myelitis, demyelinating disease, aseptic meningitis, some acute confusional states, and psychotic episodes. Thrombotic syndromes are generally due to antiphospholipid antibodies; some examples include seizures and strokes.

A neurologic manifestation is more likely to be attributed to SLE if the timing of the NP event occurs within 6 months of the onset of SLE, but it cannot be necessarily excluded if the timing is unclear. Also, it is more probable to be due to SLE if there is high SLE disease activity with other SLE systemic manifestations, abnormal brain imaging, abnormal cerebrospinal fluid (CSF) analysis, and aPL positivity [56]. For treatment of neuropsychiatric SLE [55], see Fig. 3.5.

3.3.5 Catastrophic Antiphospholipid Syndrome (CAPS)

Antiphospholipid syndrome (APS) is a systemic autoimmune disorder characterized by thrombosis, pregnancy morbidity, and non-thrombotic manifestations in patients with persistently positive antiphospholipid antibodies (aPL), namely the lupus anticoagulant (LA) test, anticardiolipin antibodies (aCL), and anti–β_2-glycoprotein I antibodies (aβ_2GPI) [57]. The manifestations of APS that may be

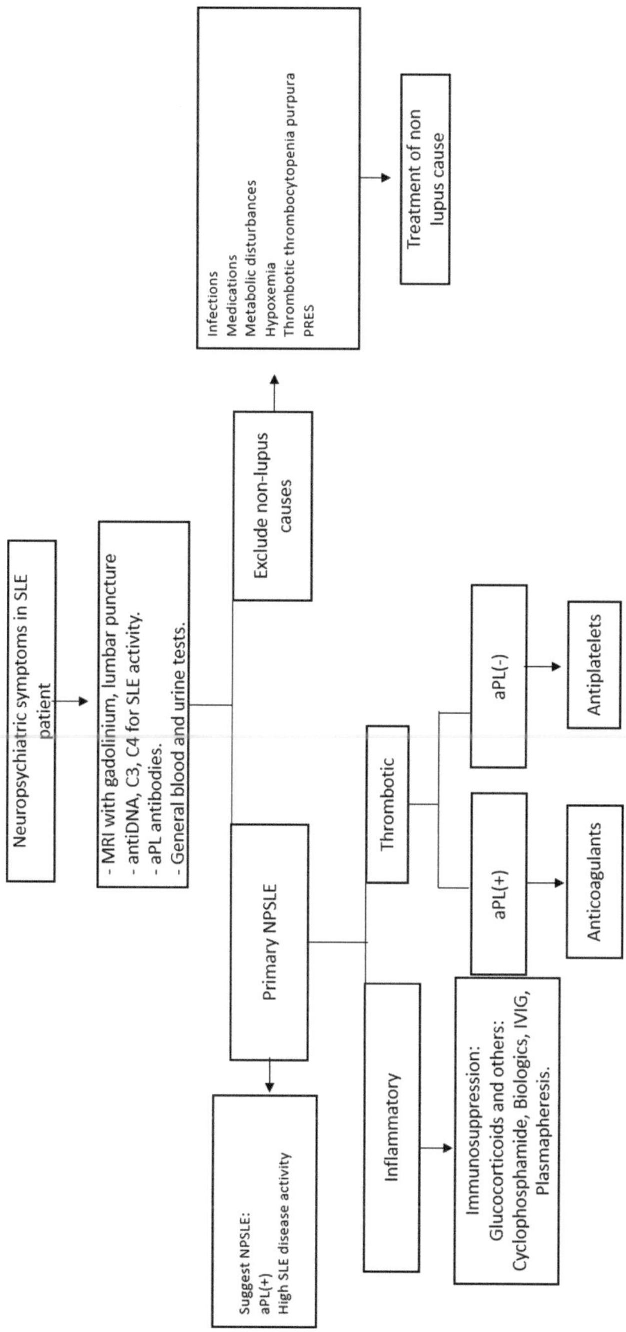

Fig. 3.5 Diagnostic and treatment algorithm to manage neuropsychiatric SLE

seen more frequently in ICU patients are diffuse alveolar hemorrhage and catastrophic APS (CAPS). The diagnosis and treatment of diffuse alveolar hemorrhage in APS do not differ from that in SLE. Except that in DAH by APS, the use of Rituximab is recommended without much available evidence [58]. We refer the reader to that section.

Catastrophic antiphospholipid syndrome (CAPS) is a rare, life-threatening form of APS characterized by thrombotic complications, usually microvascular as well as large-vessel thrombosis, affecting multiple organs with multiorgan failure, that develop simultaneously or over a short period. Approximately 1% of patients with APS develop CAPS, and half of the patients debut with CAPS without having a previous diagnosis of APS [57].

The hallmark of CAPS is multisystem involvement with multiorgan failure (often with evidence of ischemic changes on imaging), acute onset in less than a week, presence of microthrombosis, and large vessel thrombosis, which may occur despite adequate anticoagulation in patients with established APS diagnosis. There is general microangiopathic hemolytic anemia with characteristic thrombocytopenia and blood smear with schistocytes. All of this with concomitant aPL. This contrasts with APS, where there is typically a single, large-vessel thrombotic event or a series of events separated in time, such as an initial pulmonary embolus followed by a deep vein thrombosis months later associated with inadequate anticoagulation [57]. In CAPS, the kidneys are the organ more often affected (74%), followed by the lungs (55%), the brain (56%), the heart (53%), and the skin (45%) [59]. However, other organs can be affected.

Ordering a blood smear to search for schistocytes and hemolysis testing such as reticulocyte count, lactate dehydrogenase (LDH), and haptoglobin is suggested. Also, specific testing for aPL: LA, aCL, and aβ_2GPI, and testing to exclude alternative differential diagnosis: ADAMTS13 activity for TTP, complement testing for complement-mediated thrombotic microangiopathy.

Classification criteria for CAPS have been proposed and validated for research purposes [60].

Definite CAPS is present if all four criteria are present:

1. Involvement of $\geq$3 organs, systems, or tissues.
2. Manifestations develop simultaneously or over <1 week.
3. Small vessel occlusion is confirmed histologically in at least one organ or tissue.
4. The presence of aPL (aCL, aβ_2GPI, and LA) is documented twice, at least 12 weeks apart.

CAPS is defined as probable only if three of the four requirements are met. The main differential diagnosis of CAPS includes other TMAs and sepsis, which need to be ruled out.

A combination of anticoagulation, glucocorticoids, IVIG, and/or plasma exchange (triple therapy) is independently associated with higher survival. Rituximab has been suggested in refractory cases and those with thrombocytopenia [59].

3.3.6 Macrophagic Activation Syndrome (MAS)

Macrophagic activation syndrome (MAS) is a form of secondary hemophagocytosis lymphohistiocytosis (HLH) occurring as a complication of a rheumatic disease [61]. It is characterized by hemophagocytosis and multi-organ damage [62]. The three most common rheumatologic conditions that cause MAS are Systemic Juvenile Idiopathic Arthritis (sJIA), Adult-onset Still disease (AOSD), and Systemic Lupus Erythematosus (SLE) [63].

There is no single diagnostic test for MAS. Patients present with fever of unknown origin, systemic inflammation, high ferritin, and multilinear cytopenias in the context of systemic autoimmune disease. In the ICU, MAS should be considered in deteriorating critically ill patients with a disproportionate inflammatory response (e.g., persistent fever, unresponsiveness to vasopressors, need for extracorporeal life support), cytopenias, and organ failure not responding to appropriate therapy, antimicrobial treatment, and aggressive supportive care [64]. Hyperferritinemia assessed using the threshold of >500 μg/L has a high sensitivity (96.2%) [65], while values >10,000 microgram/L is usually considered pathognomonic, and > 5000 is highly suggestive for diagnosis, especially if CRP, aspartate aminotransferase (AST), alanine aminotransferase (ALT), and lactate dehydrogenase (LDH) are elevated [66]. Notably, procalcitonin (PCT) can be frequently elevated in MAS, making the differential diagnosis with severe sepsis more challenging.

The diagnosis can be supported by the HLH-2004 Diagnostic Criteria if at least 5 of 8 criteria are present [67] (Table 3.4) or by using the online HScore calculator, which has been designed to aid in diagnosing secondary cause HLH. HScore estimates the probability of HLH [68]. An HScore ≥250 confers a 99% probability of HLH, whereas a score of ≤90 confers a < 1% probability of HLH. Other clinical and laboratory features supporting the diagnosis are in Table 3.5 [63].

Table 3.4 Hemophagocytic lymphohistiocytosis (HLH): HLH-4 Classification Criteria

Criteria	Parameters	Frequency
Fever	≥ 38.5 C	>95% of cases
High ferritin	≥ 500 mg/L	>95% of cases
Splenomegaly		>70% of cases
Cytopenia (affecting ≥2 of 3 lineages)	Hemoglobin <9 g/dl, platelets <100.000, neutrophils <1000	>95% of cases
High triglycerides and/or low fibrinogen	Triglycerides >265 mg/dl, fibrinogen <150 mg/dl	60% cases
Hemophagocytosis	In bone marrow and other tissues	
High soluble IL-2 receptor (sCD25)	>2400 U/ml or > 2 SD above laboratory normal sCD25 > 10.000 is specific	
Low NK cell activity	Low or absent NK cell activity (according to local laboratory reference)	

Table 3.5 Clinical and laboratory findings in macrophagic activation syndrome

Clinical features	
Neurological involvement	65% of cases. Encephalopathy, Seizures, Encephalitis, PRES
Renal involvement	88% of cases. Renal failure. Nephrotic syndrome
Peripheral adenopathies	33% of cases
Rash	25% cases. Non-specific cutaneous involvement. Erythematous rashes, purpura, petechiae
Laboratory	
ESR/CRP discordance	Low/normal ESR or falling ESR with high CRP. Procalcitonin (PCT) could also be elevated
High AST/ALT/LDH	95% of cases
Coagulopathy	60% of cases. High D-Dimer, disseminated intravascular coagulation

Conventionally, GC is the first-line treatment. High-dose pulse methylprednisolone (1 g/d for 3–5 consecutive days) is a frequent initial approach. Early use of high-dose GC may be successful alone, but over half of the reported adult cases are steroid-resistant. In conjunction with GC, the joint use of anakinra, an IL-1–blocking therapy, is recommended in doses of 2 to 6 mg/kg up to 10 mg/kg per day subcutaneously in divided doses [69]. Cyclosporine (2–7 mg/kg per day) can be added in patients with an insufficient immediate response. Finally, in patients with severe active disease or CNS involvement, despite GC, Anakinra, and/or cyclosporine, a reduced dose of etoposide (50–100 mg/m^2 once weekly) may be very effective [64]. In SLE cases, there are successful cases treated with IVIG, cyclophosphamide, and rituximab [65]. Neutralizing IFNγ with emapalumab was efficacious in inducing remission of MAS secondary to sJIA or AOSD in patients who had failed high-dose glucocorticoids [70].

3.3.7 Interstitial Lung Disease (ILD) Related to Rheumatic Diseases (RD) in ICU

Interstitial lung disease (ILD) occurs in patients with rheumatic diseases (RD) and is more frequent in those with systemic sclerosis (SSc), idiopathic inflammatory myopathies (IIM), and rheumatoid arthritis (RA); however, it has been reported in other conditions (Table 3.6) [71].

Interstitial pneumonia with autoimmune features (IPAF) is a term recently proposed for the subset of patients with ILD and clinical or serological features consistent with an RD who do not meet any diagnostic criteria for a specific RD [72].

The histopathologic and imaging classification of RD-ILD follows idiopathic interstitial pneumonia (IIPs). It includes usual interstitial pneumonia (UIP), nonspecific interstitial pneumonia (NSIP), organizing pneumonia (OP), acute interstitial pneumonia (AIP), and lymphoid interstitial pneumonia (LIP) [73].

ILD diagnosis is based on HRCT or lung biopsy, with biopsy performed rarely in the context of acute disease. At the same time, pulmonary function tests and

Table 3.6 Rheumatic disease-associated interstitial lung disease (RD-ILD)

	Rheumatic disease (RD) serologies	Prevalence of ILD in RD patients	ILD patterns	Risk factors for ILD
SSc-ILD	Anti-Scl-70 Anticentromere Anti-RNA polymerase III A nucleolar pattern of ANA immunofluorescence (IF)	35–52%	NSIP>UIP	Diffuse cutaneous SSc, Scl-70+, nucleolar pattern of ANA IF, male sex, older age, cardiac involvement, and high Rodnan skin score
IIM-ILD	Myositis-specific autoantibodies (e.g., anti-MDA5, anti-Mi2 and anti-synthetase antibodies) Myositis-associated autoantibodies (e.g., anti-Ro-52, anti-Ku and PM-Sc, U1RNPl)	19–40% 69–100% in anti-synthetase syndrome	NSIP > OP > AIP > UIP	Anti-synthetase antibodies, anti-MDA-5 antibodies, clinically amyopathic dermatomyositis (CADM) PM-Scl, Ku, Ro52/SSA, and U1RNP

(continued)

Table 3.6 (continued)

	Rheumatic disease (RD) serologies	Prevalence of ILD in RD patients	ILD patterns	Risk factors for ILD
RA-ILD	Rheumatoid factor (RF) Anti-citrullinated peptide antibodies (ACPA)	3–40%	UIP > NSIP > OP	Older age, male sex, smoking, high titers of RF and ACPA, and RA disease activity
IPAF	ANA ≥1:320 titer any pattern ANA nucleolar pattern (any titer) ANA centromere pattern (any titer) RF ≥2× upper limit of normal Anti-CCP Anti-dsDNA Anti-Ro/SSA Anti-La/SSB Anti-ribonucleoprotein (RNP) Anti-Smith Anti-Scl-70 Anti-synthetases antibodies Anti-PM-Scl Anti-MDA-5	100%	NSIP, OP, NSIP with OP	All the patients have ILD
ANCA-associated vasculitis-ILD	MPO-ANCA PR3-ANCA	Up to 23% in GPA; up to 45% in MPA; unknown for EGPA	UIP, NSIP	Older age, MPO-ANCA positivity, genetic *MCU5B* variant
Primary Sjogren syndrome-ILD	ANA ≥1: 160 titer RF Anti-Ro/SSA Anti-La/SSB	13–20%	NSIP, UIP, LIP	Older age, male sex, smoking, disease duration, non-sicca onset of disease, anti-Ro-52, increased CRP

Adapted from [71]

arterial blood gases are used to evaluate the extent of the disease and the impairment level of pulmonary function. Since RD may be accompanied by several complications, such as infections or secondary pulmonary hypertension, the diagnostic workup includes bronchoscopy with bronchoalveolar lavage studies, heart ultrasound, and right heart catheterization.

Common accompanying clinical signs that can help make the diagnosis of RD are the findings of fissuring and hyperkeratosis of the palms and lateral fingers (mechanic hands), fingertip ulcerations, cutaneous ulcers, palmar papules, arthritis, palmar telangiectasia, Raynaud phenomenon, unexplained rash on the extensor surfaces of digits (Gottron sign), muscle weakness, among others [72].

In the ICU, the RD-ILD can be seen in two different scenarios.

- *Scenario 1: Debut of a rapidly progressive interstitial lung disease (RPILD).* Usually occurs in a patient with no previous diagnosis of RD. RPILD is defined as severe ILD within 1 month after the onset of respiratory symptoms [74]. The histopathologic and HRCT pattern is usually AIP, but sometimes it could be OP [73]. Regarding the causes of RD-RPILD, the first option is due to an IIM, usually MDA-5 antibodies, and the second is anti-synthetase antibodies [75].
  Anti-MDA-5 disease can present in RPILD form with catastrophic respiratory failure in 50–80% of the patients [76]. This rapidly progressive form is often associated with clinically amyopathic dermatomyositis (CADM), i.e., no muscle weakness or CK increase. Risk factors, such as anti-MDA5 antibody titer, lactate dehydrogenase (LDH) level, and serum ferritin level, have been linked to the development of RPILD.
- *Scenario 2: Acute exacerbations in a patient already diagnosed with RD-ILD.* The second scenario is acute exacerbations in a patient diagnosed with RD-ILD. Acute exacerbations are characterized by rapid worsening of respiratory symptoms, hypoxemia, and new bilateral ground-glass opacities or consolidations on HRCT [77]. Other causes are infection, microaspiration, or DMARD treatment side effects (e.g., methotrexate pneumonia). There are "idiopathic exacerbations," which are frequent in patients with idiopathic pulmonary fibrosis but can also occur in RA-ILD and less frequent in SSc-ILD [78].
  The differential diagnosis of RD-ILD includes Idiopathic pulmonary pneumonia, chronic hypersensitivity pneumonitis, occult aspiration, drug reaction, and infections [78].

We will focus on treating RD-ILD in the two acute scenarios presented above:

- *Scenario 1*: Pulses of methylprednisolone (e.g., methylprednisolone 1 gram daily for 3 days) followed by systemic corticosteroids along with an immunosuppressant agent (tacrolimus, mycophenolate mofetil, cyclophosphamide, or rituximab) have been used. Due to the severity of the condition, giving combinations of these therapies is recommended. Administered early, appears to give the highest survival rates [79].
- *Scenario 2*: Acute exacerbations of RD-ILD could be difficult to differentiate from an infection. Bronchoalveolar lavage is recommended to exclude infections and to count immune cells. Broad-spectrum antibiotics and the temporary with-

drawal of DMARDs are often used in these cases. High-dose steroids, intravenous cyclophosphamide, or rituximab have been proposed, but evidence in support of these strategies is limited [78]. In the case of RA-ILD, medications to treat RA, such as inhibitors of TNF and IL-6, are associated with progression of both pre-existing ILD and acute exacerbation [80, 81]. Although little evidence is available, the British Society of Rheumatology has previously advised against TNF inhibitors in patients with pre-existing ILD and suggested that their withdrawal should be considered in patients with worsening or new features of ILD [82].

3.3.8 Scleroderma Renal Crisis

The most important renal manifestation of systemic sclerosis (SSc) is scleroderma renal crisis (SRC). SRC is a life-threatening complication of SSc that almost always occurs within the first 5 years of disease onset. It is usually characterized by malignant hypertension and acute kidney injury, occurring in ~5% of all SSc patients [83].

The clinical spectrum of SRC is broad, from presenting as new onset accelerated arterial hypertension and rapidly progressive oliguric renal failure to more modest elevations in blood pressure and renal dysfunction, and at times (10% of the cases) normotensive presentations [83].

The typical presentation is that of a stable patient who abruptly develops severe arterial hypertension and kidney injury with accelerated oliguric renal failure. Other findings include microscopic hematuria and proteinuria; red blood cell casts are occasionally seen in the urine. The plasma renin level is extremely high in essential malignant hypertension. Also, there is thrombotic microangiopathy with microangiopathic hemolytic anemia and thrombocytopenia. In up to one-fifth of cases, SRC may be the presenting feature of SSc [84].

The diagnosis is clinical. SRC must be distinguished from other forms of thrombotic microangiopathy, particularly thrombotic thrombocytopenic purpura (TTP) and hemolytic uremic syndrome (HUS). A renal biopsy should not delay therapy. When the biopsy is performed, typical findings of thrombotic microangiopathy are found, with a major compromise of small vessels (arcuate and interlobular arteries) rather than glomerular alterations [84].

SRC is a medical emergency that requires aggressive treatment. Successful treatment of SRC depends upon its initiation before irreversible kidney damage has occurred [85]. The mainstay of therapy in SRC is effective and prompt blood pressure control. The principal goal is to return the patient to their previous baseline blood pressure within 72 h. The optimal antihypertensive agent is an ACE inhibitor. If this blood pressure goal cannot be achieved with ACE inhibitor therapy alone, other antihypertensive agents should be added, but maximizing the ACE inhibitor dose is the chief priority.

When prescribing ACE inhibitors in SRC, it is important to achieve effective angiotensin blockade as soon as possible and avoid interruptions in therapy. Both short- and long-acting ACE inhibitors have been used, and the dose can and should be increased to the maximal dose or until adequate blood pressure control is achieved. It has been suggested to initiate treatment with captopril, which has a shorter half-life than other ACE inhibitors. The ACE inhibitor should never be stopped, even in rising serum creatinine. The captopril can be used up to 300–450 mg/day, usually divided into three daily doses.

Set of Multiple Questions

What of the following could be the cause of diffuse alveolar hemorrhage?

1. Chemicals/toxics
2. ANCA-associated vasculitis
3. Systemic lupus erythematosus
4. Infection
5. **All the previous**

Rapidly progressive glomerulonephritis (GN) is most frequently due to:

1. Immune-complex mediated GN
2. Anti-GBM GN
3. **Pauci-immune GN**
4. Hypovolemic shock
5. None of the previous

Which of the following is the most specific test for the diagnosis of primary CNS vasculitis?

1. CSF analysis showing increased leucocyte count and total protein concentration
2. MRI showing multiple cerebral infarctions involving different anatomic territories
3. Cerebral angiography showing segments of stenotic or occluded artery alternating with normal or dilated segments
4. **Biopsy of CNS tissue showing vasculitis**
5. Elevation of CRP

What is the recommended therapy for cerebral sinus thrombosis secondary to Behçet's disease?

1. **High-dose glucocorticoids eventually combined with immunosuppressants**
2. Anticoagulation
3. Plasmapheresis
4. Intravenous Immunoglobulin (IVIG)
5. Colchicine

What immunology laboratory tests rule out an immunologic cause of diffuse alveolar hemorrhage?

(a) **Antinuclear antibodies (ANA), double-stranded (ds) DNA antibodies, complement levels, antiphospholipid (aPL) antibodies, ANCA antibodies, and anti-glomerular basement (GMB) antibodies**
(b) ANA, HLA B-27, aPL antibodies, ANCA antibodies, rheumatoid factor (RF), and anti-cyclic citrullinated peptide (anti-CCP)
(c) RF, ANA, dsDNA, complement levels, ANCA antibodies, and anti-GBM antibodies
(d) ANA, dsDNA antibodies, complement levels, aPL antibodies, RF, and anti-CCP
(e) Anti-Ro antibodies, dsDNA antibodies, aPL antibodies, ANCA antibodies, RF, and anti-CCP

Which of the following tests is most specific for the diagnosis of systemic lupus erythematosus?

(a) Antinuclear antibody
(b) **Anti-double-stranded DNA**
(c) Anti-single-stranded DNA.
(d) Anti-Ro/SSA and anti-La/SSB
(e) Complement levels

A 40-year-old woman with a known diagnosis of primary antiphospholipid syndrome (APS), in whom anticoagulation with warfarin is suspended due to elective hip surgery. She subsequently presents with anemia, elevated LDH, indirect bilirubin, reticulocyte count, and low haptoglobin. The smear shows abundant schistocytes. He also presented with thrombocytopenia and multiorgan failure. In a period of less than a week, she presents cerebral and renal infarcts. The serology for lupus is negative. What is the recommended therapy for her?

(a) Anticoagulation, cyclophosphamide, and intravenous immunoglobulin
(b) Cyclophosphamide, anticoagulation, and glucocorticoids
(c) **Glucocorticoids, anticoagulation, and plasmapheresis**
(d) Plasmapheresis, Anti-TNF, and glucocorticoids
(e) Cyclophosphamide, plasmapheresis, and glucocorticoids

Female 40 years old with a recent diagnosis of diffuse systemic sclerosis presents in the emergency room with severe arterial hypertension and kidney injury with accelerated oliguric renal failure. After performing other basic laboratory tests, you conclude it is a scleroderma renal crisis.

What is the most important drug you would start?

(a) Thiazide diuretics
(b) **Angiotensin-converting enzyme (ACE) inhibitors**

(c) High doses of glucocorticoids
(d) Plasmapheresis
(e) Calcium channel blockers

References

1. Raza T. Rheumatology in ICU. Qatar Med J. 2020;2019(2 – Qatar Critical Care Conference Proceedings)
2. Kollef MH, Enzenauer RJ. Predicting outcome from intensive care for patients with rheumatologic diseases. J Rheumatol. 1992;19(8):1260–2.
3. Godeau B, Boudjadja A, Dhainaut JF, Schlemmer B, Chastang C, Brunet F, et al. Outcome of patients with systemic rheumatic disease admitted to medical intensive care units. Ann Rheum Dis. 1992;51(5):627–31.
4. Janssen NM, Karnad DR, Guntupalli KK. Rheumatologic diseases in the intensive care unit: epidemiology, clinical approach, management, and outcome. Crit Care Clin. 2002;18(4):729–48.
5. Chevet B, Cornec D, Casal Moura M, Cornec-Le Gall E, Fervenza FC, Warrington KJ, et al. Diagnosing and treating ANCA-associated vasculitis: an updated review for clinical practice. Rheumatology (Oxford). 2023;62(5):1787–803.
6. Aguiar CL, Erkan D. Catastrophic antiphospholipid syndrome: how to diagnose a rare but highly fatal disease. Ther Adv Musculoskelet Dis. 2013;5(6):305–14.
7. Berti A, Specks U. The survival of patients with alveolar hemorrhage secondary to Antineutrophil cytoplasmic antibody-associated Vasculitis. J Rheumatol. 2021;48(3):314–7.
8. Walsh M, Merkel PA, Peh CA, Szpirt WM, Puéchal X, Fujimoto S, et al. Plasma exchange and glucocorticoids in severe ANCA-associated Vasculitis. N Engl J Med. 2020;382(7):622–31.
9. Lara AR, Schwarz MI. Diffuse alveolar hemorrhage. Chest. 2010;137(5):1164–71.
10. Cornec D, Cornec-Le Gall E, Fervenza FC, Specks U. ANCA-associated vasculitis – clinical utility of using ANCA specificity to classify patients. Nat Rev Rheumatol. 2016;12(10):570–9.
11. Cartin-Ceba R, Diaz-Caballero L, Al-Qadi MO, Tryfon S, Fervenza FC, Ytterberg SR, et al. Diffuse alveolar hemorrhage secondary to Antineutrophil cytoplasmic antibody-associated Vasculitis: predictors of respiratory failure and clinical outcomes. Arthritis Rheumatol. 2016;68(6):1467–76.
12. Kronbichler A, Bajema I, Geetha D, Säemann M. Novel aspects in the pathophysiology and diagnosis of glomerular diseases. Ann Rheum Dis. 2023;82(5):585–93.
13. Duong MD, Reidy KJ. Acute postinfectious glomerulonephritis. Pediatr Clin N Am. 2022;69(6):1051–78.
14. Jennette JC. Rapidly progressive crescentic glomerulonephritis. Kidney Int. 2003;63(3):1164–77.
15. Falk RJ, Nachman PH, Hogan SL, Jennette JC. ANCA glomerulonephritis and vasculitis: a Chapel Hill perspective. Semin Nephrol. 2000;20(3):233–43.
16. Couser WG. Rapidly progressive glomerulonephritis: classification, pathogenetic mechanisms, and therapy. Am J Kidney Dis. 1988;11(6):449–64.
17. Fanouriakis A, Kostopoulou M, Cheema K, Anders HJ, Aringer M, Bajema I, et al. 2019 update of the joint European league against rheumatism and European renal association-European dialysis and transplant association (EULAR/ERA-EDTA) recommendations for the management of lupus nephritis. Ann Rheum Dis. 2020;79(6):713–23.
18. Hellmich B, Sanchez-Alamo B, Schirmer JH, Berti A, Blockmans D, Cid MC, et al. EULAR recommendations for the management of ANCA-associated vasculitis: 2022 update. Ann Rheum Dis. 2023;

19. Rovin BH, Adler SG, Barratt J, Bridoux F, Burdge KA, Chan TM, et al. Executive summary of the KDIGO 2021 Guideline for the Management of Glomerular Diseases. Kidney Int. 2021;100(4):753–79.
20. Jennette JC, Falk RJ, Bacon PA, Basu N, Cid MC, Ferrario F, et al. 2012 revised international Chapel Hill consensus conference nomenclature of Vasculitides. Arthritis Rheum. 2013;65(1):1–11.
21. Salvarani C, Cantini F, Boiardi L, Hunder GG. Polymyalgia rheumatica and giant-cell arteritis. N Engl J Med. 2002;347(4):261–71.
22. Soriano A, Muratore F, Pipitone N, Boiardi L, Cimino L, Salvarani C. Visual loss and other cranial ischaemic complications in giant cell arteritis. Nat Rev Rheumatol. 2017;13(8):476–84.
23. Salvarani C, Giannini C, Miller DV, Hunder G. Giant cell arteritis: involvement of intracranial arteries. Arthritis Rheum. 2006;55(6):985–9.
24. Hellmich B, Agueda A, Monti S, Buttgereit F, de Boysson H, Brouwer E, et al. 2018 update of the EULAR recommendations for the management of large vessel vasculitis. Ann Rheum Dis. 2020;79(1):19–30.
25. Pugh D, Karabayas M, Basu N, Cid MC, Goel R, Goodyear CS, et al. Large-vessel vasculitis. Nat Rev Dis Primers. 2022;7(1):93.
26. Muratore F, Crescentini F, Spaggiari L, Pazzola G, Casali M, Boiardi L, et al. Aortic dilatation in patients with large vessel vasculitis: a longitudinal case control study using PET/CT. Semin Arthritis Rheum. 2019;48(6):1074–82.
27. Mason JC. Takayasu arteritis–advances in diagnosis and management. Nat Rev Rheumatol. 2010;6(7):406–15.
28. Watanabe Y, Miyata T, Tanemoto K. Current clinical features of new patients with Takayasu arteritis observed from cross-country research in Japan: age and sex specificity. Circulation. 2015;132(18):1701–9.
29. Comarmond C, Biard L, Lambert M, Mekinian A, Ferfar Y, Kahn JE, et al. Long-term outcomes and prognostic factors of complications in Takayasu arteritis: a multicenter study of 318 patients. Circulation. 2017;136(12):1114–22.
30. Pagnoux C, Seror R, Henegar C, Mahr A, Cohen P, Le Guern V, et al. Clinical features and outcomes in 348 patients with polyarteritis nodosa: a systematic retrospective study of patients diagnosed between 1963 and 2005 and entered into the French Vasculitis Study Group Database. Arthritis Rheum. 2010;62(2):616–26.
31. Marvisi C, Muratore F, Cabassi C, Galli E, Boiardi L, Piana S, et al. What to know about biopsy sampling and pathology in Vasculitis? Curr Rheumatol Rep. 2022;24(9):279–91.
32. Chung SA, Gorelik M, Langford CA, Maz M, Abril A, Guyatt G, et al. 2021 American College of Rheumatology/Vasculitis Foundation Guideline for the Management of Polyarteritis Nodosa. Arthritis Rheumatol. 2021;73(8):1384–93.
33. Salvarani C, Brown RD Jr, Hunder GG. Adult primary central nervous system vasculitis. Lancet. 2012;380(9843):767–77.
34. Salvarani C, Brown RD Jr, Calamia KT, Christianson TJ, Huston J 3rd, Meschia JF, et al. Rapidly progressive primary central nervous system vasculitis. Rheumatology (Oxford). 2011;50(2):349–58.
35. Zuccoli G, Pipitone N, Haldipur A, Brown RD Jr, Hunder G, Salvarani C. Imaging findings in primary central nervous system vasculitis. Clin Exp Rheumatol. 2011;29(1 Suppl 64):S104–9.
36. Salvarani C, Brown RD Jr, Christianson T, Miller DV, Giannini C, Huston J 3rd, et al. An update of the Mayo Clinic cohort of patients with adult primary central nervous system vasculitis: description of 163 patients. Medicine (Baltimore). 2015;94(21):e738.
37. Alibaz-Oner F, Karadeniz A, Ylmaz S, Balkarl A, Kimyon G, Yazc A, et al. Behçet disease with vascular involvement: effects of different therapeutic regimens on the incidence of new relapses. Medicine (Baltimore). 2015;94(6):e494.
38. Tascilar K, Melikoglu M, Ugurlu S, Sut N, Caglar E, Yazici H. Vascular involvement in Behçet's syndrome: a retrospective analysis of associations and the time course. Rheumatology (Oxford). 2014;53(11):2018–22.

39. Saadoun D, Wechsler B, Desseaux K, Le Thi HD, Amoura Z, Resche-Rigon M, et al. Mortality in Behçet's disease. Arthritis Rheum. 2010;62(9):2806–12.
40. Hatemi G, Christensen R, Bang D, Bodaghi B, Celik AF, Fortune F, et al. 2018 update of the EULAR recommendations for the management of Behçet's syndrome. Ann Rheum Dis. 2018;77(6):808–18.
41. Akman-Demir G, Serdaroglu P, Tasçi B. Clinical patterns of neurological involvement in Behçet's disease: evaluation of 200 patients. The Neuro-Behçet Study Group. Brain. 1999;122(Pt 11):2171–82.
42. Uluduz D, Midi I, Duman T, Colakoglu S, Tüfekci A, Bakar M, et al. Behçet's disease as a causative factor of cerebral venous sinus thrombosis: subgroup analysis of data from the VENOST study. Rheumatology (Oxford). 2019;58(4):600–8.
43. Zhou Q, Yang D, Ombrello AK, Zavialov AV, Toro C, Zavialov AV, et al. Early-onset stroke and vasculopathy associated with mutations in ADA2. N Engl J Med. 2014;370(10):911–20.
44. Ombrello AK, Qin J, Hoffmann PM, Kumar P, Stone D, Jones A, et al. Treatment strategies for deficiency of adenosine deaminase 2. N Engl J Med. 2019;380(16):1582–4.
45. Beck DB, Ferrada MA, Sikora KA, Ombrello AK, Collins JC, Pei W, et al. Somatic mutations in UBA1 and severe adult-onset autoinflammatory disease. N Engl J Med. 2020;383(27):2628–38.
46. Boyadzhieva Z, Ruffer N, Kötter I, Krusche M. How to treat VEXAS-syndrome: a systematic review on effectiveness and safety of current treatment strategies. Rheumatology (Oxford). 2023;
47. Al-Adhoubi NK, Bystrom J. Systemic lupus erythematosus and diffuse alveolar hemorrhage, etiology and novel treatment strategies. Lupus. 2020;29(4):355–63.
48. Stoots SA, Lief L, Erkan D. Clinical insights into diffuse alveolar hemorrhage in antiphospholipid syndrome. Curr Rheumatol Rep. 2019;21(10):56.
49. Kazzaz NM, Coit P, Lewis EE, McCune WJ, Sawalha AH, Knight JS. Systemic lupus erythematosus complicated by diffuse alveolar haemorrhage: risk factors, therapy and survival. Lupus Sci Med. 2015;2(1):e000117.
50. Davidson A. What is damaging the kidney in lupus nephritis? Nat Rev Rheumatol. 2016;12(3):143–53.
51. Littlejohn E, Marder W, Lewis E, Francis S, Jackish J, McCune WJ, et al. The ratio of erythrocyte sedimentation rate to C-reactive protein is useful in distinguishing infection from flare in systemic lupus erythematosus patients presenting with fever. Lupus. 2018;27(7):1123–9.
52. Kidney Disease: Improving Global Outcomes (KDIGO) Glomerular Diseases Work Group. KDIGO 2021 clinical practice guideline for the Management of Glomerular Diseases. Kidney Int. 2021;100(4s):S1–s276.
53. Song D, Wu LH, Wang FM, Yang XW, Zhu D, Chen M, et al. The spectrum of renal thrombotic microangiopathy in lupus nephritis. Arthritis Res Ther. 2013;15(1):R12.
54. Go RS, Winters JL, Leung N, Murray DL, Willrich MA, Abraham RS, et al. Thrombotic Microangiopathy care pathway: a consensus statement for the Mayo Clinic complement alternative pathway-thrombotic Microangiopathy (CAP-TMA) Disease-Oriented Group. Mayo Clin Proc. 2016;91(9):1189–211.
55. Bertsias GK, Ioannidis JP, Aringer M, Bollen E, Bombardieri S, Bruce IN, et al. EULAR recommendations for the management of systemic lupus erythematosus with neuropsychiatric manifestations: report of a task force of the EULAR standing committee for clinical affairs. Ann Rheum Dis. 2010;69(12):2074–82.
56. Bortoluzzi A, Scirè CA, Bombardieri S, Caniatti L, Conti F, De Vita S, et al. Development and validation of a new algorithm for attribution of neuropsychiatric events in systemic lupus erythematosus. Rheumatology (Oxford). 2015;54(5):891–8.
57. Cervera R, Bucciarelli S, Plasín MA, Gómez-Puerta JA, Plaza J, Pons-Estel G, et al. Catastrophic antiphospholipid syndrome (CAPS): descriptive analysis of a series of 280 patients from the "CAPS Registry". J Autoimmun. 2009;32(3–4):240–5.
58. Erkan D. Expert perspective: management of microvascular and catastrophic antiphospholipid syndrome. Arthritis Rheumatol. 2021;73(10):1780–90.

59. Cervera R, Rodríguez-Pintó I, Legault K, Erkan D. 16th international congress on antiphospholipid antibodies task force report on catastrophic antiphospholipid syndrome. Lupus. 2020;29(12):1594–600.
60. Asherson RA, Cervera R, de Groot PG, Erkan D, Boffa MC, Piette JC, et al. Catastrophic antiphospholipid syndrome: international consensus statement on classification criteria and treatment guidelines. Lupus. 2003;12(7):530–4.
61. Grom AA, Horne A, De Benedetti F. Macrophage activation syndrome in the era of biologic therapy. Nat Rev Rheumatol. 2016;12(5):259–68.
62. Henter JI, Samuelsson-Horne A, Aricò M, Egeler RM, Elinder G, Filipovich AH, et al. Treatment of hemophagocytic lymphohistiocytosis with HLH-94 immunochemotherapy and bone marrow transplantation. Blood. 2002;100(7):2367–73.
63. Ramos-Casals M, Brito-Zerón P, López-Guillermo A, Khamashta MA, Bosch X. Adult haemophagocytic syndrome. Lancet. 2014;383(9927):1503–16.
64. La Rosée P, Horne A, Hines M, von Bahr Greenwood T, Machowicz R, Berliner N, et al. Recommendations for the management of hemophagocytic lymphohistiocytosis in adults. Blood. 2019;133(23):2465–77.
65. Gavand PE, Serio I, Arnaud L, Costedoat-Chalumeau N, Carvelli J, Dossier A, et al. Clinical spectrum and therapeutic management of systemic lupus erythematosus-associated macrophage activation syndrome: a study of 103 episodes in 89 adult patients. Autoimmun Rev. 2017;16(7):743–9.
66. Üsküdar Cansu D, Üsküdar Teke H, Cansu GB, Korkmaz C. Evaluation of hyperferritinemia causes in rheumatology practice: a retrospective, single-center experience. Rheumatol Int. 2021;41(9):1617–24.
67. Henter JI, Horne A, Aricó M, Egeler RM, Filipovich AH, Imashuku S, et al. HLH-2004: diagnostic and therapeutic guidelines for hemophagocytic lymphohistiocytosis. Pediatr Blood Cancer. 2007;48(2):124–31.
68. Fardet L, Galicier L, Lambotte O, Marzac C, Aumont C, Chahwan D, et al. Development and validation of the HScore, a score for the diagnosis of reactive hemophagocytic syndrome. Arthritis Rheumatol. 2014;66(9):2613–20.
69. Carter SJ, Tattersall RS, Ramanan AV. Macrophage activation syndrome in adults: recent advances in pathophysiology, diagnosis and treatment. Rheumatology (Oxford). 2019;58(1):5–17.
70. De Benedetti F, Grom AA, Brogan PA, Bracaglia C, Pardeo M, Marucci G, et al. Efficacy and safety of emapalumab in macrophage activation syndrome. Ann Rheum Dis. 2023;82(6):857–65.
71. Panagopoulos P, Goules A, Hoffmann-Vold AM, Matteson EL, Tzioufas A. Natural history and screening of interstitial lung disease in systemic autoimmune rheumatic disorders. Ther Adv Musculoskelet Dis. 2021;13:1759720x211037519.
72. Fischer A, Antoniou KM, Brown KK, Cadranel J, Corte TJ, du Bois RM, et al. An official European Respiratory Society/American Thoracic Society research statement: interstitial pneumonia with autoimmune features. Eur Respir J. 2015;46(4):976–87.
73. Travis WD, Costabel U, Hansell DM, King TE Jr, Lynch DA, Nicholson AG, et al. An official American Thoracic Society/European Respiratory Society statement: update of the international multidisciplinary classification of the idiopathic interstitial pneumonias. Am J Respir Crit Care Med. 2013;188(6):733–48.
74. Xu L, You H, Wang L, Lv C, Yuan F, Li J, et al. Identification of three different phenotypes in anti-melanoma differentiation-associated gene 5 antibody-positive dermatomyositis patients: implications for prediction of rapidly progressive interstitial lung disease. Arthritis Rheumatol. 2023;75(4):609–19.
75. Pinal-Fernandez I, Casal-Dominguez M, Huapaya JA, Albayda J, Paik JJ, Johnson C, et al. A longitudinal cohort study of the anti-synthetase syndrome: increased severity of interstitial lung disease in black patients and patients with anti-PL7 and anti-PL12 autoantibodies. Rheumatology (Oxford). 2017;56(6):999–1007.

76. Alenzi FM. Myositis specific autoantibodies: a clinical perspective. Open Access Rheumatol. 2020;12:9–14.
77. Winthrop KL, Novosad SA, Baddley JW, Calabrese L, Chiller T, Polgreen P, et al. Opportunistic infections and biologic therapies in immune-mediated inflammatory diseases: consensus recommendations for infection reporting during clinical trials and postmarketing surveillance. Ann Rheum Dis. 2015;74(12):2107–16.
78. Luppi F, Sebastiani M, Salvarani C, Bendstrup E, Manfredi A. Acute exacerbation of interstitial lung disease associated with rheumatic disease. Nat Rev Rheumatol. 2022;18(2):85–96.
79. McPherson M, Economidou S, Liampas A, Zis P, Parperis K. Management of MDA-5 antibody positive clinically amyopathic dermatomyositis associated interstitial lung disease: a systematic review. Semin Arthritis Rheum. 2022;53:151959.
80. Pearce F, Johnson SR, Courtney P. Interstitial lung disease following certolizumab pegol. Rheumatology (Oxford). 2012;51(3):578–80.
81. Akiyama M, Kaneko Y, Yamaoka K, Kondo H, Takeuchi T. Association of disease activity with acute exacerbation of interstitial lung disease during tocilizumab treatment in patients with rheumatoid arthritis: a retrospective, case-control study. Rheumatol Int. 2016;36(6):881–9.
82. Ding T, Ledingham J, Luqmani R, Westlake S, Hyrich K, Lunt M, et al. BSR and BHPR rheumatoid arthritis guidelines on safety of anti-TNF therapies. Rheumatology (Oxford). 2010;49(11):2217–9.
83. Butler EA, Baron M, Fogo AB, Frech T, Ghossein C, Hachulla E, et al. Generation of a Core set of items to develop classification criteria for scleroderma renal crisis using consensus methodology. Arthritis Rheumatol. 2019;71(6):964–71.
84. Cole A, Ong VH, Denton CP. Renal disease and systemic sclerosis: an update on scleroderma renal crisis. Clin Rev Allergy Immunol. 2023;64(3):378–91.
85. Nagaraja V. Management of scleroderma renal crisis. Curr Opin Rheumatol. 2019;31(3):223–30.

Part II

The Central Nervous System

Neuro-Immune Response and Brain-Peripheral Crosstalk: The Role of the Complement System

4

Domenico Mercurio, Simone Bellavia, Stefano Fumagalli, and Elisa R. Zanier

4.1 Background

The central nervous system (CNS), to support its functions, establishes many interactions with the immune system. These interactions are based on a brain-peripheral crosstalk, which originates during development, continues in adulthood, and modifies in pathological states. The CNS is populated by tissue-resident immune cells of myeloid origin, including parenchymal microglia and extraparenchymal CNS-associated macrophages (CAMs), the latter being located at selective CNS barriers, like the blood-brain barrier (BBB), the choroid plexus (ChP), and the meninges [1]. Microglia and CAMs originate from common prenatal erythromyeloid progenitors (EMPs), but then follow different differentiation paths during the development of the CNS. Animal and human studies [2] showed that meningeal macrophages and microglia derive from common progenitors in the yolk sac, which exploit the forming vascular network to settle in the brain, where they are long-lived. Perivascular and ChP CAMs derive from EMPs invading the brain in the embryo, then need further maturation steps after birth upon receiving differentiation signals from the surrounding endothelial cells, which form a differentiation *niche* [3]. In particular, arterial vascular smooth muscle cells mediate the establishment of perivascular macrophages through an integrin-dependent mechanism, involving an integrin activation regulator called *Tln1*, whose deletion was reported to halve the perivascular macrophages at post-natal day 14 in mice [3]. It is therefore clear that a crosstalk between a CNS structure, like the vasculature, and blood-borne EMPs is needed to

D. Mercurio · S. Bellavia · S. Fumagalli (✉) · E. R. Zanier
Department of Acute Brain and Cardiovascular Injury, Istituto di Ricerche Farmacologiche Mario Negri IRCCS, Milan, Italy
e-mail: domenico.mercurio@marionegri.it; simone.bellavia@marionegri.it; stefano.fumagalli@marionegri.it; elisa.zanier@marionegri.it

D. Battaglini et al. (eds.), *Organ System Crosstalk in Critical Illness*,
https://doi.org/10.1007/978-3-032-01024-7_4

drive the specification of selective brain resident myeloid populations during development and in early post-natal phases.

In adulthood, this type of crosstalk is continued, but likely attenuated since the CNS limitans, like the blood-brain barrier (BBB), restrict the access of immune cells to the brain. However, damage to the brain barriers may change the scenario, making the brain-peripheral crosstalk a key pathophysiological process. The cerebral blood vessels represent the main interface between the brain and the periphery; as such, cerebrovascular pathologies cause a neuro-immune response where the two compartments, i.e., the brain and the circulation, are mutually affected. Ischemic stroke is a brain pathology with a defined vascular cause—a blockage of blood supply to the brain—thus offering many examples of a neuro-immune response involving a brain-peripheral crosstalk. In this chapter, we will discuss how systemic inflammation increases the risk of ischemic stroke and, vice versa, how the pathology stimulates a humoral inflammatory pathway.

4.2 How Peripheral Inflammation Increases the Risk of Stroke, the Case of Atherosclerosis

Atherosclerosis is a systemic and multifocal inflammatory disease characterized by chronic, lipid-driven vascular inflammation. Atherosclerosis involves the formation in the arteries of lesions that are characterized by inflammation, lipid accumulation, cell death, and fibrosis. Over time, these lesions, which are known as atherosclerotic plaques or atheroma, mature and gain new characteristics [4] such as the accumulation of calcium minerals and a fibrous structure [5]. Although clinical complications of atherosclerosis can arise from plaques causing flow-limiting stenoses (i.e., vessel narrowing), the most severe clinical events follow the rupture of a plaque, which exposes the prothrombotic material in the plaque to the blood and causes sudden thrombotic occlusion of the artery at the site of disruption. In the heart, atherosclerosis can lead to myocardial infarction and heart failure; whereas in the arteries that perfuse the brain, it can cause ischemic stroke and transient ischemic attacks [4].

4.3 From Attenuated Risk of Infections to Increased Sterile Inflammation of Non-communicable Diseases

Atherosclerosis represents the major cause of cardiovascular diseases (CVDs). CVDs, which include coronary heart disease, hypertension, and stroke, are the leading cause of global mortality and a major contributor to disability [6]. Prevalent cases of total CVD nearly doubled from 271 million (95% confidence interval [CI]: 257 to 285 million) in 1990 to 523 million (95% CI: 497 to 550 million) in 2019, and the number of CVD deaths steadily increased from 12.1 million (95% CI:11.4 to 12.6 million) in 1990, reaching 18.6 million (95% CI: 17.1 to 19.7 million) in 2019. In this period, the global trends for DALYs also increased significantly, doubling from 17.7 million (95% CI: 12.9 to 22.5 million) to 34.4 million (95% CI:

24.9 to 43.6 million) [6]. Although atherosclerotic cardiovascular disease was once limited to industrialized nations, it has now become a global problem due to an "epidemiological transition" [7, 8]. Increased sanitation, vaccination, and the treatment of acute infections have diminished the prevalence of communicable diseases in developing countries, and more individuals now survive to experience chronic diseases typical of the elderly, such as atherosclerosis. The adoption of less healthy dietary patterns may also have contributed to this, thus causing many people to live longer, but less healthy, suffering the consequences of atherosclerosis, including myocardial infarction, ischemic cardiomyopathy (which is the commonest cause of heart failure), strokes (which often rob people of their independence, mobility, cognition or ability to communicate), and peripheral arterial disease, which limits activity and jeopardizes limbs. These conditions contribute to the "morbidity extension" in the developing world: although many individuals escape early death, they must bear the burden not only of chronic cardiovascular diseases but also of arthritis, depression, and other long-term impediments to a healthy life. Today, the major pool of risk for developing cardiovascular disease occurs not in Western countries but in the more populous developing world [5]. The global spread of non-communicable diseases creates an urgent need to understand the genesis of this malady, advance in its management, develop prospects for alleviating its burden, and improve people's lifestyle.

Emerging evidence has spurred a considerable evolution of concepts relating to atherosclerosis, which, as said, represents a typical condition of an aging population. Traditionally, atherosclerosis was regarded as a cholesterol storage disease caused by the retention of lipoproteins including low-density lipoprotein (LDL) in the intimal space of arteries. Indeed, plasma lipoprotein levels constitute the major risk factor for atherosclerosis. If the entire population had maintained LDL concentrations akin to those of a neonate (or to those of adults of most other animal species), atherosclerosis would well be an orphan disease [9]. However, atherogenesis seems to be a far more complex process than simple lipid deposition. In fact, despite effective interventions for the control of LDL, as well as blood pressure and other traditional risk factors, a considerable residual risk remains for atherosclerotic cardiovascular disease [10]. Recent research has challenged and expanded on the traditional risk factors. With global trends toward a decrease in LDL and the introduction of highly effective therapies for lowering LDL (i.e., statins), as well as inexpensive and efficacious antihypertensive drugs, dyslipidemia and hypertension are less atherogenic today than they were in previous years. Beyond these traditional risk factors, a convincing body of experimental and clinical data indicates that sterile inflammation participates fundamentally in atherogenesis [4].

Sterile inflammation is defined as the inflammatory response in absence of an exogenous pathogen, as observed in diseased conditions. It might arise as an endogenous protective mechanism to limit disease progression, but, in the context of atherosclerosis, it does not supplant or demote lipid risk; rather, inflammatory responses provide a series of pathways that link lipids and other traditional risk factors to atherosclerosis. For example, obesity and its attendant dysmetabolism, often manifested by insulin resistance and diabetes, now drive an increasing proportion of cardiovascular disease risk worldwide. Adipose tissue abounds with cells that produce proinflammatory mediators which contribute mechanistically to the link between obesity, insulin resistance, and atherosclerotic risk [11]. Moreover, environmental factors, such as air pollution, noise, disturbed sleep, and other stressors, have gained increasing recognition as contributors to the risk of atherosclerotic events in part through the activation of inflammatory pathways [12–14]. Additionally, it has been recently showed that clonal hematopoiesis, relatively common in older individuals, is strongly associated with atherosclerosis [15]. One likely explanation is that the clones, particularly of monocytes and neutrophils, gain proinflammatory phenotypes in aging subjects, promoting long-term effects like atherosclerotic lesion growth, as reported in experimental models [16, 17]. In sum, there has been a significant shift in the ranking of risk factors for atherosclerosis: some factors, in particular LDL blood levels and hypertension, have receded in their importance since they are better managed with current therapies, and others, like obesity, physical inactivity, low level of high-density lipoprotein (HDL), and an elevation in triglyceride-rich lipoproteins (TGLR) in the blood, have gained more attention. This is in part due to socioeconomic and behavioral factors, such as the increasing prosperity with the attendant shift from traditional dietary habits to unhealthy ones, especially in developing countries [8, 18].

4.4 Initiation and Complications of Atherosclerosis

The atherosclerotic process tends to occur in regions of vasculature such as bifurcations and inner curvatures where the shear stress caused by a turbulent blood flow results in low-grade inflammation [19]. This event involves different cell types and effector molecules that modify the morphology of the plaque. In its morphological evolution, the atherosclerotic plaque expands outward radially, in an abluminal (away from the lumen) direction, preserving the caliber of the arterial lumen. During the process, smooth muscle cells (SMCs) release proteinases degrading the arterial extracellular matrix, such as matrix metalloproteinase 3 (MMP3), causing the remodeling of the arterial wall [20, 21]. Eventually, the growing atherosclerotic plaque begins to encroach upon the arterial lumen, leading to the formation of flow-limiting lesions and a progressive occlusion (stenosis) of the vessel. Plaques grown till an occlusive state, i.e., >70% of stenosis, may remain symptomatically silent for years, as the blood flow is not completely prevented. Indeed, more than stenosis, it is plaque vulnerability that raises the risk of an acute cardiovascular event.

The thrombotic complications of atherosclerosis are the most common cause of acute events including ischemic stroke [22]. These thromboembolic complications are typical of fragile, rupture-prone plaques, which have been termed "vulnerable" [23]. The typically vulnerable plaque has a large lipid core filled with macrophage foam cells and debris of dead cells. A thin fibrous cap (<60 μm), rich in extracellular matrix macromolecules, such as interstitial collagens, typically overlies the lipid-rich necrotic core of the plaque. These morphological characteristics gave rise to the nomenclature thin-capped fibroatheroma (TCFA). The rupture of the so-called vulnerable plaque exposes blood with its coagulation factors to thrombogenic material residing within the plaque.

Recent observations suggest a complex interplay between local mechanical triggers and both an innate and an adaptive immune response as driving forces in plaque erosion. Many studies support a key role for turbulent local fluid dynamics as well as consequently altered endothelial shear stress as "first hit" initiators of the cascade that drives plaque erosion [24–29]. During atherogenesis, disturbed flow primes lesion-specific overexpression of various toll-like receptors, including toll-like receptor 2 (TLR2) [30, 31], especially in endothelial cells and macrophages [32–35]. Exogenous but also endogenous ligands such as agonists released during tissue damage or apoptosis, cholesterol crystals, or hyaluronic acid activate TLRs [32–35]. Through myeloid differentiation primary response gene 88 (MyD88) and other signaling adapters, TLR ligation results in the activation of interferon response factor (IRF) family members and nuclear factor-kB (NF-kB), leading to the expression of leukocyte adhesion molecules and chemoattractants, activation of interferon and pro-inflammatory cytokine pathways, and generation of MMPs [34–36]. A general deficiency of MyD88, TLR2, or TLR4 significantly reduced atherosclerosis and vascular inflammation in mice and humans [35]. At sites of disturbed flow conditions predisposed to plaque erosion [25, 27–29], NF-kB activation through TLR2 has been proposed to facilitate disruption of endothelial cell (EC)-to-extracellular matrix contact, EC apoptosis, and the desquamation of the endothelial monolayer that is characteristic of eroded plaque [31, 32, 36]. In addition, neutrophils adhere to areas of endothelial activation and denudation, and potentiate EC death [31, 36] and release NETs [37] which have been crucially implicated in the pathophysiology of plaque erosion [31, 36, 38, 39]. NETs sustain a low-level proinflammatory response on the luminal endothelium [38, 40] and promote pathological thrombosis by induction of prothrombotic endothelial tissue factor [41] and by facilitating platelet adhesion, activation, and aggregation [42]. This interplay between endothelial dysfunction, TLR overexpression, and neutrophil accumulation and activation is accompanied by a local enrichment of both $CD4^+$ and $CD8^+$ T-lymphocytes [24]. Effector mediators secreted by cytotoxic T cells, such as granzyme A, granulysin, and perforin, were shown to further promote EC death enhancing plaque erosion [24]. Furthermore, along with these inflammatory mechanisms, increasing evidence suggests that the complement system plays a crucial role in plaque erosion. The deposition of cholesterol crystals (CC) within plaques retrieves the pattern recognition molecules from the complement system inducing an inflammatory response. The complement system initiates a cascade of reactions leading to opsonization and phagocytosis of CC, recognized as danger signals and mediated by increased CRP in the inflamed area [43] and by the recruitment of inflammatory cells such as neutrophils.

4.5 The Complement System and Its Involvement in the Risk of Ischemic Stroke

The complement system is a humoral component of innate immunity that is activated upon the recognition of danger signals, such as exogenous pathogen-associated molecular patterns (PAMPs) [44–46] and, in case of endogenous diseased conditions, damage-associated molecular patterns (DAMPs). DAMPs include glycoproteins and proteins from the extracellular matrix, intracellular proteins, DNA or RNA fragments, and heat-shock proteins, all produced when tissue homeostasis is altered by a pathological condition. On activation, the complement system acts upstream as a major coordinator of inflammation, phagocytosis, and cell death, thus critically contributing to pathophysiological processes [45]. Different signals lead to the activation of different complement pathways. The classical (CP) is activated by antibodies, C-reactive protein, apoptotic cells, and nucleic acids, the lectin (LP) is activated on recognition of carbohydrate patterns, and the alternative (AP) is constitutively active and working as an amplifying loop of complement. In addition, specific agents like tissue factor and enzymes can activate complement components directly. All activation mechanisms generate cleaved active fragments by cascade-like proteolytic reactions [45, 47]. The initial activation pathways converge at C3 by the generation of a C3-convertase, which cleaves inactive C3 into active C3 fragments (C3a and C3b). From there on, through the generation of a C5- convertase and active C5 fragments (C5a and C5b), the assembly of the terminal C5b-9 generates the membrane attack complex, a structure promoting cell lysis or sublytic cell activation. Irrespective of the final steps, the whole cascade includes biologically active molecules able to orchestrate inflammation and opsonization, a chemotactic stimulus for phagocytosis. These latter functions can occur through complement-independent mechanisms [48, 49].

Gathering evidence extends the role of LP over the well-known complement cascade activation, placing it at a crossroads of the interplay between inflammation and coagulation, referred to as thromboinflammation. The complement and coagulation systems are major proteolytic cascade systems. They have common evolutionary origins, and their interaction is warranted by their sharing of (1) the same compartment (blood), (2) activation time (first line of defense), and (3) common components throughout the cascades [48]. Thus, the LP controls and coordinates multiple inflammatory cascades, and should be regarded as a hub in vascular injury, able to impact stroke injury progression as well as vascular events preceding stroke symptoms. In this regard, the LP is implicated in thrombotic processes that are risk factors for stroke, as documented in previous studies on atherosclerotic patients [43, 50]. As previously detailed, atherosclerosis depends on processes such as the oxidative modification of lipoproteins in the arterial walls, representing danger stressors offering targets for LP initiators [51]. In support of LP involvement in atherosclerosis, higher ficolin-2 and ficolin-3 serum levels were reported in asymptomatic patients with severe carotid atherosclerosis than in healthy controls suggesting that they both accumulate during the atherosclerotic process [52]. Recent evidence showed that ficolin-2 accumulates in patients with a growing plaque, especially if the plaque is loading cholesterol crystals and immune cells [53]. In line with this, ficolin-2 has been shown to target cholesterol crystals in vitro [54] and in human plaque specimens [53], offering chemotactic stimuli for immune cells (monocytes/granulocytes) that are recruited to the plaques' necrotic core and cause a vulnerable morphological evolution of the plaque [53, 55, 56]. High blood ficolin-2 levels were reported to be independent predictors of a future major adverse cardiovascular event in atherosclerotic patients followed-up for 18 months after endarterectomy.

4.6 The Complement System and Its Detrimental Effects Following Acute Brain Injury

As said, the complement system can be activated after the sensing of DAMPs, thus driving sterile inflammation in diseased conditions, including cerebrovascular injury. Among the complement system activation cascades, the LP has been reported as that predominantly involved in stroke. Studies in experimental models [57–59] and in patients [52, 57, 60, 61] documented a prominent pathogenic role of LP molecules. Glycoproteins exposed on the surface of damaged brain cells, like apoptotic or necrotic cells and stressed endothelium, are typical DAMPs recognized by LP initiator molecules, which include mannose-binding lectin (MBL), ficolins (ficolin-1, 2 and 3), and collectins (CL-11 and 12, Fig. 4.1). The LP initiators act as soluble pattern recognition molecules. They circulate in normal conditions complexed with MBL-associated serine proteases (MASPs: MASP-1 and MASP-3, encoded by the *MASP1* gene and generated by alternative splicing, and MASP-2, encoded by the *MASP2* gene). The binding of these complexes to DAMPs initiates complement activation through the conversion of zymogen MASPs into their enzymatically active state [51]. MBL was the first LP recognition molecule to be identified and described structurally [62]. It is mainly synthesized in the liver, and its circulating levels are genetically determined. In humans, genetic variants cause MBL deficiency in about 20–30% of the general population [61, 63–65]. Interestingly, stroke patients with MBL deficiency have smaller infarctions and better outcomes [57, 60] lending support to the hypothesis of a key pathogenic role of LP in this condition. In line with the clinical evidence, MBL deficiency in ischemic mice was associated with preserved cerebrovascular functions following stroke. The detrimental effects of MBL depended on multiple thrombo-inflammatory events that the lectin mediated (Fig. 4.2). Early after ischemia (6 h), platelets bound to MBL, which in turn drove their activation in a calcium-dependent manner. Active

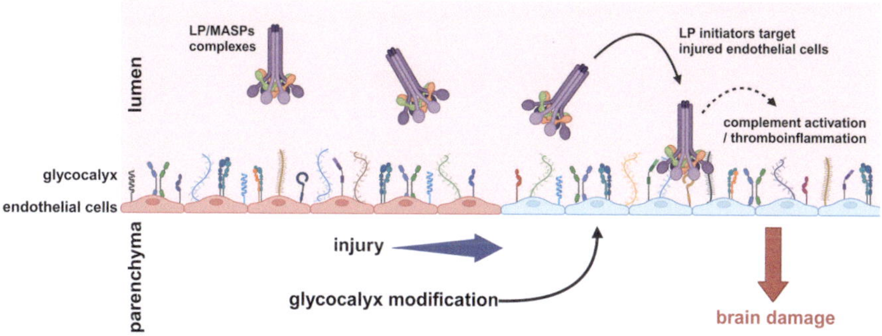

Fig. 4.1 The LP initiators act as soluble pattern recognition molecules. They circulate in normal conditions complexed with MBL-associated serine proteases (MASPs), specifically MASP-1, MASP-2, and MASP-3. After an injury, the endothelium undergoes modifications that expose the damage-associated molecular patterns (DAMPs). The binding of LP/MASPs complexes to DAMPs initiates complement activation and leads to the activation of thrombo-inflammatory mechanisms

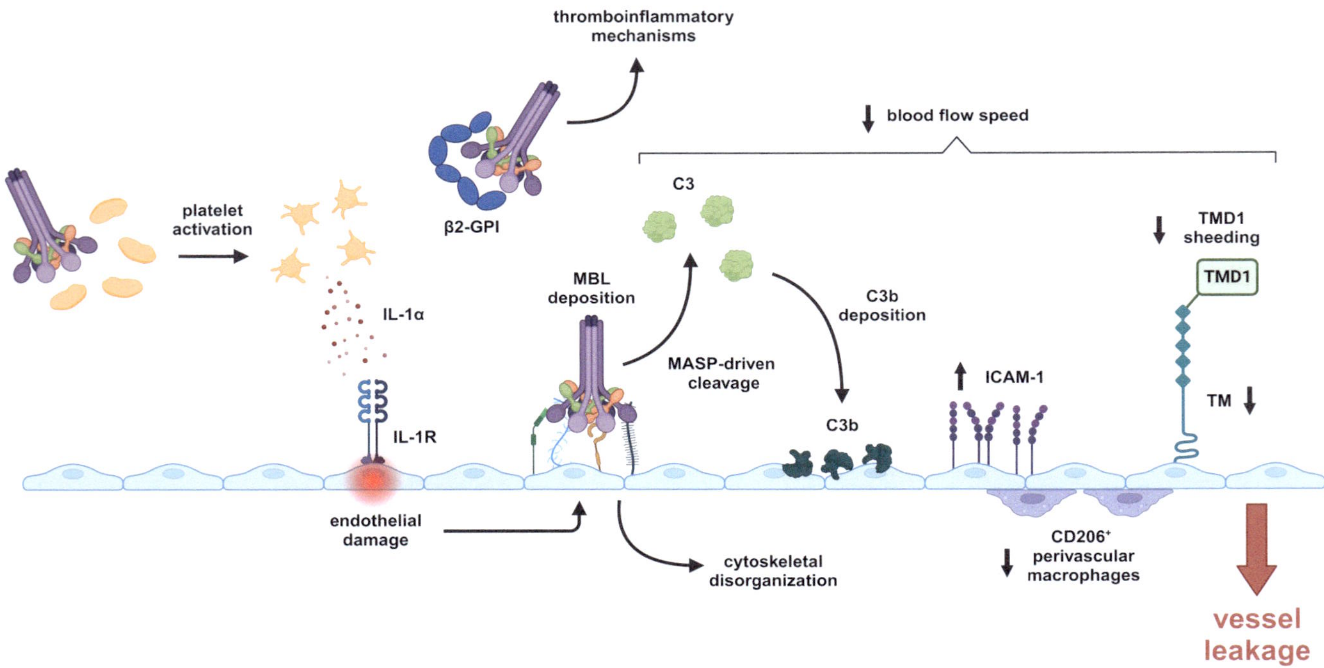

Fig. 4.2 MBL and IL-1α interplay on the ischemic endothelium and its consequences. Early after ischemia (6 h), circulating MBL drives platelet activation by a direct action on platelets [49]. Activated platelets release IL-1α, which on binding to its receptor (IL-1R) contributes to endothelial damage [105], β2-GPI tags stressed neurons and participates, in association with the complement system, to their clearing through phagocytosis [106]. Damaged endothelial cells drive MBL deposition, which results in further direct endothelial damage (i.e., cytoskeletal disorganization, [66] complement activation, increase of Intercellular Adhesion Molecule 1 (ICAM-1) expression on vessels—favoring focal no-reflow, [107] decrease of thrombomodulin (TM) expression on the endothelium and of its circulating shedded domain (TMD1), and decrease of CD206-positive perivascular macrophages in the brain—a population involved in blood-brain barrier (BBB) structural maintenance). All these events contribute to reduction of cerebral blood flow and increase of BBB leakage, both representing secondary vascular injuries to the initial ischemic onset

platelets released IL-1α that, on binding to its receptor (IL-1R1), caused brain vascular inflammation, increasing the endothelium expression of ICAM-1, VCAM-1, and CXCL1, as well as enhancing neutrophil trans-endothelial migration, thus facilitating vascular injury. Later on, at 24 h after the ischemic onset, damaged endothelial cells induced MBL deposition, triggering the complement activation and favoring a pro-inflammatory activation of the endothelium.

MBL-deficient ischemic mice had decreased endothelial expression of ICAM-1 and increased recruitment of $CD206^+$ macrophages to the sites of injury. These latter macrophages may limit BBB leakage and inflammation, promoting pro-healing processes after brain injury. Also, MBL-deficient mice expressed elevated endothelial levels of the anticoagulant and anti-inflammatory protein thrombomodulin and increased shedding of its fragment TMD1 compared to wild-type mice. TMD1 possesses several protective actions like it prevents excessive blood clotting by inhibiting the thrombin-induced conversion of fibrinogen into fibrin and inhibiting complement activation [49].

In addition to the findings observed in human subjects and murine models, a detrimental role of MBL has also been demonstrated in an in vitro ischemia model using brain microvascular endothelial cells exposed to serum-derived MBL. Specifically, it has been observed that, following hypoxic stimulation, MBL was taken up by endothelial cells where it was associated with cytoskeletal disorganization and cell death. While the exact mechanisms triggered by internalized MBL are not known, one possible explanation could be that MBL recognized molecules such as cytokeratins, which are among its targets, and interfered with their correct assembly. This latter mechanism seemed to be independent of complement activation [66].

Similar to MBL, ficolins can activate the LP on binding with their targets, thus promoting a downstream complement activation. Ficolins share with MBL proinflammatory, procoagulant, and prothrombotic properties and thus contribute to vascular events. Ficolin-1 is primarily synthesized and presented on the surface of peripheral monocytes and neutrophils, promoting neutrophil adhesion, aggregation, and migration [67–71]. Ficolin-2 and -3 are mainly produced by the liver and circulate in the bloodstream. Emerging clinical evidence implicates ficolins in the progression of brain damage in stroke, as indicated by their lower circulating levels early (within 6 h from onset) after stroke. Ficolins' circulating levels are reduced as a result of their consumption exceeding production/release, which can be regarded as an index of their use to target the DAMPs in the acute phases of stroke [61]. Ficolin-1 and ficolin-3 blood levels, measured respectively at 6 h and 12 h after stroke, seem to be independent predictors of the 3-month outcome of ischemic stroke patients, suggesting that they might be sensitive prognostic markers [52, 61]. Less data are available on collectin-11 (CL-11), the LP initiator molecule discovered more recently, in ischemic injury. It is mainly produced by the kidneys, and its structure is similar to MBL, including a carbohydrate-binding motif [72]. High CL-11 plasma levels have been found in patients with disseminated intravascular coagulation because of derangement of the coagulation system after substantial activation of innate immunity [73].

Other types of acute brain injuries cause vascular damage, with subsequent involvement of the LP. Complement activation following intracerebral hemorrhage (ICH) was first observed in a rodent model, where an increased activation of the complement cascade and formation of the membrane attack complex (MAC) in the perihematomal region were observed at 24 and 72 h post-hemorrhage [74]. More recent studies reported elevated levels of the complement components C3a and C5a in the perihematomal region, affecting neurons, glia, and endothelial cells, in a time range from days 1 to 5 post-ICH [75]. ICH also induces the activation of the LP, with circulating ficolin-3 being consumed at a higher extent in patients with severe compared to mild subarachnoid hemorrhage (SAH), as defined per the World Federation of Neurosurgical Societies (WFNS) grading scale [64]. Supporting the involvement of the LP in ICH, an increased brain presence of MASP-2 was reported in patients developing SAH following severe traumatic brain injury, as compared to those not showing traumatic SAH [76]. In addition, the LP activation has been reported as a consequence of mild TBI too, with circulating ficolin-2, −3, and MASP-2 levels observed to be higher in patients with an unfavorable outcome at 90 days (classified as Glasgow outcome scale extended, GOSE, 1–4) [77].

4.7 The Crosstalk Between the Complement System and Toll-Like Receptors

In addition to the complement system, another critically important pattern recognition system in the peripheral immune response is the Toll-like receptor (TLR) system. TLRs are pattern recognition receptors (PRRs) localized on a variety of different cell types including neutrophils, monocytes/macrophages, mast cells, T- and B-cells, but also endothelial and smooth muscle cells [78]. The TLRs are dependent on interaction with a broad range of extracellular accessory proteins and cofactors to elucidate full-scale intracellular signaling and induction of proinflammatory gene transcription and cytokine release [79]. CD14 is a key molecule in TLR signaling. It is present as a soluble protein in the blood and as a membrane-bound protein on myeloid cells. This accessory molecule enhances LPS responsiveness by facilitating the transfer of LPS from LPS-binding protein to TLR4–MD2 complexes [80]. CD14 works also as an accessory molecule in relation to other TLRs (TLR2, TLR3, TLR7, and TLR9) and has the ability to bind a variety of microbial products [81]. Thus, CD14 is a unique upstream and promiscuous molecule, implicated in different TLRs-signaling reacting with a number of ligands with low affinity, and transferring the ligand to receptors with a higher degree of specificity and affinity [80].

There is an extensive cross-talk between the complement system and TLRs [82–84] ostensibly to coordinate immune and inflammatory responses through synergistic or antagonistic (regulatory) interactions. However, over-activation or dysregulation of either system may lead—often synergistically—to exaggerated inflammation and host tissue injury [85]. In this regard, future therapies for inflammatory or autoimmune diseases could focus on inhibiting complement and TLRs systems; indeed, combined inhibition may be more effective than inhibition of each system alone. For instance, in a human whole-blood model, the combined inhibition of complement and TLRs blocked *Escherichia coli*-induced cytokine responses more effectively than the single inhibition [86, 87]. In addition, the combined inhibition of CD14 and the complement components C3 and C5 attenuated the systemic inflammatory response, as observed in murine and porcine polymicrobial sepsis, as well as in a baboon and a human whole-blood model of Escherichia Coli sepsis [86, 88–90]. Ischemic stroke is characterized by a highly interconnected and multiphasic neuropathological cascade of events in which an intense and protracted inflammatory response plays a crucial role in worsening brain injury. As discussed above, the complement system plays a detrimental role in ischemia/reperfusion injuries, as reviewed by [91–93], including ischemic stroke [48, 49, 66, 94]. Notably, TLR4 and TLR2, both using CD14 as a co-receptor, have been found to be involved in ischemia-reperfusion injury [95], particularly in cardiac injury and in ischemia-induced neuronal damage [96].

4.8 Neuroprotective Therapeutic Approaches Targeting the LP

LP proteins are part of a humoral pathway, whose downstream detrimental mechanisms start on the luminal side of the brain vessels. As such, LP proteins, including MBL, ficolins, and MASPs, offer easily accessible pharmacological targets, which means no need of crossing the brain limitans, often hampering a successful clinical application of anti-inflammatory agents. After complement's first discovery in 1880s–1890s, only in more recent years a so-called "clinical complement revolution" has highlighted the clinical significance of the complement system. Hence, clinical applications of complement modulation were developed and are now already in practice [97]. As an example, genetic conditions caused by complement protein deficiencies, which regards the three activation pathways of complement, are treated by the exogenous administration of recombinant complement proteins. This is the case for hereditary angioedema, caused by C1-inhibitor deficiency and treated by the prophylactic administration of recombinant C1-inhibitor. This latter molecule showed a potent inhibitory effect on the LP, which was indeed neuroprotective in an experimental model of ischemic stroke [98]. Further means to target the LP focused on its initiator molecules, like MBL, by providing poly-mannosylated compounds, which could be neuroprotective in a model of ischemic stroke [59] or of traumatic brain injury [99]. Alternative strategies to inhibit the LP activation targeted the MBL-associated serine proteases, with antibodies against MASP-2 able to ameliorate the sensorimotor deficits after experimental stroke [100] or the long-term cognitive deficits in experimental traumatic brain injury [101]. In addition to acute brain injuries, it has been recently shown that inhibiting MASP-2 could reduce brain microglial reactivity and vascular inflammation following covid-19 infection, as reported using a murine model of SARS-CoV-2 [102]. The LP activation is caused by the highly glycosylated spike protein of the virus, with MBL-driven LP activation playing a major role in determining the severity of the disease [103]. In line with this, the anti-MASP-2 demonstrated a significant benefit in the treatment of patients who were critically ill with Covid-19 in a phase 2 open-label clinical study [104].

References

1. Amann L, Masuda T, Prinz M. Mechanisms of myeloid cell entry to the healthy and diseased central nervous system. Nat Immunol. 2023;24:393–407. https://doi.org/10.1038/s41590-022-01415-8.
2. Goh I, Botting RA, Rose A, Webb S, Engelbert J, Gitton Y, Stephenson E, Quiroga Londoño M, Mather M, Mende N, et al. Yolk sac cell atlas reveals multiorgan functions during human early development. Science. 2023;381:eadd7564. https://doi.org/10.1126/science.add7564.
3. Masuda T, Amann L, Monaco G, Sankowski R, Staszewski O, Krueger M, Del Gaudio F, He L, Paterson N, Nent E, et al. Specification of CNS macrophage subsets occurs postnatally in defined niches. Nature. 2022;604:740–8. https://doi.org/10.1038/s41586-022-04596-2.
4. Hansson GK, Libby P. The immune response in atherosclerosis: a double-edged sword. Nat Rev Immunol. 2006;6:508–19. https://doi.org/10.1038/nri1882.
5. Libby P, Buring JE, Badimon L, Hansson GK, Deanfield J, Bittencourt MS, Tokgözoğlu L, Lewis EF. Atherosclerosis. Nat Rev Dis Primer. 2019;5:56. https://doi.org/10.1038/s41572-019-0106-z.
6. Roth GA, Mensah GA, Johnson CO, Addolorato G, Ammirati E, Baddour LM, Barengo NC, Beaton AZ, Benjamin EJ, Benziger CP, et al. Global burden of cardiovascular diseases and risk factors, 1990–2019. J Am Coll Cardiol. 2020;76:2982–3021. https://doi.org/10.1016/j.jacc.2020.11.010.
7. Braunwald's Heart Disease, Single Volume, 12th Edition – 9780323824675 https://evolve.elsevier.com/cs/product/9780323824675?role=student.
8. Dai H, Much AA, Maor E, Asher E, Younis A, Xu Y, Lu Y, Liu X, Shu J, Bragazzi NL. Global, regional, and national burden of ischaemic heart disease and its attributable risk factors, 1990-2017: results from the Global Burden of Disease Study 2017. Eur Heart J Qual Care Clin Outcomes. 2022;8:50–60. https://doi.org/10.1093/ehjqcco/qcaa076.
9. Goldstein JL, Brown MS. A century of cholesterol and coronaries: from plaques to genes to statins. Cell. 2015;161:161–72. https://doi.org/10.1016/j.cell.2015.01.036.
10. Ridker PM. How common is residual inflammatory risk? Circ Res. 2017;120:617–9. https://doi.org/10.1161/CIRCRESAHA.116.310527.
11. Ross R, Neeland IJ, Yamashita S, Shai I, Seidell J, Magni P, Santos RD, Arsenault B, Cuevas A, Hu FB, et al. Waist circumference as a vital sign in clinical practice: a consensus statement from the IAS and ICCR Working Group on Visceral Obesity. Nat Rev Endocrinol. 2020;16:177–89. https://doi.org/10.1038/s41574-019-0310-7.
12. Münzel T. Up in the air: links between the environment and cardiovascular disease. Cardiovasc Res. 2019;115:e144–6. https://doi.org/10.1093/cvr/cvz134.
13. Brook RD, Newby DE, Rajagopalan S. Air pollution and cardiometabolic disease: an update and call for clinical trials. Am J Hypertens. 2017;31:1–10. https://doi.org/10.1093/ajh/hpx109.
14. Drager LF, McEvoy RD, Barbe F, Lorenzi-Filho G, Redline S, INCOSACT Initiative (International Collaboration of Sleep Apnea Cardiovascular Trialists). Sleep apnea and cardiovascular disease: lessons from recent trials and need for team science. Circulation. 2017;136:1840–50. https://doi.org/10.1161/CIRCULATIONAHA.117.029400.
15. Jaiswal S, Natarajan P, Silver AJ, Gibson CJ, Bick AG, Shvartz E, McConkey M, Gupta N, Gabriel S, Ardissino D, et al. Clonal hematopoiesis and risk of atherosclerotic cardiovascular disease. N Engl J Med. 2017;377:111–21. https://doi.org/10.1056/NEJMoa1701719.

16. Fidler TP, Xue C, Yalcinkaya M, Hardaway B, Abramowicz S, Xiao T, Liu W, Thomas DG, Hajebrahimi MA, Pircher J, et al. The AIM2 inflammasome exacerbates atherosclerosis in clonal haematopoiesis. Nature. 2021;592:296–301. https://doi.org/10.1038/s41586-021-03341-5.
17. Tyrrell DJ, Goldstein DR. Ageing and atherosclerosis: vascular intrinsic and extrinsic factors and potential role of IL-6. Nat Rev Cardiol. 2021;18:58–68. https://doi.org/10.1038/s41569-020-0431-7.
18. Libby P. The changing landscape of atherosclerosis. Nature. 2021;592:524–33. https://doi.org/10.1038/s41586-021-03392-8.
19. Jongstra-Bilen J, Haidari M, Zhu S-N, Chen M, Guha D, Cybulsky MI. Low-grade chronic inflammation in regions of the normal mouse arterial intima predisposed to atherosclerosis. J Exp Med. 2006;203:2073–83. https://doi.org/10.1084/jem.20060245.
20. Galis ZS, Muszynski M, Sukhova GK, Simon-Morrissey E, Unemori EN, Lark MW, Amento E, Libby P. Cytokine-stimulated human vascular smooth muscle cells synthesize a complement of enzymes required for extracellular matrix digestion. Circ Res. 1994;75:181–9. https://doi.org/10.1161/01.res.75.1.181.
21. Alexander MR, Moehle CW, Johnson JL, Yang Z, Lee JK, Jackson CL, Owens GK. Genetic inactivation of IL-1 signaling enhances atherosclerotic plaque instability and reduces outward vessel remodeling in advanced atherosclerosis in mice. J Clin Invest. 2012;122:70–9. https://doi.org/10.1172/JCI43713.
22. Lusis AJ. Atherosclerosis. Nature. 2000;407:233–41. https://doi.org/10.1038/35025203.
23. Bentzon JF, Otsuka F, Virmani R, Falk E. Mechanisms of plaque formation and rupture. Circ Res. 2014;114:1852–66. https://doi.org/10.1161/CIRCRESAHA.114.302721.
24. Leistner DM, Kränkel N, Meteva D, Abdelwahed YS, Seppelt C, Stähli BE, Rai H, Skurk C, Lauten A, Mochmann H-C, et al. Differential immunological signature at the culprit site distinguishes acute coronary syndrome with intact from acute coronary syndrome with ruptured fibrous cap: results from the prospective translational OPTICO-ACS study. Eur Heart J. 2020;41:3549–60. https://doi.org/10.1093/eurheartj/ehaa703.
25. Kwon JE, Lee WS, Mintz GS, Hong YJ, Lee SY, Kim KS, Hahn J-Y, Kumar KS, Won H, Hyeon SH, et al. Multimodality intravascular imaging assessment of plaque Erosion versus plaque rupture in patients with acute coronary syndrome. Korean Circ J. 2016;46:499–506. https://doi.org/10.4070/kcj.2016.46.4.499.
26. Yamamoto E, Thondapu V, Poon E, Sugiyama T, Fracassi F, Dijkstra J, Lee H, Ooi A, Barlis P, Jang I-K. Endothelial shear stress and plaque erosion: a computational fluid dynamics and optical coherence tomography study. JACC Cardiovasc Imaging. 2019;12:374–5. https://doi.org/10.1016/j.jcmg.2018.07.024.
27. Vergallo R, Papafaklis MI, Yonetsu T, Bourantas CV, Andreou I, Wang Z, Fujimoto JG, McNulty I, Lee H, Biasucci LM, et al. Endothelial shear stress and coronary plaque characteristics in humans: combined frequency-domain optical coherence tomography and computational fluid dynamics study. Circ Cardiovasc Imaging. 2014;7:905–11. https://doi.org/10.1161/CIRCIMAGING.114.001932.
28. Thondapu V, Mamon C, Poon EKW, Kurihara O, Kim HO, Russo M, Araki M, Shinohara H, Yamamoto E, Dijkstra J, et al. High spatial endothelial shear stress gradient independently predicts site of acute coronary plaque rupture and erosion. Cardiovasc Res. 2021;117:1974–85. https://doi.org/10.1093/cvr/cvaa251.
29. McElroy M, Kim Y, Niccoli G, Vergallo R, Langford-Smith A, Crea F, Gijsen F, Johnson T, Keshmiri A, White SJ. Identification of the haemodynamic environment permissive for plaque erosion. Sci Rep. 2021;11:7253. https://doi.org/10.1038/s41598-021-86501-x.
30. Mullick AE, Soldau K, Kiosses WB, Bell TA, Tobias PS, Curtiss LK. Increased endothelial expression of Toll-like receptor 2 at sites of disturbed blood flow exacerbates early atherogenic events. J Exp Med. 2008;205:373–83. https://doi.org/10.1084/jem.20071096.
31. Franck G, Mawson T, Sausen G, Salinas M, Masson GS, Cole A, Beltrami-Moreira M, Chatzizisis Y, Quillard T, Tesmenitsky Y, et al. Flow perturbation mediates neutrophil recruit-

ment and potentiates endothelial injury via TLR2 in mice: implications for superficial erosion. Circ Res. 2017;121:31–42. https://doi.org/10.1161/CIRCRESAHA.117.310694.
32. Komarova YA, Huang F, Geyer M, Daneshjou N, Garcia A, Idalino L, Kreutz B, Mehta D, Malik AB. VE-cadherin signaling induces EB3 phosphorylation to suppress microtubule growth and assemble adherens junctions. Mol Cell. 2012;48:914–25. https://doi.org/10.1016/j.molcel.2012.10.011.
33. Scheibner KA, Lutz MA, Boodoo S, Fenton MJ, Powell JD, Horton MR. Hyaluronan fragments act as an endogenous danger signal by engaging TLR21. J Immunol. 2006;177:1272–81. https://doi.org/10.4049/jimmunol.177.2.1272.
34. Mullaly SC, Kubes P. Toll gates and traffic arteries: from endothelial TLR2 to atherosclerosis. Circ Res. 2004;95:657–9. https://doi.org/10.1161/01.RES.0000144806.19585.5b.
35. Falck-Hansen M, Kassiteridi C, Monaco C. Toll-like receptors in atherosclerosis. Int J Mol Sci. 2013;14:14008–23. https://doi.org/10.3390/ijms140714008.
36. Quillard T, Araújo HA, Franck G, Shvartz E, Sukhova G, Libby P. TLR2 and neutrophils potentiate endothelial stress, apoptosis and detachment: implications for superficial erosion. Eur Heart J. 2015;36:1394–404. https://doi.org/10.1093/eurheartj/ehv044.
37. Libby P, Pasterkamp G, Crea F, Jang I-K. Reassessing the mechanisms of acute coronary syndromes. Circ Res. 2019;124:150–60. https://doi.org/10.1161/CIRCRESAHA.118.311098.
38. Fahed AC, Jang I-K. Plaque erosion and acute coronary syndromes: phenotype, molecular characteristics and future directions. Nat Rev Cardiol. 2021;18:724–34. https://doi.org/10.1038/s41569-021-00542-3.
39. Quillard T, Franck G, Mawson T, Folco E, Libby P. Mechanisms of erosion of atherosclerotic plaques. Curr Opin Lipidol. 2017;28:434–41. https://doi.org/10.1097/MOL.0000000000000440.
40. Warnatsch A, Ioannou M, Wang Q, Papayannopoulos V. Inflammation. Neutrophil extracellular traps license macrophages for cytokine production in atherosclerosis. Science. 2015;349:316–20. https://doi.org/10.1126/science.aaa8064.
41. Folco EJ, Mawson TL, Vromman A, Bernardes-Souza B, Franck G, Persson O, Nakamura M, Newton G, Luscinskas FW, Libby P. Neutrophil extracellular traps induce endothelial cell activation and tissue factor production through interleukin-1α and Cathepsin G. Arterioscler Thromb Vasc Biol. 2018;38:1901–12. https://doi.org/10.1161/ATVBAHA.118.311150.
42. Fuchs TA, Brill A, Duerschmied D, Schatzberg D, Monestier M, Myers DD, Wrobleski SK, Wakefield TW, Hartwig JH, Wagner DD. Extracellular DNA traps promote thrombosis. Proc Natl Acad Sci USA. 2010;107:15880–5. https://doi.org/10.1073/pnas.1005743107.
43. Pilely K, Fumagalli S, Rosbjerg A, Genster N, Skjoedt M-O, Perego C, Ferrante AMR, De Simoni M-G, Garred P. C-reactive protein binds to cholesterol crystals and co-localizes with the terminal complement complex in human atherosclerotic plaques. Front Immunol. 2017;8:1040. https://doi.org/10.3389/fimmu.2017.01040.
44. Fumagalli S, Perego C, Pischiutta F, Zanier ER, De Simoni M-G. The ischemic environment drives microglia and macrophage function. Front Neurol. 2015;6 https://doi.org/10.3389/fneur.2015.00081.
45. Orsini F, De Blasio D, Zangari R, Zanier ER, De Simoni M-G. Versatility of the complement system in neuroinflammation, neurodegeneration and brain homeostasis. Front Cell Neurosci. 2014;8 https://doi.org/10.3389/fncel.2014.00380.
46. Ricklin D, Reis ES, Lambris JD. Complement in disease: a defence system turning offensive. Nat Rev Nephrol. 2016;12:383–401. https://doi.org/10.1038/nrneph.2016.70.
47. Alawieh A, Elvington A, Tomlinson S. Complement in the homeostatic and ischemic brain. Front Immunol. 2015;6:417. https://doi.org/10.3389/fimmu.2015.00417.
48. Fumagalli S, De Simoni M-G. Lectin complement pathway and its bloody interactions in brain ischemia. Stroke. 2016;47:3067–73. https://doi.org/10.1161/STROKEAHA.116.012407.
49. Orsini F, Fumagalli S, Császár E, Tóth K, De Blasio D, Zangari R, Lénárt N, Dénes Á, De Simoni M-G. Mannose-binding lectin drives platelet inflammatory phenotype and vascular damage after cerebral ischemia in mice via IL (interleukin)-1α. Arterioscler Thromb Vasc Biol. 2018;38:2678–90. https://doi.org/10.1161/ATVBAHA.118.311058.

50. Fumagalli S, Perego C, Zangari R, De Blasio D, Oggioni M, De Nigris F, Snider F, Garred P, Ferrante AMR, De Simoni M-G. Lectin pathway of complement activation is associated with vulnerability of atherosclerotic plaques. Front Immunol. 2017;8:288. https://doi.org/10.3389/fimmu.2017.00288.
51. Wallis R, Mitchell DA, Schmid R, Schwaeble WJ, Keeble AH. Paths reunited: initiation of the classical and lectin pathways of complement activation. Immunobiology. 2010;215:1–11. https://doi.org/10.1016/j.imbio.2009.08.006.
52. Füst G, Munthe-Fog L, Illes Z, Széplaki G, Molnar T, Pusch G, Hirschberg K, Szegedi R, Széplaki Z, Prohászka Z, et al. Low ficolin-3 levels in early follow-up serum samples are associated with the severity and unfavorable outcome of acute ischemic stroke. J Neuroinflammation. 2011;8:185. https://doi.org/10.1186/1742-2094-8-185.
53. Carbone F, Valente A, Perego C, Bertolotto M, Pane B, Spinella G, Palombo D, De Simoni M-G, Montecucco F, Fumagalli S. Ficolin-2 serum levels predict the occurrence of acute coronary syndrome in patients with severe carotid artery stenosis. Pharmacol Res. 2021;166:105462. https://doi.org/10.1016/j.phrs.2021.105462.
54. Pilely K, Rosbjerg A, Genster N, Gal P, Pál G, Halvorsen B, Holm S, Aukrust P, Bakke SS, Sporsheim B, et al. Cholesterol crystals activate the lectin complement pathway via Ficolin-2 and mannose-binding lectin: implications for the progression of atherosclerosis. J Immunol. 2016;196:5064–74. https://doi.org/10.4049/jimmunol.1502595.
55. Moore KJ, Tabas I. Macrophages in the pathogenesis of atherosclerosis. Cell. 2011;145:341–55. https://doi.org/10.1016/j.cell.2011.04.005.
56. Koelwyn GJ, Corr EM, Erbay E, Moore KJ. Regulation of macrophage immunometabolism in atherosclerosis. Nat Immunol. 2018;19:526–37. https://doi.org/10.1038/s41590-018-0113-3.
57. Cervera A, Planas AM, Justicia C, Urra X, Jensenius JC, Torres F, Lozano F, Chamorro A. Genetically-defined deficiency of mannose-binding lectin is associated with protection after experimental stroke in mice and outcome in human stroke. PLoS One. 2010;5:e8433. https://doi.org/10.1371/journal.pone.0008433.
58. Gesuete R, Storini C, Fantin A, Stravalaci M, Zanier ER, Orsini F, Vietsch H, Mannesse MLM, Ziere B, Gobbi M, et al. Recombinant C1 inhibitor in brain ischemic injury. Ann Neurol. 2009;66:332–42. https://doi.org/10.1002/ana.21740.
59. Orsini F, Villa P, Parrella S, Zangari R, Zanier ER, Gesuete R, Stravalaci M, Fumagalli S, Ottria R, Reina JJ, et al. Targeting mannose-binding lectin confers long-lasting protection with a surprisingly wide therapeutic window in cerebral ischemia. Circulation. 2012;126:1484–94. https://doi.org/10.1161/CIRCULATIONAHA.112.103051.
60. Osthoff M, Katan M, Fluri F, Schuetz P, Bingisser R, Kappos L, Steck AJ, Engelter ST, Mueller B, Christ-Crain M, et al. Mannose-binding lectin deficiency is associated with smaller infarction size and favorable outcome in ischemic stroke patients. PLoS One. 2011;6:e21338. https://doi.org/10.1371/journal.pone.0021338.
61. Zangari R, Zanier ER, Torgano G, Bersano A, Beretta S, Beghi E, Casolla B, Checcarelli N, Lanfranconi S, Maino A, et al. Early ficolin-1 is a sensitive prognostic marker for functional outcome in ischemic stroke. J Neuroinflammation. 2016;13:16. https://doi.org/10.1186/s12974-016-0481-2.
62. Matsushita M, Fujita T. Activation of the classical complement pathway by mannose-binding protein in association with a novel C1s-like serine protease. J Exp Med. 1992;176:1497–502. https://doi.org/10.1084/jem.176.6.1497.
63. Garred P, Larsen F, Seyfarth J, Fujita R, Madsen HO. Mannose-binding lectin and its genetic variants. Genes Immun. 2006;7:85–94. https://doi.org/10.1038/sj.gene.6364283.
64. Zanier ER, Zangari R, Munthe-Fog L, Hein E, Zoerle T, Conte V, Orsini F, Tettamanti M, Stocchetti N, Garred P, et al. Ficolin-3–mediated lectin complement pathway activation in patients with subarachnoid hemorrhage. Neurology. 2014;82:126–34. https://doi.org/10.1212/WNL.0000000000000020.
65. Eisen DP, Dean MM, Boermeester MA, Fidler KJ, Gordon AC, Kronborg G, Kun JFJ, Lau YL, Payeras A, Valdimarsson H, et al. Low serum mannose-binding lectin level increases

the risk of death due to pneumococcal infection. Clin Infect Dis. 2008;47:510–6. https://doi.org/10.1086/590006.
66. Neglia L, Fumagalli S, Orsini F, Zanetti A, Perego C, De Simoni M-G. Mannose-binding lectin has a direct deleterious effect on ischemic brain microvascular endothelial cells. J Cereb Blood Flow Metab. 2019; https://doi.org/10.1177/0271678X19874509.
67. Endo Y, Matsushita M, Fujita T. New insights into the role of ficolins in the lectin pathway of innate immunity. Int Rev Cell Mol Biol. 2015;316:49–110. https://doi.org/10.1016/bs.ircmb.2015.01.003.
68. Honoré C, Rørvig S, Munthe-Fog L, Hummelshøj T, Madsen HO, Borregaard N, Garred P. The innate pattern recognition molecule Ficolin-1 is secreted by monocytes/macrophages and is circulating in human plasma. Mol Immunol. 2008;45:2782–9. https://doi.org/10.1016/j.molimm.2008.02.005.
69. Liu Y, Endo Y, Iwaki D, Nakata M, Matsushita M, Wada I, Inoue K, Munakata M, Fujita T. Human M-ficolin is a secretory protein that activates the lectin complement pathway. J Immunol (Baltim Md: 1950). 2005;175:3150–6. https://doi.org/10.4049/jimmunol.175.5.3150.
70. Rørvig S, Honore C, Larsson L-I, Ohlsson S, Pedersen CC, Jacobsen LC, Cowland JB, Garred P, Borregaard N. Ficolin-1 is present in a highly mobilizable subset of human neutrophil granules and associates with the cell surface after stimulation with fMLP. J Leukoc Biol. 2009;86:1439–49. https://doi.org/10.1189/jlb.1008606.
71. Zhang J, Yang L, Ang Z, Yoong SL, Tran TTT, Anand GS, Tan NS, Ho B, Ding JL. Secreted M-ficolin anchors onto monocyte transmembrane G protein-coupled receptor 43 and cross talks with plasma C-reactive protein to mediate immune signaling and regulate host defense. J Immunol (Baltim Md: 1950). 2010;185:6899–910. https://doi.org/10.4049/jimmunol.1001225.
72. Selman L, Hansen S. Structure and function of collectin liver 1 (CL-L1) and collectin 11 (CL-11, CL-K1). Immunobiology. 2012;217:851–63. https://doi.org/10.1016/j.imbio.2011.12.008.
73. Takahashi K, Ohtani K, Larvie M, Moyo P, Chigweshe L, Van Cott EM, Wakamiya N. Elevated plasma CL-K1 level is associated with a risk of developing disseminated intravascular coagulation (DIC). J Thromb Thrombolysis. 2014;38:331–8. https://doi.org/10.1007/s11239-013-1042-5.
74. Hua Y, Xi G, Keep RF, Hoff JT. Complement activation in the brain after experimental intracerebral hemorrhage. J Neurosurg. 2000;92:1016–22. https://doi.org/10.3171/jns.2000.92.6.1016.
75. Holste K, Xia F, Garton HJL, Wan S, Hua Y, Keep RF, Xi G. The role of complement in brain injury following intracerebral hemorrhage: a review. Exp Neurol. 2021;340:113654. https://doi.org/10.1016/j.expneurol.2021.113654.
76. De Blasio D, Fumagalli S, Orsini F, Neglia L, Perego C, Ortolano F, Zanier ER, Picetti E, Locatelli M, Stocchetti N, et al. Human brain trauma severity is associated with lectin complement pathway activation. J Cereb Blood Flow Metab. 2019;39:794–807. https://doi.org/10.1177/0271678X18758881.
77. Osthoff M, Walder B, Delhumeau C, Trendelenburg M, Turck N. Association of Lectin Pathway Protein Levels and Genetic Variants Early after injury with outcomes after severe traumatic brain injury: a prospective cohort study. J Neurotrauma. 2017;34:2560–6. https://doi.org/10.1089/neu.2016.4941.
78. Chang ZL. Important aspects of toll-like receptors, ligands and their signaling pathways. Inflamm Res. 2010;59:791–808. https://doi.org/10.1007/s00011-010-0208-2.
79. Barratt-Due A, Pischke SE, Nilsson PH, Espevik T, Mollnes TE. Dual inhibition of complement and toll-like receptors as a novel approach to treat inflammatory diseases—C3 or C5 emerge together with CD14 as promising targets. J Leukoc Biol. 2017;101:193–204. https://doi.org/10.1189/jlb.3VMR0316-132R.
80. Barratt-Due A, Pischke SE, Brekke O-L, Thorgersen EB, Nielsen EW, Espevik T, Huber-Lang M, Mollnes TE. Bride and groom in systemic inflammation – The bells ring for comple-

ment and Toll in cooperation. Immunobiology. 2012;217:1047–56. https://doi.org/10.1016/j.imbio.2012.07.019.

81. Lee CC, Avalos AM, Ploegh HL. Accessory molecules for Toll-like receptors and their function. Nat Rev Immunol. 2012;12:168–79. https://doi.org/10.1038/nri3151.
82. Kolev M, Le Friec G, Kemper C. Complement–tapping into new sites and effector systems. Nat Rev Immunol. 2014;14:811–20. https://doi.org/10.1038/nri3761.
83. Song W-C. Crosstalk between complement and toll-like receptors. Toxicol Pathol. 2012;40:174–82. https://doi.org/10.1177/0192623311428478.
84. Raby A-C, Holst B, Davies J, Colmont C, Laumonnier Y, Coles B, Shah S, Hall J, Topley N, Köhl J, et al. TLR activation enhances C5a-induced pro-inflammatory responses by negatively modulating the second C5a receptor, C5L2. Eur J Immunol. 2011;41:2741–52. https://doi.org/10.1002/eji.201041350.
85. Hajishengallis G, Lambris JD. More than complementing tolls: complement–toll-like receptor synergy and crosstalk in innate immunity and inflammation. Immunol Rev. 2016;274:233–44. https://doi.org/10.1111/imr.12467.
86. Lau C, Nygård S, Fure H, Olstad OK, Holden M, Lappegård KT, Brekke O-L, Espevik T, Hovig E, Mollnes TE. CD14 and complement crosstalk and largely mediate the transcriptional response to Escherichia coli in human whole blood as revealed by DNA microarray. PLoS One. 2015;10:e0117261. https://doi.org/10.1371/journal.pone.0117261.
87. Brekke O-L, Christiansen D, Fure H, Pharo A, Fung M, Riesenfeld J, Mollnes TE. Combined inhibition of complement and CD14 abolish E. coli-induced cytokine-, chemokine- and growth factor-synthesis in human whole blood. Mol Immunol. 2008;45:3804–13. https://doi.org/10.1016/j.molimm.2008.05.017.
88. Huber-Lang M, Barratt-Due A, Pischke SE, Sandanger Ø, Nilsson PH, Nunn MA, Denk S, Gaus W, Espevik T, Mollnes TE. Double blockade of CD14 and complement C5 abolishes the cytokine storm and improves morbidity and survival in Polymicrobial sepsis in mice. J Immunol Author Choice. 2014;192:5324–31. https://doi.org/10.4049/jimmunol.1400341.
89. Skjeflo EW, Sagatun C, Dybwik K, Aam S, Urving SH, Nunn MA, Fure H, Lau C, Brekke O-L, Huber-Lang M, et al. Combined inhibition of complement and CD14 improved outcome in porcine polymicrobial sepsis. Crit Care. 2015;19:415. https://doi.org/10.1186/s13054-015-1129-9.
90. Keshari RS, Silasi R, Popescu NI, Regmi G, Chaaban H, Lambris JD, Lupu C, Mollnes TE, Lupu F. CD14 inhibition improves survival and attenuates thrombo-inflammation and cardiopulmonary dysfunction in a baboon model of Escherichia coli sepsis. J Thromb Haemost. 2021;19:429–43. https://doi.org/10.1111/jth.15162.
91. Gorsuch WB, Chrysanthou E, Schwaeble WJ, Stahl GL. The complement system in ischemia-reperfusion injuries. Immunobiology. 2012;217:1026–33. https://doi.org/10.1016/j.imbio.2012.07.024.
92. Banz Y, Rieben R. Role of complement and perspectives for intervention in ischemia-reperfusion damage. Ann Med. 2012;44:205–17. https://doi.org/10.3109/07853890.2010.535556.
93. Liang C-F, Liu JT, Wang Y, Xu A, Vanhoutte PM. Toll-like receptor 4 mutation protects obese mice against endothelial dysfunction by decreasing NADPH oxidase isoforms 1 and 4. Arterioscler Thromb Vasc Biol. 2013;33:777–84. https://doi.org/10.1161/ATVBAHA.112.301087.
94. Neglia L, Oggioni M, Mercurio D, De Simoni M-G, Fumagalli S. Specific contribution of mannose-binding lectin murine isoforms to brain ischemia/reperfusion injury. Cell Mol Immunol. 2020;17:218–26. https://doi.org/10.1038/s41423-019-0225-1.
95. Arumugam TV, Okun E, Tang S-C, Thundyil J, Taylor SM, Woodruff TM. Toll-like receptors in ischemia-reperfusion injury. Shock (Augusta Ga). 2009;32:4–16. https://doi.org/10.1097/SHK.0b013e318193e333.
96. Hamanaka J, Hara H. Involvement of Toll-like receptors in ischemia-induced neuronal damage. Cent Nerv Syst Agents Med Chem. 2011;11:107–13. https://doi.org/10.2174/187152411796011312.

97. Garred P, Tenner AJ, Mollnes TE. Therapeutic targeting of the complement system: from rare diseases to pandemics. Pharmacol Rev. 2021;73:792–827. https://doi.org/10.1124/pharmrev.120.000072.
98. Mercurio D, Piotti A, Valente A, Oggioni M, Ponstein Y, Van Amersfoort E, Gobbi M, Fumagalli S, De Simoni M-G. Plasma-derived and recombinant C1 esterase inhibitor: binding profiles and neuroprotective properties in brain ischemia/reperfusion injury. Brain Behav Immun. 2021;93:299–311. https://doi.org/10.1016/j.bbi.2021.01.002.
99. De Blasio D, Fumagalli S, Longhi L, Orsini F, Palmioli A, Stravalaci M, Vegliante G, Zanier ER, Bernardi A, Gobbi M, et al. Pharmacological inhibition of mannose-binding lectin ameliorates neurobehavioral dysfunction following experimental traumatic brain injury. J Cereb Blood Flow Metab. 2017;37:938–50. https://doi.org/10.1177/0271678X16647397.
100. Orsini F, Chrysanthou E, Dudler T, Cummings WJ, Takahashi M, Fujita T, Demopulos G, De Simoni M-G, Schwaeble W. Mannan binding lectin-associated serine protease-2 (MASP-2) critically contributes to post-ischemic brain injury independent of MASP-1. J Neuroinflammation. 2016;13:213. https://doi.org/10.1186/s12974-016-0684-6.
101. Mercurio D, Pischiutta F, Seminara S, Tribuzio F, Lisi I, Pasetto L, Bonetto V, De Simoni M-G, Schwaeble W, Yaseen S, et al. Inhibition of mannan-binding lectin associated serine protease (MASP)-2 reduces the cognitive deficits in a mouse model of severe traumatic brain injury. J Neuroinflammation. 2024;21:141. https://doi.org/10.1186/s12974-024-03133-4.
102. Ali YM, Carnell GW, Fumagalli S, Mercurio D, Seminara S, Lynch NJ, Khatri P, Arachchilage CH, Mascheroni L, Kaminski C, et al. Inhibition of the lectin pathway of complement activation reduces acute respiratory distress syndrome severity in a mouse model of SARS-CoV-2 infection. J Infect Dis. 2023;jiad462 https://doi.org/10.1093/infdis/jiad462.
103. Stravalaci M, Pagani I, Paraboschi EM, Pedotti M, Doni A, Scavello F, Mapelli SN, Sironi M, Perucchini C, Varani L, et al. Recognition and inhibition of SARS-CoV-2 by humoral innate immunity pattern recognition molecules. Nat Immunol. 2022;23:275–86. https://doi.org/10.1038/s41590-021-01114-w.
104. Rambaldi A, Gritti G, Micò MC, Frigeni M, Borleri G, Salvi A, Landi F, Pavoni C, Sonzogni A, Gianatti A, et al. Endothelial injury and thrombotic microangiopathy in COVID-19: treatment with the lectin-pathway inhibitor narsoplimab. Immunobiology. 2020;225:152001. https://doi.org/10.1016/j.imbio.2020.152001.
105. Thornton P, McColl BW, Greenhalgh A, Denes A, Allan SM, Rothwell NJ. Platelet interleukin-1alpha drives cerebrovascular inflammation. Blood. 2010;115:3632–9. https://doi.org/10.1182/blood-2009-11-252643.
106. Grossi C, Artusi C, Meroni P, Borghi MO, Neglia L, Lonati PA, Oggioni M, Tedesco F, De Simoni M-G, Fumagalli S. β2 glycoprotein I participates in phagocytosis of apoptotic neurons and in vascular injury in experimental brain stroke. J Cereb Blood Flow Metab. 2021;41:2038–53. https://doi.org/10.1177/0271678X20984551.
107. del Zoppo GJ, Mabuchi T. Cerebral microvessel responses to focal ischemia. J Cereb Blood Flow Metab. 2003;23:879–94. https://doi.org/10.1097/01.WCB.0000078322.96027.78.

New Insights in Septic Encephalopathy

5

Sara Albertinetti and Ines Lakbar

5.1 Introduction

Sepsis is a life-threatening organ dysfunction caused by a dysregulated immune response to infection. This systemic inflammatory state leads to extended tissue damage and multiple organ failure that can progress to septic shock and death. The definition of sepsis has evolved considerably over the past decades, now including the Sequential Organ Failure Assessment (SOFA) score, a tool to assess several organ dysfunctions. In the emergency room, a shorter version of the SOFA score, named the quick SOFA (qSOFA) score, is often employed as a rapid screening tool to identify patients who may be at risk for sepsis. The qSOFA is comprised of three components: altered mental status (commonly manifested as confusion), a systolic blood pressure of 100 mm Hg or lower, and a respiratory rate of 22 breaths per minute or higher. The inclusion of confusion as one of these key elements underscores its importance as an early clinical marker. Altered mental status is frequently observed early in the disease process and is considered as an early manifestation of septic encephalopathy [1].

Sepsis-associated encephalopathy (SAE) is a significant neurological complication which affects 70% of septic patients, characterized by diffuse brain dysfunction in the absence of CNS infection. It represents a risk factor for mortality, and survivors often face long-term disabilities [2]. It is increasingly recognized for its

S. Albertinetti
Department of Surgical Sciences and Integrated Diagnostics, University of Genova, Genoa, Italy

Anesthesia and Intensive Care, IRCCS Ospedale Policlinico San Martino, Genoa, Italy

I. Lakbar (✉)
Anesthesiology and Intensive Care; Anesthesia and Critical Care Department B, Saint Eloi Teaching Hospital, PhyMedExp, University of Montpellier, Montpellier, France
e-mail: ines.lakbar@chu-montpellier.fr

D. Battaglini et al. (eds.), *Organ System Crosstalk in Critical Illness*,
https://doi.org/10.1007/978-3-032-01024-7_5

complex pathophysiological mechanisms, which include metabolic and inflammatory factors, blood-brain barrier (BBB) dysfunction, and neurodegeneration. The condition manifests with a wide range of clinical presentations, from mild delirium to coma, and poses notable challenges in diagnosis and management, making it a critical area of research in intensive care medicine [3].

Understanding the pathophysiology of SAE is essential for effective clinical management. Inflammation and endothelial dysfunction lead to compromised BBB integrity, contributing to cerebral ischemia and neuronal injury. High levels of inflammatory cytokines have been observed, which may exacerbate neuroinflammation and cognitive impairment. Current clinical strategies focus on the prompt identification of underlying infections, supportive care, and the use of sedatives to manage agitation, highlighting the necessity of a multidisciplinary approach in treating affected patients.

Recent research underscores the importance of translational mechanisms in the treatment of SAE, including the application of intravenous antimicrobials designed to penetrate the BBB and the exploration of biomarkers that may facilitate diagnosis and treatment efficacy. Innovations such as intrathecal dosing are being considered for effectively targeting resistant pathogens, while potential immunomodulatory therapies are under investigation to mitigate neuroinflammation.

The purpose of this chapter is to navigate from well-established concepts of physiopathology to the most innovative and latest research and treatment strategies.

5.2 Pathophysiology

SAE is a complex condition which involves a range of pathophysiological mechanisms that ultimately lead to brain dysfunction and injury. The pathophysiology of SAE has not yet been fully established; it is likely to be multifactorial and mostly independent from the presence of microorganisms or toxins within the cerebral tissue [4]. Several likely mechanisms have been proposed, affecting both brain cell function and signaling—including neuroinflammation, ischemic processes, mitochondrial and endothelial dysfunction, neurotransmitter imbalances, and disturbances in calcium homeostasis—as well as brain perfusion and oxygenation. These alterations can be further exacerbated by external factors such as renal or hepatic dysfunction, dysglycemia, fever, and neurotropic drugs. The interaction between neurodegenerative and neurovascular mechanisms leads to variable clinical presentations, influenced by sepsis severity, preexisting neurological conditions, and individual brain vulnerability [5–7].

5.2.1 Neuroinflammation

Systemic inflammation can affect the brain primarily through two pathways: the circumventricular organs, structures lacking a BBB and located near neuroendocrine and brainstem regions, and the vagus nerve, which detects peripheral inflammation and activates cholinergic anti-inflammatory and autonomic responses [8, 9].

In SAE, neuroinflammation plays a central role. Both peripheral and local inflammatory responses lead to the activation of microglia and astroglia which undergo morphological, immunological, and metabolic changes acquiring neurotoxic properties. This leads to increased release of cytokines (e.g., tumor necrosis factor (TNF)-α, interleukin (IL)-1β, IL-6, High Mobility Group Box (HMGB1)), reactive oxygen species, and chemokines, causing BBB disruption, neuronal dysfunction, and cell death, particularly in vulnerable brain regions. These inflammatory mediators also exacerbate systemic immune activation and metabolic dysregulation [10]. High levels of inflammatory cytokines, such as TNF-α and IL-1β, are often observed in brain tissue during sepsis, highlighting the role of neuroinflammation in disease progression [11].

5.2.2 Astrocytes and Blood-Brain Barrier Dysfunction

Neuroinflammation triggers neutrophil infiltration and astrocyte activation via toll-like receptors, with downstream effects including aquaporin-4 overexpression and increased prostaglandin and nitric oxide synthesis. These changes disrupt brain water balance, activate the hypothalamic–pituitary–adrenal axis, and contribute to symptoms like fever, behavioral changes, and neuronal death [12].

Astrocytes, key regulators of BBB function, brain water homeostasis, and synaptic transmission, are increasingly recognized as central players in SAE pathogenesis. Their dysfunction alters neurovascular and synaptic stability. Inflammatory stimuli, such as lipopolysaccharide (LPS), inhibit gap junction communication and open hemichannels, impairing neuron–glia signaling. While animal models consistently show astrogliosis in SAE, human evidence is limited to morphological studies, lacking functional insights into astrocyte-neuron interactions [13, 14].

In SAE, the integrity of BBB is significantly compromised. Increased BBB permeability, especially in the cerebral cortex and hippocampus [15], allows immune cell infiltration and the release of cytotoxic mediators, contributing to brain inflammation, edema, and neurological damage. Clinical conditions such as white matter lesions and posterior reversible encephalopathy syndrome (PRES) further highlight the impact of BBB dysfunction in SAE.

Markers like C-type natriuretic peptide (NT-proCNP), reflecting endothelial injury, and altered cerebrovascular indices on transcranial Doppler suggest impaired autoregulation and correlate with disease severity, particularly in pediatric patients [16, 17].

5.2.3 Neurodegeneration and Cognitive Dysfunction

The neurodegenerative changes observed in SAE include notable structural and functional brain changes, with the hippocampus being particularly vulnerable.

Among the most prominent findings are brain atrophy and neuronal loss, especially in the cerebral cortex and hippocampal regions—areas intimately involved in memory processing and cognitive integration. The hippocampus, in particular, shows marked susceptibility due to its high metabolic demand and dense concentration of glutamatergic synapses, which make it especially prone to oxidative stress and excitotoxic injury during systemic inflammation [6].

These changes are often correlated with cognitive dysfunction, as indicated by various behavioral assessments in animal models [6]. Morphologically, electron microscopy has revealed acute cellular injuries in neurons, including mitochondrial swelling and endoplasmic reticulum expansion, which may underlie the cognitive impairments associated with SAE.

These ultrastructural abnormalities suggest impaired cellular energy metabolism and calcium dysregulation, key mechanisms contributing to synaptic failure and neuronal apoptosis.

Furthermore, neuroinflammatory cascades, driven by elevated cytokines like IL-1β and TNF-α, exacerbate hippocampal damage by promoting microglial activation and glutamate-mediated excitotoxicity. The cumulative impact of these events likely underpins the long-term cognitive deficits observed in SAE survivors, aligning hippocampal damage as a central feature in the pathophysiology of sepsis-induced cognitive decline.

5.2.4 Mitochondrial Dysfunction: Energy Metabolism and Perfusion

A significant reduction in cerebral blood flow (CBF) has been linked to SAE, which, in addition to increased metabolic and bioenergetics demands, directly affects cellular metabolism and contributes to oxidative stress and mitochondrial dysfunction [18]. Disruptions in cerebral perfusion and autoregulation are critical factors in the pathogenesis of SAE, involving mechanisms such as abnormal vasoconstriction and inflammatory insults.

Alterations in glycolysis and energy metabolism were also reported in SAE, further emphasizing the importance of maintaining adequate cerebral perfusion for preventing neuronal injury [19]. The resulting energy deficit due to a decrease in adenosine triphosphate (ATP) production, the generation of oxygen/nitrogen reactive species, and the increased superoxide dismutase activity has been shown in various brain regions of septic animals, thus leading glial cells and neurons to apoptosis [19].

5.2.5 Neurotransmitter Dysfunction

All the inflammatory and metabolic changes described above have been proposed to lead to alterations in cerebral neurotransmission, which cause aberrant neuronal function and, thereby, SAE [20, 21]. In fact, changes in neurotransmitter pathways (acetylcholine, GABA, norepinephrine, serotonin, dopamine, and glutamate) are closely related to delirium [2, 22]. Variations in neurotransmitters concentration in the synaptic cleft (increasing in release and decreasing in uptake) [23] is the basis for excitotoxic processes, a pathological mechanism resulting from neuroinflammation, ischemia, nitric oxide (NO) production [21], increased indoleamine-2,3 dioxygenase (IDO) activity but also systemic disorders such as hypoxemia, dysglycemia, drug toxicity, electrolyte disorders and circulating neurotoxic aromatic amino acids (AAA) excess (ammonium, tyrosine, tryptophan and phenylalanine). Neurotoxic AAA, neurotransmitters' precursors, are released in excess due to extensive muscular proteolysis and reduced hepatic clearance during sepsis, but their role in neurotransmitter imbalance is still controversial. Encephalopathic septic patients have greater elevation of aromatic amino acids in plasma than non-encephalopathic patients [24]. In CNS, aromatic amino acids can act as false neurotransmitters or they can reduce cerebral concentrations of dopamine, serotonin, and norepinephrine, leading to abnormalities in neurotransmission [25].

A small number of CNS structures such as amygdala, nucleus tractus solitarii, and locus coeruleus are particularly vulnerable to sepsis and are responsible for neuronal apoptosis [26].

Excitotoxicity through glutamate receptors induces functional disorders but also cell death, which may be responsible for clinical and electrophysiological features of SAE [27]. Analysis of the cerebrospinal fluid of SAE patients showed decreased levels of ascorbate, an antioxidant produced by astrocytes, that plays an important role in neuroprotection [28].

Various neurotransmitter pathways seem to be impaired during sepsis, notably dopaminergic, β-adrenergic, gamma Aminobutyric acid (GABA), and the cholinergic ones [29]. Hypocholinergia has been postulated to cause delirium [30, 31], and a dopamine/choline imbalance might be particularly involved in SAE [32], but its incidence or its duration are reduced with cholinergic drugs such as rivastigmine or antidopaminergic drugs such as haloperidol [29]. On the other side, the use of GABA-agonists such as midazolam or lorazepam increases the risk of delirium [33], whereas the effect of dexmedetomidine, a selective agonist of $\alpha 2$-adrenoceptors expressed in the locus coeruleus, on delirium, is still unclear [34, 35].

5.2.6 Iatrogenic Factors

Various drugs commonly administered to septic patients have been demonstrated to be neurotoxic, including antibiotics and sedatives. Antibiotics overdose has been shown to be associated with delirium; moreover, many antibiotics have a neurotoxic effect, both in overdose and at therapeutic doses. It is now known that benzodiazepines induce delirium, especially when administered in an ICU setting where environment and sleep deprivation play an important role. It is possible to apply prevention and early delirium recognition tools, such as the ABCDE bundle, which includes: Assess, Prevent, and Manage Pain, Both Spontaneous Awakening Trials

(SAT) and Spontaneous Breathing Trials (SBT), Choice of analgesia and sedation, Delirium: Assess, Prevent, and Manage, Early mobility and Exercise, and Family engagement and empowerment [29, 36].

5.2.7 Calcium Homeostasis

SAE is linked to elevated intracellular calcium levels, and disruptions in calcium homeostasis are known to impair learning, memory, and cognitive functions [12].

5.2.8 Interaction Between Brain and Peripheral Organs in Sepsis

5.2.8.1 Brain and Gut Microbiota

The gut-brain axis is a bidirectional neuroendocrine and immune communication network that regulates not only gastrointestinal functions but also emotional responses, immune activity, brain development, and overall physiological homeostasis. Its integrity is essential for cognitive and behavioral regulation, and its disruption has been linked to numerous psychiatric and neurological disorders.

In sepsis, patients often show profound disturbances in gut microbiota composition (i.e., drop in diversity, loss of protective bacteria taxa and consequent pathobiont proliferation, selection of anaerobes, and more virulent bacteria) resulting in a condition known as dysbiosis. Although the underlying mechanisms are not fully understood, growing evidence links gut microbiota alterations to the development of SAE [37]. Animal studies using fecal microbiota transplantation (FMT) have shown that microbiota from SAE-resistant mice can reduce systemic and cerebral inflammation after sepsis, decreasing IL-1β and TNF-α levels in both serum and brain tissues, and improving survival. These findings highlight the role of gut microbes in modulating neuroinflammatory responses.

The gut microbiota may also influence SAE through intestinal epithelial cells (IECs), which release immunologically active exosomes carrying proteins, DeoxyriboNucleic Acid (DNA), and cytokines, thereby modulating immune responses [38, 39].

5.2.8.2 Brain and Liver Metabolite

Studies show that an intermediate metabolite of fat oxidation metabolism in the liver, the ketone body β-hydroxybutyrate (BHB), exerts neuroprotective effects and helps prevent cognitive impairment after sepsis [40].

Cirrhosis is an established independent risk factor for both sepsis and sepsis-related mortality. In ICU setting, patients with cirrhosis are more vulnerable to sepsis and its complications than the general population, due to increased intestinal microbiota translocation, systemic immune dysregulation, and a hyperdynamic circulatory state characterized by elevated cardiac output and reduced systemic vascular resistance. SAE and hepatic encephalopathy (HE) are two common neurological complications in these patients, often coexisting and presenting diagnostic challenges due to overlapping clinical features. HE is a severe reversible metabolic complication of sepsis-induced liver cirrhosis, demonstrating clinical manifestations of minor cognitive dysfunction such as personality changes, memory decline, attention deficit, and other neurological changes, including lethargy, delirium, and coma. Additionally, bacterial infections can act as precipitating events in the onset of hepatic encephalopathy (HE). Several authors have suggested that SAE may share metabolic mechanisms with HE, given their similar neuropsychiatric presentations, which can range from confusion and delirium to coma [41].

5.3 Diagnosis and Monitoring

SAE is basically a diagnosis of exclusion, with no specific clinical manifestations, and requires ruling out conditions that may be responsible for an altered level of consciousness, such as CNS direct infection, multisystem organ failure (MOF), stroke, intracranial hemorrhage, head trauma, meningoencephalitis, endocarditis, embolism, drug side effects, or other metabolic disturbance.

When SAE is suspected, the first step is the assessment of the mental status, which can be subtle, especially in early stages, particularly if we consider the widespread use of sedatives in this population. Once CNS pathologies potentially responsible for the alteration of mental status have been excluded, the evaluation must aim at finding the source of the infection and the responsible infectious agent [25, 42].

5.3.1 Clinical Presentation

SAE is the combination of extracranial infection with clinical signs of neurological dysfunction [29], which can vary widely among patients. It may manifest as a rapid change in cognitive status or level of consciousness, with symptoms ranging from mild delirium (50%, mainly hypoactive) to coma (46%) [43, 44]. Convulsive seizures (10%) and focal neurological signs (18%) are less common but warrant further investigation to rule out potential brain injury. SAE can also be associated with nonepileptic myoclonus, tremor, or asterixis [45].

In children, symptoms such as vomiting, headache, and neck pain may be present, but hypotonia and irritability are also common.

There are no pathognomonic signs or symptoms of SAE: changes in the mental status of a septic patient can be related to other causes like vitamin or other nutritional deficiency, electrolyte disturbances, drug administration, overdose, withdrawal, etc.

The physician must look for sepsis in any patient who presents with change in consciousness or behavior.

There are several validated scores to identify delirium and monitor the cognitive status in patients with SAE, even if the most appropriate screening tool for ICU is still controversial. In non-sedated and RASS >-3 patients, Confusion Assessment Method for the Intensive Care Unit (CAM-ICU) and Intensive Care Delirium

Screening Checklist (ICSDC) can be used for diagnosing delirium showing very high sensitivity and positive predictive value. It assesses a wide range of responses, while the Assessment to Intensive Care Environment (ATICE) score assesses awakening, comprehension, and calmness by evaluating eye-opening to a variety of stimuli [46].

Glasgow Coma Scale (GCS), RASS (Richmond Agitation-Sedation Scale), and Full Outline of UnResponsiveness (FOUR) can be used for monitoring coma. In deeply sedated patients, the score can be helpful for detecting brainstem dysfunction [47].

Once the neurological dysfunction is identified, a complete neurological examination is essential to rule out other causes of encephalopathy: it must evaluate the motor and sensory response, the cranial nerves' function, the reflexes, while in sedated patients the evaluation of eye movement, pupil morphology, cough and corneal reflexes, and response to painful stimuli assumes particular importance [48].

It is also necessary to pay attention to the pharmacological regimen, as several commonly used drugs, such as benzodiazepines, anticonvulsants, opioids, anticholinergics, and even certain antibiotics, corticosteroids, and antiarrhythmics, are frequently associated with neurological impairment [15]. Moreover, a history of overdose or withdrawal from psychoactive medications may be responsible for the altered state of consciousness.

A detailed physical examination is important to explore the source of infection. It should be associated with a comprehensive metabolic panel of analyses to search for evidence of organ dysfunction of other abnormalities that may be responsible for the change in sensorium. Serologies and proper cultures (blood, respiratory, urine, CSF culture and analysis) help to identify the pathological organism behind SAE, even if sometimes the recognition could be challenging.

5.3.2 Imaging

Neuroimaging and neuromonitoring in septic patients are potentially of great help for diagnosis, management, and prognostication. A multimodal monitoring approach is increasingly adopted in this context and should be tailored to the patient's clinical condition [49].

The neuroradiological correlates of SAE's symptoms are poorly known due to the lack of studies on SAE in septic-shock patients. Sanz et al. conducted brain imaging in 49 pediatric septic shock patients, identifying ischemia and cerebritis (i.e., cerebral edema or damage associated with infection) as the most common acute brain lesions [50]. In contrast, Sandquist et al. examined neuroimaging in septic pediatric patients with a focus on long-term rather than acute changes. They found that the most frequent abnormality was brain volume loss (39%), likely representing the chronic outcome of earlier lesions such as ischemia or infarction [17, 51].

When neuroimaging is indicated, CT scan should be the first-line examination due to its ease of access and ability to quickly rule out intracranial pathologies such as ischemic or hemorrhagic injuries, particularly in patients presenting with seizures or focal neurological signs [52]. However, MRI offers greater sensitivity for detecting microvascular injuries, embolic events, cerebral edema, and conditions like PRES.

Neuroimaging findings in SAE patients are variable: while some individuals exhibit normal brain MRI scans despite having SAE, others present with a wide range of abnormalities [53, 54].

An important prospective study performed in septic shock patients with acute brain dysfunction showed abnormal MRI in half of them, with ischemic stroke and diffuse or confluent white matter hyperdensities (leukoencephalopathy) as the two most frequent lesions. The evidence of ischemia suggests the importance of cerebral perfusion impairment and microcirculatory dysfunction; leukoencephalopathy confirms the presence of a group of pathologic processes including BBB dysfunction with vasogenic edema, axon loss, lacunar infarcts, and gliosis. They also demonstrated that ischemia is associated with increased mortality and mid-term neurologic disability [55].

Sepsis can be complicated by PRES, with vasogenic edema in typical location, including cerebellum, occipital, parietal, frontal, and temporal lobes [56] [57].

Finelli et al. described the presence of bilateral basal ganglia, thalamic, cerebellar, brainstem, and cerebral MRI abnormalities in a case of SAE [58]. A neuroimaging study in critically ill patients who suffered from delirium showed that a longer duration of delirium was associated with a smaller brain volume 3 months after hospital discharge and an increased cognitive impairment at 12 months [59].

Because SAE may result from an imbalance between cerebral energy demand and blood flow, optimizing cerebral perfusion by identifying personalized mean arterial pressure targets represents a promising strategy. However, well-defined therapeutic targets for these tools have yet to be established. Bedside transcranial doppler (TCD) ultrasonography can be employed to noninvasively measure and monitor blood velocity in the major cerebral vessels, potentially offering indirect information about cerebral blood flow, cerebral autoregulation, and cerebrovascular reactivity to carbon dioxide ($PaCO_2$) [60].

The three main parameters obtainable through this method include flow direction, velocities, and indices for arterial resistance, with elevated pulsatility index (PI) (>1.2) and resistive index (RI) indicating autoregulatory failure in 78% of SAE cases. In particular, PI was reported to increase during adult and children sepsis and was related to illness severity; PI and RI may together predict SAE development and associated mortality [17, 61, 62].

However, it cannot be used as a diagnostic tool since the alteration of cerebral perfusion is not a constant characteristic of SAE and because the technique remains highly operator dependent [63].

Cerebral oxygenation can be non-invasively assessed with near-infrared spectroscopy (NIRS), which measures hemoglobin oxygen saturation in the frontal cortex and helps detect perfusion and circulatory changes. Temporal variations in NIRS-derived cerebral oxygenation, combined with mean arterial pressure, may aid in evaluating cerebral autoregulation and guiding optimal MAP targets [64].

However, NIRS is limited by influence from extracranial circulation and only reflects anterior brain regions [65]. Due to limited evidence in septic patients, further research is needed before adopting NIRS as a standard monitoring tool.

Positive emission tomography (PET) imaging using translocator protein (TSPO) ligands holds promise for quantifying microglial activation, though clinical data remain sparse [66].

5.3.3 Biomarkers

Serum biomarkers may be useful in both diagnosis and monitoring of SAE as they reflect damage to different structures involved in the pathophysiological processes. Aspecific markers like C-reactive protein and procalcitonin indicate systemic inflammation and may correlate with SAE occurrence [29].

Although limited data exist on specific brain injury biomarkers in SAE, some of them have shown potential. Biomarkers such as NT-proCNP (endothelial dysfunction), S100β (microglial activation), and NSE or neurofilament (brain injury with axonal damage) have been linked to SAE, though none are currently used in routine clinical practice [67, 68]. High Mobility Group Box 1 (HMGB1) and Zonula Occludens-1 (ZO-1) are also being studied for associations with cognitive impairment and organ dysfunction [69].

Among these, S100β and NSE are the most promising ones: their serum levels are elevated in patients with brain dysfunction and correlate with neuroimaging findings, suggesting their potential as bedside tools or triggers for further neuroimaging investigation. Notably, elevated S100β is linked to more severe sepsis and higher early ICU mortality [55].

These biomarkers can be measured in plasma or CSF; however, their sensitivity and specificity remain poor, as they reflect brain processes and not the nature of pathology [70]. Thus, while potentially helpful, the use of these biomarkers is not yet part of standard daily clinical practice, and their clinical utility remains investigational. The search for more accurate and reliable biomarkers remains an important area for future research.

Serum microRNAs (miR-124, miR-155) show preliminary diagnostic potential, with miR-124's neural specificity offering advantages over protein biomarkers in distinguishing sepsis-related delirium from other encephalopathies [71].

5.3.4 Neurophysiological Features

Continuous electroencephalography (cEEG) monitoring detects early spectral abnormalities, though sedation limits its utility in ventilated patients. Somatosensory evoked potentials (SEPs), though technically challenging in ICUs, reveal delayed latencies correlating with axonal injury severity.

5.3.4.1 Electroencephalography

Several studies demonstrate the sensitivity of EEG as a diagnostic, monitoring, and prognostic tool in SAE. In those patients, Young et al. identified EEG features consistent with a potentially reversible encephalopathy and developed an electrophysiological classification of SAE severity, distinguishing EEG patterns and correlating them with mortality percentages. It includes four grades, with a direct correlation between the severity of EEG abnormalities and mortality [72]:

- Grade 0: normal EEG (0% mortality)
- Grade 1: predominant theta activity (19% mortality)
- Grade 2: predominant delta activity (36% mortality)
- Grade 3: predominant triphasic activity (50% mortality)
- Grade 4: suppression (67% mortality)

Slowing of the EEG background or the emergence of left–right asymmetry may serve as early indicators of neurological deterioration, prompting timely initiation of further diagnostic investigations [73].

In a prospective study based on standard 20-min EEG recordings involving 110 septic patients performed within the first 3 days following ICU admission, Azabou et al. identified predominant delta and theta rhythms in 33% and 48%, respectively. Triphasic waves were observed in 6% of cases, while suppression patterns were detected in fewer than 3%. Additionally, low voltage and absence of reactivity were reported in 65% and 25% of patients, respectively [74].

The reported incidence of pseudo-epileptic discharges (PEDs) ranges from 19% to 48%, while epileptic seizures occur in approximately 9–50% of cases [75].

cEEG monitoring can detect non-convulsive seizures in up to 20–30% of these patients, allowing for the timely administration of antiepileptic treatment aimed at preventing secondary cerebral injury [2].

Quantitative EEG analysis can also be employed to calculate the burst-suppression ratio (BSR), a pattern that may result from excessive sedation, associated with an increased risk of delirium [76].

There is no strong correlation between clinical manifestation and EEG findings. Thus, clinical seizures are exceptionally reported in septic patients, indicating that electrographic seizures are mostly nonconvulsive [45]. Although electrographic seizures are more commonly observed in patients presenting with delirium at the time of EEG recording, most comatose and delirious septic patients do not exhibit epileptic activity. Furthermore, EEG abnormalities may be present even in the absence of clinical neurological deterioration [77].

These findings suggest that EEG alterations are more likely to reflect disease severity rather than pathogenicity. Moreover, sepsis has been associated with a modest increase in the long-term risk of epilepsy. Currently, there is no evidence supporting the use of prophylactic antiepileptic therapy, nor are there clear guidelines for the management of electrographic seizures in septic patients [29].

5.3.4.2 Somatosensory-Evoked Potentials

SEPs can be useful for evaluating SAE in sedated critically ill patients as their latencies are only minimally affected by sedatives, unlike EEG.

In a study involving 68 septic patients, impairment of subcortical and cortical SEPs pathways was observed in 34% and 84% of cases, respectively [78, 79].

5.4 Management Strategies

Despite progress in understanding sepsis, no specific treatment for SAE is currently available. Nevertheless, several practical considerations should be considered in the management of these patients. Continuous monitoring of vital signs, serum drug levels, and neurological status is essential for detecting complications related to neurotoxic agents or secondary brain injuries.

Management focuses on early recognition and treatment of delirium, identification of the underlying infection and causative organism, timely and appropriate antibiotic therapy, and supportive care (i.e., fluid resuscitation and vasopressors to maintain hemodynamic stability). Intravenous antibiotics should be started promptly after cultures, as early treatment is associated with reduced mortality [80].

SAE management also involves correcting neurotoxic factors and targeted management of seizures, delirium, and coma. Early withdrawal of sedative agents may help reduce the risk of delirium and facilitate timely neurological assessment.

In case of severe agitation or dysautonomia, sedatives like propofol or dexmedetomidine may be utilized to mitigate secondary brain injury, although care must be taken as some sedatives, like midazolam, are associated with exacerbated encephalopathy [15].

Non-pharmacological strategies to reduce the risk of delirium may also be helpful in patients with SAE. These include reinforcement of normal circadian rhythms avoiding sleep deprivation, early mobilization, aid to orientation (emphasizing date, place, and reason for hospitalization), discontinuation of sedation, adequate lighting and noise reduction, encouragement of oral fluids to prevent dehydration, management of physical and psychological discomfort, and identification and avoidance of prodelirious drugs (i.e., drugs with anticholinergic, histaminergic, or other psychotropic properties) [81].

There is no specific recommendation on pharmacological management of sepsis-associated delirium, except avoiding or discontinuing sedation whenever possible [82].

Patients experiencing systemic inflammatory processes often exhibit increased sensitivity to benzodiazepines, making their use inadvisable in such cases. In the MENDS trial, dexmedetomidine, an alpha-2 adrenergic agonist, has shown advantages over lorazepam in septic patients as those treated with dexmedetomidine experienced more delirium-free days, shorter time on mechanical ventilation, and a lower 28-day mortality rate compared to those receiving lorazepam [34]. Furthermore, dexmedetomidine contributes to improved outcomes by the inhibition of neuronal apoptosis and the reduction of the sepsis-associated inflammatory response [83]. However, a recent large-scale study found that early goal-directed sedation using dexmedetomidine did not provide significant benefits in critically ill patients [35]. Until further evidence is available, dexmedetomidine is the preferred sedative over benzodiazepines for patients with SAE requiring sedation.

Ketamine may offer neuroprotective benefits in SAE, although it has not yet been evaluated in interventional trials.

Since seizures are relatively uncommon in SAE (less than 10%), the routine prophylactic use of antiepileptic drugs is not recommended. However, early EEG monitoring is advised in comatose or sedated patients to allow prompt seizure detection and timely intervention when needed.

Although statins, and in particular rivastigmine, was theoretically promising due to its potential microglial effects, it has not demonstrated any benefit in reducing delirium in ICU patients [84, 85].

Steroids may be administered to patients with sepsis and have also been shown to reduce the incidence of post-traumatic stress disorder. However, their use has been associated with an increased risk of acquired neuromuscular weakness, particularly critical illness myopathy (CIM). Additionally, steroid administration may itself contribute to the development of psychosis [25].

Although strict glucose control in the ICU has been shown to reduce morbidity and mortality, maintaining tight glycemic targets in septic and critically ill patients may increase the risk of neurologic complications related to hypoglycemia, such as seizures and encephalopathy. Moreover, recent clinical trials, such as the NICE-SUGAR trial, have clearly demonstrated that patients receiving strict glucose control (target blood glucose level 81–108 mg/dL) experienced a higher incidence of severe hypoglycemia and significantly increased 90-day mortality compared to a conventional target control (<180 mg/dL) [86]. Avoiding hyperglycemia and hypoglycemia can therefore protect neuronal cells from apoptosis.

The use of recombinant activated protein C (drotrecogin alfa) has been suggested to reduce neural damage in human sepsis, as evaluated by serum measurements of S100b [87].

However, although initially promising, it is no longer available as a therapeutic option and cannot be used in septic patients.

Experimental studies have suggested potential benefits of other agents, such as minocycline and intravenous immunoglobulins; however, no human data are currently available to support their use [88].

Furthermore, the role of nutritional support, specifically the adequacy of vitamins such as B6, folic acid, and vitamin D, has been emphasized as vital for brain resistance against infections.

It has been shown that minimizing fluctuations in urea levels at the start of renal replacement therapy can lower the risk of developing dialysis disequilibrium syndrome and subsequent brain edema.

Additionally, careful monitoring of anticoagulation parameters may help reduce the incidence of intracerebral hemorrhage [89].

5.5 Future Perspectives: Emerging Therapeutic Approaches

Diagnosing and treating SAE are equally challenging tasks. Since no definitive treatment for SAE is currently available, there is still a need for potential future therapies targeting CNS abnormalities such as microcirculatory dysfunction, blood–brain barrier disruption, and impaired neurotransmission. Although several strategies have shown promise in both human and animal models of SAE, clinical trials are essential to validate their safety and efficacy.

5.5.1 Neuroprotection

- *Melatonin*: Siemiński et al. [90] explored the potential neuroprotective role of melatonin in SAE. Beyond its role in circadian rhythm regulation, this neurohormone exhibits strong antioxidant and anti-inflammatory properties, has a beneficial impact on BBB integrity, and helps improve mitochondrial function. The authors highlight experimental and early clinical data suggesting that melatonin may mitigate neuroinflammation and oxidative stress in SAE. These findings position melatonin as a promising candidate for future preventive and therapeutic interventions, though further clinical validation is required.
- *Branched chain amino acids*: Their role was evaluated by Freund, who obtained positive results in septic encephalopathic patients treated with branched chain amino acid-enriched solution. There were normalization of plasma amino acid pattern and regression of encephalopathic signs in septic patients who were given a solution containing 35% of branched-chain amino acids [91].
- *Glutamate release inhibitor riluzole and antioxidant ascorbate*: They have been found to be beneficial in animal models of SAE [92, 93].
- *N-Acetylcysteine (NAC)*: Preclinical studies have shown that NAC can restore normal cortical ATP levels in porcine models of sepsis.
- *Intravenous lidocaine*: A recent retrospective cohort study published in 2025 evaluated the efficacy of intraoperative intravenous lidocaine administration in SAE management [94]. The study found that patients receiving lidocaine had significantly shorter ICU stays and higher rates of favorable prognosis compared to the control group.

5.5.2 Immunomodulation

Recent studies have highlighted the potential of immunomodulatory therapies in the management of SAE. These may include cytokine inhibitors and other agents targeting inflammatory pathways, which could attenuate the neuroinflammatory response associated with sepsis [95].

- *Anti-C5a antibodies*: Complement component C5a is a potent inflammatory mediator implicated in the pathogenesis of SAE. In experimental models, C5a contributes to BBB disruption, neuroinflammation, and pituitary dysfunction. The use of anti-C5a antibody, through complement cascade modulation, reduces BBB damage in a cecal ligation and puncture (CLP) model in rats, and C5a or C5aR blockade apparently improves mortality in experimental studies [12, 96].

  TRPV1 antagonists: Transient receptor potential vanilloid 1 (TRPV1) is a thermosensitive cation channel expressed on neurons and glial cells throughout the brain, activated by various physical and chemical stimuli. Its activity increases in response to proinflammatory signals, making it a target of interest for pain and inflammation treatments. Despite this, using TRPV1 antagonists as a broad anti-inflammatory strategy has shown limited clinical success due to side effects. Moreover, its modulation can yield either pro- or anti-inflammatory outcomes depending on the cytokine environment, which may worsen sepsis outcome, raising concerns about their safety in vulnerable populations [97].

  Recent evidence suggests that TRPV1 may have both anti-inflammatory and neuroprotective effects, having an overall protective role in sepsis outcome, with TRPV1 antagonism showing complex impacts on neuroinflammation and epigenetic regulation [98].

  Notably, TRPV1 blockade may promote a shift of microglia toward an anti-inflammatory phenotype and contribute to neuroprotection by regulating intracellular calcium levels. Additionally, TRPV1 antagonists may influence genes related to synaptic and cognitive functions through the inhibition of histone deacetylase 2 (HDAC2) [99, 100].

  However, no clinical trials have evaluated the efficacy of TRPV1 antagonists in SAE. Some compounds like vitexin, which modulate TRPV1 and oxidative stress, have shown anti-inflammatory effects in preclinical models, but their clinical relevance remains unclear [101].
- *JNK inhibitors*: In sepsis, activation of the JNK pathway leads to persistent release of inflammatory cytokines, increased oxidative stress, and the development of pathophysiological changes associated with septic encephalopathy.

  A 2025 study published in *Metabolic Brain Disease* investigated the effects of SP600125, a selective JNK inhibitor, in a mouse model of sepsis induced by CLP. The treatment significantly reduced cognitive deficits, neuronal injury, neuroinflammation, and oxidative stress, apoptosis, and improved morphological characteristics of brain tissue in a dose-dependent manner. These findings suggest that inhibiting the c-Jun N-terminal kinase (JNK) pathway may provide neuroprotective effects and represent a promising therapeutic strategy for managing SAE [102].

  Similarly, a study published in *Mediators of Inflammation* highlighted the potential of JNK pathway inhibition to modulate systemic inflammation in sepsis [103].

- *α7nAChR agonists*: α7 nicotinic acetylcholine receptor (α7nAChR) agonists play a pivotal role in the cholinergic anti-inflammatory pathway. In vitro studies have shown that α7nAChR agonists can significantly reduce microglial activation and the expression of pro-inflammatory cytokines such as TNF-α, IL-1β, and IL-6 in human immune cells, while also decreasing neuronal apoptosis and toxicity following lipopolysaccharide (LPS) stimulation in animal models [104].

  Furthermore, studies suggest that α7nAChR agonists may suppress immune responses of human monocytes by downregulating the expressions of CD14, TLR4, intercellular adhesion molecule 1, and CD40, indicating a potential role in modulating systemic inflammation [105]. These findings suggest that α7nAChR agonists may offer neuroprotective benefits in SAE, attenuating neuroinflammation and cognitive deficits associated with sepsis [106].

5.6 Conclusions

In conclusion, SAE represents one of the most severe neurological complications in septic patients, with significant implications for both mortality and long-term recovery. Its clinical manifestations, ranging from mild delirium to deep coma, reflect the complexity of its pathophysiology, which involves neuroinflammation, BBB dysfunction, neurodegenerative damage, and alterations in cerebral energy metabolism. Recent research has highlighted key mechanisms such as microglia activation and neutrophil infiltration, which promote neuronal damage and central nervous system inflammation. Although no specific biomarker for SAE diagnosis currently exists, the use of markers such as S100β, NSE, and neurofilament, combined with monitoring techniques like EEG, near infrared spectroscopy (NIRS), and brain imaging, may improve the ability to detect and track the condition early. Therapeutic strategies, still under investigation, include immunomodulatory approaches and optimization of cerebral perfusion. Further exploration of these aspects, alongside a multidisciplinary approach to sepsis management, could significantly improve neurological outcomes for patients with SAE.

References

1. Evans L, Rhodes A, Alhazzani W, Antonelli M, Coopersmith CM, French C, et al. Surviving sepsis campaign: international guidelines for management of sepsis and septic shock 2021. Intensive Care Med. 2021;47(11):1181–247. https://doi.org/10.1007/s00134-021-06506-y. Epub 2021 Oct 2. PMID: 34599691; PMCID: PMC8486643.
2. Robba C, Crippa IA, Taccone FS. Septic encephalopathy. Curr Neurol Neurosci Rep. 2018;18(12):82. https://doi.org/10.1007/s11910-018-0895-6. PMID: 30280261.
3. Ito H, Hosomi S, Koyama Y, Matsumoto H, Imamura Y, Ogura H, et al. Sepsis-associated encephalopathy: a mini-review of inflammation in the brain and body. Front Aging Neurosci [Internet]. 2022 [cited 2025 Feb 18]; 14. Available from: https://www.frontiersin.org/journals/aging-neuroscience/articles/10.3389/fnagi.2022.912866/full

4. Siami S, Annane D, Sharshar T. The encephalopathy in sepsis. Crit Care Clin. 2008;24(1):67–82, viii. https://doi.org/10.1016/j.ccc.2007.10.001. PMID: 18241779
5. Zhan RZ, Fujiwara N, Shimoji K. Regionally different elevation of intracellular free calcium in hippocampus of septic rat brain. Shock. 1996;6(4):293–7. https://doi.org/10.1097/00024382-199610000-00012.
6. Heming N, Mazeraud A, Verdonk F, Bozza FA, Chrétien F, Sharshar T. Neuroanatomy of sepsis-associated encephalopathy. Crit Care. 2017;21(1):65. https://doi.org/10.1186/s13054-017-1643-z. PMID: 28320461; PMCID: PMC5360026.
7. Flierl MA, Rittirsch D, Huber-Lang MS, Stahel PF. Pathophysiology of septic encephalopathy–an unsolved puzzle. Crit Care. 2010;14(3):165. https://doi.org/10.1186/cc9035. Epub 2010 Jun 16. PMID: 20565858; PMCID: PMC2911737.
8. Wuerfel E, Infante-Duarte C, Glumm R, Wuerfel JT. Gadofluorine M-enhanced MRI shows involvement of circumventricular organs in neuroinflammation. J Neuroinflammation. 2010;7:70.
9. Borovikova LV, Ivanova S, Zhang M, Yang H, Botchkina GI, Watkins LR, et al. Vagus nerve stimulation attenuates the systemic inflammatory response to endotoxin. Nature. 2000;405:458–62.
10. Mehdi SF, Qureshi MH, Pervaiz S, Kumari K, Saji E, Shah M, et al. Endocrine and metabolic alterations in response to systemic inflammation and sepsis: a review article. Mol Med. 2025;31(1):16. https://doi.org/10.1186/s10020-025-01074-z. PMID: 39838305; PMCID: PMC11752782.
11. DiSabato DJ, Quan N, Godbout JP. Neuroinflammation: the devil is in the details. J Neurochem. 2016;139(Suppl 2):136–53. https://doi.org/10.1111/jnc.13607. Epub 2016 May 4. PMID: 26990767; PMCID: PMC5025335.
12. Zampieri FG, Park M, Machado FS, Azevedo LC. Sepsis-associated encephalopathy: not just delirium. Clinics (Sao Paulo). 2011;66(10):1825–31. https://doi.org/10.1590/s1807-59322011001000024. PMID: 22012058; PMCID: PMC3180153.
13. Retamal MA, Froger N, Palacios-Prado N, Ezan P, Sáez PJ, Sáez JC, Giaume C. Cx43 hemichannels and gap junction channels in astrocytes are regulated oppositely by proinflammatory cytokines released from activated microglia. J Neurosci. 2007;27:13781–92. https://doi.org/10.1523/JNEUROSCI.2042-07.2007.
14. Howarth C. The contribution of astrocytes to the regulation of cerebral blood flow. Front Neurosci. 2014;8 https://doi.org/10.3389/fnins.2014.00103.
15. Sonneville R, Verdonk F, Rauturier C, Klein IF, Wolff M, Annane D, et al. Understanding brain dysfunction in sepsis. Ann Intensive Care. 2013;3:15.
16. Schütze S, Drevets DA, Tauber SC, Nau R. Septic encephalopathy in the elderly – biomarkers of potential clinical utility. Front Cell Neurosci [Internet]. 2023 [cited 2025 Feb 18];17. Available from: https://www.frontiersin.org/journals/cellular-neuroscience/articles/10.3389/fncel.2023.1238149/full.
17. Algebaly H, ElSherbini S, Galal A, Hamdi R, Baz A, Elbeleidy A. Transcranial Doppler can predict development and outcome of sepsis-associated encephalopathy in pediatrics with severe sepsis or septic shock. Front Pediatr. 2020;8:450.
18. Bozza FA, D'Avila JC, Ritter C, Sonneville R, Sharshar T, Dal-Pizzol F. Bioenergetics, mitochondrial dysfunction, and oxidative stress in the pathophysiology of septic encephalopathy. Shock. 2013;39(Suppl 1):10–6. https://doi.org/10.1097/SHK.0b013e31828fade1.
19. Azevedo LC. Mitochondrial dysfunction during sepsis. Endocr Metab Immune Disord Drug Targets. 2010;10(3):214–23. https://doi.org/10.2174/187153010791936946.
20. van Gool WA, van de Beek D, Eikelenboom P. Systemic infection and delirium: when cytokines and acetylcholine collide. Lancet. 2010;375(9716):773–5. https://doi.org/10.1016/S0140-6736(09)61158-2.
21. Jacob A, Brorson JR, Alexander JJ. Septic encephalopathy: inflammation in man and mouse. Neurochem Int. 2011;58(4):472–6. https://doi.org/10.1016/j.neuint.2011.01.004.
22. Zhang Q-H, Sheng Z-Y, Yao Y-M. Septic encephalopathy: when cytokines interact with acetylcholine in the brain. Mil Med Res. 2014; https://doi.org/10.1186/2054-9369-1-20.

23. Sharshar T, Annane D, de la Gradmaison GL, Brouland JP, Hopkinson NS, Gray F. The neuropathology of septic shock. Brain Pathol. 2004;14:21–33.
24. Basler T, Meier-Hellmann A, Bredle D, Reinhart K. Amino acid imbalance early in septic encephalopathy. Intensive Care Med. 2002;28(3):293–8. https://doi.org/10.1007/s00134-002-1217-6.
25. Chaudhry N, Duggal AK. Sepsis associated encephalopathy. Adv Med. 2014;2014:762320. https://doi.org/10.1155/2014/762320. Epub 2014 Sep 30. PMID: 26556425; PMCID: PMC4590973.
26. Sharshar T, Gray F, Lorin de la Grandmaison G, et al. Apoptosis of neurons in cardiovascular autonomic centres triggered by inducible nitric oxide synthase after death from septic shock. Lancet. 2003;362:1799–805. https://doi.org/10.1016/S0140-6736(03)14899-4.
27. Viviani B, Boraso M, Marchetti N, Marinovich M. Perspectives on neuroinflammation and excitotoxicity: a neurotoxic conspiracy? Neurotoxicology. 2014;43:10–20. https://doi.org/10.1016/j.neuro.2014.03.004.
28. Voigt K, Kontush A, Stuerenburg HJ, Muench-Harrach D, Hansen HC, Kunze K. Decreased plasma and cerebrospinal fluid ascorbate levels in patients with septic encephalopathy. Free Radic Res. 2002;36:735–9. https://doi.org/10.1080/10715760290032557.
29. Mazeraud A, Righy C, Bouchereau E, Benghanem S, Bozza FA, Sharshar T. Septic-associated encephalopathy: a comprehensive review. Neurotherapeutics. 2020;17(2):392–403. https://doi.org/10.1007/s13311-020-00862-1. PMID: 32378026; PMCID: PMC7283452.
30. Hshieh TT, Fong TG, Marcantonio ER, Inouye SK. Cholinergic deficiency hypothesis in delirium: a synthesis of current evidence. J Gerontol A Biol Sci Med Sci. 2008;63(7):764–72. https://doi.org/10.1093/gerona/63.7.764.
31. Soejima Y, Fujii Y, Ishikawa T, Takeshita H, Maekawa T. Local cerebral glucose utilization in septic rats. Crit Care Med. 1990;18(4):423–7. https://doi.org/10.1097/00003246-199004000-00015.
32. Bleck TP. Dopamine antagonists in ICU delirium. N Engl J Med. 2018;379:2569–70. https://doi.org/10.1056/NEJMe1813382.
33. Pandharipande PP, Girard TD, Jackson JC, et al. Long-term cognitive impairment after critical illness. N Engl J Med. 2013;369:1306–16. https://doi.org/10.1056/NEJMoa1301372.
34. Pandharipande PP, Pun BT, Herr DL, et al. Effect of sedation with dexmedetomidine vs lorazepam on acute brain dysfunction in mechanically ventilated patients: the MENDS randomized controlled trial. JAMA J Am Med Assoc. 2007;298(22):2644–53. https://doi.org/10.1001/jama.298.22.2644.
35. Shehabi Y, Howe BD, Bellomo R, et al. Early sedation with dexmedetomidine in critically ill patients. N Engl J Med. 2019;380 https://doi.org/10.1056/NEJMoa1904710.
36. Marra A, Ely EW, Pandharipande PP, Patel MB. The ABCDEF bundle in critical care. Crit Care Clin. 2017;33(2):225–43. https://doi.org/10.1016/j.ccc.2016.12.005. PMID: 28284292; PMCID: PMC5351776.
37. Adelman MW, Woodworth MH, Langelier C, Busch LM, Kempker JA, Kraft CS, Martin GS. The gut microbiome's role in the development, maintenance, and outcomes of sepsis. Crit Care. 2020;24(1):278. https://doi.org/10.1186/s13054-020-02989-1. PMID: 32487252; PMCID: PMC7266132.
38. Wang X, Wen X, Yuan S, Zhang J. Gut-brain axis in the pathogenesis of sepsis-associated encephalopathy. Neurobiol Dis. 2024;195:106499. https://doi.org/10.1016/j.nbd.2024.106499. Epub 2024 Apr 7. PMID: 38588753.
39. Fang H, Wang Y, Deng J, Zhang H, Wu Q, He L, et al. Sepsis-induced gut dysbiosis mediates the susceptibility to sepsis-associated encephalopathy in mice. mSystems. 2022;7:e0139921. https://doi.org/10.1128/msystems.01399-21.
40. Zhang J, Chen S, Hu X, Huang L, Loh P, Yuan X, Liu Z, Lian J, Geng L, Chen Z, Guo Y, Chen B. The role of the peripheral system dysfunction in the pathogenesis of sepsis-associated encephalopathy. Front Microbiol. 2024;15:1337994. https://doi.org/10.3389/fmicb.2024.1337994. PMID: 38298892; PMCID: PMC10828041.

41. Li J, Yang D, Ge S, et al. Identifying hub genes of sepsis-associated and hepatic encephalopathies based on bioinformatic analysis—focus on the two common encephalopathies of septic cirrhotic patients in ICU. BMC Med Genet. 2024;17:19. https://doi.org/10.1186/s12920-023-01774-7.
42. Gofton TE, Bryan, Young G. Sepsis-associated encephalopathy. Nat Rev Neurol. 2012;8(10):557–66. https://doi.org/10.1038/nrneurol.2012.183.
43. Sonneville R, Benghanem S, Jeantin L, de Montmollin E, Doman M, Gaudemer A, et al. The spectrum of sepsis-associated encephalopathy: a clinical perspective. Crit Care. 2023;27:386.
44. Ely EW, Shintani A, Truman B, Speroff T, Gordon SM, Harrell FE, Inouye SK, Bernard GR, Dittus RS. Delirium as a predictor of mortality in mechanically ventilated patients in the intensive care unit. JAMA. 2004;291:1753–62.
45. Gilmore EJ, Gaspard N, Choi HA, Cohen E, Burkart KM, Chong DH, Claassen J, Hirsch LJ. Acute brain failure in severe sepsis: a prospective study in the medical intensive care unit utilizing continuous EEG monitoring. Intensive Care Med. 2015;41:686–94.
46. De Jonghe B, Cook D, Griffith L, et al. Adaptation to the Intensive Care Environment (ATICE): development and validation of a new sedation assessment instrument. Crit Care Med. 2003;31(9):2344–54. https://doi.org/10.1097/01.CCM.0000084850.16444.94.
47. Riker RR, Fugate JE, Participants in the International Multidisciplinary Consensus Conference on Multimodality Monitoring. Clinical monitoring scales in acute brain injury: assessment of coma, pain, agitation, and delirium. Neurocrit Care. 2014;21(Suppl 2):S27–37.
48. Ebersoldt M, Sharshar T, Annane D. Sepsis-associated delirium. Intensive Care Med. 2007;33(6):941–50. https://doi.org/10.1007/s00134-007-0622-2.
49. Oddo M, Taccone FS. How to monitor the brain in septic patients? Minerva Anestesiol. 2015;81:776–88.
50. Sanz D, D'Arco F, Robles CA, Brierley J. Incidence and pattern of brain lesions in paediatric septic shock patients. Br J Radiol. 2018;91(1084):20170861. https://doi.org/10.1259/bjr.20170861.
51. Sandquist MK, Clee MS, Patel SK, Howard KA, Yunger T, Nagaraj UD, Jones BV, Fei L, Vadivelu S, Wong HR. High frequency of neuroimaging abnormalities among pediatric patients with sepsis who undergo neuroimaging. Pediatr Crit Care Med. 2017;18(7):607–13. https://doi.org/10.1097/PCC.0000000000001173. PMID: 28498230; PMCID: PMC5503765.
52. Luitse MJ, van Asch CJ, Klijn CJ. Deep coma and diffuse white matter abnormalities caused by sepsis-associated encephalopathy. Lancet. 2013;381(9884):2222.
53. Sharshar T, Carlier R, Bernard F, Guidoux C, Brouland JP, Nardi O, de la Grandmaison GL, Aboab J, Gray F, Menon D, Annane D. Brain lesions in septic shock: a magnetic resonance imaging study. Intensive Care Med. 2007;33(5):798–806. https://doi.org/10.1007/s00134-007-0598-y. Epub 2007 Mar 22. PMID: 17377766.
54. Wilson JX, Young GB. Progress in clinical neurosciences: sepsis-associated encephalopathy: evolving concepts. Can J Neurol Sci. 2003;30(2):98–105. https://doi.org/10.1017/S031716710005335X).
55. Polito A, Eischwald F, Maho AL, Polito A, Azabou E, Annane D, Chrétien F, Stevens RD, Carlier R, Sharshar T. Pattern of brain injury in the acute setting of human septic shock. Crit Care. 2013;17(5):R204. https://doi.org/10.1186/cc12899. PMID: 24047502; PMCID: PMC4057119.
56. Racchiusa S, Mormina E, Ax A, Musumeci O, Longo M, Granata F. Posterior reversible encephalopathy syndrome (PRES) and infection: a systematic review of the literature. Neurol Sci. 2019;40:915–22. https://doi.org/10.1007/s10072-018-3651-4.
57. Bartynski WS, Boardman JF, Zeigler ZR, Shadduck RK, Lister J. Posterior reversible encephalopathy syndrome in infection, sepsis, and shock. Am J Neuroradiol. 2006;27(10):2179–90.
58. Finelli PF, Uphoff DF. Magnetic resonance imaging abnormalities with septic encephalopathy. J Neurol Neurosurg Psychiatry. 2004;75(8):1189–91. https://doi.org/10.1136/jnnp.2003.030833.
59. Gunther ML, Morandi A, Krauskopf E, et al. The association between brain volumes, delirium duration, and cognitive outcomes in intensive care unit survivors: the VISIONS

cohort magnetic resonance imaging study. Crit Care Med. 2012;40(7):2022–32. https://doi.org/10.1097/CCM.0b013e318250acc0.
60. Robba C, Cardim D, Sekhon M, Budohoski K, Czosnyka M. Transcranial doppler: a stethoscope for the brain-neurocritical care use. J Neurosci Res. 2018;96(4):720–30.
61. Pierrakos C, Attou R, Decorte L, Kolyviras A, Malinverni S, Gottignies P, Devriendt J, De Bels D. Transcranial Doppler to assess sepsis-associated encephalopathy in critically ill patients. BMC Anesthesiol. 2014;14:45. https://doi.org/10.1186/1471-2253-14-45. PMID: 24944522; PMCID: PMC4061318.
62. Crippa IA, Subira C, Vincent JL, Fernandez RF, Hernandez SC, Cavicchi FZ, et al. Impaired cerebral autoregulation is associated with brain dysfunction in patients with sepsis. Crit Care. 2018;22:327. https://doi.org/10.1186/s13054-018-2258-8.
63. Schramm P, Klein KU, Falkenberg L, et al. Impaired cerebrovascular autoregulation in patients with severe sepsis and sepsis-associated delirium. Crit Care. 2012;16:R181. https://doi.org/10.1186/cc11665.
64. Vasko A, Siro P, Laszlo I, Szatmari S, Molnar L, Fulesdi B, et al. Assessment of cerebral tissue oxygen saturation in septic patients during acetazolamide provocation – a near infrared spectroscopy study. Acta Physiol Hung. 2014;101:32–9.
65. Minati L, Kress IU, Visani E, Medford N, Critchley HD. Intra- and extra-cranial effects of transient blood pressure changes on brain near-infrared spectroscopy (NIRS) measurements. J Neurosci Methods. 2011;197(2):283–8.
66. Cumbers GA, Harvey-Latham ED, Kassiou M, Werry EL, Danon JJ. Emerging TSPO-PET radiotracers for imaging Neuroinflammation: a critical analysis. Semin Nucl Med. 2024;54(6):856–74. ISSN 0001-2998.
67. Lei J, Zhai J, Qi J, Sun C. Identification of sepsis-associated encephalopathy biomarkers through machine learning and bioinformatics approaches. Sci Rep. 2024;14:31717.
68. Ehler J, Saller T, Wittstock M, et al. Diagnostic value of NTproCNP compared to NSE and S100B in cerebrospinal fluid and plasma of patients with sepsis-associated encephalopathy. Neurosci Lett. 2019;692:167–73.
69. Barichello T, Generoso JS, Singer M, Dal-Pizzol F. Biomarkers for sepsis: more than just fever and leukocytosis—a narrative review. Crit Care. 2022;26:14.
70. Nguyen DN, Spapen H, Su F, et al. Elevated serum levels of S-100β protein and neuron-specific enolase are associated with brain injury in patients with severe sepsis and septic shock. Crit Care Med. 2006;34(7):1967–74. https://doi.org/10.1097/01.CCM.0000217218.51381.49.
71. Wang HJ, Zhang PJ, Chen WJ, Feng D, Jia YH, Xie LX. Four serum microRNAs identified as diagnostic biomarkers of sepsis. J Trauma Acute Care Surg. 2012;73(4):850–4. https://doi.org/10.1097/TA.0b013e31825a7560.
72. Young GB, Bolton CF, Archibald YM, Austin TW, Wells GA. The electroencephalogram in sepsis-associated encephalopathy. J Clin Neurophysiol. 1992;9:145–52.
73. Hosokawa K, Gaspard N, Su F, Oddo M, Vincent JL, Taccone FS. Clinical neurophysiological assessment of sepsis-associated brain dysfunction: a systematic review. Crit Care. 2014;18:674.
74. Azabou E, Magalhaes E, Braconnier A, et al. Early standard electroencephalogram abnormalities predict mortality in septic intensive care unit patients. PLoS One. 2015;10:e0139969. https://doi.org/10.1371/journal.pone.0139969.
75. Foreman B, Mahulikar A, Tadi P, et al. Generalized periodic discharges and "triphasic waves": a blinded evaluation of inter-rater agreement and clinical significance. Clin Neurophysiol. 2016;127:1073–80. https://doi.org/10.1016/j.clinph.2015.07.018.
76. Andresen JM, Girard TD, Pandharipande PP, Davidson MA, Ely EW, Watson PL. Burst suppression on processed electroencephalography as a predictor of postcoma delirium in mechanically ventilated ICU patients. Crit Care Med. 2014;42(10):2244–51. https://doi.org/10.1097/CCM.0000000000000522. PMID: 25072756; PMCID: PMC4493889.
77. Oddo M, Carrera E, Claassen J, Mayer SA, Hirsch LJ. Continuous electroencephalography in the medical intensive care unit. Crit Care Med. 2009;37:2051–6. https://doi.org/10.1097/CCM.0b013e3181a00604.

78. Zauner C, Gendo A, Kramer L, Funk GC, Bauer E, Schenk P, Ratheiser K, Madl C. Impaired subcortical and cortical sensory evoked potential pathways in septic patients. Crit Care Med. 2002;30:1136–9.
79. Azabou E, Rohaut B, Heming N, et al. Early impairment of intracranial conduction time predicts mortality in deeply sedated critically ill patients: a prospective observational pilot study. Ann Intensive Care. 2017;7:63.
80. Gaieski DF, Mikkelsen ME, Band RA, et al. Impact of time to antibiotics on survival in patients with severe sepsis or septic shock in whom early goal-directed therapy was initiated in the emergency department. Crit Care Med. 2010;38(4):1045–53. https://doi.org/10.1097/CCM.0b013e3181cc4824.
81. Inouye SK, Bogardus ST Jr, Charpentier PA, et al. A multicomponent intervention to prevent delirium in hospitalized older patients. N Engl J Med. 1999;340(9):669–76. https://doi.org/10.1056/NEJM199903043400901.
82. Mehta S, Burry L, Cook D, et al. Daily sedation interruption in mechanically ventilated critically ill patients cared for with a sedation protocol: a randomized controlled trial. JAMA. 2012;308:1985–92. https://doi.org/10.1001/jama.2012.13872.
83. Zhang X, Yan F, Feng J, Qian H, Cheng Z, Yang Q, et al. Dexmedetomidine inhibits inflammatory reaction in the hippocampus of septic rats by suppressing NF-κB pathway. PLoS One. 2018;13(5):e0196897.
84. Needham DM, Colantuoni E, Dinglas VD, Hough CL, Wozniak AW, Jackson JC, Morris PE, Mendez-Tellez PA, Ely EW, Hopkins RO. Rosuvastatin versus placebo for delirium in intensive care and subsequent cognitive impairment in patients with sepsis-associated acute respiratory distress syndrome: an ancillary study to a randomised controlled trial. Lancet Respir Med. 2016;4:203–12. https://doi.org/10.1016/S2213-2600(16)00005-9.
85. Reis PA, Alexandre PCB, D'Avila JC, Siqueira LD, Antunes B, Estato V, et al. Statins prevent cognitive impairment after sepsis by reverting neuroinflammation, and microcirculatory/endothelial dysfunction. Brain Behav Immun. 2017;60:293–303.
86. NICE-SUGAR Study Investigators, Finfer S, Chittock DR, et al. Intensive versus conventional glucose control in critically ill patients. N Engl J Med. 2009;360:1283–97. https://doi.org/10.1056/NEJMoa0810625.
87. Spapen H, Nguyen DN, Troubleyn J, Huyghens L, Schiettecatte J. Drotrecogin alfa (activated) may attenuate severe sepsis-associated encephalopathy in clinical septic shock. Crit Care. 2010;14:R54.
88. Esen F, Senturk E, Ozcan PE, Ahishali B, Arican N, Orhan N, Ekizoglu O, Kucuk M, Kaya M. Intravenous immunoglobulins prevent the breakdown of the blood-brain barrier in experimentally induced sepsis. Crit Care Med. 2012;40(4):1214–20. https://doi.org/10.1097/CCM.0b013e31823779ca.
89. Pandharipande P, Cotton BA, Shintani A, Thompson J, Pun BT, Morris JA Jr, et al. Prevalence and risk factors for development of delirium in surgical and trauma intensive care unit patients. J Trauma. 2008;65:34–41.
90. Sieminski M, Szaruta-Raflesz K, Szypenbejl J, Krzyzaniak K. Potential neuroprotective role of melatonin in sepsis-associated encephalopathy due to its scavenging and anti-oxidative properties. Antioxidants (Basel). 2023;12(9):1786. https://doi.org/10.3390/antiox12091786. PMID: 37760089; PMCID: PMC10525116.
91. Freund HR, Ryan JA Jr, Fischer JE. Amino acid derangements in patients with sepsis: treatment with branched chain amino acid rich infusions. Ann Surg. 1978;188(3):423–30. https://doi.org/10.1097/00000658-197809000-00017.
92. Toklu HZ, Uysal MK, Kabasakal L, Sirvanci S, Ercan F, Kaya M. The effects of riluzole on neurological, brain biochemical, and histological changes in early and late term of sepsis in rats. J Surg Res. 2009;152(2):238–48. https://doi.org/10.1016/j.jss.2008.03.013.
93. Wilson JX. Mechanism of action of vitamin C in sepsis: ascorbate modulates redox signaling in endothelium. Biofactors. 2009;35(1):5–13. https://doi.org/10.1002/biof.7.

94. Zhang Y-X, Ma L, Yiliaikebaier M, Zhang W, Li R-X, Wang Y, et al. Intravenous lidocaine for the treatment of sepsis-associated encephalopathy: a retrospective cohort study. Neurol Res. 2025;47:115–21.
95. Bode C, Weis S, Sauer A, Wendel-Garcia P, David S. Targeting the host response in sepsis: current approaches and future evidence. Crit Care. 2023;27:478.
96. Guo RF, Riedemann NC, Ward PA. Role of C5a-C5ar interaction in sepsis. Shock. 2004;21:1–7. https://doi.org/10.1097/01.shk.0000105502.75189.5e.
97. Quezado ZM, Szallasi A. TRPV1 antagonists may exacerbate sepsis in aged mice: should we be nervous? Cell Cycle. 2012;11(4):647–8. https://doi.org/10.4161/cc.11.4.19280. Epub 2012 Feb 15. PMID: 22313731.
98. Bodkin JV, Fernandes ES. TRPV1 and SP: key elements for sepsis outcome? Br J Pharmacol. 2013;170(7):1279–92. https://doi.org/10.1111/bph.12056. PMID: 23145480; PMCID: PMC3838676.
99. Devesa I, Planells-Cases R, Fernández-Ballester G, González-Ros JM, Ferrer-Montiel A, Fernández-Carvajal A. Role of the transient receptor potential vanilloid 1 in inflammation and sepsis. J Inflamm Res. 2011;4:67–81. https://doi.org/10.2147/JIR.S12978. Epub 2011 May 24. PMID: 22096371; PMCID: PMC3218746.
100. Escelsior A, Sterlini B, Belvederi Murri M, Valente P, Amerio A, di Brozolo MR, da Silva BP, Amore M. Transient receptor potential vanilloid 1 antagonism in neuroinflammation, neuroprotection and epigenetic regulation: potential therapeutic implications for severe psychiatric disorders treatment. PsychiatrGenet. 2020;30(2):39–48. https://doi.org/10.1097/YPG.0000000000000249.
101. Cao H, Wang X, Zhang B, Ren M. The protective effect of vitexinin septic encephalopathy by reducing leukocyte-endothelial adhesion and inflammatory response. Ann Palliat Med. 2020;9(4):2079–89. https://doi.org/10.21037/apm-20-1211. Epub 2020 Jul 14. PMID: 32692224.
102. Gagnani R, Singh H, Suri M, et al. JNK inhibition mitigates sepsis-associated encephalopathy via attenuation of neuroinflammation, oxidative stress and apoptosis. Metab Brain Dis. 2025;40:148. https://doi.org/10.1007/s11011-025-01563-4.
103. Pizzino G, Bitto A, Pallio G, Irrera N, Galfo F, Interdonato M, Mecchio A, De Luca F, Minutoli L, Squadrito F, Altavilla D. Blockade of the JNK signalling as a rational therapeutic approach to modulate the early and late steps of the inflammatory cascade in polymicrobial sepsis. Mediators Inflamm. 2015;2015:591572. https://doi.org/10.1155/2015/591572. Epub 2015 Mar 22. PMID: 25873765; PMCID: PMC4385695.
104. Gao F, Weihong D, Guo C, Geng P, Liu W, Jin X. α7nACh receptor, a promising target to reduce BBB damage by regulating inflammation and autophagy after ischemic stroke. Biomed Pharmacother. 2024;179
105. Ren C, Yao RQ, Zhang H, Feng YW, Yao YM. Sepsis-associated encephalopathy: a vicious cycle of immunosuppression. J Neuroinflammation. 2020;17(1):14. https://doi.org/10.1186/s12974-020-1701-3. PMID: 31924221; PMCID: PMC6953314.
106. Kim TH, Kim SJ, Lee SM. Stimulation of the α7 nicotinic acetylcholine receptor protects against sepsis by inhibiting Toll-like receptor via phosphoinositide 3-kinase activation. J Infect Dis. 2014;209(10):1668–77. https://doi.org/10.1093/infdis/jit669. Epub 2013 Dec 1. Erratum in: J Infect Dis. 2015 Mar 1;211(5):851. 10.1093/infdis/jiu824. PMID: 24298024.

Stroke Inflammatory Blood-Brain Barrier Dysfunction

6

Syed Ameen Ahmad, Olivia Liu, Isabella Blackman, Paul Nyquist, Aaron Shoskes, and Sung-Min Cho

Abbreviations

AIS	Acute ischemic stroke
AMD3100	Plerixafor
ATP	Adenosine triphosphate
BBB	Blood-brain barrier
BDNF	Brain-derived neurotrophic factor
C1C2	Claudin-1 peptide
Ca^{2+}	Calcium
CCL2	C-C motif chemokine ligand 2
CCR5	C-C chemokine receptor type 5
cGAS-STING	Cyclic GMP-AMP synthase-stimulator of IFN genes
CIRP	Cold-inducible RNA-binding protein
CNS	Central nervous system
COX	Cyclooxygenase
CSF	Cerebrospinal fluid
CT	Computerized tomography
CXCR	C-X-C motif chemokine receptor
CXCL	C-X-C motif chemokine ligand
DAMPs	Danger-associated molecular patterns
eNOS	Endothelial NOS

S. A. Ahmad · O. Liu · I. Blackman · P. Nyquist · S.-M. Cho (✉)
Department of Neurosciences Critical Care, Departments of Neurology, Neurosurgery, Anesthesiology and Critical Care Medicine, Johns Hopkins University School of Medicine, Baltimore, MD, USA
e-mail: csungmi1@jhmi.edu

A. Shoskes
Department of Neurology, University of Utah, Salt Lake City, UT, USA

D. Battaglini et al. (eds.), *Organ System Crosstalk in Critical Illness*, https://doi.org/10.1007/978-3-032-01024-7_6

FLAIR	Fluid-attenuated inversion recovery
HIF-1 α	Hypoxia-inducible factor 1-alpha
HMGBP1	High mobility group box protein 1
HSP	Heat shock proteins
HT	Hemorrhagic transformation
ICH	Intracerebral hemorrhage
ICP	Intracranial pressure
IFN-β	Interferon-beta
IFN-γ	Interferon-gamma
IL	Interleukin
iNOS	Inducible nitric oxide synthase
ICAM- 1	Intracellular adhesion molecule-1
IVT	Intravenous thrombolysis
LRP	Low-density lipoprotein-related receptor-related protein
M1	Microglia 1
M2	Microglia 2
MAPK	Mitogen-activated protein kinase
MCAO	Middle cerebral artery occlusion
MCP-1	Monocyte chemoattractant protein-1
MMPs	Matrix metalloproteinases
mRS	Modified Rankin Score
MRI	Magnetic resonance imaging
mRNA	Messenger ribonucleic acid
Myd88	Myeloid differentiation primary response 88
NADPH	Nicotinamide adenine dinucleotide phosphate
NGF	Nerve growth factor
NO	Nitric oxide
NOS	Nitric oxide synthase
nNOS	Neuronal NOS
NOX	NADPH oxidase
NETs	Neutrophil extracellular traps
NF-kB	Nuclear factor kappa-light-chain enhancer of activated B cells
NLRP3	NLR family pyrin domain containing 3
Nrf2	Nuclear factor-erythroid-related factor-2
NVU	Neurovascular unit
OHS	Oxford handicap score
PDGF	Platelet-derived growth factor
PD-L1	Programmed cell death ligand 1
pro-CPU	Procarboxypeptidase U (pro-CPU)
RNS	Reactive nitrogen species
ROS	Reactive oxygen species
SAH	Subarachnoid hemorrhage
S100B	Calcium-binding protein B
T2DM	Type II diabetes mellitus
TGF-β	Transforming growth factor-beta

TIA	Transient ischemic attack
TLR	Toll-like receptor
TNF-α	Tumor necrosis factor-alpha
tPA	Tissue plasminogen activator
Tregs	Regulatory T cells
VCAM-1	Vascular adhesion protein-1
ZO	Zonula occludens

6.1 Introduction: Blood-Brain Barrier Overview

Stroke is the third most common contributor to mortality worldwide and represents the most significant contributor to long-term disability in adults [1]. Despite advances in treatment, the risk of death after stroke remains high, with a cumulative all-cause mortality of 10.5% at 30 days and 39.8% at 5 years [2]. Among those who survive, one-third will still not have regained functional independence by 1 year after the event and many will require long-term care [3].

One structure critical to a complete understanding of the pathophysiology of stroke is the blood-brain barrier (BBB). The BBB is located in the central nervous system (CNS) vasculature and forms the interface between the brain and the systemic vasculature. The BBB is linked to the neurovascular unit (NVU), which is composed of the tightly linked endothelial cells and smooth muscle cells comprising intracerebral blood vessels, perivascular astrocytes, and microglia as well as their associated neurons [4]. The BBB plays an important role in microvascular permeability, ion balance, nutrient transport, and cerebral hemodynamics [5, 6]. By restricting the passage of most non-lipophilic molecules and regulating the passage of glucose, amino acids, and other important nutrients, the BBB promotes CNS homeostasis and preserves healthy neuronal function [5–10].

Acute ischemic stroke (AIS) can lead to BBB disruption resulting in increased inflammation, cerebral edema, and neuronal degeneration [11, 12]. Evidence demonstrates that widespread BBB dysfunction occurs after ischemic infarct, and increased BBB permeability is associated with poor functional outcomes [13–15]. Disruption of the BBB may be a potential contributor to parenchymal injury and may be an important clinical target. However, despite the physiologic importance of the BBB, there is a paucity of data regarding the frequency and clinical influence of BBB dysfunction in AIS. Understanding the changes in the BBB after AIS may improve the early identification of high-risk patients, selection of appropriate treatments, development of new therapies, and potential improvement in patient outcomes.

Herein, we describe the pathophysiology of inflammatory BBB dysfunction following AIS, the imaging modalities for assessing that dysfunction, the risk factors, and long-term outcomes, as well as ongoing investigations into BBB-specific therapeutics.

6.2 Pathophysiology

BBB endothelial cells have distinct characteristics. Most importantly, they lack membrane fenestrations and have high levels of tight junction connections—such as claudins and zonula occludens (ZO)—resulting in the impermeability of the BBB [16]. In AIS, these tight junctions are altered, leading to increases in solute permeability and inflammatory cell infiltration [17]. There are unique changes that occur throughout the different stages of AIS (Fig. 6.1).

6.2.1 Ischemic Stroke: Hyperacute Stage

Several mechanisms underlie BBB disruption during AIS. Insufficient blood flow leads to the deprivation of oxygen and glucose to the brain, resulting in neuronal cell death from metabolic stress. This step reflects the beginning of the pathophysiology involved in BBB dysregulation and repair (Fig. 6.2). In the hyperacute stage (within 12–24 h of initial insult), cell death results in the release of danger-associated molecular patterns (DAMPs) from dead and dying cells. These DAMPs include high mobility group box protein 1 (HMGBP1), adenosine triphosphate (ATP), heat shock proteins (HSP), cold shock domain proteins, purines, peroxiredoxins, calcium-binding protein B (S100B), and mitochondrial DAMPs [18]. Immediately after AIS, high levels of DAMPs from necrotic tissue trigger the inflammatory process by activating receptors such as toll-like receptors (TLR)2 and TLR4 on immune cells—thus activating microglia and stimulating the release of pro-inflammatory cytokines like tumor necrosis factor-alpha (TNF-α), interferon-gamma (IFN-γ), interleukin (IL)-1 β, and IL-6 [19, 20]. Additionally, released blood products from erythrocyte degradation—such as methemoglobin, heme, hemin, and oxyhemoglobin—also act as DAMPs on TLRs [21]. Blood product DAMPs correlate with high TNF-α and IL-1 β levels, formation of neutrophil extracellular traps (NETs), and chemotaxis of neutrophils via secretion of IL-8 [22–27].

The activation of microglia and recruitment of neutrophils induce the accretion of matrix metalloproteinases (MMPs). MMPs are proteolytic enzymes that degrade all components of the extracellular matrix (ECM) and the tight junctions of the BBB [28]. MMP-2 levels are increased during the early BBB opening, while MMP-9 levels are increased during the later BBB opening (24–48 h after AIS) [29]. In addition to microglia and neutrophils, MMPs can also be activated from the generation

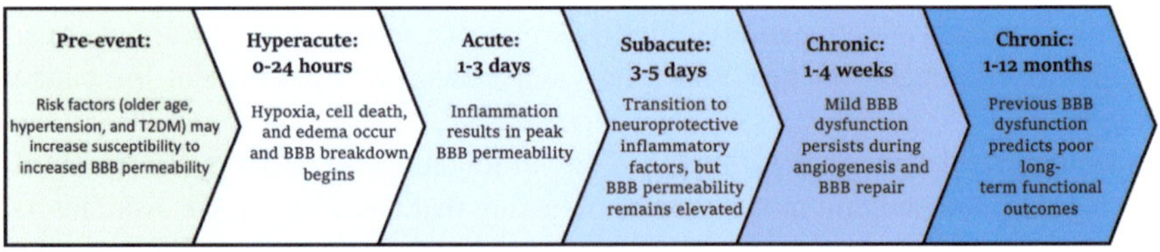

Fig. 6.1 Timeline of acute ischemic stroke (AIS) broken down into different phases

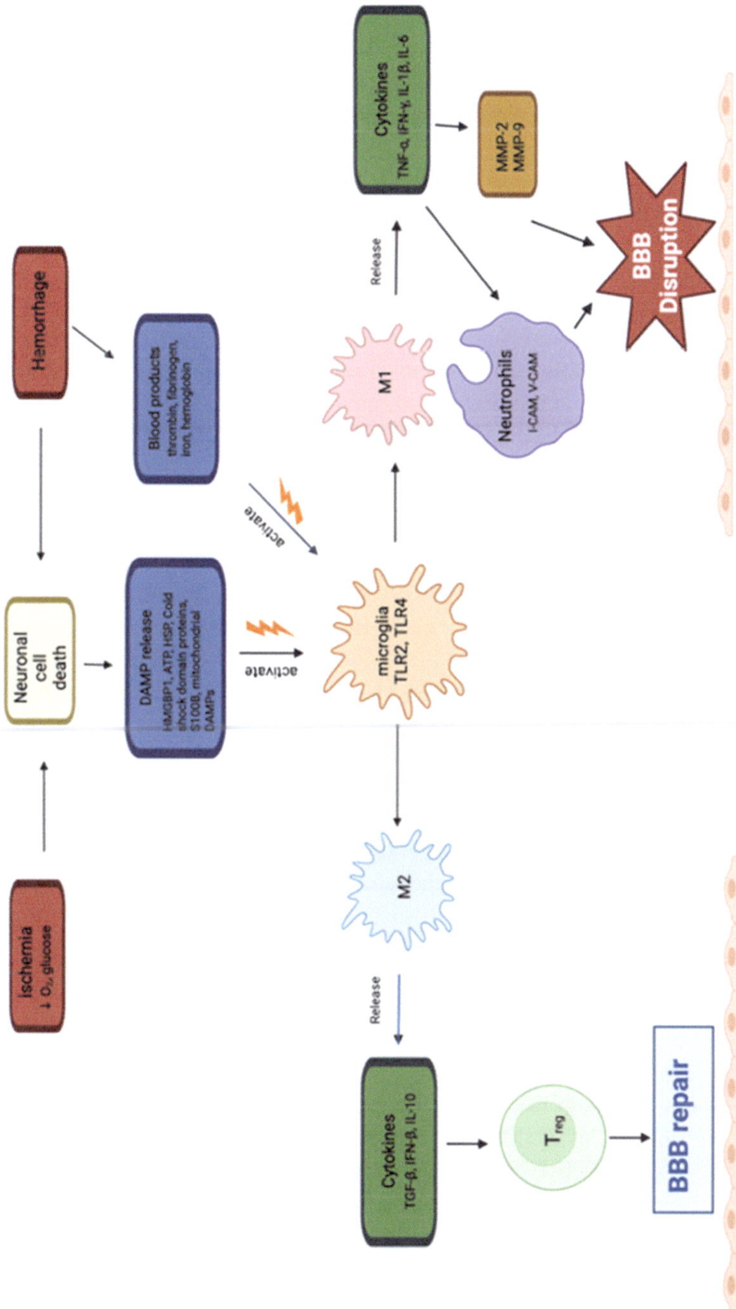

Fig. 6.2 Visual representation of pathophysiology involved in inflammatory blood-brain barrier (BBB) dysfunction following acute ischemic stroke. Neuronal cell death leads to the release of danger-associated molecular patterns (DAMPs), which activate and polarize microglia into either the microglia 1 (M1) pro-inflammatory state or the microglia 2 (M2) anti-inflammatory state. M1 activation leads to the accretion of matrix metalloproteinases (MMPs), and ultimately BBB disruption

of reactive oxygen species (ROS) due to ischemic mitochondrial dysfunction. In particular, the nicotinamide adenine dinucleotide phosphate (NADPH) oxidase (NOX) family is a major source of ROS that induces MMP-9 expression, loss of tight junctions, and disruption of the BBB in AIS [30].

In all, MMPs play a vital role in the initial pathogenesis of BBB disruption following AIS through a variety of different mechanisms.

6.2.2 Ischemic Stroke: Acute Phase

In the acute phase of stroke (24–72 h after onset), the DAMP-induced activation of microglia and neutrophils rapidly increases and peaks. Upregulation of adhesion molecules such as intracellular adhesion molecule-1 (ICAM-1) and vascular adhesion molecule-1 (VCAM) allows for leukocyte infiltration [31]. Once these leukocytes cross the BBB, they exacerbate inflammation and increase infarct size [30, 32]. In particular, microglia have different phenotypes once activated that take on different functions and secrete different factors. The classically activated microglia 1 (M1) phenotype contributes to the release of pro-inflammatory, deleterious cytokines such as TNF- α, IL-1 β, and IL-6 and furthers damage to tissue [33].

Elevated TNF-α levels lead to the migration of pericytes and release of MMP-9 via a mitogen-activated protein kinase (MAPK)-mediated pathway, thus leading to pericyte loss and increased permeability of the BBB [34]. Similarly, IL-1 β induces ICAM-1 expression, secretion of MMP-9, and infiltration of T cells, macrophages, and neutrophils through the damaged BBB [35, 36]. Finally, IL-6 plays a vital role, as it is an adverse prognostic marker after AIS and is positively correlated with levels of MMP-2 and MMP-9 [37]. In all, these pro-inflammatory cytokines work to exacerbate the initial BBB damage from the hyperacute stage via similar mechanisms, such as the increased release of MMP-9. Of note, in the acute stage of stroke, endothelial damage and dysfunction of tight junctions lead to increased permeability of vessels, reperfusion injury, and higher chance of hemorrhagic transformation (HT) [38].

6.2.3 Ischemic Stroke: Subacute Phase

In the subacute stage of stroke (3–5 days after onset), microglia continue to be activated at high rates, but there is a shift in phenotype from inflammatory M1 to the neuroprotective microglia 2 (M2) phenotype. These M2 cells release anti-inflammatory cytokines such as IL-10, IFN- β, and transforming growth factor-beta (TGF- β), which assist in the repair of BBB damage [39, 40]. M2 cells also produce trophic factors such as brain-derived neurotrophic factor (BDNF) and nerve growth factor (NGF) to help BBB remodeling after AIS [41].

These anti-inflammatory cytokines work toward the goal of restoring BBB integrity. For instance, IL-10 suppresses the recruitment of inflammatory cells and reduces infarct size [42–44]. IFN-β also reduces neutrophil infiltration and stabilizes the BBB by downregulating MMP-9, decreasing paracellular permeability, and increasing tight-junction stability [45–48]. Finally, TGF-β reduces neutrophil infiltration and contributes to neurogenesis after stroke, thus enhancing recovery [49]. Overall, microglia play both damaging and protective roles on the BBB following AIS. Modulation of this balance between phenotypes is essential in promoting BBB repair.

Apart from microglia, regulatory T cells (Tregs) are also an important class of lymphocytes in mediating the deleterious effects of stroke in the recovery phase. Tregs are increased in the subacute phase, performing a protective role through the induction of IL-10 and suppression of effector T cell secretion of TNF-α and IFN-γ [50–52]. They also interact with C-C Chemokine receptor type 5 (CCR5) to inhibit MMP-9 [53].

6.2.4 Ischemic Stroke: Chronic Phase

During the chronic phase of stroke (6 weeks onwards), the BBB undergoes repair processes to restore its function. Tight junction proteins are upregulated and reorganized, thus increasing BBB integrity. Vascular endothelial growth factor (VEGF)-mediated angiogenesis, beginning in the days after the initial injury, is one of the first steps in improving blood flow to the ischemic area [54]. Vascular remodeling initially results in increased and possibly deleterious vascular permeability of newly formed vessels, followed by maturation with improved BBB integrity [55]. This angiogenesis is also accompanied by increased endothelial progenitor cell circulation and upregulation of tight junction proteins [8, 56]. However, the integrity of the BBB may not be fully restored [57]. Disorganization of newly expressed tight junction proteins impedes the full repair, thus leading to a risk of HT in the recovery phase of ischemic stroke [58].

6.2.5 Hemorrhagic Stroke

Hemorrhagic stroke is less common than AIS, with intracerebral hemorrhage (ICH) and subarachnoid hemorrhage (SAH) contributing approximately to 10% and 3% of strokes, respectively [59]. ICH disrupts the BBB through mechanisms similar to AIS. In ICH, blood products—such as thrombin, fibrinogen, iron, and hemoglobin—are released and act as DAMPs to elicit inflammatory cytokines that contribute directly to BBB disruption [60–63]. Apart from this, increased intracranial pressure (ICP) and mass effect lead to secondary ischemia, neuronal death, and the release of DAMPs that are also seen in AIS—including HMGB1, S100B, HSP, and mitochondrial DAMPs [64, 65]. Thus, the DAMPs released from ICH and AIS converge on similar mechanisms—leading to the activation of microglia, production of cytokines, extravasation of leukocytes, activation of MMP-9, and eventual degradation of the BBB. The BBB dysfunction in SAH is beyond the scope of this review.

6.3 Neuroimaging and Diagnostic Overview of BBB Breakdown

Multiple imaging modalities have been proposed to approximate BBB permeability and dysfunction after AIS. Changes in permeability can be evaluated via intravenous contrast agents (such as gadolinium chelates and iodinated contrast media) and their associated efflux rate from plasma into tissue [66]. Utilizing a combination of T1/T2-weighted magnetic resonance imaging (MRI) signal intensities and dynamic computerized tomography (CT) can yield clinically relevant pharmacokinetic data and permeability measures that can help to ascertain the degree of BBB dysfunction and predict complications (Figs. 6.3 and 6.4) [67–69]. This is clinically significant, as the degree of BBB breakdown following AIS is associated with initial stroke severity and infarct evolution/growth [70]. In a prospective study of 57 patients diagnosed with transient ischemic attacks (TIAs) or minor strokes, dynamic-contrast enhanced MRI demonstrated that the quantity of brain volume with BBB dysfunction (as assessed by degree of permeability) was significantly higher compared to healthy controls. Interestingly, BBB dysfunction localization in MRI corresponded to the clinical presentation in 72% of patients, and patients who developed recurrent ischemic strokes within the four-year study period had significantly higher quantities of brain volume with BBB dysfunction at their initial presentation [71].

These imaging studies approximating BBB breakdown are also clinically significant because they can help to predict complications, such as HT. For instance, in a retrospective analysis of 32 patients with AIS, admission BBB permeability (as assessed by delayed-acquisition perfusion CT data) above the threshold was 100% sensitive and 79% specific to predict symptomatic HT and malignant cerebral edema [72]. Likewise, in a retrospective analysis of 26 patients with AIS, dynamic

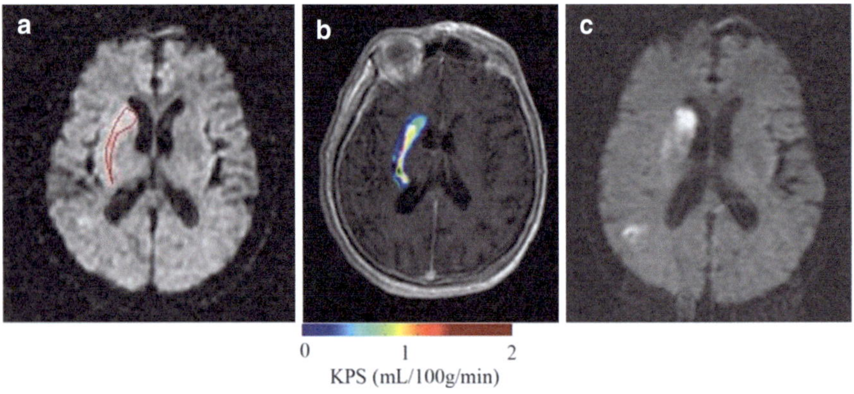

Fig. 6.3 Figure taken with permission from Kassner and Merali [68] and the *Stroke* journal. Magnetic resonance imaging (MRI) in a patient with acute ischemic stroke (AIS) can ascertain permeability metrics to predict complications. (**a**) Baseline subcortical infarct. (**b**) Increased blood-brain barrier (BBB) permeability (utilizing KPS) in the infarcted area. (**c**) Imaging taken ~30 h after baseline which demonstrates hemorrhagic transformation

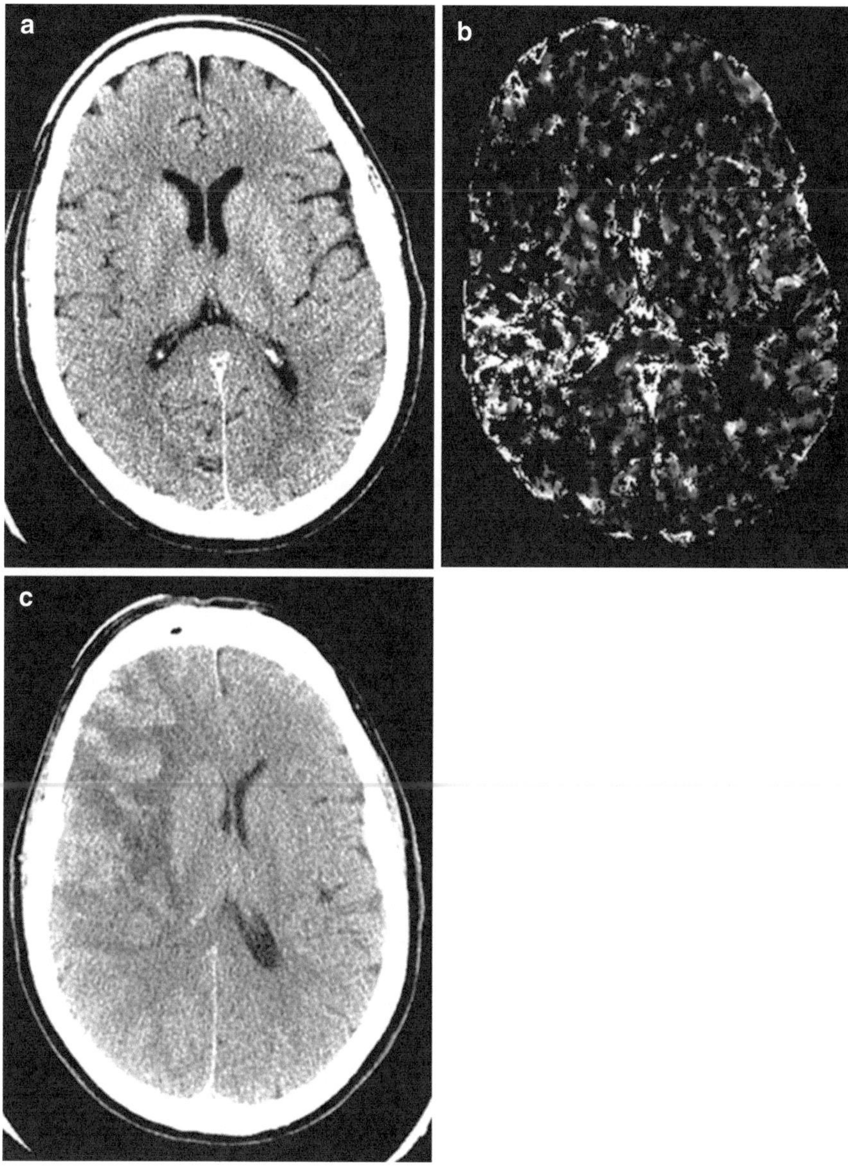

Fig. 6.4 Figure taken with permission from Kassner and Merali [68] and the *Stroke* journal. Computed tomography (CT) in a patient with acute ischemic stroke (AIS) who received thrombolytic therapy. (**a**) Baseline infarct. (**b**) Increased blood-brain barrier (BBB) permeability (utilizing increased intensity on permeability CT image) in the infarcted area. (**c**) Imaging taken after baseline and administration of thrombolytic therapy demonstrates parenchymal hematoma. (CT images courtesy of Dr. Richard Aviv, Sunnybrook Health Sciences Centre)

susceptibility contrast MRI metric for permeability (relative recirculation, (*r*R) and dynamic contrast-enhanced MRI estimates of BBB permeability (KPS) yielded a sensitivity of 91% and 91% and a specificity of 87% and 80%, respectively, to predict HT [73].

This clinical significance of imaging also holds true for treated AIS patients, where the development of subsequent complications is not rare—such as in the case of patients treated with intravenous thrombolysis (IVT) and mechanical thrombectomy (MT). For example, in a prospective study of 171 patients, CT perfusion could reliably associate pre-treatment BBB permeability and post-treatment HT with administration of IVT or endovascular thrombectomy [74].

Focusing on IVT, measuring BBB permeability via MRI perfusion imaging before and after IVT has been shown to be highly predictive of neurological complications following IVT, such as HT or malignant cerebral edema [72, 75, 76]. In one prospective study of 33 IVT-treated AIS patients, investigators found that post-contrast T1 parenchymal enhancement after IVT is associated with HT of AIS. Further, one of four patients who had enhancement of cerebrospinal fluid (CSF) on fluid-attenuated inversion recovery (FLAIR) developed HT—suggesting that CSF signal may be clinically useful in predicting HT [77]. Post-contrast enhancement in FLAIR sequence was strongly associated with BBB alterations 3 h from the onset of ischemia, mainly reflecting vasogenic edema [13]. In addition to IVT, multiple thrombectomy passes/attempts (a known predictor of worse outcomes in patients undergoing MT) were associated with increased odds of detecting BBB permeability on subsequent MRI [78]. In one study, investigators found 56/210 (26.7%) AIS patients developed BBB disruption after MT [79]. Notably, blood restoration of the infarcted area was found to be associated with decreased BBB permeability and a lesser chance of HT [75]. Taken together, in addition to the severity of the initial stroke itself, the BBB permeability following AIS may be a surrogate marker for predicting poor neurological outcomes. Thus, neuroimaging data early after AIS may help to identify patients at high risk of HT and malignant edema.

6.4 Risk Factors and Outcomes of BBB Breakdown in AIS

6.4.1 Risk Factors

Many comorbid conditions can contribute to the risk of AIS and poor functional outcome after AIS such as hyperglycemia and Type II diabetes mellitus (T2DM), hypertension, atrial fibrillation, older age, and hyperlipidemia [59]. In animal studies, diabetic mice showed an increased BBB breakdown after AIS and more severe neurological deficits than normo-glycemic controls [80]. In addition, hypertensive rats have differential expression of tight junction proteins after AIS [81]. Although the effect of these risk factors after stroke has not been extensively studied in humans, they are associated with increased baseline BBB dysfunction. For instance, T2DM is associated with increased BBB permeability on T1-weighted MRI likely through tight junction degradation [82]. Hypertension has also been correlated with

BBB permeability and tight junction dysfunction [83, 84]. Even healthy aging has a number of effects on BBB integrity, including age-dependent breakdown in the hippocampus of Alzheimer's disease patients and increased blood/CSF albumin ratio (a biomarker for BBB leakage) in gray and white matter [85, 86].

6.4.2 Outcomes

Assessing BBB dysfunction with neuroimaging studies can help to better characterize the outcomes such as stroke recovery, functional outcomes, recurrent stroke risk, and cognitive outcomes.

In a study of 84 AIS patients treated with IVT, higher BBB permeability as measured by MRI at 1 and 5 days was significantly associated with worse functional outcomes as measured by modified Rankin Score (mRS) at 30 and 90 days—independent of age, stroke volume, or stroke severity. Interestingly, they also found that for each percentage increase in BBB permeability at 5 days, there was a 76% decrease in the chance of achieving a good functional outcome following AIS [14]. Similarly, in a sample of 110 patients following AIS, BBB disruption was associated with poor outcomes (mRS >2) obtained at 30 or 90 days follow-ups [87].

Evaluating for BBB permeability immediately following an AIS has the potential not only to prognosticate long-term functional outcomes, but also to help identify the chance of stroke recovery and recurrent stroke risk. In a study of 70 patients with AIS, poor functional outcome, defined as Oxford Handicap Score (OHS) 3–6, was associated with increased basal ganglia BBB permeability and higher white matter hyperintensity scores at a median clinical follow-up time of 39 months. Evaluating white matter hyperintensity is clinically relevant since it has been found that BBB leakage and interstitial fluid were higher in white matter hyperintensity versus normal appearing white matter in patients with non-disabling lacunar and cortical strokes. Of these 70 patients, 25 of them had clinical and imaging evidence of recurrent neurological events—including 2 cases of clinically diagnosed recurrent AIS, 23 cases of new focal weakness, and 4 new clinically silent infarcts seen on follow-up MRIs [15].

Furthermore, in a study of 201 patients, BBB leakage into white matter hyperintensity predicted a lower cognition at 1 year [88]. The BBB disruption has also been implicated in the pathogenesis of major depressive disorder. Since post-stroke depression is common and affects approximately one-third of stroke survivors, assessing for BBB dysfunction may also play a vital role in combating the development of psychiatric conditions like depression [89, 90].

6.5 Potential Targeted Therapeutics

Therapeutics that attenuate disruption of the BBB following AIS have many different targets including inflammatory cells, junctional proteins, as well as other novel avenues.

For inflammatory cells, animal studies have demonstrated that disrupting neutrophil rolling and adhesion with anti-ICAM-1 and P-selectin antibodies can help improve BBB leakage following AIS [91–93]. P-selectin has been an area of focus as it is a mediator of early phase leukocyte recruitment and contributor to BBB dysfunction following AIS. For example, middle cerebral artery occlusion (MCAO) in P-selectin knockout mice had less BBB dysfunction at 24 h after AIS in comparison to wildtype mice [93]. Thus, targeting early mediators of inflammation could help to decrease the BBB disruption associated with AIS.

In addition to neutrophils, suppression of the nuclear factor kappa-light-chain enhancer of activated B cells (NF-κ B) pathway

(and thus attenuation of microglia and pro-inflammatory cytokines) has also been an area of investigation. The NF-κ B pathway is a major inflammatory signaling pathway that regulates both innate and adaptive immune responses. The drug adjudin was found to suppress the NF- κ B pathway. In a transient MCAO model in mice, investigators found that administration of adjudin decreased microglia signaling on fluorescence microscopy in the brain, reducing transcription of key pro-inflammatory cytokines such as TNF-α, IL1-β, and IL-6. The presence of microglia and these cytokines was found to be linked with BBB disruption, as mice treated with adjudin had significantly reduced IgG leakage on immunofluorescence staining indicating less BBB breakdown [94]. Other drugs that act similarly to adjudin, such as curcumin, which works by downregulating NF- κ B and upregulating nuclear factor-erythroid-related factor-2 (Nrf2), was also found to support the idea that BBB disruption is attenuated by suppressing the NF-κ B pathway [95]. Apart from this pathway, fingolimod, a sphingosine 1-phosphate antagonist typically used in the treatment of multiple sclerosis, enhances the integrity of the BBB in rats [96]. Cyclooxygenase (COX) enzymes downstream of the NF-κ B pathway are other potential therapeutic targets. Post-AIS treatment with the COX-2 inhibitor nimesulide has been found to reduce BBB disruption (as measured by Evans blue extravasation) in rats [97]. Similarly, indomethacin, a non-selective COX inhibitor, was found to reduce BBB damage 24 hours following intracerebral injection of TNF-α by attenuating MMP-9 expression [98]. MMP-9 is of a particular focus as a potential target for therapeutics due to the key role it plays in BBB disruption following AIS. Several studies demonstrated that the use of MMP-9 neutralizing antibodies, MMP-9 inhibitors, and MMP-9 gene silencing helps to maintain the integrity of the BBB [99–101].

Manipulating the polarization of microglia is also a potential therapeutic strategy for stroke patients since it can lead to a reduction of pro-inflammatory cytokines. For instance, stroke models have demonstrated that anti-IL-6 antibodies attenuate increases in BBB permeability and modulate the expression of tight junction proteins [102]. Through inhibiting microglia activation with small molecules such as adjudin, levels of proinflammatory cytokines can be decreased and BBB damage can be attenuated.

Apart from these inflammatory and immune mechanisms, another group of therapeutics targets junctional cells. For instance, adherens junctions and tight junctions are calcium dependent [103], and one animal study with rats demonstrated calcium channel blockers (nimodipine and nifedipine) preserve the microvascular integrity, suggesting that these agents can play a role in reducing BBB disruption [104]. Another example of targeting junctional proteins comes from an animal study—where mice were treated with electroacupuncture with the goal of reducing BBB dysfunction following ischemia-reperfusion injury. They found that the expression of tight junction proteins, such as ZO-1 and claudin-5, were increased, while aquaporin 4 (a water channel protein which increases BBB permeability) was decreased [105]. Similarly, mice treated with conivaptan (which blocks V2 receptors) following MCAO and reperfusion had lower rates of BBB disruption and cerebral edema [106].

The tight junction proteins claudins and occludins have been another target for therapeutics. Investigators have found that during the BBB leakage associated with the chronic phase of stroke, there was upregulation of claudin-1 and downregulation of claudin-5—resulting in decreased claudin-5 and ZO-1 interaction and impaired tight junction complexes. Notably, targeting claudin-1 with a specific claudin-1 peptide (C1C2) improved endothelial brain permeability and recovery during the chronic stroke phase [107]. However, these results are inconclusive, as some studies have reported that knocking out claudin-3 (which maintains claudin-1 expression) leads to increased permeability of the BBB via increased tight junction complexity [108]. Future studies should continue to elucidate these trends to analyze how tight junction proteins may be targeted as an area of therapeutic focus.

Although less common, some studies aim to target the BBB in less conventional ways. Transcranial Doppler ultrasound (TCD) can temporarily open the BBB and induce microglia toward the M2 phenotype to help reduce destruction of the BBB [109, 110]. Non-invasive vagus nerve stimulation during MCAO has been shown to protect tight junction protein disruption in microvessels, as well as reducing MMP-2 and MMP-9 expression—thus protecting the BBB and reducing the infarct size in the ischemic brain [111]. In other studies, investigators have found that des-acylated ghrelin reduced BBB disruption, infarct and swelling, and apoptosis in mice after transient MCAO [112].

However, many of these studies were performed in animal models, and there may be incongruence between the controlled conditions of experimental animal stroke and the diverse manifestations of stroke in human populations [113]. Many factors, such as model selection, differing neuroprotective effects of the anesthetic used, and lack of objective evaluation criteria to know if infarction actually occurs, are some of the many variables that may explain why animal studies fail to translate to human outcomes [114]. Nonetheless, there are studies and clinical trials that have investigated immunomodulation in stroke with differing levels of success. Fingolimod was found to reduce inflammatory lymphocyte entry into the brain, decrease microvascular permeability, limit infarct size, and increase neurological rehabilitation [115]. ApTOLL, a TLR4 antagonist, has been found to mediate DAMP-induced inflammatory damage in the APRIL clinical trial [116]. Furthermore, the MultiStem Administration for Stroke Treatment and Enhanced Recovery Study (MASTERS) trial investigated the use of multipotent adult progenitor stem cells to suppress the immune response and limit BBB disruption in a spleen-dependent and

IL-6-suppressing manner. While the MASTERS trial did not show significant improvement, the MASTERS 2 trial is investigating stem cells in AIS with a narrower enrollment window [117, 118]. Imatinib also has neuroprotective potential in AIS. In vivo studies have shown that imatinib attenuates BBB injury in AIS in rats by increasing levels of ZO-1 [119], and a clinical trial is underway to investigate the use of Imatinib in patients [120]. In summary, these studies show great promise for managing the BBB disruption via immunomodulation in the context of AIS.

6.6 Conclusions

The BBB breakdown occurs after AIS resulting in secondary immune-mediated damage. This breakdown is mediated by DAMPs released from ischemic and dying cells, which activate MMPs and immune cells. This dysfunction can be detected using MRI and CT imaging and is associated with reduced neurologic outcome and increased risk of complications like HT or cerebral edema. Being able to evaluate changes in the BBB with neuroimaging and biomarkers is particularly relevant in treatment management where providers may be able to provide better prognoses, predict outcomes, and develop new therapeutics.

Understanding the role of BBB dysfunction after AIS offers insight into the pathophysiology of neuron damage and new avenues for treatment, but much work remains to clarify and manipulate the complex inflammatory interactions.

Disclosures The authors have nothing to disclose

References

1. WHO Mortality Database – WHO [Internet]. [cited 2023 Aug 11]. Available from: https://www.who.int/data/data-collection-tools/who-mortality-database.
2. Koton S, Schneider ALC, Rosamond WD, Shahar E, Sang Y, Gottesman RF, et al. Stroke incidence and mortality trends in US Communities, 1987 to 2011. JAMA. 2014;312(3):259–68.
3. Wolfe CDA. The impact of stroke. Br Med Bull. 2000;56(2):275–86.
4. Abbott NJ, Rönnbäck L, Hansson E. Astrocyte–endothelial interactions at the blood–brain barrier. Nat Rev Neurosci. 2006;7(1):41–53.
5. Abbott NJ, Patabendige AAK, Dolman DEM, Yusof SR, Begley DJ. Structure and function of the blood–brain barrier. Neurobiol Dis. 2010;37(1):13–25.
6. Lo EH, Rosenberg GA. The neurovascular unit in health and disease. Stroke. 2009;40(3 Suppl):S2–3.
7. Huber JD, Egleton RD, Davis TP. Molecular physiology and pathophysiology of tight junctions in the blood–brain barrier. Trends Neurosci. 2001;24(12):719–25.
8. Jiang X, Andjelkovic AV, Zhu L, Yang T, Bennett MVL, Chen J, et al. Blood-brain barrier dysfunction and recovery after ischemic stroke. Prog Neurobiol. 2018;163–164:144–71.
9. Obermeier B, Daneman R, Ransohoff RM. Development, maintenance and disruption of the blood-brain barrier. Nat Med. 2013;19(12):1584–96.
10. Oldendorf WH, Cornford ME, Brown WJ. The large apparent work capability of the blood-brain barrier: a study of the mitochondrial content of capillary endothelial cells in brain and other tissues of the rat. Ann Neurol. 1977;1(5):409–17.

11. Daneman R, Prat A. The blood–brain barrier. Cold Spring Harb Perspect Biol [Internet]. 2015 Jan [cited 2023 Jun 21];7(1). Available from: https://www.ncbi.nlm.nih.gov/pmc/articles/PMC4292164/.
12. Profaci CP, Munji RN, Pulido RS, Daneman R. The blood–brain barrier in health and disease: important unanswered questions. J Exp Med. 2020;217(4):e20190062.
13. Giraud M, Cho TH, Nighoghossian N, Maucort-Boulch D, Deiana G, Østergaard L, et al. Early blood brain barrier changes in acute ischemic stroke: a sequential MRI study. J Neuroimaging. 2015;25(6):959–63.
14. Nadareishvili Z, Simpkins AN, Hitomi E, Reyes D, Leigh R. Post-stroke blood-brain barrier disruption and poor functional outcome in patients receiving thrombolytic therapy. Cerebrovasc Dis. 2019;47(3–4):135–42.
15. Wardlaw JM, Doubal FN, Valdes-Hernandez M, Wang X, Chappell FM, Shuler K, et al. Blood-brain barrier permeability and long term clinical and imaging outcomes in cerebral small vessel disease. Stroke. 2013;44(2) https://doi.org/10.1161/STROKEAHA.112.669994.
16. Kniesel U, Wolburg H. Tight junctions of the blood-brain barrier. Cell Mol Neurobiol. 2000;20(1):57–76.
17. Abdullahi W, Tripathi D, Ronaldson PT. Blood-brain barrier dysfunction in ischemic stroke: targeting tight junctions and transporters for vascular protection. Am J Phys Cell Phys. 2018;315(3):C343–56.
18. Gülke E, Gelderblom M, Magnus T. Danger signals in stroke and their role on microglia activation after ischemia. Ther Adv Neurol Disord. 2018;11:175628641877425.
19. Yu Y, Tang D, Kang R. Oxidative stress-mediated HMGB1 biology. Front Physiol. 2015;6:93.
20. Tian X, Liu C, Shu Z, Chen G. Review: therapeutic targeting of HMGB1 in stroke. Curr Drug Deliv. 2017;14(6):785–90.
21. Gladwin MT, Ofori-Acquah SF. Erythroid DAMPs drive inflammation in SCD. Blood. 2014;123(24):3689–90.
22. Kwon M, Woo S, Kurland D, Yoon S, Palmer A, Banerjee U, et al. Methemoglobin is an endogenous toll-like receptor 4 ligand—relevance to subarachnoid hemorrhage. IJMS. 2015;16(12):5028–46.
23. Dutra FF, Bozza MT. Heme on innate immunity and inflammation. Front Pharmacol [Internet] 2014 May 27 [cited 2023 May 4];5. Available from: http://journal.frontiersin.org/article/10.3389/fphar.2014.00115/abstract.
24. Dutra FF, Alves LS, Rodrigues D, Fernandez PL, De Oliveira RB, Golenbock DT, et al. Hemolysis-induced lethality involves inflammasome activation by heme. Proc Natl Acad Sci USA [Internet] 2014 Sep 30 [cited 2023 May 4];111(39). Available from: https://pnas.org/doi/full/10.1073/pnas.1405023111.
25. Butt OI, Buehler PW, D'Agnillo F. Blood-brain barrier disruption and oxidative stress in Guinea pig after systemic exposure to modified cell-free hemoglobin. Am J Pathol. 2011;178(3):1316–28.
26. Smiley ST, King JA, Hancock WW. Fibrinogen stimulates macrophage chemokine secretion through toll-like receptor 4. J Immunol. 2001;167(5):2887–94.
27. Seeger FH, Blessing E, Gu L, Bornhold R, Denger S, Kreuzer J. Fibrinogen induces chemotactic activity in endothelial cells: fibrinogen and chemotaxis. Acta Physiol Scand. 2002;176(2):109–15.
28. Yang Y, Rosenberg GA. Blood-brain barrier breakdown in acute and chronic cerebrovascular disease. Stroke. 2011;42(11):3323–8.
29. Lucivero V, Prontera M, Mezzapesa DM, Petruzzellis M, Sancilio M, Tinelli A, et al. Different roles of matrix metalloproteinases-2 and -9 after human ischaemic stroke. Neurol Sci. 2007;28(4):165–70.
30. Gidday JM, Gasche YG, Copin JC, Shah AR, Perez RS, Shapiro SD, et al. Leukocyte-derived matrix metalloproteinase-9 mediates blood-brain barrier breakdown and is

proinflammatory after transient focal cerebral ischemia. Am J Phys Heart Circ Phys. 2005;289(2):H558–68.
31. Yang JT, Lee TH, Lee IN, Chung CY, Kuo CH, Weng HH. Dexamethasone inhibits ICAM-1 and MMP-9 expression and reduces brain edema in intracerebral hemorrhagic rats. Acta Neurochir. 2011;153(11):2197–203.
32. Rallidis LS, Vikelis M, Panagiotakos DB, Rizos I, Zolindaki MG, Kaliva K, et al. Inflammatory markers and in-hospital mortality in acute ischaemic stroke. Atherosclerosis. 2006;189(1):193–7.
33. Xiong XY, Liu L, Yang QW. Functions and mechanisms of microglia/macrophages in neuro-inflammation and neurogenesis after stroke. Prog Neurobiol. 2016;142:23–44.
34. Shaftel SS, Carlson TJ, Olschowka JA, Kyrkanides S, Matousek SB, O'Banion MK. Chronic interleukin-1beta expression in mouse brain leads to leukocyte infiltration and neutrophil-independent blood brain barrier permeability without overt neurodegeneration. J Neurosci. 2007;27(35):9301–9.
35. Block F, Peters M, Nolden-Koch M. Expression of IL-6 in the ischemic penumbra. Neuroreport. 2000;11(5):963–7.
36. Zhang J, Sadowska GB, Chen X, Park SY, Kim JE, Bodge CA, et al. Anti–IL-6 neutralizing antibody modulates blood-brain barrier function in the ovine fetus. FASEB J. 2015;29(5):1739–53.
37. Shaafi S, Sharifipour E, Rahmanifar R, Hejazi S, Andalib S, Nikanfar M, et al. Interleukin-6, a reliable prognostic factor for ischemic stroke. Iran J Neurol. 2014;13(2):70–6.
38. Krueger M, Bechmann I, Immig K, Reichenbach A, Härtig W, Michalski D. Blood–brain barrier breakdown involves four distinct stages of vascular damage in various models of experimental focal cerebral ischemia. J Cereb Blood Flow Metab. 2015;35(2):292–303.
39. Yang C, Hawkins KE, Doré S, Candelario-Jalil E. Neuroinflammatory mechanisms of blood-brain barrier damage in ischemic stroke. Am J Phys Cell Phys. 2019;316(2):C135–53.
40. Zhang Y, Gao Z, Wang D, Zhang T, Sun B, Mu L, et al. Accumulation of natural killer cells in ischemic brain tissues and the chemotactic effect of IP-10. J Neuroinflammation. 2014;11(1):79.
41. Liesz A, Suri-Payer E, Veltkamp C, Doerr H, Sommer C, Rivest S, et al. Regulatory T cells are key cerebroprotective immunomodulators in acute experimental stroke. Nat Med. 2009;15(2):192–9.
42. Veldhuis WB, Floris S, van der Meide PH, Vos IMP, de Vries HE, Dijkstra CD, et al. Interferon-beta prevents cytokine-induced neutrophil infiltration and attenuates blood-brain barrier disruption. J Cereb Blood Flow Metab. 2003;23(9):1060–9.
43. Veldhuis WB, Derksen JW, Floris S, Van Der Meide PH, De Vries HE, Schepers J, et al. Interferon-beta blocks infiltration of inflammatory cells and reduces infarct volume after ischemic stroke in the rat. J Cereb Blood Flow Metab. 2003;23(9):1029–39.
44. Ma M, Ma Y, Yi X, Guo R, Zhu W, Fan X, et al. Intranasal delivery of transforming growth factor-beta1 in mice after stroke reduces infarct volume and increases neurogenesis in the subventricular zone. BMC Neurosci. 2008;9:117.
45. Pang L, Ye W, Che XM, Roessler BJ, Betz AL, Yang GY. Reduction of inflammatory response in the mouse brain with adenoviral-mediated transforming growth factor-ss1 expression. Stroke. 2001;32(2):544–52.
46. Shen W, Li S, Chung SH, Zhu L, Stayt J, Su T, et al. Tyrosine phosphorylation of VE-cadherin and claudin-5 is associated with TGF-β1-induced permeability of centrally derived vascular endothelium. Eur J Cell Biol. 2011;90(4):323–32.
47. Glabinski AR, Tani M, Aras S, Stoler MH, Tuohy VK, Ransohoff RM. Regulation and function of central nervous system chemokines. Int J Dev Neurosci. 1995;13(3–4):153–65.
48. Chen Y, Hallenbeck JM, Ruetzler C, Bol D, Thomas K, Berman NEJ, et al. Overexpression of monocyte chemoattractant protein 1 in the brain exacerbates ischemic brain injury and is associated with recruitment of inflammatory cells. J Cereb Blood Flow Metab. 2003;23(6):748–55.

49. Wang Y, Huang J, Li Y, Yang GY. Roles of chemokine CXCL12 and its receptors in ischemic stroke. Curr Drug Targets. 2012;13(2):166–72.
50. Yan J, Greer JM, Etherington K, Cadigan GP, Cavanagh H, Henderson RD, et al. Immune activation in the peripheral blood of patients with acute ischemic stroke. J Neuroimmunol 2009;206(1–2):112–7.
51. Hua Y, Wu J, Keep RF, Nakamura T, Hoff JT, Xi G. Tumor necrosis factor-alpha increases in the brain after intracerebral hemorrhage and thrombin stimulation. Neurosurgery. 2006;58(3):542–50; discussion 542–550
52. Barone FC, Arvin B, White RF, Miller A, Webb CL, Willette RN, et al. Tumor necrosis factor-alpha. A mediator of focal ischemic brain injury. Stroke. 1997;28(6):1233–44.
53. Yang GY, Gong C, Qin Z, Liu XH, Lorris BA. Tumor necrosis factor alpha expression produces increased blood-brain barrier permeability following temporary focal cerebral ischemia in mice. Brain Res Mol Brain Res. 1999;69(1):135–43.
54. Plate KH, Beck H, Danner S, Allegrini PR, Wiessner C. Cell type specific upregulation of vascular endothelial growth factor in an MCA-occlusion model of cerebral infarct. J Neuropathol Exp Neurol. 1999;58(6):654–66.
55. Moisan A, Favre IM, Rome C, Grillon E, Naegele B, Barbieux M, et al. Microvascular plasticity after experimental stroke: a molecular and MRI study. Cerebrovasc Dis. 2014;38(5):344–53.
56. Yang Y, Thompson JF, Taheri S, Salayandia VM, McAvoy TA, Hill JW, et al. Early inhibition of MMP activity in ischemic rat brain promotes expression of tight junction proteins and angiogenesis during recovery. J Cereb Blood Flow Metab. 2013;33(7):1104–14.
57. Rahman AA, Amruta N, Pinteaux E, Bix GJ. Neurogenesis after stroke: a therapeutic perspective. Transl Stroke Res. 2021;12(1):1–14.
58. Ögren J, Irewall AL, Bergström L, Mooe T. Intracranial hemorrhage after ischemic stroke: incidence, time trends, and predictors in a Swedish Nationwide cohort of 196 765 patients. Circ Cardiovasc Qual Outcomes. 2015;8(4):413–20.
59. Tsao CW, Aday AW, Almarzooq ZI, Anderson CAM, Arora P, Avery CL, et al. Heart disease and stroke statistics—2023 update: a report from the American Heart Association. Circulation. 2023;147(8):e93–621.
60. Keep RF, Xiang J, Ennis SR, Andjelkovic A, Hua Y, Xi G, et al. Blood-brain barrier function in intracerebral hemorrhage. Acta Neurochir Suppl. 2008;105:73–7.
61. Ye F, Garton HJL, Hua Y, Keep RF, Xi G. The role of thrombin in brain injury after hemorrhagic and ischemic stroke. Transl Stroke Res. 2020; https://doi.org/10.1007/s12975-020-00855-4.
62. Yang S, Chen Y, Deng X, Jiang W, Li B, Fu Z, et al. Hemoglobin-induced nitric oxide synthase overexpression and nitric oxide production contribute to blood-brain barrier disruption in the rat. J Mol Neurosci. 2013;51(2):352–63.
63. Zhao F, Hua Y, He Y, Keep RF, Xi G. Minocycline-induced attenuation of iron overload and brain injury after experimental intracerebral hemorrhage. Stroke. 2011;42(12):3587–93.
64. Prabhakaran S, Naidech AM. Ischemic brain injury after intracerebral hemorrhage. Stroke. 2012;43(8):2258–63.
65. Balança B, Desmurs L, Grelier J, Perret-Liaudet A, Lukaszewicz AC. DAMPs and RAGE pathophysiology at the acute phase of brain injury: an overview. Int J Mol Sci. 2021;22(5):2439.
66. Candelario-Jalil E, Dijkhuizen RM, Magnus T. Neuroinflammation, stroke, blood-brain barrier dysfunction, and imaging modalities. Stroke. 2022;53(5):1473–86.
67. Cuenod CA, Balvay D. Perfusion and vascular permeability: basic concepts and measurement in DCE-CT and DCE-MRI. Diagn Interv Imaging. 2013;94(12):1187–204.
68. Kassner A, Merali Z. Assessment of blood–brain barrier disruption in stroke. Stroke. 2015;46(11):3310–5.
69. Sourbron SP, Buckley DL. Classic models for dynamic contrast-enhanced MRI. NMR Biomed. 2013;26(8):1004–27.
70. Reschke M, Salvador E, Schlegel N, Burek M, Karnati S, Wunder C, et al. Isosteviol sodium (STVNA) reduces pro-inflammatory cytokine IL-6 and GM-CSF in an in vitro murine stroke model of the Blood–Brain Barrier (BBB). Pharmaceutics. 2022;14(9):1753.

71. Serlin Y, Ofer J, Ben-Arie G, Veksler R, Ifergane G, Shelef I, et al. Blood-brain barrier leakage. Stroke. 2019;50(5):1266–9.
72. Hom J, Dankbaar JW, Soares BP, Schneider T, Cheng SC, Bredno J, et al. Blood-brain barrier permeability assessed by perfusion CT predicts symptomatic hemorrhagic transformation and malignant edema in acute ischemic stroke. Am J Neuroradiol. 2011;32(1):41–8.
73. Wu S, Thornhill RE, Chen S, Rammo W, Mikulis DJ, Kassner A. Relative recirculation: a fast, model-free surrogate for the measurement of blood-brain barrier permeability and the prediction of hemorrhagic transformation in acute ischemic stroke. Investig Radiol. 2009;44(10):662.
74. Arba F, Piccardi B, Palumbo V, Biagini S, Galmozzi F, Iovene V, et al. Blood-brain barrier leakage and hemorrhagic transformation: the Reperfusion Injury in Ischemic StroKe (RISK) study. Eur J Neurol. 2021;28(9):3147–54.
75. Simpkins AN, Dias C, Leigh R, Benson RT, Hsia AW, Latour LL, et al. Identification of reversible disruption of the human blood–brain barrier following acute ischemia. Stroke. 2016;47(9):2405–8.
76. Maïer B, Tsai AS, Einhaus JF, Desilles JP, Ho-Tin-Noé B, Gory B, et al. Neuroimaging is the new "spatial omic": multi-omic approaches to neuro-inflammation and immuno-thrombosis in acute ischemic stroke. Semin Immunopathol. 2023;45(1):125–43.
77. Hjort N, Wu O, Ashkanian M, Sølling C, Mouridsen K, Christensen S, et al. MRI detection of early blood-brain barrier disruption. Stroke. 2008;39(3):1025–8.
78. Luby M, Hsia AW, Nadareishvili Z, Cullison K, Pednekar N, Adil MM, et al. Frequency of blood-brain barrier disruption post-endovascular therapy and multiple Thrombectomy passes in acute ischemic stroke patients. Stroke. 2019;50(8):2241–4.
79. Shi ZS, Duckwiler GR, Jahan R, Tateshima S, Szeder V, Saver JL, et al. Early blood-brain barrier disruption after mechanical thrombectomy in acute ischemic stroke. J Neuroimaging. 2018;28(3):283–8.
80. Zhang Z, Yan J, Shi H. Role of hypoxia inducible factor 1 in hyperglycemia-exacerbated blood-brain barrier disruption in ischemic stroke. Neurobiol Dis. 2016;95:82–92.
81. Hom S, Fleegal MA, Egleton RD, Campos CR, Hawkins BT, Davis TP. Comparative changes in the blood-brain barrier and cerebral infarction of SHR and WKY rats. Am J Phys Regul Integr Comp Phys. 2007;292(5):R1881–92.
82. Starr JM, Wardlaw J, Ferguson K, MacLullich A, Deary IJ, Marshall I. Increased blood–brain barrier permeability in type II diabetes demonstrated by gadolinium magnetic resonance imaging. J Neurol Neurosurg Psychiatry. 2003;74(1):70–6.
83. Mohammadi MT, Dehghani GA. Acute hypertension induces brain injury and blood–brain barrier disruption through reduction of claudins mRNA expression in rat. Pathol Res Pract. 2014;210(12):985–90.
84. Fan Y, Yang X, Tao Y, Lan L, Zheng L, Sun J. Tight junction disruption of blood–brain barrier in white matter lesions in chronic hypertensive rats. Neuroreport. 2015;26(17):1039–43.
85. Montagne A, Barnes SR, Sweeney MD, Halliday MR, Sagare AP, Zhao Z, et al. Blood-brain barrier breakdown in the aging human hippocampus. Neuron. 2015;85(2):296–302.
86. Verheggen ICM, de Jong JJA, van Boxtel MPJ, Gronenschild EHBM, Palm WM, Postma AA, et al. Increase in blood–brain barrier leakage in healthy, older adults. GeroScience. 2020;42(4):1183–93.
87. Latour LL, Kang DW, Ezzeddine MA, Chalela JA, Warach S. Early blood–brain barrier disruption in human focal brain ischemia. Ann Neurol. 2004;56(4):468–77.
88. Wardlaw JM, Makin SJ, Valdés Hernández MC, Armitage PA, Heye AK, Chappell FM, et al. Blood-brain barrier failure as a core mechanism in cerebral small vessel disease and dementia: evidence from a cohort study. Alzheimers Dement. 2017;13(6):634–43.
89. Wu S, Yin Y, Du L. Blood–brain barrier dysfunction in the pathogenesis of major depressive disorder. Cell Mol Neurobiol. 2022;42(8):2571–91.
90. Towfighi A, Ovbiagele B, El Husseini N, Hackett ML, Jorge RE, Kissela BM, et al. Poststroke depression: a scientific statement for healthcare professionals from the American Heart Association/American Stroke Association. Stroke. 2017;48(2):e30–43.

91. Qiu Y-M, Zhang C-L, Chen A-Q, Wang H-L, Zhou Y-F, Li Y-N, et al. Immune cells in the BBB disruption after acute ischemic stroke: targets for immune therapy? Front Immunol [Internet]. 2021 [cited 2023 May 4];12. Available from: https://www.frontiersin.org/articles/10.3389/fimmu.2021.678744.
92. Vemuganti R, Dempsey RJ, Bowen KK. Inhibition of intercellular adhesion Molecule-1 protein expression by antisense oligonucleotides is neuroprotective after transient middle cerebral artery occlusion in rat. Stroke. 2004;35(1):179–84.
93. Jin AY, Tuor UI, Rushforth D, Kaur J, Muller RN, Petterson JL, et al. Reduced blood brain barrier breakdown in P-selectin deficient mice following transient ischemic stroke: a future therapeutic target for treatment of stroke. BMC Neurosci. 2010;11(1):12.
94. Liu T, Zhang T, Yu H, Shen H, Xia W. Adjudin protects against cerebral ischemia reperfusion injury by inhibition of neuroinflammation and blood-brain barrier disruption. J Neuroinflammation. 2014;11(1):107.
95. Li W, Suwanwela NC, Patumraj S. Curcumin by down-regulating NF-kB and elevating Nrf2, reduces brain edema and neurological dysfunction after cerebral I/R. Microvasc Res. 2016;106:117–27.
96. Cannon RE, Peart JC, Hawkins BT, Campos CR, Miller DS. Targeting blood-brain barrier sphingolipid signaling reduces basal P-glycoprotein activity and improves drug delivery to the brain. Proc Natl Acad Sci USA. 2012;109(39):15930–5.
97. Candelario-Jalil E, González-Falcón A, García-Cabrera M, León OS, Fiebich BL. Post-ischaemic treatment with the cyclooxygenase-2 inhibitor nimesulide reduces blood–brain barrier disruption and leukocyte infiltration following transient focal cerebral ischaemia in rats. J Neurochem. 2007;100(4):1108–20.
98. Candelario-Jalil E, Taheri S, Yang Y, Sood R, Grossetete M, Estrada EY, et al. Cyclooxygenase inhibition limits blood-brain barrier disruption following intracerebral injection of tumor necrosis factor-alpha in the rat. J Pharmacol Exp Ther. 2007;323(2):488–98.
99. Ji Y, Gao Q, Ma Y, Wang F, Tan X, Song D, et al. An MMP-9 exclusive neutralizing antibody attenuates blood-brain barrier breakdown in mice with stroke and reduces stroke patient-derived MMP-9 activity. Pharmacol Res. 2023;190:106720.
100. Nagel S, Su Y, Horstmann S, Heiland S, Gardner H, Koziol J, et al. Minocycline and hypothermia for reperfusion injury after focal cerebral ischemia in the rat—effects on BBB breakdown and MMP expression in the acute and subacute phase. Brain Res. 2008;1188:198–206.
101. Bonoiu A, Mahajan SD, Ye L, Kumar R, Ding H, Yong KT, et al. MMP-9 gene silencing by a quantum dot–siRNA nanoplex delivery to maintain the integrity of the blood brain barrier. Brain Res. 2009;1282:142–55.
102. Kraus J, Voigt K, Schuller AM, Scholz M, Kim KS, Schilling M, et al. Interferon-beta stabilizes barrier characteristics of the blood-brain barrier in four different species in vitro. Mult Scler. 2008;14(6):843–52.
103. Brown RC, Davis TP. Calcium modulation of Adherens and tight junction function. Stroke. 2002;33(6):1706–11.
104. Farkas E, De Jong GI, Apró E, Keuker JIH, Luiten PGM. Calcium antagonists decrease capillary wall damage in aging hypertensive rat brain. Neurobiol Aging. 2001;22(2):299–309.
105. Jung YS, Lee SW, Park JH, Seo HB, Choi BT, Shin HK. Electroacupuncture preconditioning reduces ROS generation with NOX4 down-regulation and ameliorates blood-brain barrier disruption after ischemic stroke. J Biomed Sci. 2016;23(1):32.
106. Zeynalov E, Jones SM, Seo JW, Snell LD, Elliott JP. Arginine-vasopressin receptor blocker Conivaptan reduces brain edema and blood-brain barrier disruption after experimental stroke in mice. PLoS One. 2015;10(8):e0136121.
107. Sladojevic N, Stamatovic SM, Johnson AM, Choi J, Hu A, Dithmer S, et al. Claudin-1-Dependent Destabilization of the Blood–Brain Barrier in Chronic Stroke. J Neurosci 2019;39(4):743–757.

108. Winkler L, Blasig R, Breitkreuz-Korff O, Berndt P, Dithmer S, Helms HC, et al. Tight junctions in the blood–brain barrier promote edema formation and infarct size in stroke – ambivalent effects of sealing proteins. J Cereb Blood Flow Metab. 2021;41(1):132–45.
109. Gómez-de Frutos MC, Laso-García F, García-Suárez I, Diekhorst L, Otero-Ortega L, Alonso de Leciñana M, et al. The role of ultrasound as a diagnostic and therapeutic tool in experimental animal models of stroke: a review. Biomedicine. 2021;9(11):1609
110. Guo J, Lo WLA, Hu H, Yan L, Li L. Transcranial ultrasound stimulation applied in ischemic stroke rehabilitation: a review. Front Neurosci. 2022;16:964060.
111. Yang Y, Yang LY, Orban L, Cuylear D, Thompson J, Simon B, et al. Non-invasive vagus nerve stimulation reduces blood-brain barrier disruption in a rat model of ischemic stroke. Brain Stimul. 2018;11(4):689–98.
112. Ku JM, Taher M, Chin KY, Barsby T, Austin V, Wong CHY, et al. Protective actions of des-acylated ghrelin on brain injury and blood–brain barrier disruption after stroke in mice. Clin Sci. 2016;130(17):1545–58.
113. Matur AV, Candelario-Jalil E, Paul S, Karamyan VT, Lee JD, Pennypacker K, et al. Translating Animal Models of Ischemic Stroke to the Human Condition. Transl Stroke Res [Internet]. 2022 Sep 20 [cited 2023 Aug 5]; Available from: https://doi.org/10.1007/s12975-022-01082-9.
114. Xu S-Y, Pan S-Y. The failure of animal models of neuroprotection in acute ischemic stroke to translate to clinical efficacy. Med Sci Monit Basic Res. 2013;19:37–45.
115. Fu Y, Zhang N, Ren L, Yan Y, Sun N, Li YJ, et al. Impact of an immune modulator fingolimod on acute ischemic stroke. Proc Natl Acad Sci USA. 2014;111(51):18315–20.
116. Hernández-Jiménez M, Abad-Santos F, Cotgreave I, Gallego J, Jilma B, Flores A, et al. APRIL: a double-blind, placebo-controlled, randomized, phase Ib/IIa clinical study of ApTOLL for the treatment of acute ischemic stroke. Front Neurol. 2023;14:1127585.
117. Hess DC, Wechsler LR, Clark WM, Savitz SI, Ford GA, Chiu D, et al. Safety and efficacy of multipotent adult progenitor cells in acute ischaemic stroke (MASTERS): a randomised, double-blind, placebo-controlled, phase 2 trial. Lancet Neurol. 2017;16(5):360–8.
118. Athersys, Inc. MultiStem® Administration for Stroke Treatment and Enhanced Recovery Study (MASTERS-2) [Internet]. clinicaltrials.gov; 2022 Feb [cited 2023 Aug 4]. Report No.: NCT03545607. Available from: https://clinicaltrials.gov/study/NCT03545607.
119. Wang J, Bai T, Wang N, Li H, Guo X. Neuroprotective potential of imatinib in global ischemia-reperfusion-induced cerebral injury: possible role of Janus-activated kinase 2/signal transducer and activator of transcription 3 and connexin 43. Korean J Physiol Pharmacol. 2020;24(1):11–8.
120. Ahmed N. Imatinib in acute Ischaemic stroke: a phase 3, randomized, double-blind, placebo controlled, parallel-arm efficacy trial of Imatinib in acute Ischaemic stroke [Internet]. clinicaltrials.gov; 2020 Sep [cited 2023 Aug 4]. Report No.: NCT03639922. Available from: https://clinicaltrials.gov/study/NCT03639922.

Molecular Crosstalk in Traumatic Brain Injury

7

Daniel Agustin Godoy, Manuel Quintana Diaz, and Maximiliano Rovegno

7.1 Introduction

Traumatic brain injury (TBI) refers to brain damage generated as a result of a traumatic insult [1, 2]. It constitutes a serious public health problem worldwide [1, 2]. It does not respect sex or age, and its production mechanisms are multiple and varied [1, 2]. TBI is a highly prevalent entity, with an estimated rate of almost two million cases annually in the United States alone, with the sad privilege of being the third cause of death and the first cause of severe disabling sequelae, especially in the young adult population [1, 2]. TBI is an entity characterized by its wide injury spectrum, dynamism, and unpredictable evolution [1, 2].

7.2 Pathophysiology of TBI

TBI is a heterogeneous disease with a complex pathophysiology [3–5]. The brain parenchyma damage occurs as a result of the external energy applied to and absorbed by the different cranial structures (scalp, skull, brain parenchyma, cerebrospinal fluid (CSF), and blood vessels) [6]. There are different types of applied mechanical loads: coup or direct impact, kickback, acceleration-deceleration forces, rotation, translation, angulation, and penetrating injuries with or without expansive waves

D. A. Godoy (✉)
Unidad de Cuidados Neurointensivos, Sanatorio Pasteur, Human Resources and Planning (Government of Catamarca), Catamarca, Argentina

M. Q. Diaz
Department of Critical Care, Autonomic University of Madrid, La Paz University Hospital, Madrid, Spain

M. Rovegno
Department of Critical Care, Pontifical Catholic University of Chile, Santiago, Chile

D. Battaglini et al. (eds.), *Organ System Crosstalk in Critical Illness*,
https://doi.org/10.1007/978-3-032-01024-7_7

[6]. These mechanisms can transmit energy over the static or moving (dynamic) skull [6]. The nature, intensity, and duration of the aforementioned forces determine the pattern and extent of the damage. At the same time, the lesional type will depend on the location and severity of the applied mechanical load [6]. Traditionally two types of injury were recognized: primary followed by secondary insults [1, 2, 4, 5]; however, the advancement of pathophysiological knowledge allows us to identify, in the evolutive profile of TBI, two additional types of insults: tertiary and quaternary (Fig. 7.1) [7, 8].

7.2.1 Primary Injury

It occurs immediately after impact [1, 9]. At the cellular level, its development can continue during the first hours of the injury [1, 9]. Primary damage is irreversible and can only be avoided through education and the rigorous implementation of primary prevention campaigns [1]. The immediate consequences of the primary injury will be different types of lesions; they can be functional or structural, reversible or irreversible, focal or diffuse [9].

Microscopically, primary damage is characterized by cellular necrosis, lacerations, tears, and axon retraction, with or without the concomitant presence of vascular rupture and/or torsion (hemorrhages; Fig. 7.2) [9].

At the same time, the primary injury triggers a series of molecular cascades of damage that feed back in a continuum and can cause local (brain) or systemic damage (pulmonary, cardiac, renal, intestinal crosstalk), highlighting inflammatory phenomena, oxidative stress, excitotoxicity, and oxygen free radical liberation, which will be detailed in more depth later in this chapter (Fig. 7.3) [9].

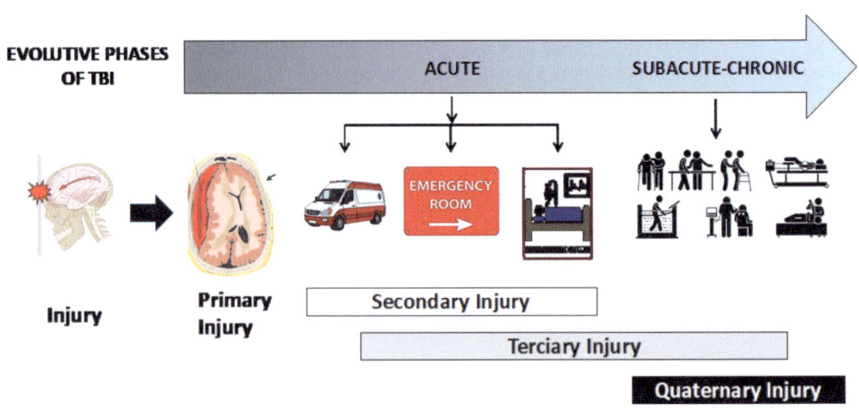

Fig. 7.1 Evolutive phases and injury types after TBI

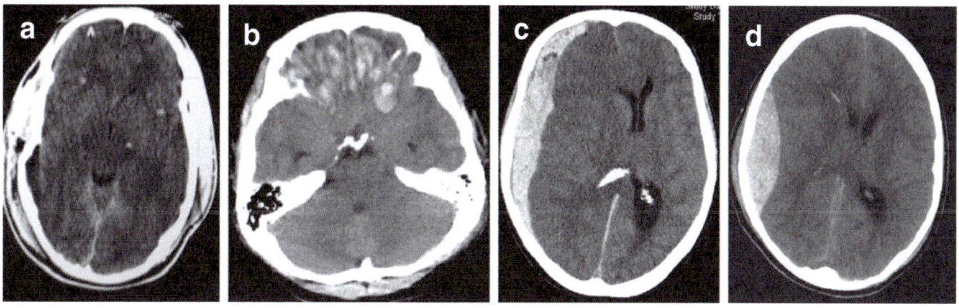

Fig. 7.2 Examples of primary injuries. (**a**) Diffuse axonal injury; (**b**) contusions; (**c**) acute subdural hematoma; (**d**) acute epidural hematoma

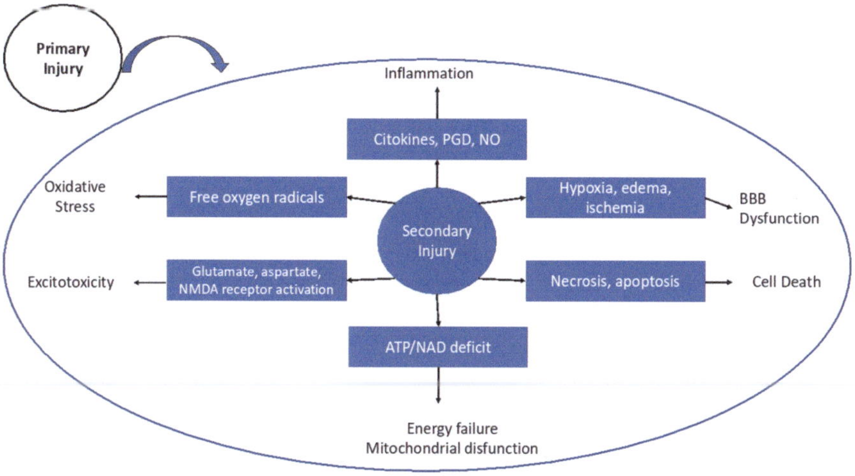

Fig. 7.3 Cascade of events that are triggered after the primary injury and cause secondary injury. *PGS* prostaglandins, *NO* nitric oxide, *NMDA* N-methyl aspartate, *ATP* adenosine triphosphate

7.2.2 Secondary Injury

Secondary injury occurs immediately after the primary injury as a consequence of the different molecular pathophysiological phenomena triggered at different levels and brain-organ crosstalk [1, 3, 4, 10]. This leads to altering the intracranial physiological balance at all levels, causing elevation of the intracranial pressure (ICP) and compromising oxygenation, metabolism, and energy utilization by the brain parenchyma among other deleterious phenomena [1, 3, 4]. At the same time, alterations in systemic physiology (arterial hypotension, hypoxemia, hypocapnia, fever) exacerbate the aforementioned damage mechanisms [1, 3, 4, 10].

Secondary injury contributes to worsening or perpetuating the primary injury [1, 3, 4]. Unlike primary injury, secondary injury is reversible and, more importantly, capable of early detection and correction, especially in the acute phase [1, 3, 4]. If present, secondary insults have a negative impact on the final outcome [1, 11, 12].

Table 7.1 Secondary insults

Systemic	Intracranial
Arterial hypotension	Intracranial hypertension
Hypoxemia	Ischemia
Fever	Brain hypoxia
Hypocapnia	Edema
Hypercapnia	Hematomas
Hypoglycemia	Swelling
Hyperglycemia	Vasospasm
Hyponatremia	Disseminated cortical depression
Hypernatremia	Seizures
Severe anemia	Hyperemia
Coagulation alteration	Infections
Systemic inflammatory response	Paroxysmal sympathetic hyperactivity

Preventing and correcting secondary insults is the current basis of TBI therapy [1, 3, 4]. The different secondary insults are shown in Table 7.1.

7.2.3 Tertiary Injury

TBI has a systemic impact, especially in its most severe forms [1, 3, 4]. The brain-systemic organ crosstalk is a complex biological communication mediated via cellular, soluble molecules, and neurohormonal actions, based on a two-way pathway [12]. The communication between the brain and the rest of body organs involves nerves, endocrine, inflammatory, and immunity systems, as well as the emotional and cognitive centers of the brain [12]. Particularly, TBI is complicated by neuroinflammation and neurodegeneration causing multiorgan inflammation, microbial dysbiosis, gastrointestinal dysfunction and dysmotility, liver dysfunction, acute kidney injury, and pulmonary and cardiac dysfunction [12].

In its evolutionary profile and beginning in the acute phase, extending to the subacute-chronic period, tertiary injury can manifest [7, 8]. We call tertiary injury all those situations that add more damage in a multifactorial manner, triggered as a consequence of the brain-organ crosstalk or the patient's care [7, 8, 12]. These injury mechanisms generally occur during TBI therapy, including:

- Brain-organ crosstalk
- Complications arising from prolonged stay in the intensive care unit
- Adverse effects of drugs or blood products
- injuries induced by mechanical ventilation
- Infections associated or not with invasive devices
- Complications of multifactorial origin

The potentially harmful impact of tertiary injury has not yet been accurately determined; however, despite the reversible and preventable nature of this type of injury, it should not be underestimated. For this reason, it is key to deeply analyze the risk-benefit relationship of each treatment measure to be instituted.

Therefore, it is essential to establish specific protocols that allow the control of the appearance and progression of this injury type.

7.2.4 Quaternary Injury

The consequences and/or the outcome of TBI show great interindividual variability, even if it is the same type of injury. This variability can be explained in part by the severity of the injury, the age of the individual, and previous health state, but in the vast majority of situations, the reasons remain unelucidated. In this context, genetics can potentially guide us to find the secondary individual response to TBI [8, 13, 14].

The advances in medical genetics over the last years have increased our understanding of many biological processes.

Although the moment in which it begins is not clear, the quaternary injury manifests itself during the subacute and chronic period of TBI and is fundamentally characterized by a series of pathophysiological events that prevent the repair, counteracting, or ameliorating of the primary damage [8, 13, 14].

The pathophysiological mechanisms of the quaternary lesion manifest when the cellular damage process appears to have stopped and have important genetic influence [8, 13, 14]. Among these mechanisms are:

- Persistence of the inflammatory phenomenon
- Absence of mitigation of cell death processes (necrosis, apoptosis)
- Incomplete cleaning of detritus or waste generated during the injury process
- Aberrant immune response
- Glial neurotoxicity

Previous post-TBI studies have shown that individuals carrying the e4 isoform of apolipoprotein E are associated with the presence of alterations in cognitive function and subsequent development of Alzheimer's disease with worse long-term functional outcome [15].

7.3 Molecular Mechanism of Secondary Damage

7.3.1 Overview

TBI is a leading cause of mortality and mobility worldwide. The annual incidence of TBI is estimated at around 69 million, where the highest burden of disease occurs in Southeast Asia and the Western Pacific regions [16].

Mainly, secondary to road traffic collisions [16]. Many survivors have significant disabilities, increasing the economic impact associated with the disease. Also, individuals >75 years old have experienced a growing mortality trend because of population aging and falls in developed countries [17]. TBI is defined as an alteration of brain function, or other evidence of brain pathology (e.g., imaging, laboratory), caused by external force [18].

7.3.2 Secondary Damage Concept

After trauma has occurred in the brain tissue, a complex process of damage progression occurs, which becomes independent of the initial injury and involves local and systemic factors that will lead to a greater extension of the original injury [4–6]. Secondary injury mechanisms are also initiated at the moment of the traumatic incident but are believed to continue for many years through a series of cellular, physiological, and molecular processes impacting all kinds of cells in the brain [4–6]. Blood-brain barrier (BBB) disturbance, excitotoxicity, mitochondrial dysfunction, oxidative stress, inflammation, and cell loss are the principal identified mechanisms orchestrating secondary injury mechanisms [19]. This resulting damage is known as secondary. Among the systemic factors, the presence of hypotension and hypoxia stands out, which separately double the probability of a poor neurological outcome [11]. Other systemic factors are hyper- and hypocapnia, hyponatremia, anemia, hypoglycemia, and fever. Local factors correspond to a series of cellular and tissue biological mechanisms that account for the amplification of the lesion, on which we will focus our attention [4, 5, 11].

7.3.3 Molecular Mechanisms of Brain Damage

7.3.3.1 Excitotoxicity

Glutamate is the main neurotransmitter of excitatory synapses in the brain and is essential in synaptic plasticity as a substrate for learning and memory processes [19]. Glutamate is stored in synaptic vesicles within the presynaptic terminal [19]. Post stimulation, it is released into the inter-synaptic space where it binds to its receptors present both in the postsynaptic neuron and in the astrocytes that form the glial component of the tripartite synapse (presynaptic neuron, astrocyte, postsynaptic neuron) [20]. After minutes of trauma, there is an acute rise in extracellular glutamate levels [19].

Because of massive depolarization secondary to trauma, ischemia, and spreading depression, glutamate activates ionotropic and metabotropic receptors in postsynaptic neurons [19]. Among the first are α-amino-3-hydroxy-5-methyl-4-isoxazolepropionic acid (AMPA) receptor, kainic acid (KA) receptors, both permeable to Na^+ and K^+, and N-methyl-D-aspartate (NMDA) receptors permeable to Ca2+ [21]. The massive increment in glutamate in turn induces increased Na^+ and Ca^{2+} influx to the cell, and the resulting intracellular Ca^{2+} overload triggers cell damage mechanisms that finally lead to apoptosis through caspase activation [19, 21]. Astrocytes represent the main defense against excitotoxicity [19, 21–23]. They reuptake the extracellular glutamate through their glutamate transporter 1 (GLT-1) and the glutamate-aspartate transporter (GLAST). Also, they can metabolize the glutamate to glutamine and buffer it through their connexin-based channels. Indeed, astrocytes are highly interconnected through connexin-based channels, forming a functional syncytium. These syncytia allow astrocytes to spatially buffer K^+, H^+, and glutamate in the brain [22]. However, if the increase in glutamate persists together with ATP shortage, the astrocytes can invert the glutamate transport, thereby increasing the excitotoxic damage [23].

7.3.3.2 Ischemia

The human brain is a highly metabolically active organ. It receives 15% of cardiac output and consumes 25% of oxygen transport but weights 2.5% of the total body [24]. This framework renders the brain exquisitely sensitive to reduction in blood flow. Ischemia is defined as a reduction of blood flow to less than 20 ml/100 gr tissue/min. Since the postmortem series published by Graham and Adams, it has been recognized as part of the injury mechanism after trauma. They studied 171 consecutive patients who died as a result of TBI, where 91% had ischemic damage considered as severe in 37% of them [25]. Ischemia can be focal, arriving from space-occupying lesions, either extra-axial hematomas or cerebral contusions, where distortion of surrounding parenchyma threatens tissue perfusion. Also, it can be global due to brain edema, intracranial hypertension, and herniations. Whatever the origin of injury focal or global, an ischemic cascade involves a reduction of cerebral blood flow (CBF) resulting in decreased energy production, which in turn causes failure of ionic pumps, mitochondrial injury, and massive neuronal depolarization.

Increased cellular levels of Na^+, Cl^-, and Ca^{2+} ions result in the activation of phospholipases and proteases including caspases, followed by the generation and release of prostaglandins and leukotrienes, breakdown of DNA and the cytoskeleton, and ultimately, destruction of the cell membrane. First, xenon computed tomography (CT) to study regional CBF and the most recent positron emission tomography (PET)-CT studies have shown ischemic brain areas in patients with moderate-severe TBI, many times surrounding lesions as cerebral contusions [26]. These ischemic findings have been named traumatic penumbra to differentiate it from classic ischemic penumbra seen in stroke pathology. PET-CTs used an intravenous infusion of $[^{18}F]$ fluorodeoxyglucose (FDG) and $[^{15}O]H_2O$, combined with single breath inhalation of $[^{15}O]CO$ and $[^{15}O]O_2$ to study the regional cerebral metabolic rate of glucose (CMR_{glc}), CBF, the cerebral metabolic rate of oxygen ($CMRO_2$), and oxygen extraction fraction (OEF), respectively [26]. Findings compatible with ischemia are decreases in CBF, with low or maintained $CMRO_2$ together with increases in OEF and even CMR_{glc}, because of a switch to non-oxidative glucose metabolism [26].

7.3.3.3 Inflammation

Primary brain tissue injury together with secondary damage causes cell death and the release of damage-associated molecular pattern molecules (DAMPs); these danger signals can trigger the inflammasome and innate immune system [19, 27]. Examples of DAMPs are adenosine triphosphate (ATP), S100B proteins,

High-Mobility Group Box protein (HMGB1), and even segments of deoxyribonucleic acid (DNA) or ribonucleic acid (RNA) [27]. Inflammation involves glial cells, microglia, astrocytes, and peripheric leucocytes [19]. The microglia, the innate immune system cells resident in the central nervous system (CNS), are one of the first to react to these danger signals. Minutes after the injury, microglia are activated, undergo morphological changes, transform into a phagocytic cell, and secrete cytokines [19, 28]. Astrocytes, the most abundant cells in the CNS, actively participate in the immune response after injury. They recruit peripheral immune cells and regulate the activity of microglia through the secretion of cytokines and chemokines. Surviving astrocytes undergo a phenotypic change known as reactive astrocytosis, characterized by hypertrophy, hyperplasia, and increased expression of glial fibrillary acidic protein, an intermediate filament of their cytoskeleton [29]. Endothelial cells, also activated in the CNS, together with coagulation allow invasion of peripheral myeloid cells (mainly neutrophils) and lymphocytes [19].

All of them enhance the progression of inflammation, contributing to damage to the brain parenchyma and its vasculature including degradation of the blood-brain barrier (BBB) [19].

During a TBI not only the parenchyma is affected also cerebral vasculature. There metalloproteinases are activated in BBB, disrupting the junctions between astrocytes and endothelial cells, degrading the basal lamina [19]. Meanwhile, proinflammatory cytokines induce an increase in the expression of adhesion molecules, especially Intercellular Adhesion Molecule-1 (ICAM-1) in the endothelial cells of the neurovascular unit. This disruption of the BBB acts as a gateway for peripheral inflammatory infiltration [19]. After TBI, neutrophils invade the tissue, being the first infiltrating immune cells, followed by monocytes [30]. Both subtypes bind to the endothelium and migrate through the vessel wall toward injured tissue. Here, neutrophils cause secondary damage as a result of the release of inflammatory factors such as reactive oxygen species (ROS), proteases, and metalloproteinases, with maximum activity between 3 to 7 days after injury [30]. Unlike neutrophils, lymphocytes are recruited in later stages of brain injury (3–7 days post-injury) [30]. It has been described that different subtypes of lymphocytes infiltrate the CNS, such as Cluster of Differentiation (CD)4$^+$ T cells, CD8$^+$ T cells, regulatory T cells, and γδT cells [31].

7.3.3.4 Apoptosis, Oxidative Stress, and Mitochondrial Dysfunction

A central element in the induction of neuronal death that occurs due to the overactivation of the glutamate receptor is the increase in the concentration of intracellular Ca^{2+} ($Ca^{2+}{}_i$) [19]. This acute increase of $Ca^{2+}{}_i$ can overload mitochondrial Ca^{2+} stores. It triggers the formation of a non-selective pore, through the outer and inner mitochondrial membrane, known as the mitochondrial permeability transition pore (mPTP) [32].

The formation of mPTP is a point of no return because the loss of membrane potential becomes irreversible. The formation of the outer membrane permeabilization channel formed by BAX/BAK proteins (MOMP) will lead to the release of mitochondrial proteins such as cytochrome c (cyt c), SMAC/diablo complex, and apoptosis-inducing factor (AIF), which trigger cell death pathways, both caspase dependent and independent [33].

Mitochondria are the most important intracellular organelles to control oxidative stress. Then its compromise renders cells vulnerable to ROS.

Neurons have an elevated metabolic rate and have significant amounts of unsaturated fatty acids and polyunsaturated fatty acids (PUFAs). They also have a limited defense against oxidative stress. A risky combination after TBI involving excitotoxic mitochondrial dysfunction releasing ROS- superoxide (O2•−), hydrogen peroxide (H_2O_2), peroxyl (ROO^-) radical, and the hydroxyl radical (•OH). These radicals react with lipids, proteins, and nucleic acids. Also, O2•− reacts with nitric oxide to generate peroxynitrite (ONOO−), a reactive nitrogen specie with a longer half-life than O2•− [34].

ROS-induced cell damage is defined by lipid peroxidation where electrons transfer from membrane lipids (mainly PUFAs) to free radicals, resulting in a chain reaction forming high quantities of lipid peroxyl radical, lipid hydroperoxide, and peroxyl-fatty acid radicals. Advancing oxide reduction reaction produces neurotoxic aldehydes such as 4-hydroxynonenal (4-HNE) and 2-propenal (acrolein). Lipid peroxidation is measured by malondialdehyde (MDA) levels [35]. This is a reactive aldehyde capable of reacting with proteins, DNA, and lipids, forming covalent protein adducts and DNA adducts, respectively. Another source of oxidative stress already mentioned is that coming from inflammatory cells: microglia, neutrophils, and monocytes can release ROS. Regardless of its origin, oxidative stress is toxic for cells promoting a full spectrum of damage from cell death to synapsis dysfunction persisting over time [36].

7.3.3.5 Edema

Nearly 50% of deaths due to severe TBI are associated with the development of cerebral [37]. Klatzo, using a cold trauma model, described two subtypes of cerebral edema depending on its origin: cytotoxic and vasogenic [38]. The first occurs due to cellular damage, the failure of ion pumps, and the activation of channels that lead to cellular swelling, while the second occurs due to an increase in the permeability of the BBB. In extreme cases of cellular swelling, oncotic death occurs as a result of the massive entry of H_2O and ions that finally fracture the plasma membrane. During pure cytotoxic edema, there is no increase in cerebral water content, since only a redistribution of water occurs from the interstitial to the intracellular space. In TBI, it has been proposed that cytotoxic edema is predominant [39]. However, there is a temporal evolution and an interrelationship between the different subtypes of cerebral edema.

Katamaya, using a controlled cortical contusion model in rats, demonstrated an increase in osmolarity and water content of the bruised tissue 6–12 h post-trauma [40]. During the following days, secondary cellular damage causes cytotoxic edema, where astrocytes are of special importance, in part because they are 10 times more numerous than neurons. Marmarou studied the apparent diffusion coefficients and water content using MRI in a cohort of 44 patients with severe TBI [39]. Demonstrating that cytotoxic edema was the predominant component in diffuse TBI [39]. Finally, with a bimodal behavior, BBB damage predominates in the pericontusional areas during the first 24 h after TBI [39]. However, after 5 days, a progression of vasogenic edema occurs due to rupture of the BBB [41]. Here, the development of inflammation becomes important, as well as the increase in the expression of metalloproteinases and mediators such as vascular endothelial growth factor (VEGF-A), which degrade the extracellular matrix and increase the permeability of the BBB [41].

7.3.3.6 Cortical Spreading Depression

Cortical spreading depression (CSD), first described by Leao in 1944 [42], is a slowly propagating wave of cellular depolarization (2–5 mm/min) involving neurons and astrocytes in brain tissue [43]. CSD causes almost complete depolarization and breakdown of ionic gradients across the cell membrane, suppression of electrical activity, cellular swelling, distortion of dendritic spines (beading), and changes in regional blood flow [44, 45]. Acute brain injuries such as stroke, TBI, and subarachnoid hemorrhage (SAH) may be complicated by CSDs [46]. Unfortunately, CSDs are not detected by conventional monitoring in clinical care. Furthermore, a prospective observational study using electrocorticography found more than 50% of CSD incidence in ICU patients recovering from TBI, SAH, and Strokes [46]. CSDs are repetitive and produce a metabolic overload that enhances secondary damage [47, 48].

Indeed, the incidence of CSD was independently associated with poor neurologic outcomes in a cohort of severe TBI patients [49].

7.4 Brain-Systemic Organs Crosstalk

7.4.1 Introduction

The brain is not isolated, but anatomically and functionally interacts with each and every compartment (neck, thorax, abdomen) and organ of the body (heart, lungs, kidneys, etc.), through a complex and extensive bilateral biological communication network that basically involves the emotional and cognitive brain centers, nerves, humoral mediators, inter and intracellular signaling and hormones; the endocrine, immune and autonomic nervous systems being its main actors [4, 5, 50–53].

In general, this interaction has as its main objective to achieve and maintain physiological homeostasis in the body; however, sometimes the balance is broken and the original function is distorted and becomes injurious, causing dysfunction of the brain and other body organs [50–53].

7.4.2 Pathophysiology

Acute brain injury, regardless of the etiology (traumatic, ischemic, hemorrhagic), triggers a cascade of events that, due to the interaction between the brain and systemic organs, can potentially lead to the development of systemic organic dysfunctions [50–53]. At the same time, these dysfunctions contribute to the development of secondary systemic insults that perpetuate or aggravate the primary brain injury, closing a vicious circle with a strong negative impact on the brain and system.

The pathophysiological mechanisms of brain-systemic damage are generally the consequence of an imbalance in the biological response to injury, characterized mainly by [50–53]:

- Overactivity of the autonomic nervous system, mainly sympathetic
- Stimulation of the hypothalamus-pituitary-adrenal axis
- Immune dysregulation

These situations, in turn, cause:

- Massive release of catecholamines and cortisol
- Increased sympathetic tone
- Release of inflammatory mediators and cell damage (cytokines, chemokines, free oxygen radicals, etc.)

The factors mentioned constitute the fundamental substrates for the development of systemic dysfunction [50–53]. In the following, we will briefly point out the impact of brain injury on different organs of the body, which will be treated in greater depth in subsequent chapters of this work (Fig. 7.4).

7.4.3 Specifics Brain-Organ Crosstalk

7.4.3.1 Brain-Heart Crosstalk

Heart and brain are deeply interconnected by afferent and efferent fibers of the autonomic nervous system [54–57].

Cardiac dysfunction is common in the setting of severe head trauma even in individuals without previous involvement. The prevalence of cardiac dysfunction reported in current literature is 15 to 70% [54–57].

Myocarditis secondary to massive catecholamine elevation, modification of the structure, metabolism, and functionality of adrenoreceptors, and inflammation are the prominent mechanisms of injury. Increased levels of troponin and B-type natriuretic peptide are the markers usually found [54–57].

Spasm of coronary epicardial arteries, endothelial dysfunction, direct cytotoxicity, and micro-thrombosis contribute to the genesis of systolic, diastolic, or global cardiac dysfunction (stress cardiomyopathy) [54–57]. Pathological studies have clearly described “contraction band necrosis [53].”

7.4.3.2 Brain-Gastrointestinal Crosstalk

The digestive tract is connected to the brain by an extensive enteric neuronal network belonging to the autonomic nervous system responsible for modulating gastrointestinal function at different levels such as [55, 58–60]:

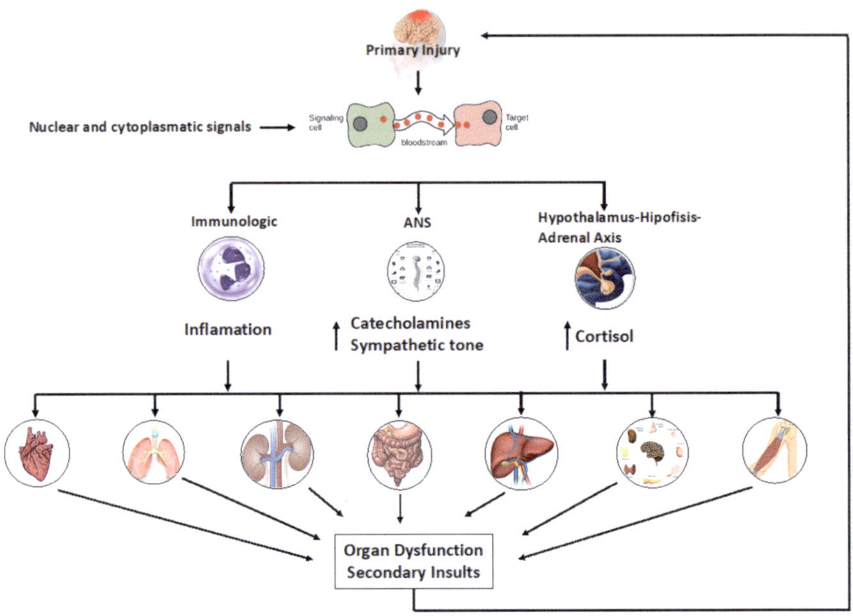

Fig. 7.4 Common mechanism of brain-distant organ crosstalk in acute brain conditions. Inflammation, increased sympathetic tone, and catecholamine arise in response to traumatic brain injury and may act in different organs simultaneously, leading to their dysfunction and generation of secondary insults that negatively impact in primary injury

- Gut motility regulation
- Release and local hormonal and humoral secretion (gastrin, pepsin, motilin, substance P)
- Control of vascular smooth muscle tone and splanchnic perfusion
- Establishment of an intraluminal microenvironment (pH, microbiota)
- Maintenance of immune function and integrity of the gastrointestinal mucosa

Acute brain injury, especially during the first week and as a consequence of the triggering of the inflammatory cascade together with the massive increase in adrenergic discharge, can alter gastrointestinal homeostasis, causing [55, 58–60]:

- Gastroparesis, gastroesophageal reflux, ileus, micro-aspirations of gastric contents, food intolerance
- Bacterial overgrowth at the stomach level
- Alteration of the microbiota
- Compromise of splanchnic perfusion and ischemia
- Increased permeability of the gastrointestinal mucosa and bacterial translocation
- Increased intra-abdominal pressure
- Constipation/diarrhea

The alterations indicated have deleterious consequences for the injured brain since they predispose to the development of deleterious complications, including [55, 58–60]:

- Gastrointestinal hemorrhages
- Hydro-electrolytic imbalances
- Respiratory dysfunction (atelectasis, respiratory distress, prolonged mechanical ventilation)
- Infections such as pneumonia, sepsis
- Malnutrition
- Intracranial hypertension

7.4.3.3 Brain-Liver Crosstalk

At the hepatic level, brain injury, fundamentally mediated by the activation of the sympathetic system, triggers alterations in protein metabolism (hypoalbuminemia, coagulation factor deficiency), lipid metabolism (fatty acids necessary for cell repair), and carbohydrate metabolism (hyperglycemia, hypoglycemia), clearly established secondary insults that negatively impact brain function [53, 61, 62].

At the same time, the ability to maintain the detoxification (encephalopathy) and immunological mechanisms necessary to modulate the inflammatory response and to prevent local and distant infections is compromised [53, 61, 62].

7.4.3.4 Brain-Respiratory Crosstalk

The respiratory system is highly susceptible to complications after acute brain injury. This interaction is the most studied [51–53].

The loss of consciousness and the loss of reflexes that protect the airway (cough, swallowing) with the consequent aspiration of gastric contents, plus the alteration of ventilatory mechanics, predispose to the development of atelectasis, pneumonia, and compromised gas exchange (hypoxemia, hypercapnia, hypocapnia) [51–53]. Consequently, the need for an artificial airway and mechanical ventilation alters the usual mechanisms of immunological defense while changing the physiological conditions of ventilation to a positive pressure regime, which under certain circumstances can perpetuate and potentiate pulmonary and systemic inflammation [51–53]. The increase in catecholamine levels causes a state of pulmonary microcirculation hypertension, which together with the inflammatory increase in the permeability of the alveolar-capillary barrier constitute the key substrates for the development of neurogenic pulmonary edema [51–53].

Additionally, the brain-digestive interaction changes the conditions of the intestinal microbiota, causing pathogenic bacterial overgrowth, a substrate for the development of ventilator-associated pneumonia [51–53].

7.4.3.5 Brain-Bone and Muscle Crosstalk

The combination of the mechanism of the biological response to injury already discussed above acts at the level of the Beta receptors of osteoblasts and osteoclasts, decreasing bone formation and increasing bone resorption [51, 52].

At the muscular level, protein catabolism, inflammation, overactivity of the autonomic nervous system, and free oxygen radicals contribute to the decrease in muscle mass and atrophy [51, 52]. Five to 20% of victims of severe cranial trauma present heteropic ossification [51, 52].

7.4.3.6 Brain-Renal Crosstalk

Renal perfusion compromise secondary to increased sympathetic tone and pro-inflammatory mediators with the addition of vasopressin, atrial natriuretic peptide, and the renin-angiotensin-aldosterone system dysfunction, alter renal physiology causing [51–53]:

- Acute kidney injury
- Specific syndromes (inappropriate secretion of antidiuretic hormone, cerebral salt wasting, diabetes insipidus)

which in turn mark the genesis of

- Hydro-electrolytic imbalances (hyponatremia, hypovolemia, hypernatremia)
- Alterations in acid-base homeostasis
- Plasma osmolarity disorders

all of which are seriously detrimental to the injured brain, predisposing it to the development

- Cerebral edema
- Intracranial hypertension
- Cerebral tissue hypoxia

7.4.3.7 Brain-Endocrine System Crosstalk

As a consequence of the increase in circulating catecholamines, inflammation, ischemia, or direct structural damage caused by the primary injury, the endocrine system presents alterations at different levels, either as a result of the inhibition of synthesis or the release of different hormonal axis [51, 52]. Nearly, 25–50% of individuals who suffer cranial trauma will develop pituitary dysfunction. Its impact in the acute stage is unknown with certainty. Among the most prominent syndromes are [51, 52]:

- Pan hypopituitarism
- Central diabetes insipidus
- Euthyroid sick syndrome

- Hypercortisolism

7.4.3.8 Anatomical Brain-Thorax-Abdomen Interaction

Both the afferent arterial blood flow (carotid arteries) and the efferent venous flow (jugular veins) to and from the brain parenchyma travel along the neck toward the thorax, maintaining a communication between both cavities [4, 5, 63]. For its part, the abdomen is in close interaction with the thorax through the diaphragm and the corresponding orifices through which both the aorta and the inferior vena cava pass [4, 5, 63].

Considering the anatomical communication between the skull, thorax, and abdomen, any pressure increase in extracranial body compartments can affect the intracranial pressure (ICP) and cerebral perfusion pressure (CPP), so the pressure increase in one body compartment can affect pressure in another body compartment [4, 5, 63]. ICP has been shown to have a complex relationship with both intra-abdominal pressure (IAP) and intrathoracic pressure (ITP) [4, 5, 63].

If ITP or IAP increases, ICP and CPP can be compromised by the following principal mechanisms [4, 5, 63]:

- Cerebral venous drainage compromise
- Decreased mean arterial pressure

Increased IAP increases ITP through diaphragm elevation, inducing higher peak airway pressures while decreasing functional residual capacity, lung volume, and chest wall compliance [4, 5, 63]. Positive pressure causes an increase in intrapleural pressure, which in turn increases pulmonary artery pressure and right ventricular afterload. Increased IAP also decreases cardiac compliance and cardiac output, all of which could potentially decrease CPP and exacerbate ICP increase if the venous return is limited [4, 5, 63]. Fluid resuscitation may increase IAP and also contribute to ITP and ICP increase (Fig. 7.5) [4, 5, 63].

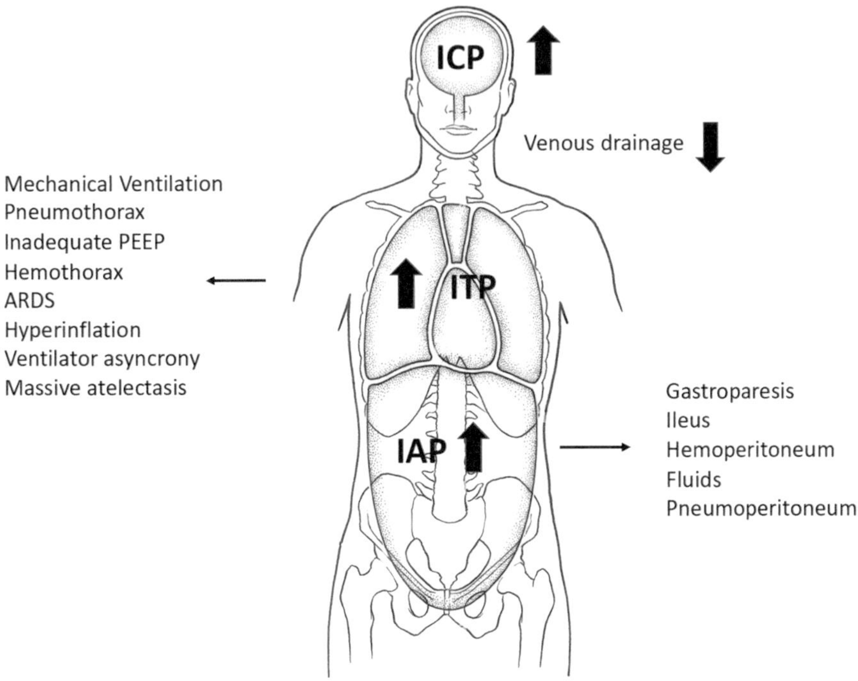

Fig. 7.5 Interplay between intra-abdominal (IAP), intrathoracic (ITP), and intracranial pressure (ICP). Any increase in IAP or ITP decreases venous drainage to the heart increasing cerebral venous pressure and ICP

References

1. Stocchetti N, Carbonara M, Citerio G, Ercole A, Skrifvars MB, Smielewski P, et al. Severe traumatic brain injury: targeted management in the intensive care unit. Lancet Neurol. 2017;16:452–64.
2. Badiwhala JH, Wilson JR, Fehlings MG. Global burden of traumatic brain and spinal cord injury. Lancet Neurol. 2019;18:24–5.
3. Wang K, Cui D, Gao L. Traumatic brain injury: a review of characteristics, molecular basis and management. Front Biosci. 2016;21:890–9.
4. Godoy DA, Khan AA, Rubiano AM. Management of severe traumatic brain injury: a practical approach. In: Rabinstein A, editor. Neurological emergencies. Cham: Springer; 2020. p. 245–70.
5. Godoy DA, Videtta W, Di Napoli M. Practical approach to posttraumatic intracranial hypertension according to pathophysiologic reasoning. Neurol Clin. 2017;35:613–40. https://doi.org/10.1016/j.ncl.2017.06.002.
6. Gennarelli TA. Mechanisms of brain injury. J Emerg Med. 1993;11(Suppl 1):5–11.
7. Chesnut RM. A conceptual approach to managing severe traumatic brain injury in a time of uncertainly. Ann N Y Acad Sci. 2015;1345:99–107.
8. Godoy DA, Murillo-Cabezas F. Evolutionary conceptualization of the injury mechanisms in traumatic brain injury. Med Intensiva (Engl Ed). 2022;46:90–3. https://doi.org/10.1016/j.medine.2021.11.009.

9. Kaur P, Sharma S. Recent advances in pathophysiology of traumatic brain injury. Curr Neuropharmacol. 2018;16:1224–38. https://doi.org/10.2174/1570159X15666170613083606.
10. Battaglini D, De Rosa S, Godoy DA. Crosstalk between the nervous system and systemic organs in acute brain injury. Neurocrit Care. 2023;40 https://doi.org/10.1007/s12028-023-01725-1.
11. Chesnut RM, Marshall LF, Klauber MR, et al. The role of secondary brain injury in determining outcome from severe head injury. J Trauma. 1993;34:216–22. https://doi.org/10.1097/00005373-199302000-00006.
12. McHugh GS, Engel DC, Butcher I, Steyerberg EW, Lu J, Mushkudiani N, et al. Prognostic value of secondary insults in traumatic brain injury: results from the IMPACT study. J Neurotrauma. 2007;24:287–93. https://doi.org/10.1089/neu.2006.0031.
13. Puccio AM, Alexander S. Chapter 4 genomics, transcriptomics, and epigenomics in traumatic brain injury research. Annu Rev Nurs Res. 2015;33:75–109. https://doi.org/10.1891/0739-6686.33.75.
14. Kals M, Kunzmann K, Parodi L, Radmanesh F, Wilson L, Izzy S, et al. Genetic associations in Neurotrauma (GAIN) consortium (with contribution from the CENTER-TBI, TRACK-TBI, CABI, MGB, and TBIcare studies). A genome-wide association study of outcome from traumatic brain injury. EBioMedicine. 2022;77:103933. https://doi.org/10.1016/j.ebiom.2022.103933.
15. Li L, Bao Y, He S, Wang G, Guan Y, Ma D, et al. The association between apolipoprotein E and functional outcome after traumatic brain injury: a meta-analysis. Medicine. 2015;94:e2028.
16. Dewan MC, Rattani A, Gupta S, Baticulon RE, Hung Y-C, Punchak M, Agrawal A, Adeleye AO, Shrime MG, Rubiano AM, Rosenfeld JV, Park KB. Estimating the global incidence of traumatic brain injury. J Neurosurg. 2018;130:1080–97.
17. Shaik NF, Law CA, Elser H, Schneider ALC. Trends in traumatic brain injury mortality in the US. JAMA Neurol. 2023;28:3670–82.
18. Menon DK, Schwab K, Wright DW, Maas AI. Position statement: definition of traumatic brain injury. Arch Phys Med Rehabil. 2010;91:1637–40.
19. Jarrahi A, Braun M, Ahluwalia M, Gupta RV, Wilson M, Munie S, Ahluwalia P, Vender JR, Vale FL, Dhandapani KM, et al. Revisiting traumatic brain injury: from molecular mechanisms to therapeutic interventions. Biomedicine. 2020;8:389.
20. Perea G, Navarrete M, Araque A. Tripartite synapses: astrocytes process and control synaptic information. Trends Neurosci. 2009;32:421–31.
21. Mira RG, Cerpa W. Building a bridge between NMDAR-mediated excitotoxicity and mitochondrial dysfunction in chronic and acute diseases. Cell Mol Neurobiol. 2021;41:1413–30.
22. Fields RD, Stevens-Graham B. New insights into neuron-glia communication. Science. 2002;298(5593):556–62.
23. Allen NJ, Káradóttir R, Attwell D. Reversal or reduction of glutamate and GABA transport in CNS pathology and therapy. Pflugers Arch. 2004;449:132–42.
24. Zauner A, Daugherty WP, Bullock MR. Warner DS (2002) Brain oxygenation and energy metabolism: part I-biological function and pathophysiology. Neurosurgery. 2002;51:289–301. discussion 302
25. Graham DI, Adams JH, Doyle D. Ischaemic brain damage in fatal non-missile head injuries. J Neurol Sci. 1978;39:213–34.
26. Abate MG, Trivedi M, Fryer TD, Smielewski P, Chatfield DA, Williams GB, Aigbirhio F, Carpenter TA, Pickard JD, Menon DK, Coles JP. Early derangements in oxygen and glucose metabolism following head injury: the ischemic penumbra and pathophysiological heterogeneity. Neurocrit Care. 2008;9:319–25.
27. Liesz A, Dalpke A, Mracsko E, Antoine DJ, Roth S, Zhou W, Yang H, Na S-Y, Akhisaroglu M, Fleming T, Eigenbrod T, Nawroth PP, Tracey KJ, Veltkamp R. DAMP signaling is a key pathway inducing immune modulation after brain injury. J Neurosci. 2015;35:583–98.
28. Ransohoff RM, Perry VH. Microglial physiology: unique stimuli, specialized responses. Annu Rev Immunol. 2009;27:119–45.
29. Laird MD, Vender JR, Dhandapani KM. Opposing roles for reactive astrocytes following traumatic brain injury. Neurosignals. 2008;16:154–64.

30. Roth TL, Nayak D, Atanasijevic T, Koretsky AP, Latour LL, McGavern DB. Transcranial amelioration of inflammation and cell death after brain injury. Nature. 2014;505:223–8.
31. Xie L, Yang S-H. Interaction of astrocytes and T cells in physiological and pathological conditions. Brain Res. 2015;1623:63–73.
32. Szabó I, Zoratti M. The giant channel of the inner mitochondrial membrane is inhibited by cyclosporin A. J Biol Chem. 1991;266:3376–9.
33. Lamade AM, Anthonymuthu TS, Hier ZE, Gao Y, Kagan VE, Bayır H. Mitochondrial damage & lipid signaling in traumatic brain injury. Exp Neurol. 2020;329:113307.
34. Fesharaki-Zadeh A. Oxidative stress in traumatic brain injury. Int J Mol Sci. 2022;23:13000.
35. Cornelius C, Crupi R, Calabrese V, Graziano A, Milone P, Pennisi G, Radak Z, Calabrese EJ, Cuzzocrea S. Traumatic brain injury: oxidative stress and neuroprotection. Antioxid Redox Signal. 2013;19:836–53.
36. Arundine M, Tymianski M. Molecular mechanisms of glutamate-dependent neurodegeneration in ischemia and traumatic brain injury. Cell Mol Life Sci. 2004;61:657–68.
37. Miller JD, Becker DP, Ward JD, Sullivan HG, Adams WE, Rosner MJ. Significance of intracranial hypertension in severe head injury. J Neurosurg. 1977;47:503–16.
38. Klatzo I, Presidental address. Neuropathological aspects of brain edema. J Neuropathol Exp Neurol. 1967;26:1–14.
39. Marmarou A, Signoretti S, Fatouros PP, Portella G, Aygok GA, Bullock MR. Predominance of cellular edema in traumatic brain swelling in patients with severe head injuries. J Neurosurg. 2006;104:720–30.
40. Katayama Y, Mori T, Maeda T, Kawamata T. Pathogenesis of the mass effect of cerebral contusions: rapid increase in osmolality within the contusion necrosis. Acta Neurochir Suppl. 1998;71:289–92.
41. Jha RM, Kochanek PM, Simard JM. Pathophysiology and treatment of cerebral edema in traumatic brain injury. Neuropharmacology. 2019;145:230–46.
42. Leao AAP. Spreading depression of activity in the cerebral cortex. J Neurophysiol. 1944;7:359–90.
43. Sugaya E, Takato M, Noda Y. Neuronal and glial activity during spreading depression in cerebral cortex of cat. J Neurophysiol. 1975;38:822–41.
44. Kraig RP, Nicholson C. Extracellular ionic variations during spreading depression. Neuroscience. 1978;3:1045–59.
45. Pietrobon D, Moskowitz M. Chaos and commotion in the wake of cortical spreading depression and spreading depolarizations. Nat Rev Neurosci. 2014;15:379–93.
46. Dreier JP. The role of spreading depression, spreading depolarization and spreading ischemia in neurological disease. Nat Med. 2011;17:439–47.
47. Hertle DN, Dreier JP, Woitzik J, Hartings JA, Bullock R, Okonkwo DO, Shutter LA, Vidgeon S, Strong AJ, Kowoll C, Dohmen C, Diedler J, Veltkamp R, Bruckner T, Unterberg AW, Sakowitz OW. Effect of analgesics and sedatives on the occurrence of spreading depolarizations accompanying acute brain injury. Brain. 2012;135:2390–8.
48. Zhao HT, Tuohy MC, Chow D, Kozberg MG, Kim SH, Shaik MA, Hillman EMC. Neurovascular dynamics of repeated cortical spreading depolarizations after acute brain injury. Cell Rep. 2021;37:109794.
49. Hinzman JM, Andaluz N, Shutter LA, Okonkwo DO, Pahl C, Strong AJ, Dreier JP, Hartings JA. Inverse neurovascular coupling to cortical spreading depolarizations in severe brain trauma. Brain. 2014;137:2960–72.
50. Khalid F, Yang GL, McGuire JL, Robson MJ, Foreman B, Ngwenya LB, Lorenz JN. Autonomic dysfunction following traumatic brain injury: translational insights. Neurosurg Focus. 2019;47:E8. https://doi.org/10.3171/2019.8.FOCUS19517.
51. McDonald SJ, Sharkey JM, Sun M, Kaukas LM, Shultz SR, Turner RJ, et al. Beyond the brain: peripheral interactions after traumatic brain injury. J Neurotrauma. 2020;37:770–81. https://doi.org/10.1089/neu.2019.6885.
52. Rachfalska N, Putowski Z, Krzych ŁJ. Distant organ damage in acute brain injury. Brain Sci. 2020;10:1019. https://doi.org/10.3390/brainsci10121019.

53. Battaglini D, De Rosa S, Godoy DA. Crosstalk between the nervous system and systemic organs in acute brain injury. Neurocrit Care. 2024;40:337–48. Erratum in: Neurocrit Care. 2024; 40: 379–381
54. Mazzeo AT, Micalizzi A, Mascia L, Scicolone A, Siracusano L. Brain–heart crosstalk: the many faces of stress-related cardiomyopathy syndromes in anaesthesia and intensive care. Br J Anaesth. 2014;112:803–15.
55. Battaglini D, Robba C, Lopes da Silva A, dos Santos SC, Leme Silva P, Dal Pizzol F, Pelosi P, Rocco PRM. Brain–heart interaction after acute ischemic stroke. Crit Care. 2020;24:163.
56. El-Menyar A, Goyal A, Latifi R, Al-Thani H, Frishman W. Brain-heart interactions in traumatic brain injury. Cardiol Rev. 2017;25:279–88.
57. Dimitri GM, Beqiri E, Placek MM, Czosnyka M, Stocchetti N, Ercole A, Smielewski P, Li P, Collaborators CENTER-TBI. Modeling brain-heart crosstalk information in patients with traumatic brain injury. Neurocrit Care. 2022;36:738–50.
58. Carabotti M, Scirocco A, Maselli MA, Severi C. The gut-brain axis: interactions between enteric microbiota, central and enteric nervous systems. Ann Gastroenterol. 2018;28:203–9.
59. Holtmann G, Talley NJ. The stomach–brain axis. Best Pract Res Clin Gastroenterol. 2014;28:967–79.
60. Battaglini D, Pimentel-Coelho PM, Robba C, dos Santos CC, Cruz FF, Pelosi P, Rocco PRM. Gut microbiota in acute ischemic stroke: from pathophysiology to therapeutic implication. Front Neurol. 2020;11:598.
61. Matsubara Y, Kiyohara H, Teratani T, Mikami Y, Kanai T. Organ and brain crosstalk: the liver-brain axis in gastrointestinal, liver, and pancreatic diseases. Neuropharmacology. 2022;205:108915.
62. Villapol S. Consequences of hepatic damage after traumatic brain injury: current outlook and potential therapeutic targets. Neural Regen Res. 2016;11:226.
63. Wilson MH. Monro-Kellie 2.0: the dynamic vascular and venous pathophysiological components of intracranial pressure. J Cereb Blood Flow Metab. 2016;36:1338–50.

Melatonin and the Brain-Heart Crosstalk 8

Dorota Siwicka and Wojciech Dabrowski

8.1 Introduction

Brain damage and its consequences are a serious social health problem, commonly associated with longer hospital stay and mortality. A spectrum of potential pathologies may result from traumatic brain injury (TBI) or non-traumatic brain injury (non-TBI), as a result of factors such as enormous stress and emotional experiences, severe general diseases, or a spectrum of post-operative diseases. Recently, head injuries, especially in intensive care conditions, are perceived more like a multifactorial syndrome resulting in multi-organ dysfunction [1].

Brain damage, mainly associated with crucial biochemical, hormonal, immunological, and metabolic disturbances, contributes to BI (brain injury)-related damage to extracerebral organs. These connections are commonly known as brain–multiorgan interactions.

Current treatment recommendations for different brain injuries, especially in intensive care units, are based mainly on clinical symptoms, and disturbances in several biochemical and hormonal pathways, especially tryptophan metabolism, are still underestimated. Tryptophan is metabolized in two pathways: kynurenine and serotonin. Melatonin is the final metabolite of serotonin pathway. Several studies have documented the effective role of melatonin in the central nervous system and extracerebral organs metabolism including the cardiac system. Therefore, the role of melatonin and brain heart axis deserve special attention.

D. Siwicka (✉) · W. Dabrowski
Department of Anaesthesiology and Intensive Care, Medical University of Lublin, Lublin, Poland

D. Battaglini et al. (eds.), *Organ System Crosstalk in Critical Illness*, https://doi.org/10.1007/978-3-032-01024-7_8

8.2 The Brain-Heart Interaction

The interaction between the brain and the heart was first described in 1942 by Walter Cannon [2].

"Brain-heart axis" refers to the bidirectional interaction between the brain and the heart. It involves complex pathways involving the autonomic nervous system, hormones, and other factors such as cytokines [3].

The organization of the autonomic nervous system is divided into the afferent (central) part, integrating centers, and the efferent (centrifugal) part. Receptors that are crucial for the autonomic regulation of the circulatory system are: arterial baroreceptors, mechanoreceptors located in the wall of the heart chambers, cardiac chemoreceptors, vascular chemoreceptors, and central chemoreceptors (central chemodetectors) and propioceptors. Nerve impulses generated as a result of receptor stimulation are transmitted to central integrating centers located in the hypothalamus, brainstem, and medulla oblongata. A special element integrating afferent pathways from receptors of the cardiovascular system is the nucleus of the solitary tract. In central integrating centers, information transmitted from receptors is modulated by impulses from other parts of the nervous system, including higher centers.

The centrifugal part of autonomic reflexes is organized in the form of two opposing efferent parts: sympathetic and parasympathetic.

The cardiovascular control center is located in three locations: the ventrolateral part of the medulla oblongata, the sympathetic part in the anterior region, and the parasympathetic part in the posterior region.

The first sympathetic neurons (preganglionic neurons) innervating the heart are located in the intermediate-lateral nuclei of the lateral horns of the spinal cord at the level (C8) Th1-Th4 (Th5).

Their axons leave the spinal cord through the ventral roots and, along the course of the spinal nerves, reach the sympathetic trunk, where they synapse with other sympathetic neurons (postganglionic neurons).

Axons of sympathetic postganglionic neurons reach the effector organs in the form of cardiac and vascular nerves.

Importantly, the heart is innervated parasympathetically by the vagus nerves. The rich autonomic innervation of the heart forms the cardiac plexus, which supplies innervation carried by cervical and thoracic sympathetic cardiac nerves and parasympathetic cardiac branches branching directly from the vagus nerve or indirectly from the superior and inferior laryngeal nerves. Sympathetic activation leads to the contraction of smooth muscles of blood vessels and has positive chrono-, dromo-, and inotropic effects. On the contrary, stimulation of the parasympathetic part causes feedback inhibition of the sympathetic system, has a vasodilatory effect mainly in the arteries, inhibits the sinus node, negatively affects atrioventricular conduction, as well as the contractility of cardiomyocytes (especially atrial). The main neurotransmitter in postganglionic synapses of sympathetic endings is norepinephrine, and in parasympathetic endings, acetylcholine.

In stress response, corticotropin-releasing factor (CRF) activates a cascade of mechanisms of glucocorticoid release from the adrenal cortex. Several events are evolved to control the HPA (hypothalamic-pituitary-adrenal) axis activation and integrate the stress response.

The activity of the HPA axis is controlled by the hypothalamic paraventricular nucleus—the main control center, secreting not only CRF but also vasopressin.

The inhibitory effect of glucocorticoids plays an important role in regulating the time and magnitude of glucocorticoid release. In feedback, the HPA axis regulates the level of the hypothalamus activation by a diverse group of afferent signals from limbic, mid-brain, and brain stem nuclei. The mentioned response is additionally mediated by brain stem noradrenergic neurons, sympathetic and renomedullary circuits, and parasympathetic systems.

8.3 Melatonin

Melatonin is a hormone produced naturally by the pineal gland in the brain, but also the intestines, skin, retina, testes, ovaries, glial, microglial cells, and even lymphocytes [4–7].

Melatonin is synthesized from tryptophan, which is hydroxylated to 5-hydroxytryptophan. The 5-hydroxytryptophan is decarbonized into serotonin, which is transferred to melatonin [5]. Serotonin is the precursor of melatonin via sequential acetylation to N-acetylserotonin (NAS) by AANAT or arylamine N-acetyltransferase (NAT) after methylation by hydroxyindole-O-methyltransferase (HIOMT) [8, 9].

The melatonin concentration in the blood depends on the circadian rhythm. The highest concentration is observed at night [4] Fig. 8.1.

Melatonin is metabolized by various, concurrent catabolic pathways, including enzymatic (indole and kynurenic pathways) and direct, non-enzymatic transformations [10]. The half-life of melatonin in plasma is approximately 40 minutes [11].

Melatonin degradation occurs at the site of its synthesis and in the liver, where melatonin is metabolized by cytochrome P-450 enzymes, especially the isoforms CYP1A1, CYP1A2, CYP2C19, and CYP2C9 [10].

Most circulating melatonin is metabolized in the liver to 6-hydroxymelatonin and then to 6-hydroxymelatonin sulfate. In the kynurenic pathway, melatonin is metabolized mainly to N1-acetyl-N2-formyl-5-methoxykynuramine (AFMK) and then to N1-acetyl-5-methoxykynuramine (AMK). Interestingly, both AFMK and AMK also have strong antioxidant properties [7, 12].

Melatonin is also metabolized non-enzymatically in direct reaction with reactive oxygen and nitrogen species [9, 13]. It has a high affinity for free radicals, and its best-known reaction is the interaction with the hydroxyl radical (OH–).

According to available research, the reaction of melatonin with two OH– in the presence of Fe2+ and UV leads to the formation of cyclic 3-hydroxymelatonin, which was detected in human urine [14]. The chemical structure of cyclic 3-hydroxymelatonin is similar to acetylcholinesterase inhibitors, drugs that improve brain regeneration after TBI [15].

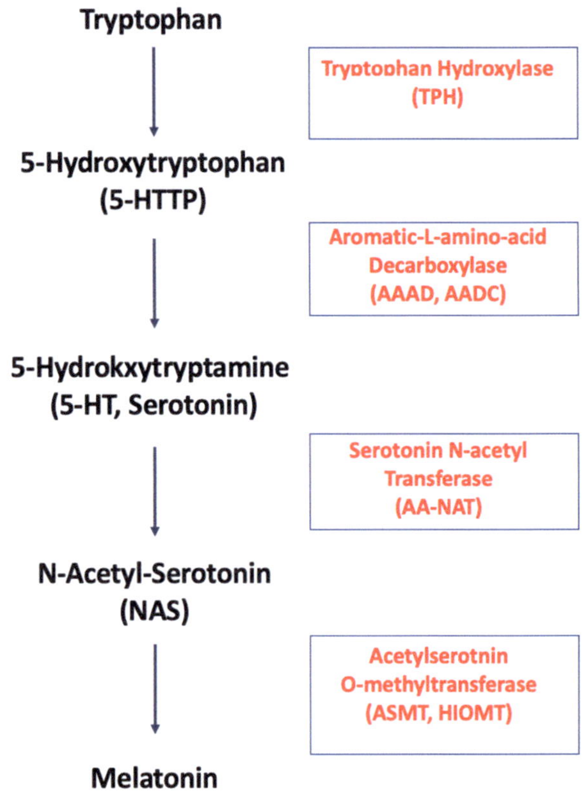

Fig. 8.1 Synthesis pathway of melatonin

Melatonin presents a broad spectrum of action because it synchronizes the circadian rhythm, regulates energy metabolism and the aging process, alleviates blood-brain barrier (BBB) disorders, and modulates the neuroinflammatory response and oxidative stress in the brain and peripheral tissues [16].

Strong antioxidant, anti-inflammatory, and anti-apoptotic properties are mainly effected at the level of cellular respiration, promoting mitochondrial oxidative phosphorylation [17]. A precursor of melatonin, N-acetylserotonin (NAS) presents also a strong antioxidant effect, especially against the peroxidation of iron, copper, H_2O_2, and lipids [18]. Both NAS and melatonin increase the antioxidant capacity, demonstrated by decreased malonaldehyde +4-hydroxynonenal (MDA + 4-HNE) and increased cellular glutathione peroxidase (GPx) levels [19].

Melatonin activity is associated with MT1 and MT2 receptors, which were found in the brain and several extracerebral organs including the heart [20].

As demonstrated above, melatonin possesses strong antioxidant and anti-inflammatory properties; however, these activities are still not well recognized, especially in extracerebral organs. A few studies described the effect of melatonin on post-ischemic cardiac function [21, 22]. Unfortunately, the effect of melatonin on brain-heart interaction has been poorly documented.

8.4 Potential Disturbances of Brain-Heart Interaction

Recent experimental data documented that hypothalamic stimulation is associated with increased sympathetic nerve impulsation to the heart and a lowered ventricular fibrillation threshold [23].

Oppenheimer et al. documented that prolonged activation of the left insula cortex is connected with bradycardia, with ST segment depression and elevated norepinephrine concentration in plasma. Importantly, stimulation of the right insula predisposes to tachycardia [24].

These results are significantly related to the results that Seifert and his research group, who found that in patients after ischemic stroke of the right insula and right inferior parietal lobe, there is importantly higher incidence of life-threatening cardiac arrhythmias and elevated troponin levels [25].

It is also worth mentioning a study based on the analysis of 730 patients with acute ischemic stroke. The authors showed that the damage of the right insula (posterior, superior, and medial parts) and the right parietal lobule was significantly related to myocardial damage [26].

This may suggest that ischemia of the right posterior insula increases the sympathetic activity of the heart and may lead to myocardial damage.

Myocardial dysfunction associated with central nervous system (CNS) damage may also be caused by excessive catecholamine release, following acute trauma or stress. Brain damage itself causes an increase in sympathetic tone, predisposing to additional release of catecholamines from synapses and adrenal glands [27].

A rapid increase in norepinephrine and epinephrine levels is noticeable already 5 minutes after the occurrence of subarachnoid hemorrhage [28]. It is important that the observed increase is associated with an increase in the concentration of troponin T in plasma and muscle creatine kinase (CK-MB). It is worth noting that the pathomechanism of myocardial damage, resulting from the increase in catecholamines, is multifactorial. These include: spasm of epicardial microarteries, increased myocardial contractility with associated transient left ventricular outflow obstruction, increased calcium overload of myocytes (Ca2+), increased production of free radicals, and myocyte apoptosis [29].

8.5 Brain Damage and Melatonin

Melatonin presents beneficial effects in various cerebral diseases, including brain trauma, ischemia, subarachnoid hemorrhage, and even COVID-19 neurological complications.

As a result of a CNS injury, daily changes in melatonin concentrations in the blood are observed. In patients with TBI, the reduction in melatonin levels depends on the severity of the injury [30, 31]. A similar effect is observed in patients treated for subarachnoid hemorrhage (SAH). An important factor in the disruption of the circadian rhythm in melatonin synthesis in this group of patients is age and the area of bleeding. According to Neumaier et al., patients with aneurysms located in the posterior part of the cerebral circulation had significantly lower blood melatonin concentrations compared to patients with aneurysms in the anterior part [32]. Additionally, the authors showed that the highest concentration of melatonin in the blood was recorded in patients with poor clinical condition, with aneurysms of the anterior communicating artery.

Melatonin significantly inhibits the release of stress hormone stimulated by adrenocorticotropes [33]. It also reduces the degree of TBI-related inflammatory response, neuronal apoptosis, and oxidative stress [34].

Moreover, melatonin supply attenuates BBB permeability and protein degradation by inhibiting the TLR4/MF-κB and matrix metalloproteinase-9 signaling pathways [35].

An experimental study has shown that melatonin reduces neuronal damage, neuroinflammation, and neurodegeneration of the brain and skin by inhibiting the hypothalamic-pituitary-adrenal (HPA) axis [36]. Moreover, prophylactic administration of melatonin inhibits endoplasmic reticulum stress and autophagy by suppressing the Jun-N-terminal kinase pathway, which is one of the main triggers of mitogen-activated protein kinase (MAPK) that induces apoptosis. It is worth noting that endoplasmic reticulum stress and autophagy are among the main molecular pathomechanisms of cerebral ischemia/reperfusion injury [37].

Decreased melatonin levels reduce anti-inflammatory and antioxidant abilities, not only in the brain, but in other crucial organs, including the heart.

Although there are no data documenting an association between melatonin deficiency and TBI-related cardiac dysfunction, maintaining an adequate blood level of melatonin may be an important strategy to reduce cerebral abnormalities or related cardiac dysfunction.

8.6 Cerebral Effect of Melatonin on TBI-Related Cardiac Dysfunction

In brain damage, melatonin has broadly understood neuroprotective properties. It reduces inflammation of the nervous system, production of free radicals, and apoptosis after different brain injuries.

Melatonin reduces the ROS (reactive oxidative species)-induced depolarization of the mitochondrial membrane potential, contributing to a decrease in mitochondrial swelling, opens the mitochondrial permeability transition pore, and releases cytochrome C.

This effect is similar to the pharmacological suppression of Ca2+ regulatory mechanisms [38].

Melatonin also plays a physiologically important role in the regulation of transient receptor potential M2 (TRPM2), which is a calcium-permeable, non-selective cation channel responsible for Ca2+ entry into neurons and astrocytes [39].

The antioxidant effect is also associated with the stimulation of antioxidant enzymes, such as superoxide dismutase and glutathione peroxidase, and the downregulation of pro-oxidant enzymes.

The antioxidant properties of AFMK are also related to electron donation, reducing and neutralizing the potential of free radicals [40]. The AMK, a conversion product of AFMK, can inhibit neuronal nitric oxide synthase (nNOS) by interacting with Ca2+-calmodulin, which plays a key role in various neural functions, including cognitive functions [41, 42]. Interestingly, many brain diseases are associated with cardiac dysfunction, and improved cognitive function alleviates cardiac disability [43].

The study by Yang et al. showed that the administration of melatonin to the paraventricular nucleus improves the activity of superoxide dismutase, corrects the level of NO^-, and reduces the level of interleukin 1β and norepinephrine. This inhibits the activity of the sympathetic nervous system, thus protecting the damaged heart muscle [44]. The authors showed that the suppression effect depends on the dose. Intravenous injection of melatonin at a dose of 1–2 mg inhibited the activity of adrenal nerves in the suprachiasmatic nucleus of the hypothalamus, while injection at a dose of 10–20 mg increased their activity [45].

Melatonin production also depends on the activity of adrenoreceptors. However, the synthesis by the pineal gland can be intensified by corticosterone only after activation of β-adrenergic receptors, as demonstrated in an animal model [46].

Melatonin inhibits the increased activity of the hypothalamus and pituitary gland, which are well-known mechanisms that limit the stimulation of the adrenal glands to release catecholamines [47].

Increased intracerebral melatonin concentrations may modulate autonomic activity in the brain and thus alleviate damage to extracerebral organs. Melatonin may also directly protect extracerebral organs. Therefore, its supplementation may also reduce cardiac dysfunction associated with brain damage.

It is worth to observe the particular role of stimulation of the hypothalamic nuclei in the development of ECG changes. The paraventricular nucleus of the hypothalamus controls the hypothalamic-pituitary-adrenal axis and stimulates the pituitary gland to secrete adrenocorticotropic hormone, which increases the risk of electrocardiographic abnormalities [48].

8.7 Direct Cardiac Protection

The cardioprotective effects of melatonin make it a promising agent for the prevention and treatment of various cardiovascular diseases.

The cardioprotective mechanisms of melatonin include:

- Antioxidant properties
- Anti-inflammatory effects
- Endothelial protection promotes the release of nitric oxide (NO)
- Mitochondrial protection and anti-apoptotic effects
- Regulation of calcium homeostasis
- Reducing the concentration of catecholamines in the blood, mainly by reducing the activity of the HPA axis

The protective effect corresponds with the antioxidant properties of melatonin and is associated with the activation of membrane melatonin receptors MT1 and MT2 [49]. The MT1 receptor in the left ventricular myocardium is activated almost immediately after the induction of ischemia, while the expression of MT2 increases during a four-week observation period. It is worth to mention that cardiac ischemia reduces plasma melatonin concentrations, which predispose to increased production and sensitivity of melatonin receptors in the left ventricle. Therefore, endogenous melatonin plays an important role in heart protection against acute ischemic damage.

Dominguez-Rodriguez et al. documented that in patients with ST-segment elevation myocardial infarction (STEMI) undergoing percutaneous coronary angioplasty, administration of melatonin statistically reduced the severity of the infarction [49]. Recent studies documented also that daily lower serum concentrations occurred in patients with hypertensive cardiomyopathy who developed heart failure and left ventricular hypertrophy. The authors hypothesized that serum melatonin concentration upon admission to hospital can be used as an independent predictor of left ventricular remodeling in patients treated for acute myocardial infarction [50, 51].

Importantly, melatonin regulates intracellular Ca2+ levels in myocytes through the connection of MT2 with intracellular proteins such as calmodulin or tubulin [52]. Modulation of membrane action potential and connexin 43 (Cx43) expression plays a crucial role in the oxidative stress modulation and arrhythmia triggers in cardiac ischemia [53].

8.8 Conclusions

Recent data suggest potential cardiac protective effects of melatonin, especially in brain heart disturbances. More studies are needed to fully understand its mechanisms and therapeutic implications for cardiovascular health.

References

1. Krishnamoorthy V, Komisarow JM, Laskowitz DT, Vavilala MS. Multiorgan dysfunction after severe traumatic brain injury: epidemiology, mechanisms, and clinical management. (1931–3543 (Electronic)).
2. Cannon WB. "Voodoo" death. Am Anthropol. 1942;44(2):169–81.
3. Hu JA-OX, Abdullah A, Nanna MA-O, Soufer RA-O. The brain-heart axis: neuroinflammatory interactions in cardiovascular disease. (1534–3170 (Electronic)).
4. Amaral FGD, Cipolla-Neto J. A brief review about melatonin, a pineal hormone. (2359–4292 (Electronic)).
5. Claustrat B, Brun J, Chazot G. The basic physiology and pathophysiology of melatonin. Sleep Med Rev. 2005;9(1):11–24.
6. Tan D-X, Reiter RJ. An evolutionary view of melatonin synthesis and metabolism related to its biological functions in plants. J Exp Bot. 2020;71(16):4677–89.
7. Tan D-X, Reiter RJ. Mitochondria: the birth place, battle ground and the site of melatonin metabolism in cells. Melatonin Res. 2019;2(1):44–66.

8. Iuvone PM, Tosini G, Pozdeyev N, Haque R, Klein DC, Chaurasia SS. Circadian clocks, clock networks, arylalkylamine N-acetyltransferase, and melatonin in the retina. Prog Retin Eye Res. 2005;24(4):433–56.
9. Slominski A, Wortsman J, Tobin DJ. The cutaneous serotoninergic/melatoninergic system: securing a place under the sun. FASEB J. 2005;19(2):176–94.
10. Reiter RJ, Mayo JC, Tan DX, Sainz RM, Alatorre-Jimenez M, Qin L. Melatonin as an antioxidant: under promises but over delivers. (1600-079X (Electronic)).
11. Fourtillan JB, Brisson AM, Gobin P, Ingrand I, Decourt JP, Girault J. Bioavailability of melatonin in humans after day-time administration of D7 melatonin. Biopharm Drug Dispos. 2000;21(1):15–22.
12. Mayo JC, Sainz RM, Tan D-X, Hardeland R, Leon J, Rodriguez C, et al. Anti-inflammatory actions of melatonin and its metabolites, N1-acetyl-N2-formyl-5-methoxykynuramine (AFMK) and N1-acetyl-5-methoxykynuramine (AMK), in macrophages. J Neuroimmunol. 2005;165(1–2):139–49.
13. Hardeland R. Melatonin and microglia. Int J Mol Sci. 2021;22(15):8296.
14. Tan D-X, Manchester LC, Reiter RJ, Plummer BF, Hardies LJ, Weintraub ST, et al. A novel melatonin metabolite, cyclic 3-Hydroxymelatonin: a biomarker of in vivo hydroxyl radical generation. Biochem Biophys Res Commun. 1998;253(3):614–20.
15. Florentino SA, Bawany MH, Ma HM. Acetylcholinesterase inhibitors to enhance recovery from traumatic brain injury: a comprehensive review and case series. Brain Inj. 2022;36(4):441–54.
16. Jiménez-Delgado A, Ortiz GG, Delgado-Lara DL, González-Usigli HA, González-Ortiz LJ, Cid-Hernández M, et al. Effect of melatonin administration on mitochondrial activity and oxidative stress markers in patients with Parkinson's disease. (1942–0994 (Electronic)).
17. Martín M, Macías M, León J, Escames G, Khaldy H, Acuña-Castroviejo D. Melatonin increases the activity of the oxidative phosphorylation enzymes and the production of ATP in rat brain and liver mitochondria. (1357–2725 (Print)).
18. Fagali N, Catalá A. The antioxidant behaviour of melatonin and structural analogues during lipid peroxidation depends not only on their functional groups but also on the assay system. Biochem Biophys Res Commun. 2012;423(4):873–7.
19. Oxenkrug G, Requintina P, Bachurin S. Antioxidant and antiaging activity of N-acetylserotonin and melatonin in the in vivo models. (0077–8923 (Print)).
20. Wongprayoon P, Govitrapong P. Melatonin receptor as a drug target for neuroprotection. Curr Mol Pharmacol. 2021;14(2):150–64.
21. Petrosillo G, Di Venosa N, Pistolese M, Casanova G, Tiravanti E, Colantuono G, Federici A, Paradies G, Ruggiero FM. Protective effect of melatonin against mitochondrial dysfunction associated with cardiac ischemia- reperfusion: role of cardiolipin. (1530–6860 (Electronic)).
22. Lochner A, Genade S, Davids A, Ytrehus K, Moolman JA. Short- and long-term effects of melatonin on myocardial post-ischemic recovery. (0742–3098 (Print)).
23. Verrier RL, Calvert A, Lown B. Effect of posterior hypothalamic stimulation on ventricular fibrillation threshold. Am J Physiol. 1975;228(3):923–7.
24. Oppenheimer SM. Neurogenic cardiac effects of cerebrovascular disease. Curr Opin Neurol. 1994;7(1):20–4.
25. Seifert F, Kallmünzer B, Gutjahr I, Breuer L, Winder K, Kaschka I, et al. Neuroanatomical correlates of severe cardiac arrhythmias in acute ischemic stroke. J Neurol. 2015;262:1182–90.
26. Ay H, Koroshetz WJ, Benner T, Vangel MG, Melinosky C, Arsava EM, et al. Neuroanatomic correlates of stroke-related myocardial injury. Neurology. 2006;66(9):1325–9.
27. Masuda T, Sato K, Yamamoto S-i, Matsuyama N, Shimohama T, Matsunaga A, et al. Sympathetic nervous activity and myocardial damage immediately after subarachnoid hemorrhage in a unique animal model. Stroke. 2002;33(6):1671–6.
28. Mazzeo AT, Micalizzi A, Mascia L, Scicolone A, Siracusano L. Brain–heart crosstalk: the many faces of stress-related cardiomyopathy syndromes in anaesthesia and intensive care. Br J Anaesth. 2014;112(5):803–15.

29. Novitzky D, Wicomb WN, Cooper DKC, Rose AG, Reichart B. Prevention of myocardial injury during brain death by total cardiac sympathectomy in the chacma baboon. Ann Thorac Surg. 1986;41(5):520–4.
30. Paparrigopoulos T, Melissaki A, Tsekou H, Efthymiou A, Kribeni G, Baziotis N, et al. Melatonin secretion after head injury: a pilot study. Brain Inj. 2006;20(8):873–8.
31. Seifman MA, Gomes K, Nguyen PN, Bailey M, Rosenfeld JV, Cooper DJ, et al. Measurement of serum melatonin in intensive care unit patients: changes in traumatic brain injury, trauma, and medical conditions. Front Neurol. 2014;5:237.
32. Neumaier F, Weiss M, Veldeman M, Kotliar K, Wiesmann M, Schulze-Steinen H, et al. Changes in endogenous daytime melatonin levels after aneurysmal subarachnoid hemorrhage–preliminary findings from an observational cohort study. Clin Neurol Neurosurg. 2021;208:106870.
33. Torres-Farfan C, Richter HG, Rojas-García P, Vergara M, Forcelledo ML, Valladares LE, et al. mt1 Melatonin receptor in the primate adrenal gland: inhibition of adrenocorticotropin-stimulated cortisol production by melatonin. J Clin Endocrinol Metabol. 2003;88(1):450–8.
34. Blum B, Kaushal S, Khan S, Kim JH, Villalba CLA. Melatonin in traumatic brain injury and cognition. Cureus. 2021;13(9):e17776.
35. Hu Y, Wang Z, Pan S, Zhang H, Fang M, Jiang H, et al. Melatonin protects against blood-brain barrier damage by inhibiting the TLR4/NF-κB signaling pathway after LPS treatment in neonatal rats. Oncotarget. 2017;8(19):31638.
36. Park G, Lee SH, Oh DS, Kim Y. Melatonin inhibits neuronal dysfunction-associated with neuroinflammation by atopic psychological stress in NC/Nga atopic-like mouse models. J Pineal Res. 2017;63(2):e12420.
37. Feng D, Wang B, Wang L, Abraham N, Tao K, Huang L, et al. Pre-ischemia melatonin treatment alleviated acute neuronal injury after ischemic stroke by inhibiting endoplasmic reticulum stress-dependent autophagy via PERK and IRE 1 signalings. J Pineal Res. 2017;62(3):e12395.
38. Jou MJ, Peng TI, Yu PZ, Jou SB, Reiter RJ, Chen JY, et al. Melatonin protects against common deletion of mitochondrial DNA-augmented mitochondrial oxidative stress and apoptosis. J Pineal Res. 2007;43(4):389–403.
39. Yürüker V, Nazıroğlu M, Şenol N. Reduction in traumatic brain injury-induced oxidative stress, apoptosis, and calcium entry in rat hippocampus by melatonin: possible involvement of TRPM2 channels. Metab Brain Dis. 2015;30:223–31.
40. Escribano BM, Colin-Gonzalez AL, Santamaría A, Túnez I. The role of melatonin in multiple sclerosis, Huntington's disease and cerebral ischemia. CNS Neurol Disord Drug Targets. 2014;13(6):1096–119.
41. Mochida S. Ca^{2+}/calmodulin and presynaptic short-term plasticity. ISRN Neurol. 2011;2011:919043.
42. León J, Escames G, Rodríguez MI, López LC, Tapias V, Entrena A, et al. Inhibition of neuronal nitric oxide synthase activity by N1-acetyl-5-methoxykynuramine, a brain metabolite of melatonin. J Neurochem. 2006;98(6):2023–33.
43. Hilal S, Chai YL, Ikram MK, Elangovan S, Yeow TB, Xin X, et al. Markers of cardiac dysfunction in cognitive impairment and dementia. Medicine. 2015;94(1):e297.
44. Yang J-B, Kang Y-M, Zhang C, Yu X-J, Chen W-S. Infusion of melatonin into the paraventricular nucleus ameliorates myocardial ischemia–reperfusion injury by regulating oxidative stress and inflammatory cytokines. J Cardiovasc Pharmacol. 2019;74(4):336–47.
45. Niijima A, Chun S-J, Shima T, Bizot-Espiard J-G, Guardiola-Lemaitre B, Nagai K. Effect of intravenous administration of melatonin on the efferent activity of the adrenal nerve. J Auton Nerv Syst. 1998;71(2–3):134–8.
46. Fernandes PA, Tamura EK, D'Argenio-Garcia L, Muxel SM, da Silveira Cruz-Machado S, Marcola M, et al. Dual effect of catecholamines and corticosterone crosstalk on pineal gland melatonin synthesis. Neuroendocrinology. 2016;104(2):126–34.
47. Weidenfeld Y, Schmidt U, Nir I. The effect of exogenous melatonin on the hypothalamic-pituitary-adrenal axis in intact and pinealectomized rats under basal and stressed conditions. J Pineal Res. 1993;14(2):60–6.

48. Whitnall MH. Regulation of the hypothalamic corticotropin-releasing hormone neurosecretory system. Prog Neurobiol. 1993;40(5):573–629.
49. Dominguez-Rodriguez A, Abreu-Gonzalez P, de la Torre-Hernandez JM, Consuegra-Sanchez L, Piccolo R, Gonzalez-Gonzalez J, et al. Usefulness of early treatment with melatonin to reduce infarct size in patients with ST-segment elevation myocardial infarction receiving percutaneous coronary intervention (from the melatonin adjunct in the acute myocardial infarction treated with angioplasty trial). Am J Cardiol. 2017;120(4):522–6.
50. Dominguez-Rodriguez A, Abreu-Gonzalez P, Arroyo-Ucar E, Reiter RJ. Decreased level of melatonin in serum predicts left ventricular remodelling after acute myocardial infarction. J Pineal Res. 2012;53(3):319–23.
51. Dominguez-Rodriguez A, Abreu-Gonzalez P, Arroyo-Ucar E, Avanzas P, Reiter RJ. Global left ventricular longitudinal strain is associated with decreased melatonin levels in patients with acute myocardial infarction: a two-dimensional speckle tracking study. Biomarkers. 2013;18(4):310–3.
52. Benítez-King G. Melatonin as a cytoskeletal modulator: implications for cell physiology and disease. J Pineal Res. 2006;40(1):1–9.
53. Sedova KA, Bernikova OG, Cuprova JI, Ivanova AD, Kutaeva GA, Pliss MG, et al. Association between antiarrhythmic, electrophysiological, and antioxidative effects of melatonin in ischemia/reperfusion. Int J Mol Sci. 2019;20(24):6331.

Subarachnoid Hemorrhage and System Crosstalk

9

Nekane Romero-García, A. Devís-Peiró,
Berta Monleón López, and Rafael Badenes

9.1 Introduction and Pathophysiology of SAH

9.1.1 Definition and Epidemiology of SAH

Subarachnoid hemorrhage (SAH) is defined as intracranial bleeding within the subarachnoid space, between the arachnoid and pia mater. Aneurysmal subarachnoid hemorrhage (aSAH) represents the most frequent cause of spontaneous SAH, accounting for 80% of global incidence. This condition affects 6.1 per 100,000 people per year and has an overall prevalence of 8.09 million cases [13]. It entails a high mortality rate, both pre- and in-hospital, of approximately 26% and 20%, respectively, in 2021, with important variations among countries [78]. Unlike other types of intracranial hemorrhage, aSAH affects patients of working age and is associated with high morbidity and socio-economic cost [22]. Only 49% of patients achieve a full recovery (Glasgow Outcome Scale, GOS, of 5) and 64% achieve independence (GOS 4–5 or modified Rankin Scale 0–2) [45]. Non-aneurysmal SAH represents only 20% and is most often caused by vascular malformations (10%), intracranial artery dissection, or traumatic brain injury (TBI) [75].

The origin of aSAH is multifactorial and comprises modifiable and non-modifiable risk factors. Modifiable risk factors include hypertension, smoking, and alcohol abuse; non-modifiable risk factors include age over 55 years, female sex,

N. Romero-García · A. Devís-Peiró · B. Monleón López
Department Anesthesiology, Critical Care and Pain Clinic, Hospital Clínic Universitari, Valencia, Spain

Department of Surgery, University of Valencia, Valencia, Spain

Biomedical Health Institute, INCLIVA VLC, Valencia, Spain

R. Badenes (✉)
Biomedical Health Institute, INCLIVA VLC, Valencia, Spain

D. Battaglini et al. (eds.), *Organ System Crosstalk in Critical Illness*,
https://doi.org/10.1007/978-3-032-01024-7_9

and family history (≥2 first-degree relatives with cerebral aneurysm, with a prevalence of 12%). Other risk factors include diabetes mellitus (only in the perimesencephalic SAH subtype) and connective tissue diseases. Risk factors for aneurysm rupture include intense physical exercise and traumatic brain injury, although only 50% of cases have an identifiable triggering factor [82]. The use of oral anticoagulants is associated in the literature with increased rebleeding, although the use of antiplatelet drugs is not well documented. The most common location of the aneurysm in aSAH is the anterior communicating artery (36%), followed by the middle cerebral artery (26%) [22].

9.1.2 Pathophysiology of SAH

The process that occurs after aneurysm rupture can be divided into three phases: acute (0–24 h), subacute or early brain injury (EBI, ≤72 h), and chronic (3–14 days). After an aneurysm rupture, the first stimulus is a rapid rise in intracranial pressure (ICP), before returning to slightly above baseline. The rise in ICP lowers cerebral perfusion pressure (CPP) and reduces cerebral blood flow (CBF). Although CPP recovers, reduced CBF and increased arterial tone persist [7]. Injury following SAH is not limited to ischemia on the territory of the ruptured vessel but is amplified by signaling cascades that include microglia- and astrocyte-mediated inflammatory response, sympathetic nervous system activation, and oxidative stress intrinsically related to neuronal apoptosis [58].

Over time, extravasated blood begins to aggravate these factors, culminating in delayed cerebral ischemia (DCI) 3–14 days after SAH. It is now believed that DCI is caused by the combined effects of large vessel vasospasm and inflammatory cascade triggered during EBI [11]. Approximately 70% of aSAH patients develop angiographic vasospasm 3–14 days after the initial rupture [44]. Angiographic narrowing is caused by clot-induced vasoconstriction, and its severity and duration are related to the thickness, density, location, and persistence of blood at the subarachnoid level. The main cause of angiographic vasospasm is the release of hemoglobin and erythrocyte content through hemolysis, which initiates several processes, such as the release of reactive oxygen species, inflammation, and endothelial injury, leading to increased endothelin-1 expression and reduced NO levels [55] (Fig. 9.1).

Cerebral autoregulation (CA), which is defined as the intrinsic capacity of brain vasculature to maintain constant cerebral blood flow (CBF) within average values of cerebral perfusion pressure, is notably impaired after SAH [40]. The main physiological mechanism underlying CBF autoregulation is known as the myogenic response, although neurogenic control via the autonomic ganglion may also play a role [81]. Myogenically active vessels, namely small- and medium-sized arteries, experience vasodilation in response to a decrease in transmural pressure, and vice versa. At the level of vascular smooth muscle cells, stretching of the membrane is sensed by mechanosensitive ion channels and triggers depolarization, L-type calcium channel opening, muscle contraction, and vasoconstriction. Several studies show that SAH increases myogenic reactivity through calcium sensitization via

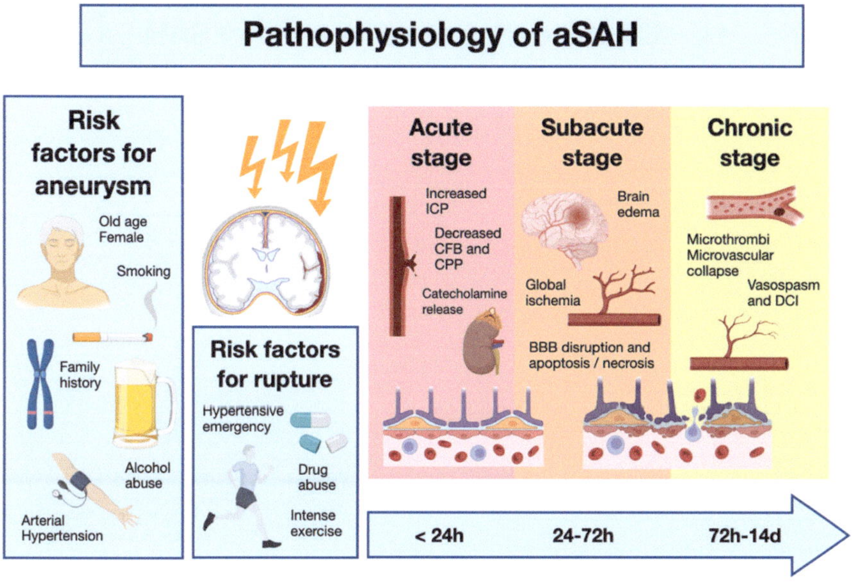

Fig. 9.1 Epidemiology and pathophysiology of SAH. (Source: Author's own elaboration)

sphingosine-1-phosphate-dependent signals, as well as changes in potassium channel expression [39, 79]. Regional ischemia and vasospasm emerge as frequent complications due to augmented vascular tone in this context. Jaeger et al. recently proved an association between impaired cerebral autoregulation, estimated through the index of brain tissue oxygen pressure reactivity, and delayed cerebral infarction and neurological outcomes in SAH patients [26].

9.1.3 Clinical Presentation, Diagnosis, and Management

The typical presentation of SAH is a sudden, severe, thunderclap headache usually accompanied by intractable nausea and vomiting in up to 70% of patients, loss of consciousness (53%), and meningeal signs such as neck stiffness or pain (35%). Some of these criteria are included in the Ottawa rule and should prompt further investigation in the context of possible SAH [22]. The various classification scales for SAH based on clinical or radiological criteria are depicted in Fig. 9.2 [10, 16, 24, 72]. The diagnosis of SAH is based on noncontrast head computed tomography (CT), which has a high sensitivity in the first few days. Once SAH is confirmed, a CT angiography or a digital subtraction angiography (DSA) should be performed to determine optimal treatment strategy according to the cause of bleeding. In diffuse SAH, DSA should always be performed to avoid missing small aneurysms or malformations [22].

Treatment goals will differ according to the stage of the disease. In the acute phase, main goals are early identification, transfer to hospital or ICU, prevention of

Classifications in aneurysmal SAH

Hunt and Hess
Clinical manifestations and mortality

Grade	Criteria	Perioperative Mortality
0	Asymptomatic, unruptured aneurysm	0-5%
I	Asymptomatic, mild headache, slight nuchal rigidity	0-5%
II	Moderate to severe headache, nuchal rigidity, no neurologic deficit other than cranial nerve palsy	2-10%
III	Drowsiness, confusion, mild focal neurologic deficit	10-15%
IV	Stupor, moderate-severe hemiparesis	60-70%
V	Coma, decerebrate posturing	70-100%

* An additional degree to be added if severe systemic disease or vasospasm

WNFS
Glasgow coma scale and motor deficit

Grade	Criteria
I	GCS 15, no motor deficit
II	GCS 13-14, no motor deficit
III	GCS 13-14, motor deficit
IV	GCS 9-12
V	GCS 8 or less

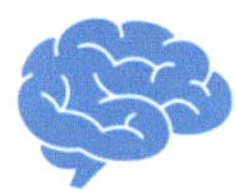

VASOGRADE
Combined. Predicts DCI.

Grade	WFNS	Modified Fisher
Green	1-2	1-2
Yellow	1-3	3-4
Red	4-5	Any

Modified Fisher scale
CT findings. Predicts vasospasm.

Grade	Criteria
0	No subarachnoid hemorrhage (SAH) No intraventricular hemorrhage (IVH)
I	Focal or diffuse thin SAH, no IHV
II	Focal or diffuse thin SAH, IVH present
III	Thick SAH*, no HV
IV	Thick SAH, VH present

* Large SAH: SAH completely filling 1 cisterna or fissure or >1mm

Fig. 9.2 Classifications used in SAH. (Source: Author's own elaboration)

further bleeding through blood pressure control and surgical or endovascular treatment, and management of associated conditions like seizures or intracranial hypertension. The main complication in this stage is rebleeding, its mortality close to 60%. In the subacute phase, the priority will be to decrease EBI; here, close hemodynamic monitoring and maintenance of CPP over 70 mmHg are key objectives, as well as optimization of oxygen transport through hemoglobin and ventilation targets. The main complications in the late stage are vasospasm and DCI, with a prevalence of 30%, most often between days 4 and 14. DCI should be suspected in case of a new-onset neurological impairment (either a focal deficit or a decrease of 2 points on the GCS scale) lasting at least 1 hour and not attributable to other causes. Usual management includes rapid diagnosis through imaging techniques (bedside transcranial doppler or CTA), euvolemia and hypertension, prevention with nimodipine, and often endovascular treatment through angioplasty [11, 22]. Although some emerging drugs may play a role in the future, such as magnesium sulfate, 3-hydroxy-3-methylglutaryl-CoA reductase inhibitors, nitric oxide donors, and endothelin-1 antagonists, their utility is yet to be confirmed [67].

9.2 System Crosstalk: Brain-Immune System Interactions

This section aims to address the complex interactions between the brain and the immune local and systemic response following SAH. Focus will be placed on cellular and humoral responses, blood-brain barrier disruption, and the impact of neuroinflammation on brain tissue damage.

9.2.1 Cellular Response After SAH

Microglial cells play a crucial role in neuroinflammation and neuroprotection in response to SAH. In the initial stages, metabolites from both hemoglobin and neuronal degradation act as damage-associated molecular patterns (DAMPs) and are detected by the tool-like receptor (TRL)-4 receptor [6]. This receptor triggers the activation of M1 microglia, upregulating the nuclear factor (NF)-κB pathway which induces the production of proinflammatory mediators. These mediators can promote neuronal apoptosis along with neutrophil and macrophage migration to the bleeding site, enhanced by overexpression of intercellular adhesion molecules (ICAM)-1 and P-selectin-glycoprotein ligand (PSGL)-1 in endothelial cells [2, 6, 67]. M1 microglia can bolster brain inflammation through upregulation of other molecules such as High mobility group box 1 protein (HMGB1) and the NOD-like receptor family, pyrin domain-containing protein 3 (NLRP3) inflammasome [2]. Continued microglia activation can be detrimental, evolving into a chronic inflammatory response.

After this initial stage, microglia shift to the M2-anti-inflammatory phenotype. These express receptors like LRP1, which are activated by ApoE, downregulate the c-Jun NH2-terminal kinase (JNK/c-Jun) inflammatory cascade [67]. M2 microglia repairing actions include blood phagocytosis, heme catabolism by HO-1, and angiogenesis [29].

Likewise, astrocytes respond to DAMPs through TLR4 by secreting pro-inflammatory mediators and recruiting peripheral immune cells. Swelling of their pericapillary processes due to excess expression of AQP-4 is key in developing cytotoxic brain edema following SAH. These alterations precede ionic alterations like K^+ and Ca^{2+} accumulation, which contribute to the disruption of neurovascular coupling promoting vasoconstriction [67]. Characteristically, after SAH, astrocyte's glutamate clearance is disrupted, implying glutamate excitotoxicity through cortical spreading depolarization leading to microvascular spasms and neuronal damage [19, 67].

Chronic inflammation leads to astrogliosis which contributes to the formation of scar tissue, brain damage, and altered cerebral vascular reactivity through increases in S100B, Glial fibrillary acidic protein (GFAP), and endothelin-1. Macrophages can contribute to tissue repair, although they can also exacerbate inflammation. Similarly, lymphocytes can modulate neuroinflammation, with T-regs playing an important role in suppressing excessive immune responses [67].

9.2.2 Humoral Response After SAH

The humoral response following SAH is characterized by an elevated production of inflammatory and anti-inflammatory cytokines both in the site of injury and systemically, with significant implications. Elevated inflammatory cytokines and chemokines may increase pulmonary capillary permeability, reduce erythropoiesis, disrupt cardiovascular functions, and induce systemic inflammation and ischemia [6].

Regarding proinflammatory cytokines, interleukin (IL-1β) is produced by numerous cells like M1-microglia, astrocytes, and macrophages and causes inflammation through the NF-κB signaling pathway, together with neurotoxic effects and immune recruitment [2].

IL-6 is produced predominantly by astrocytes and is related to increased BBB permeability. It may be involved in vasoconstriction by helping microglia to migrate to vessels and produce endothelin [6]. IL-6 is also involved in acute-phase reactants' production, such as C-reactive protein, hepcidin, and serum amyloid A, that may further promote inflammation [19]. Conversely, in the subacute phase, IL-6 stimulates endothelial cells' repair through the /phosphoinositide 3-kinase/ protein kinase B (PI3K/AKT) and Janus kinase/signal transducers and activators of transcription (JAK/STAT) pathways, protecting against neuronal apoptosis and promoting revascularization [2].

TNF-α secreted by neurons activates microglia and astrocytes which in turn can also produce it. TNF-α causes neuronal and endothelial cell apoptosis through the caspase pathway and is involved in BBB disruption through increased production of reactive oxygen species (ROS) among others [6, 67]. TNF-α also causes excitotoxicity by increasing the expression of α-Amino-3-hydroxy-5-methyl-4-isoxazolepropionic acid (AMPA) receptors [2].

Concerning anti-inflammatory cytokines, IL-4 induces macrophage/microglial shift to M2 phenotype and has a neuroprotective effect by inhibiting pro-inflammatory cytokines through different pathways like Signal transducer and activator of transcription 6 (STAT6) and Peroxisome proliferator-activated receptors (PPARγ) [50, 80]. IL-10 also reduces inflammatory cytokines through PI3K and signal transducer and activator of transcription 3 (STAT3) activation and NF-κβ pathway inhibition [2]. Nevertheless, the immunosuppressive effects of IL-10 may contribute to an increased risk of infections in these patients. Transforming growth factor (TGF)-β is another key anti-inflammatory agent involved in pro-inflammatory cytokine inhibition and T-reg cell proliferation. However, TGF-β may have detrimental effects as it generates fibrosis, which is involved in scar formation and hydrocephalus [6, 67].

The complement system also has a significative role in post-SAH inflammation. There is a rapid activation of the complement cascade triggered by different stimuli like DAMPs released by dying neurons which activate the alternative pathway. Overall, activation results in the production of C5a, C3a, and the membrane attack complex (MAC). Microglia and astrocytes express complement receptors and are activated by C3a and C5a, producing proinflammatory mediators that recruit additional immune cells and exacerbate tissue damage [2]. Besides, MAC can directly cause neuronal and glial cell lysis and could contribute to vasospasm when vascular smooth muscle cells are involved [2, 6].

9.2.3 Blood-Brain Barrier Disruption

The blood-brain barrier (BBB) is part of a neurovascular unit comprising various interacting structures. In a radial view, these include endothelial cells united via tight junctions, the basement membrane, pericytes, vascular smooth muscle cells (VSMC), astrocytes, microglia, and neuronal processes [2, 67].

In the hyperacute stage of SAH, sudden hypoxia due to decreased CBF related to increased intracranial pressure causes rupture of endothelial tight junctions, which leads to cytotoxic edema [67]. Consequently, there is apoptosis of endothelial cells and BBB disruption, which lead to increased permeability and infiltration of immune cells. This is followed by a basement membrane disruption through loss of collagen IV, culminating in vasogenic edema that further reduces CBF and triggers ischemia [27].

Blood degradation products can reach BBB through the Virchow-Robin and paravascular spaces. These molecules act as DAMPs activating perivascular glial cells and upregulating adhesion molecules [43]. Upon activation, microglia and astrocytes produce cytokines, matrix metalloproteinases, and chemokines that contribute to BBB breakdown and neuroinflammation [2]. Recruitment of immune cells further activates the inflammatory cascade, ultimately resulting in neuronal cell death, the major contributor to morbidity and mortality after SAH [67].

With regards to vasospasm, increased i-nitric oxide synthase (NOS) in endothelial cells negatively affects eNOS and NO availability, contributing to vascular smooth muscle cells (VSMC) contraction. Furthermore, cerebral vasospasm correlates in time with peak decreased expression of tight junction proteins [17].

9.2.4 Impact of Neuroinflammation on Brain Tissue Damage

Neuroinflammation is the activation of the brain's immune system in response to different stimuli, characterized by a complex and multifaceted process with multiple interactions and mediators. In the acute phase, hemorrhage-derived tissue damage triggers an inflammatory response mediated by the release of DAMPs, like HMGB-1, from apoptotic cells. DAMPs can activate immune cells which induce pro-inflammatory cytokine production amplifying the inflammatory response both locally and systemically [2].

The inflammatory response in SAH has dual implications as it can promote tissue repair and debris clearance, but can also cause secondary tissue damage through oxidative and cytotoxic pathways among others [6]. The latter contributes to post-SAH complications, such as vasospasm and cognitive impairment. Moreover, BBB disruption implies exposure of brain-specific antigens to the adaptive immune system, which can induce autoimmune disorders and chronic inflammation [6, 73]. Anti-inflammatory cytokines and Treg action may be beneficial in the acute phase of cerebral ischemia inducing immunosuppression. However, in chronic phases, derived consequences can arise, including increased risk of infections, in addition to impaired tissue repair. In contrast, some patients present sustained residual inflammation, a key factor in the development of chronic complications, such as cognitive impairment, depression, and fatigue [56].

9.3 System Crosstalk: Brain-Cardiovascular and Respiratory System Interactions

The intricate interplay between the nervous and the cardiovascular systems has been termed the *brain-heart axis*. Cardiovascular function is ultimately governed by a vast network of brain regions, both cortical and subcortical, through the autonomous nervous system (ANS). While the effects of cardiovascular disease on the brain have been extensively studied, the reverse pathway is still to be fully understood [70]. Several cardiovascular manifestations associated with neurological injury, particularly SAH, have been described, ranging from mild electrocardiogram changes to left ventricular dysfunction, or even cardiac arrest [1]. These complications are associated with a decrease in survival and increased risk of poor neurological outcomes [53]. The respiratory system is in tight relation to hemodynamic alterations and tightly related to neuro-cardiac reflexes, such as Cushing's.

9.3.1 Autonomic Dysfunction and Neuro-Cardiac Reflexes

The autonomic nervous system is subject to regulation by central nuclei located in the brainstem and the insular cortex [68], hence the autonomic disbalance that occurs in acute brain injury. Kawashara and colleagues found that sympathetic hyperactivation was present in the acute phase of SAH, quantified through heart rate variability and plasma concentration of catecholamines and cardiogenic enzymes; however, they also showed that the parasympathetic system predominated in later stages, probably as a negative feedback response to the initial sympathetic storm [3, 32]. The arterial baroreflex, which is the feedback mechanism in charge of adapting heart rate, cardiac contractility, and peripheral vascular resistance in response to variations in blood pressure, is marker of a healthy ANS. Baroreflex impairment has been described in other causes of brain injury, such as ischemic stroke or intracerebral hemorrhage, correlating with severity and unfavorable outcomes [21, 68]. The effect of autonomic disbalance is three-sided: first, it impairs cerebral perfusion; second, it increases cardiovascular risk through arrhythmogenesis, platelet aggregability, and coronary vasoconstriction; and third, it enhances secondary brain injury via cytokine production, hyperglycemia, and BBB breakdown [69]. Similarly, Nasr and colleagues found a direct correlation between baroreflex sensitivity and 3-month Glasgow Outcome Scale in aSAH [52]. Furthermore, the inverse correlation between baroreflex sensitivity (BRS) and cerebral autoregulation seems to be lost in patients who develop vasospasm [74].

Neuro-cardiac reflexes such as Cushing's, trigemino-cardiac, or vagal reflexes are present in SAH similarly to causes of acute brain injury. Cushing's reflex is triggered by the hypothalamus in response to increases in ICP and brain ischemia. At an early stage, it causes a sympathetic overdrive to increase MAP and CPP, and results in acute hypertension. The second stage is driven by carotid baroreceptors, stimulated by high blood pressure, which induce reflex bradycardia. Respiratory irregularities due to central nuclei stimulation follow [20]. Both hypotension and hypertension are frequent during the subacute and chronic phases of SAH, but the presence of Cushing's triad suggests high ICP and is related to poor prognosis [47]. In contrast, the trigemino-cardiac reflex is a purely parasympathetic reflex triggered by oxygen-sensitive neurons in the medulla oblongata. It is characterized by hypotension, bradycardia, apnea, and gastric hypermotility, and has recently gathered attention due to its possible neuroprotective role via cerebrovascular vasodilation [64].

9.3.2 Electrocardiographic Changes

Electrocardiographic changes which appear during SAH are probably related to increased central sympathetic activity and the hyperdynamic cardiovascular state. A wide range of alterations have been described, depending on the affected brain regions: high frequency heart rate variability in prefrontal cortex injury; ST depression, inverted T waves, and third-degree block in insular cortex injury; atrial fibrillation in hippocampus injury; and ventricular arrhythmias in brainstem injury [41]. Among these changes, QT prolongation and tachycardia are independently associated with angiographic vasospasm after aneurysmal SAH [25]. Ventricular arrhythmias are infrequent and increase mortality; however, QTc prolongation has not shown correlation with ventricular arrhythmias in literature [49]. ST depression and T wave inversion have successfully been used to develop normograms which improve outcome prediction after SAH [23]. Although ST changes may appear in SAH unrelated to myocardial ischemia, myocardial infarction (MI) is also a life-threatening complication of SAH, with a prevalence of 3% according to some studies [66].

9.3.3 Neurogenic Stunned Myocardium and Takotsubo Cardiomyopathy

Neurogenic stunned myocardium (NSM) is a transitory cardiac dysfunction which occurs in SAH due to the catecholaminergic storm, in relation to norepinephrine, epinephrine, dopamine, B-type natriuretic peptide and troponin Ic levels, and WFNS score [61]. It typically begins within 72 hours and manifests as systolic dysfunction with left ventricular ejection fractions $\leq$50% in up to 20% of patients, and diastolic dysfunction with mitral peak E-wave velocity by peak e′ velocity (E/e′) >14 in 2% [36]. Mild troponin increases and electrocardiographic abnormalities, such as QTc prolongation and T wave and ST segment changes, are common. In some studies, the previous use of β-blockers has been found to be a protective factor for the development of NSM after SAH [38]; however, NSM tends to parallel catecholamine concentration and spontaneously recedes during admission [61]. In contrast to Takotsubo, NSM tends to affect basal portions of the left ventricle and spare the apex [41].

Takotsubo cardiomyopathy is an entity which overlaps with NSM and may mimic acute myocardial infarction. It defines a type of transient stress-induced cardiomyopathy, characterized by left ventricular wall dyskinesia, primarily affecting the apex and mid-ventricle, in the absence of any coronary artery obstruction [28]. It is frequently accompanied by ST segment elevation or depression and T inversion on precordial leads, or both. The pathophysiology of Takotsubo is deeply related to the activation of the hypothalamic-pituitary-adrenal (HPA) axis and massive catecholaminergic release, which increases afterload through alpha receptors and contractility through beta receptors. This "apical ballooning" pathognomonic presentation is due to increased sensitivity of apex to catecholamine-mediated toxicity, when compared to basal regions of the myocardium, as it holds a more significant proportion of ß2 adrenergic receptors [41]. Although some have speculated that coronary spasm may contribute to Takotsubo, other studies have examined those patients who have undergone cardiac catheterization, and no evidence of coronary spasm was found [71]. Even though its incidence in aSAH patients is low, less than 1% according to some studies, Takotsubo cardiomyopathy is more frequent in younger female patients, in whom it markedly increases hospital stay and mortality up to 30% [12]; early diagnosis can be achieved through echocardiography. Treatment follows the guidelines for left ventricle systolic dysfunction, including angiotensin converting enzyme inhibitors, beta blockers, and diuretics [63]. In severe cases, the implantation of an intra-aortic balloon pump allows to support cardiac function until full recovery [5].

9.3.4 Neurogenic Pulmonary Edema

Neurogenic pulmonary edema (NPE) is an acute condition of respiratory distress triggered by severe injury to the CNS. Entities most frequently associated with NPE are SAH, its prevalence ranging from 2% to 42.9% according to some series [15, 51], intracerebral hemorrhage, traumatic brain injury, and epileptic seizures, although most authors agree that it is an underdiagnosed condition. The best-known precipitating factor is a sudden and severe increase in ICP, which gives rise to intense sympathetic activation and has been correlated in animal models with extravascular lung water [18]. Several other are postulated to play a role in its pathogenesis, namely direct catecholamine-induced myocardial injury and diastolic dysfunction, systolic dysfunction due to a sudden increase in afterload, alveolar endothelial damage (also known as "blast theory"), and adrenergic hypersensitivity of the pulmonary vascular bed [9]. Clinical features include abrupt respiratory distress marked with pink, frothy sputum, bilateral crackles on auscultation, and hyperdense infiltrates on chest radiograph. Once cardiogenic lung edema is ruled out, differential diagnosis should include fluid overload and aspiration pneumonia, both frequent in neurologically compromised patients [14]. NPE is not only associated with higher global mortality in aSAH, but also with higher incidence of vasospasm and worse neurological outcome [51]. Current treatment focuses on primary condition and lowering ICP; although alpha blockers may be beneficial, solid evidence is still lacking [9, 77].

9.4 System Crosstalk: Brain-Endocrine System Interactions

9.4.1 Disruption of the Hypothalamic-Pituitary-Adrenal Axis

The role of the hypothalamic-pituitary-adrenal (HPA) axis in the context of SAH has been a matter of research within the field of neuroendocrinology. Following the initial activation of the immune system in response to SAH, a posterior state of immunodepression emerges, a phenomenon that has been related with sympathetic nervous system overstimulation and HPA axis involvement [8]. Induced secretion of hypothalamic corticotropin-releasing hormone (CRH) through inflammatory cytokines, like IL-1β, leads to an increase in adrenocorticotropic hormone (ACTH) and glucocorticoid levels which have immunosuppressive properties [6].

Pituitary gland dysfunction is a notable consequence of SAH. The pituitary's unique vascular supply and the proximity of the Circle of Willis to the hypothalamic-pituitary complex make it susceptible to aneurysmal compression and vascular insufficiency [59, 60]. Ischemic injury, increased intracranial pressure, and surgical aneurysmal interventions are also potential contributors. Some authors suggest that alterations in pituitary and hypothalamus could be caused post-SAH by hypothalamic venous drainage obstruction, ischemia from vasospasm and compression, BBB disruption, among others [30].

Altered HPA axis-related laboratory values in the acute phase of SAH may initially be attributed to the body's adaptive response to critical illness and stress. Nonetheless, persistent neuroendocrine changes likely result from ischemia-induced damage [34]. The prevalence of hypopituitarism, affecting at least one axis, ranges from 37% to 55%; however, it declines over time to around 25% at 6 months [4]. Nevertheless, some studies have reported new-onset deficiencies in the chronic phase of SAH as described by Robba et al. [59].

Regarding the different axes of the anterior pituitary gland, the corticotropic axis shows transient cortisol and ACTH elevation in the initial hours post-bleeding, possibly linked to global cerebral edema and secondary cerebral hypoxia [60]. ACTH-cortisol deficiency is typical in the later phases; however, prevalence is below 2% with dynamic testing [30]. Stress response to SAH can lead to hypogonadism and hypothyroidism which could explain low levels only in early stages. Somatotropic axis dysfunction is the most common alteration due to ischemia vulnerability related to its vascularization [60]. The posterior pituitary gland exhibits hyperprolactinemia and antidiuretic hormone (ADH) abnormalities, with central diabetes insipidus being a common outcome, albeit often transient. Hyponatremia following SAH is common, and in some patients is linked to syndrome of inappropriate antidiuretic hormone secretion (SIADH) [65].

9.4.2 Adrenal Insufficiency and Cortisol Level Alterations

Adrenal insufficiency and cortisol level alterations in patients with SAH have gathered significant attention due to their potential impact on clinical outcomes. Cortisol secretion pattern in SAH is characterized by an initial peak around day 5, which has been correlated to stressful events, such as vasospasm or systemic and local inflammatory reactions, that lead to DCI. This peak is followed by a subsequent decrease in cortisol levels to a minimum around day 8, which is associated with an increased risk of poor outcomes [37]. It is noteworthy that circadian cortisol secretion is disrupted in around 50% of patients with SAH, and a substantial proportion of patients who do not respond to vasopressor therapy exhibit hypocortisolemia [76]. However, it should be emphasized that hypocortisolism does not present in all SAH patients, and when it occurs, it normally lasts no more than 1 or 2 days. The incidence of long-term, life-threatening hypocortisolism in post-SAH patients falls within the range of 2–15% of cases [37].

Patients with SAH should be evaluated for signs and symptoms of hypocortisolism, such as hyponatremia, hypotension, and hypoglycemia [30]. Some experts have even suggested the evaluation of basal hormonal testing in all SAH patients [76]. Screening aneurysmal SAH patients for signs and symptoms of adrenal insufficiency early in their hospital stay, particularly those who do not respond well to vasopressor therapy, is considered a reasonable approach. Serum total cortisol values can be affected by several factors, making it challenging to establish a cortisol cutoff for diagnosing adrenal failure in acute illness. An acute phase morning cortisol level of less than 200 nmol/L may suggest adrenal insufficiency, and glucocorticoid replacement should be established. However, under high-stress conditions related to critical illness, normal cortisol levels suggest relative hypocortisolemia. Therefore, under morning cortisol levels between 200 and 500 nmol/L coupled with adrenal insufficiency clinical signs, a glucocorticoid therapy trial should be considered [30, 37].

9.4.3 Influence of Endocrine Dysregulation on Patient Outcomes

Some authors reported a significant association between neuroendocrine dysfunction and patient outcome [30, 37]. Patients with SAH experience activation of the sympathoadrenal pathway which induces a catecholamine surge. This surge acts via the HPA axis, resulting in systemic inflammatory responses that can cause cardiac alterations, pulmonary inflammation, and acute kidney injury complications, among others [6].

Normal diurnal serum free cortisol is associated with shorter intensive care unit stays, fewer complications, and more favorable outcome in SAH [57]. Conversely, endocrine dysfunctions are associated with impaired clinical outcome and functional performance, such as low quality of life, depression, and sleeping alterations. Severe growth factor (GH) deficiency is associated with low energy and quality of life, increased body mass index, and possibly Glasgow outcome scale [33]. Neuroendocrine dysfunction can lead to variations in duration and the severity of the disease and in the response to treatment in the acute phase of SAH [60]. Prompt correction of hormone deficiencies impacts the outcome of patients with SAH; for instance, hypocortisolemia and hypothyroidism treatment is essential for stress adaptation, alongside cardiovascular and metabolic regulation [30] (Fig. 9.3).

9.5 Therapeutic Implications and Future Directions

As reviewed in Sect. 9.2, complex interactions between a wide range of neuronal cells and immune mediators are responsible for the regulation of neuroprotection and both local and systemic inflammation in SAH. The possibility to modulate the

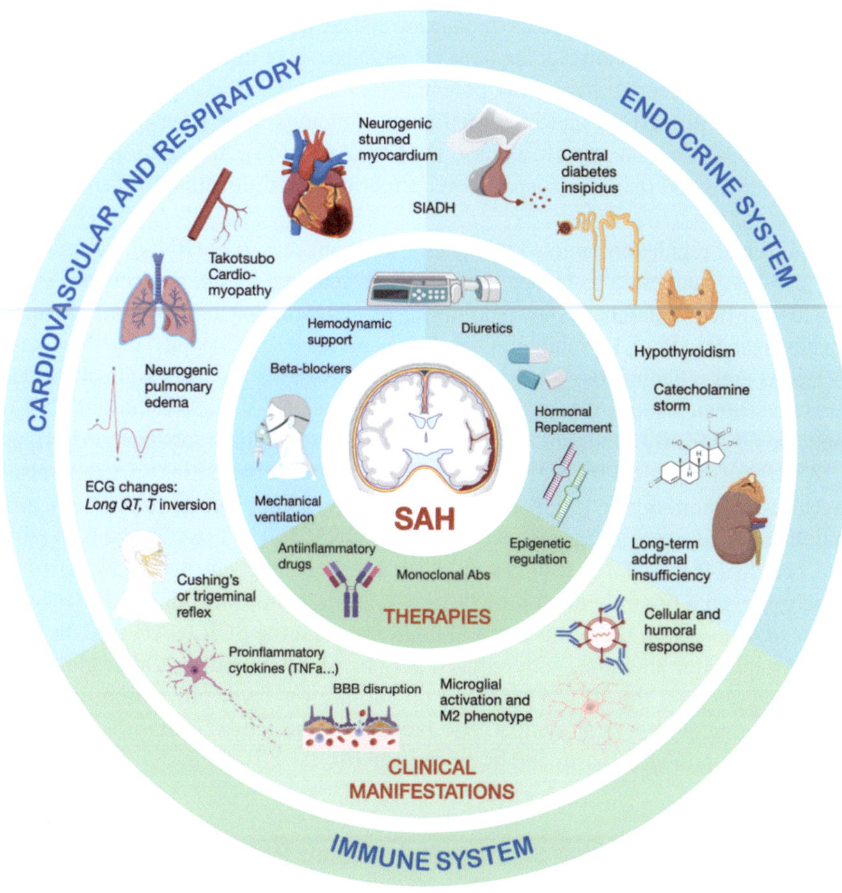

Fig. 9.3 Organ system crosstalk in SAH: Clinical manifestation and potential therapies from a systemic perspective. BBB blood-brain barrier, Ab antibodies. (Source: Author's own elaboration)

patient's anti-inflammatory or pro-inflammatory response to SAH through targeted therapies enables a more personalized and precise approach to associated alterations as they arise throughout the different chronological phases post-SAH. Multiple therapeutic targets have been identified, such as adhesion molecules involved in leukocyte recruitment and BBB disruption, Tregs which promote tissue repair, and proinflammatory cytokine and complement inhibition.

9.5.1 Anti-inflammatory Agents and Immunomodulatory Drugs

Current experimental and clinical research has been focusing on agents that could improve outcomes after SAH. Regarding non-steroidal anti-inflammatory drugs (NSAIDs), Celecoxib and NS398 are ciclo-oxygenase (COX)-2 inhibitors that effectively reduced vasospasm and neurological deficits in animal trials. Diclofenac also helped reduce inflammation and improve the clinical outcomes among patients with SAH. Corticosteroids may help in reducing vasospasm and IL-6 production and are frequently used after microsurgical clipping procedures; however, they can increase the risk of infection [6].

Epoxyeicosatrienoates are also potential therapeutic targets due to their anti-inflammatory properties, and increased serum amounts have been observed after GSK2256294 administration in a phase 1b clinical trial [48]. A recent meta-analysis revealed decreased risk of vasospasm and cerebral infarction with cilostazol administration [42].

Epigenetic regulation targeted by specific si-ribonucleic acid (RNA) and miRNA has also been suggested to reduce inflammation, neuronal injury, and cerebral vasospasm [6]. Mice models have shown promising results regarding the use of Programmed Death-Ligand1 (PD-L1) inhibition of PD-1 immune checkpoint, together with increased anti-inflammatory environments in STAT3 knockout mice. Animal models have also shown positive results for various targeted therapies, such as the anti-TNF-α monoclonal antibody adalimumab and the IL-6 receptor inhibitor tocilizumab [54].

Randomised clinical trials evaluating the use of oral simvastatin (STASH), intrathecal use of nimodipine (NEWTON2), use of magnesium sulfate (MASH II), and endothelin-1 receptor antagonist clazosentan (CONSCIOUS 1 and 2) claim no clinical benefit [46]. Positive trial results have been observed in the ALISAH trial, which showed a possible neuroprotective effect of albumin including a lower incidence of vasospasm, DCI, and cerebral infarction, and the SCIL-SAH trial on IL-1 receptor inhibitor anakinra, with reduced peripheral inflammation. Other trials currently ongoing are the INTREPID trial on cooling for fever prevention, trials on anti-inflammatory cervical sympathetic block, and the REACT trial on clazosentan's reduction in vasospasm and brain damage [6].

9.5.2 Neuroprotective Strategies and Their Potential Benefits

Neuroprotective strategies in SAH mitigate secondary injury and enhance neurological outcomes. Key interventions include controlling hypertension, administering nimodipine for vasospasm management, and treating aneurysms promptly, all of which have shown reductions in 1-year mortality as per the AHA/ASA 2023 SAH guidelines [22].

In the acute phase, high blood pressure should be prevented to avoid rebleeding, and endovascular embolization or neurosurgical clipping of aneurysms should be performed [22]. Monitoring parameters like intracranial pressure and brain tissue oxygen tension are essential for optimizing cerebral perfusion and brain oxygenation. External ventricular drain placement facilitates management of hydrocephalus and intracranial hypertension.

In the subacute phase, focus shifts to cerebral vasospasm and DCI. Clinical follow-up and transcranial Doppler measurements aid in patient monitoring [62]. Targeting a cerebral perfusion pressure of 80–120 mmHg can effectively reverse vasospasm in cases of DCI [31]. Therapeutic hypothermia, when administered early and in a mild and prolonged manner, has been associated with reduced vasospasm and DCI occurrence [35].

Preventing fever and hyperglycemia, addressing hyponatremia, and providing seizure secondary prophylaxis are integral aspects of SAH neuroprotection. Concerning anemia, higher transfusion thresholds have been associated with improved neurological outcomes, although blood transfusions may be considered with established DCI [31].

Understanding the complex crosstalk between the immune, cardiovascular, respiratory, and endocrine systems is key to improving the management and outcomes of SAH patients. This knowledge could lead to the development of targeted therapies and interventions that mitigate the secondary systemic complications of SAH, such as vasospasm and DCI, ultimately improving prognosis and minimizing neurological morbidity.

References

1. Ahmadian A, Mizzi A, Banasiak M, et al. Cardiac manifestations of subarachnoid hemorrhage. Heart Lung Vessel. 2013;5(3):168–78.
2. Alsbrook DL, Di Napoli M, Bhatia K, et al. Neuroinflammation in acute ischemic and hemorrhagic stroke. Curr Neurol Neurosci Rep. 2023;23:407–31. https://doi.org/10.1007/s11910-023-01282-2.
3. Borutta MC, Gerner ST, Moeser P, et al. Correlation between clinical severity and extent of autonomic cardiovascular impairment in the acute phase of subarachnoid hemorrhage. J Neurol. 2022;269:5541–52. https://doi.org/10.1007/s00415-022-11220-w.
4. Can A, Gross BA, Smith TR, et al. Pituitary dysfunction after aneurysmal subarachnoid hemorrhage. Neurosurgery. 2016;79:253–64. https://doi.org/10.1227/NEU.0000000000001157.
5. Catapano JS, Ducruet AF, Frisoli FA, et al. Predictors of the development of takotsubo cardiomyopathy in aneurysmal subarachnoid hemorrhage and outcomes in patients with intra-aortic balloon pumps. J Neurosurg. 2020;135(1):38–43. https://doi.org/10.3171/2020.5.JNS20536.
6. Chai C-Z, Ho U-C, Kuo L-T. Systemic inflammation after aneurysmal subarachnoid hemorrhage. Int J Mol Sci. 2023;24:10943. https://doi.org/10.3390/ijms241310943.
7. Chou SH-Y. Subarachnoid Hemorrhage. Continuum (Minneap Minn). 2021;27:1201–45. https://doi.org/10.1212/CON.0000000000001052.

8. Datta A, Saha C, Godse P, et al. Neuroendocrine regulation in stroke. Trends Endocrinol Metab. 2023;34:260–77. https://doi.org/10.1016/j.tem.2023.02.005.
9. Davison DL, Terek M, Chawla LS. Neurogenic pulmonary edema. Crit Care. 2012;16:212. https://doi.org/10.1186/cc11226.
10. de Oliveira Manoel AL, Jaja BN, Germans MR, et al. The VASOGRADE. Stroke. 2015;46:1826–31. https://doi.org/10.1161/STROKEAHA.115.008728.
11. Dodd WS, Laurent D, Dumont AS, et al. Pathophysiology of delayed cerebral ischemia after subarachnoid hemorrhage: a review. J Am Heart Assoc. 2021;10. https://doi.org/10.1161/JAHA.121.021845.
12. Elgendy AY, Elgendy IY, Mansoor H, Mahmoud AN. Clinical presentations and outcomes of Takotsubo syndrome in the setting of subarachnoid hemorrhage: a systematic review and meta-analysis. Eur Heart J Acute Cardiovasc Care. 2018;7:236–45. https://doi.org/10.1177/2048872616679792.
13. Etminan N, Chang H-S, Hackenberg K, et al. Worldwide incidence of aneurysmal subarachnoid hemorrhage according to region, time period, blood pressure, and smoking prevalence in the population. JAMA Neurol. 2019;76:588. https://doi.org/10.1001/jamaneurol.2019.0006.
14. Finsterer J. Neurological perspectives of neurogenic pulmonary edema. Eur Neurol. 2019;81:94–102. https://doi.org/10.1159/000500139.
15. Fontes RBV, Aguiar PH, Zanetti MV, et al. Acute neurogenic pulmonary edema: case reports and literature review. J Neurosurg Anesthesiol. 2003;15:144–50. https://doi.org/10.1097/00008506-200304000-00013.
16. Frontera JA, Claassen J, Schmidt JM, et al. Prediction of symptomatic vasospasmafter subarachnoid hemorrhage. Neurosurgery. 2006;59:21–7. https://doi.org/10.1227/01.neu.0000243277.86222.6c.
17. Fumoto T, Naraoka M, Katagai T, et al. The role of oxidative stress in microvascular disturbances after experimental subarachnoid hemorrhage. Transl Stroke Res. 2019;10:684–94. https://doi.org/10.1007/s12975-018-0685-0.
18. Gupta YK, Chugh A, Kacker V, et al. Development of neurogenic pulmonary edema at different grades of intracranial pressure in cats. Indian J Physiol Pharmacol. 1998;42:71–80.
19. Hartings JA, York J, Carroll CP, et al. Subarachnoid blood acutely induces spreading depolarizations and early cortical infarction. Brain. 2017;140:2673–90. https://doi.org/10.1093/brain/awx214.
20. Heymans C. The control of heart rate consequent to changes in the cephalic blood pressure and in the intracranial pressure. Am J Phys. 1928;85:498–506.
21. Hilz MJ, Moeller S, Akhundova A, et al. High NIHSS values predict impairment of cardiovascular autonomic control. Stroke. 2011;42:1528–33. https://doi.org/10.1161/STROKEAHA.110.607721.
22. Hoh BL, Ko NU, Amin-Hanjani S, et al. 2023 guideline for the management of patients with aneurysmal subarachnoid hemorrhage: a guideline from the American Heart Association/American Stroke Association. Stroke. 2023;54:e314–70. https://doi.org/10.1161/STR.0000000000000436.
23. Hong J y, You JS, Kim MJ, et al. Development and external validation of new nomograms by adding ECG changes (ST depression or tall T wave) and age to conventional scoring systems to improve the predictive capacity in patients with subarachnoid haemorrhage: a retrospective, observational study in Korea. BMJ Open. 2019;9:e024007. https://doi.org/10.1136/bmjopen-2018-024007.
24. Hunt WE, Hess RM. Surgical risk as related to time of intervention in the repair of intracranial aneurysms. J Neurosurg. 1968;28:14–20. https://doi.org/10.3171/jns.1968.28.1.0014.
25. Ibrahim GM, Macdonald RL. Electrocardiographic changes predict angiographic vasospasm after aneurysmal subarachnoid hemorrhage. Stroke. 2012;43:2102–7. https://doi.org/10.1161/STROKEAHA.112.658153.
26. Jaeger M, Soehle M, Schuhmann MU, Meixensberger J. Clinical significance of impaired cerebrovascular autoregulation after severe aneurysmal subarachnoid hemorrhage. Stroke. 2012;43:2097–101. https://doi.org/10.1161/STROKEAHA.112.659888.

27. Jurcau A, Simion A. Neuroinflammation in cerebral ischemia and ischemia/reperfusion injuries: from pathophysiology to therapeutic strategies. Int J Mol Sci. 2021;23:14. https://doi.org/10.3390/ijms23010014.
28. Kaculini C, Sy C, Lacci JV, et al. The association of Takotsubo cardiomyopathy and aneurysmal subarachnoid hemorrhage: a U.S. nationwide analysis. Clin Neurol Neurosurg. 2022;215:107211. https://doi.org/10.1016/j.clineuro.2022.107211.
29. Kaiser S, Selzner L, Weber J, Schallner N. Carbon monoxide controls microglial erythrophagocytosis by regulating CD36 surface expression to reduce the severity of hemorrhagic injury. Glia. 2020;68:2427–45. https://doi.org/10.1002/glia.23864.
30. Karaca Z, Hacioglu A, Kelestimur F. Neuroendocrine changes after aneurysmal subarachnoid haemorrhage. Pituitary. 2019;22:305–21. https://doi.org/10.1007/s11102-018-00932-w.
31. Karmakar A, Abdelwahid YM, Strandvik G. Neuroprotection in subarachnoid hemorrhage. In: Management of subarachnoid hemorrhage. Cham: Springer International Publishing; 2022. p. 41–54.
32. Kawahara E, Ikeda S, Miyahara Y, Kohno S. Role of autonomic nervous dysfunction in electrocardiographic abnormalities and cardiac injury in patients with acute subarachnoid hemorrhage. Circ J. 2003;67:753–6. https://doi.org/10.1253/circj.67.753.
33. Kreitschmann-Andermahr I, Poll E, Hutter BO, et al. Quality of life and psychiatric sequelae following aneurysmal subarachnoid haemorrhage: does neuroendocrine dysfunction play a role? Clin Endocrinol. 2007;66:833–7. https://doi.org/10.1111/j.1365-2265.2007.02821.x.
34. Krewer C, Schneider M, Schneider HJ, et al. Neuroendocrine disturbances one to five or more years after traumatic brain injury and aneurysmal subarachnoid hemorrhage: data from the German Database on Hypopituitarism. J Neurotrauma. 2016;33:1544–53. https://doi.org/10.1089/neu.2015.4109.
35. Kuramatsu JB, Kollmar R, Gerner ST, et al. Is hypothermia helpful in severe subarachnoid hemorrhage? An exploratory study on macro vascular spasm, delayed cerebral infarction and functional outcome after prolonged hypothermia. Cerebrovasc Dis. 2015;40:228–35. https://doi.org/10.1159/000439178.
36. Lång M, Jakob SM, Takala R, et al. The prevalence of cardiac complications and their impact on outcomes in patients with non-traumatic subarachnoid hemorrhage. Sci Rep. 2022;12:20109. https://doi.org/10.1038/s41598-022-24675-8.
37. Lanterna LA, Spreafico V, Gritti P, et al. Hypocortisolism in noncomatose patients during the acute phase of subarachnoid hemorrhage. J Stroke Cerebrovasc Dis. 2013;22:e189–96. https://doi.org/10.1016/j.jstrokecerebrovasdis.2012.11.002.
38. Liang CW, Chen R, Macri E, Naval N. Preadmission beta-blockers are associated with decreased incidence of neurogenic stunned myocardium in aneurysmal subarachnoid hemorrhage. J Stroke Cerebrovasc Dis. 2013;22:601–7. https://doi.org/10.1016/j.jstrokecerebrovasdis.2011.10.006.
39. Lidington D, Kroetsch JT, Bolz S-S. Cerebral artery myogenic reactivity: the next frontier in developing effective interventions for subarachnoid hemorrhage. J Cereb Blood Flow Metab. 2018;38:17–37. https://doi.org/10.1177/0271678X17742548.
40. Lidington D, Wan H, Bolz S-S. Cerebral autoregulation in subarachnoid hemorrhage. Front Neurol. 2021;12:688362. https://doi.org/10.3389/fneur.2021.688362.
41. Lionel KR. Head rules over the heart: cardiac manifestations of cerebral disorders. Indian J Crit Care Med. 2019;23:329–35. https://doi.org/10.5005/jp-journals-10071-23208.
42. Liu J, He J, Chen X, et al. Cilostazol for aneurysmal subarachnoid hemorrhage: an updated systematic review and meta-analysis. Cerebrovasc Dis. 2022;51:138–48. https://doi.org/10.1159/000518731.
43. Luo C, Yao X, Li J, et al. Paravascular pathways contribute to vasculitis and neuroinflammation after subarachnoid hemorrhage independently of glymphatic control. Cell Death Dis. 2016;7:e2160. https://doi.org/10.1038/cddis.2016.63.
44. Macdonald RL. Delayed neurological deterioration after subarachnoid haemorrhage. Nat Rev Neurol. 2014;10:44–58. https://doi.org/10.1038/nrneurol.2013.246.
45. Mahlamäki K, Rautalin I, Korja M. Case fatality rates of subarachnoid hemorrhage are decreasing with substantial between-country variation: a systematic review of population-

based studies between 1980 and 2020. Neuroepidemiology. 2022;56:402–12. https://doi.org/10.1159/000526983.
46. Marazzi TBM, Mendes PV. Updates on aneurysmal subarachnoid hemorrhage: is there anything really new? Arq Neuropsiquiatr. 2022;80:80–7. https://doi.org/10.1590/0004-282x-anp-2022-s101.
47. Marshman LAG. Cushing's 'variant' response (acute hypotension) after subarachnoid hemorrhage. Stroke. 1997;28:1445–50. https://doi.org/10.1161/01.STR.28.7.1445.
48. Martini RP, Siler D, Cetas J, et al. A double-blind, randomized, placebo-controlled trial of soluble epoxide hydrolase inhibition in patients with aneurysmal subarachnoid hemorrhage. Neurocrit Care. 2022;36:905–15. https://doi.org/10.1007/s12028-021-01398-8.
49. Michael Frangiskakis J, Hravnak M, Crago EA, et al. Ventricular arrhythmia risk after subarachnoid hemorrhage. Neurocrit Care. 2009;10:287–94. https://doi.org/10.1007/s12028-009-9188-x.
50. Miwa K, Tanaka M, Okazaki S, et al. Relations of blood inflammatory marker levels with cerebral microbleeds. Stroke. 2011;42:3202–6. https://doi.org/10.1161/STROKEAHA.111.621193.
51. Muroi C, Keller M, Pangalu A, et al. Neurogenic pulmonary edema in patients with subarachnoid hemorrhage. J Neurosurg Anesthesiol. 2008;20:188–92. https://doi.org/10.1097/ANA.0b013e3181778156.
52. Nasr N, Gaio R, Czosnyka M, et al. Baroreflex impairment after subarachnoid hemorrhage is associated with unfavorable outcome. Stroke. 2018;49:1632–8. https://doi.org/10.1161/STROKEAHA.118.020729.
53. Norberg E, Odenstedt-Herges H, Rydenhag B, Oras J. Impact of acute cardiac complications after subarachnoid hemorrhage on long-term mortality and cardiovascular events. Neurocrit Care. 2018;29:404–12. https://doi.org/10.1007/s12028-018-0558-0.
54. Ohashi SN, DeLong JH, Kozberg MG, et al. Role of inflammatory processes in hemorrhagic stroke. Stroke. 2023;54:605–19. https://doi.org/10.1161/STROKEAHA.122.037155.
55. Osgood ML. Aneurysmal subarachnoid hemorrhage: review of the pathophysiology and management strategies. Curr Neurol Neurosci Rep. 2021;21:50. https://doi.org/10.1007/s11910-021-01136-9.
56. Parikh NS, Merkler AE, Iadecola C. Inflammation, autoimmunity, infection, and stroke. Stroke. 2020;51:711–8. https://doi.org/10.1161/STROKEAHA.119.024157.
57. Poll E-M, Boström A, Bürgel U, et al. Cortisol dynamics in the acute phase of aneurysmal subarachnoid hemorrhage: associations with disease severity and outcome. J Neurotrauma. 2010;27:189–95. https://doi.org/10.1089/neu.2009.1014.
58. Reis C, Ho WM, Akyol O, et al. Pathophysiology of subarachnoid hemorrhage, early brain injury, and delayed cerebral ischemia. In: Primer on cerebrovascular diseases. Elsevier, Amsterdam, Netherlands; 2017. p. 125–30.
59. Robba C, Bacigaluppi S, Bragazzi N, et al. Clinical prevalence and outcome impact of pituitary dysfunction after aneurysmal subarachnoid hemorrhage: a systematic review with meta-analysis. Pituitary. 2016;19:522–35. https://doi.org/10.1007/s11102-016-0733-2.
60. Roe T, Welbourne J, Nikitas N. Endocrine dysregulation in aneurysmal subarachnoid haemorrhage. Br J Neurosurg. 2022;36:358–67. https://doi.org/10.1080/02688697.2022.2039378.
61. Salem R, Vallée F, Dépret F, et al. Subarachnoid hemorrhage induces an early and reversible cardiac injury associated with catecholamine release: one-week follow-up study. Crit Care. 2014;18:558. https://doi.org/10.1186/s13054-014-0558-1.
62. Sanicola HW, Stewart CE, Luther P, et al. Pathophysiology, management, and therapeutics in subarachnoid hemorrhage and delayed cerebral ischemia: an overview. Pathophysiology. 2023;30:420–42. https://doi.org/10.3390/pathophysiology30030032.
63. Sattar Y, Siew KSW, Connerney M, et al. Management of Takotsubo syndrome: a comprehensive review. Cureus. 2020. https://doi.org/10.7759/cureus.6556.
64. Schaller B. Trigeminocardiac reflex. J Neurol. 2004;251:658–65. https://doi.org/10.1007/s00415-004-0458-4.

65. Sherlock M, O'Sullivan E, Agha A, et al. The incidence and pathophysiology of hyponatraemia after subarachnoid haemorrhage. Clin Endocrinol. 2006;64:250–4. https://doi.org/10.1111/j.1365-2265.2006.02432.x.
66. Singh B. Myocardial infarction and subarachnoid hemorrhage. Frequency and impact on outcome. Neurology. 2021;96(15 Suppl 1). 73rd Annual Meeting of the American Academy of Neurology, AAN 2021.
67. Solár P, Zamani A, Lakatosová K, Joukal M. The blood–brain barrier and the neurovascular unit in subarachnoid hemorrhage: molecular events and potential treatments. Fluids Barriers CNS. 2022;19:29. https://doi.org/10.1186/s12987-022-00312-4.
68. Sykora M, Diedler J, Rupp A, et al. Impaired baroreceptor reflex sensitivity in acute stroke is associated with insular involvement, but not with carotid atherosclerosis. Stroke. 2009;40:737–42. https://doi.org/10.1161/STROKEAHA.108.519967.
69. Sykora M, Diedler J, Turcani P, et al. Baroreflex: a new therapeutic target in human stroke? Stroke. 2009;40. https://doi.org/10.1161/STROKEAHA.109.565838.
70. Tahsili-Fahadan P, Geocadin RG. Heart–Brain axis. Circ Res. 2017;120:559–72. https://doi.org/10.1161/CIRCRESAHA.116.308446.
71. Talahma M, Alkhachroum AM, Alyahya M, et al. Takotsubo cardiomyopathy in aneurysmal subarachnoid hemorrhage: institutional experience and literature review. Clin Neurol Neurosurg. 2016;141:65–70. https://doi.org/10.1016/j.clineuro.2015.12.005.
72. Teasdale GM, Drake CG, Hunt W, et al. A universal subarachnoid hemorrhage scale: report of a committee of the World Federation of Neurosurgical Societies. J Neurol Neurosurg Psychiatry. 1988;51:1457. https://doi.org/10.1136/jnnp.51.11.1457.
73. Tsygan NV, Trashkov AP, Litvinenko IV, et al. Autoimmunity in acute ischemic stroke and the role of blood-brain barrier: the dark side or the light one? Front Med. 2019;13:420–6. https://doi.org/10.1007/s11684-019-0688-6.
74. Uryga A, Nasr N, Kasprowicz M, et al. Relationship between baroreflex and cerebral autoregulation in patients with cerebral vasospasm after aneurysmal subarachnoid hemorrhage. Front Neurol. 2022;12. https://doi.org/10.3389/fneur.2021.740338.
75. van Gijn J, Rinkel GJ. Subarachnoid haemorrhage: diagnosis, causes and management. Brain. 2001;124:249–78. https://doi.org/10.1093/brain/124.2.249.
76. Weant KA, Sasaki-Adams D, Dziedzic K, Ewend M. Acute relative adrenal insufficiency after aneurysmal subarachnoid hemorrhage. Neurosurgery. 2008;63:645–50. https://doi.org/10.1227/01.NEU.0000325728.50939.15.
77. Wohns RNW, Tamas L, Pierce KR, Howe JF. Chlorpromazine treatment for neurogenic pulmonary edema. Crit Care Med. 1985;13:210–1. https://doi.org/10.1097/00003246-198503000-00016.
78. Xia C, Hoffman H, Anikpezie N, et al. Trends in the incidence of spontaneous subarachnoid hemorrhages in the United States, 2007–2017. Neurology. 2023;100:e123–32. https://doi.org/10.1212/WNL.0000000000201340.
79. Yagi K, Lidington D, Wan H, et al. Therapeutically targeting tumor necrosis factor-α/sphingosine-1-phosphate signaling corrects myogenic reactivity in subarachnoid hemorrhage. Stroke. 2015;46:2260–70. https://doi.org/10.1161/STROKEAHA.114.006365.
80. Zhang Q, Zhu W, Xu F, et al. The interleukin-4/PPARγ signaling axis promotes oligodendrocyte differentiation and remyelination after brain injury. PLoS Biol. 2019;17:e3000330. https://doi.org/10.1371/journal.pbio.3000330.
81. Zhang R, Zuckerman JH, Iwasaki K, et al. Autonomic neural control of dynamic cerebral autoregulation in humans. Circulation. 2002;106:1814–20. https://doi.org/10.1161/01.CIR.0000031798.07790.FE.
82. Zuurbier CCM, Bourcier R, Constant Dit Beaufils P, et al. Number of affected relatives, age, smoking, and hypertension prediction score for intracranial aneurysms in persons with a family history for subarachnoid hemorrhage. Stroke. 2022;53:1645–50. https://doi.org/10.1161/STROKEAHA.121.034612.

10 Inflammatory Mechanisms in Cardiac Arrest

Luisa Cappa and Chiara Robba

10.1 Introduction

Cardiac arrest is a leading cause of morbidity and mortality in industrialized countries. According to AHA, nearly 700,000 new cases of cardiac arrest occur each year in the United States [1]. Regarding the setting of Cardiac Arrest, in-hospital cardiac arrest (IHCA) accounts for more than 290,000 cases per year [2], while out-of-hospital location (OHCA) reaches more than 350,000 cases per year [3]. Survival rates for patients are, respectively, nearly 22% after IHCA and less than 15% in OHCA [4].

The pathophysiology of cardiac arrest is complex and multifaceted, involving a cascade of events that lead to widespread cellular dysfunction and death. One key player in this cascade is inflammation, which is triggered by the ischemic insult and persists into the post-resuscitation phase. This inflammatory response, while a natural part of the body's defense mechanism, can exacerbate tissue damage and contribute to poor outcomes.

The role of inflammation in cardiac arrest and its aftermath is a burgeoning area of research. Recent studies have begun to unravel the intricate cellular and molecular mechanisms involved in the inflammatory response following cardiac arrest, shedding light on potential therapeutic targets.

This chapter aims to provide an in-depth exploration of the inflammatory mechanism in cardiac arrest, its role in post-cardiac arrest damage, and its impact on long-term outcomes.

L. Cappa · C. Robba (✉)
Anaesthesia and Intensive Care, IRCCS Policlinico San Martino, Genoa, Italy

D. Battaglini et al. (eds.), *Organ System Crosstalk in Critical Illness*,
https://doi.org/10.1007/978-3-032-01024-7_10

10.2 Post-cardiac Arrest Syndrome

10.2.1 Introduction

Post-cardiac arrest syndrome (PCAS) is a complex and multifaceted condition, a consequence of the phenomenon of ischemia-reperfusion triggered by cardiac arrest, with various degrees of gravity depending on the duration of the no-flow and low-flow periods [5]. It is characterized by a combination of pathophysiological processes that lead to brain injury, myocardial dysfunction, systemic ischemia/reperfusion response, and persistent precipitating pathology. It usually manifests itself as a cardiac-circulatory dysfunction, but it can also present aspects of systemic inflammatory response syndrome (SIRS) (changes in core temperature, heart and respiratory rate) and disseminated intravascular coagulation (DIC) (with deposition of microvascular thrombi) and evolve into multi-organ failure (MOF) and shock [6]. The syndrome is a major cause of morbidity and mortality in post-cardiac arrest patients and is a significant challenge in the clinical management of these patients.

PCAS, first described in the 1950s, from a pathophysiological point of view can be divided into four phases [7]:

1. *Immediate post-arrest phase*: First 20 min after ROSC.
2. *Early post-arrest phase:* Between 20 min and 6–12 h after ROSC; during this phase, early interventions might be effective.
3. *Intermediate phase:* Between 6–12 and 72 h after ROSC; injury pathways are still active and working, and aggressive treatment has to be instituted.
4. *Recovery phase:* Beyond 3 days; during this phase, prognostication becomes more reliable [8]. An efficient and prompt cardiopulmonary resuscitation adjuvanted with appropriate clinical interventions in the post-arrest period can impact the patient outcome.

10.2.2 Pathophysiology

The pathophysiology of PCAS is complex and not completely understood, but what seems clear is that it involves the inflammatory response and that it affects multiple organ systems.

Its phases follow the different steps of cardiac arrest: no-flow, low-flow (chest compression), and return of spontaneous circulation (ROSC).

After about 20 seconds from the beginning of the no-flow phase of cardiac arrest, the decrease in the oxygen supply is counterbalanced by a reduction of the metabolic needs, lowering/interrupting the cellular function [9]. The cells keep on consuming the ATP stored, but if the circulation is not restored or the metabolic needs are not being met, we witness a shift from an aerobic metabolism to an anaerobic one, with production of lactic acid and consequent metabolic acidosis [10]. On the other hand, the decrease of ATP synthesis is responsible for the membrane depolarization and the ionic pumps dysfunction; this dysfunction leads to the opening of voltage-dependent calcium channels on the sarcolemma, generating a calcium (Ca++) current, that causes an increase in the intracellular Ca++ concentration and the fall of the mitochondrial membrane potential, ultimately leading to cellular damage [9].

These events perpetuate themselves during the no-flow and the low-flow phase of cardiac arrest, constituting the *primum movens* of the tissue damage.

Following the no-flow phase either the low-flow phase and the ROSC/post-cardiac arrest phase, with the tissue reperfusion see the synthesis and release of radical oxygen species such as hydrogen peroxide (H_2O_2), superoxide anion ($*O_2$) and radical hydroxyl (*OH). Especially the *OH causes the peroxidation of lipids on the cell membrane, inactivates cytochromes, and damages membrane transport proteins, undermining the cellular structure and causing the death of the cell [9]. The oxidative stress and the free radical-induced injury that follows it lead to cell death (necrosis/apoptosis), with the release of danger-associated molecular patterns (DAMPs) and to endothelium damage, thanks to the activation of the inflammatory cascade, initially in situ and ultimately at the systemic level. Subsequently, we have the production of proinflammatory cytokines, the activation of the complement system and of the arachidonic acid cascade, and the expression on leukocytes' endothelium of adhesion molecules. These events are all involved in the recruitment of neutrophils, accountable for the amplification of the inflammatory response [11].

The inflammatory response, leading actor in the damage of the reperfusion phases post-cardiac arrest, is held responsible for coagulation abnormalities, causing activation of coagulation factors and reduction of the levels of endogenous anticoagulants such as antithrombin and protein S and C, causing thrombosis and increasing capillary permeability, worsening the visceral damage [12].

Clinically, all these processes manifest themselves in different forms, with the main organs damaged being the brain, the lung, and the myocardium:

- *Cardio-circulatory failure, up to post-cardiac arrest shock*: Aside from a potential coronary occlusion, itself responsible for cardiac arrest and for the reduction of the heart function/contractility, we assist at an early, severe, and reversible left heart dysfunction, usually self-solving within 48–72 h [13]. It usually starts as a left ventricular dysfunction with low cardiac output, later becoming a systo-diastolic problem with concomitant low filling pressure, associated with general inflammation-induced vasodilatation. The whole situation is worsened by a relative adrenal insufficiency [7].
- *Neurological failure*: Usually seen after at least 72 h from ROSC. It is caused by a temporary increase in the cerebral vascular resistance, with consequent low blood flow, paired with low oxygen extraction. The vascular resistance usually goes back to normal in 72 h shortly followed by oxygen extraction. Clinically, patients may experience coma, seizures, myoclonus, and various other neurological signs [14]. If the damage involves the deeper brain structures, this likely to be associated with dysfunction of the hypothalamic-pituitary-adrenal axis (HPA) [15]. The prognosis of these patients is largely dependent on the extent of the brain injury and can go from almost complete recovery to severe brain injury. Though the said mechanisms are reversible, the eventual brain damage is not,

thus the neurological injury remains the leading cause of death in patients reanimated after cardiac arrest [8].

- *Respiratory dysfunction:* May be related to mechanical ventilation trauma, or lung contusions for chest compression, atelectasia, but in PCAS is mainly due to pulmonary edema. The patient may also be more prone to infections and pneumonia, either for aspiration during CPR or for tissue congestion, especially if hypothermia is used as a therapeutic means [16].
- *Others:* Acute renal failure (like respiratory dysfunction, observed in 40–50% of patients after cardiac arrest), liver insufficiency, but also digestive tract insult which often leads to bacterial translocation and endotoxemia [11].

In conclusion, PCAS is a complex syndrome with a variety of pathophysiological processes and clinical consequences. The management of these patients is challenging and requires a multidisciplinary approach.

10.3 Hypoxic-Ischemic Damage

Cardiac arrest leads to a state of global hypoxia-ischemia, where tissues and organs are deprived of essential oxygen and nutrients. This deprivation triggers a cascade of pathophysiological events that culminate in widespread tissue damage, particularly in organs with high metabolic demands such as the brain, lung, and myocardium.

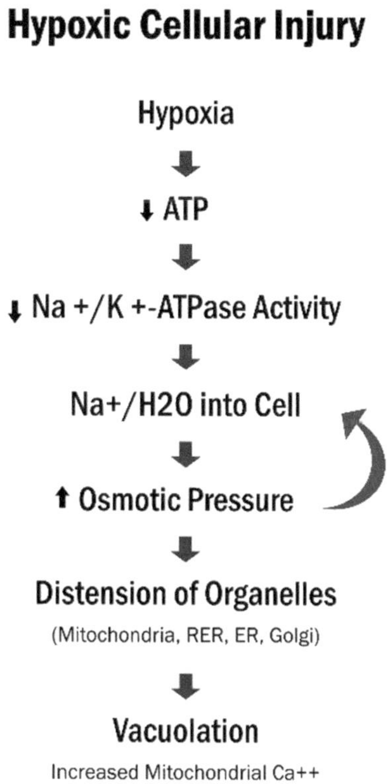

Hypoxic-ischemic damage is a critical consequence of cardiac arrest, resulting from the deprivation of oxygen and nutrients and the subsequent reperfusion injury upon the return of spontaneous circulation (ROSC). The pathophysiological mechanisms of ischemic damage and reperfusion injuries are complex and involve a cascade of cellular and molecular events [17].

During the ischemic phase, the lack of oxygen and glucose leads to a switch from aerobic to anaerobic metabolism, resulting in the production of lactic acid and a decrease in intracellular pH. This metabolic shift disrupts cellular homeostasis, leading to the dysfunction of ion pumps and the accumulation of intracellular calcium (Ca++). The excessive intracellular Ca++ can trigger apoptosis and necrosis, leading to cell death [10].

The reperfusion phase, which occurs when blood flow is restored, is paradoxically also a significant contributor to tissue damage. The sudden influx of oxygen and nutrients can lead to the overproduction of reactive oxygen species (ROS), causing oxidative stress. The reperfusion can also trigger a robust inflammatory response, characterized by the activation of immune cells, release of pro-inflammatory cytokines, and upregulation of adhesion molecules. This inflammatory response can further contribute to tissue damage and organ dysfunction [18].

10.4 Systemic Immune-Inflammatory Mechanisms

Inflammation plays a pivotal role in post-cardiac arrest damage. The ischemic insult and the subsequent reperfusion can trigger a robust inflammatory response that involves both the innate and adaptive immune systems.

The initial ischemic insult triggers the release of DAMPs (like HMGB1 heat shock proteins and mitochondrial DNA) that can activate pattern recognition receptors, such as toll-like receptors, on immune cells, leading to the activation of the immune response [19].

Neutrophils are among the first immune cells to respond to the ischemic insult. They are rapidly recruited to the site of injury, where they can release proinflammatory cytokines, produce ROS, and form neutrophil extracellular traps. These neutrophil activities can contribute to tissue damage and organ dysfunction [10].

Monocytes and macrophages also play a crucial role in the immune response worsening the immune-mediated damage.

The adaptive immune system, including T and B cells, is also involved in the immune response following cardiac arrest; however, their role is less well understood and is an area of ongoing research.

The production of ROS and proinflammatory cytokines by leukocytes amplifies the immune response, exacerbates oxidative stress, induces cell death, and contributes to tissue damage and organ dysfunction [20].

10.5 Brain Damage

10.5.1 Introduction

The brain, due to its high metabolic demand and limited energy reserves, is particularly vulnerable to hypoxic-ischemic damage.

Following cardiac arrest, the brain undergoes a series of pathophysiological changes that contribute to neuronal death and neurological dysfunction. It has been proposed a two-phase physiopathological mechanism to explain the neurological damage associated with cardiac arrest: an initial ischemic insult, followed by a second phase of damage associated with the reperfusion [17].

The first one leads to energy failure and loss of cell homeostasis, triggering excitotoxicity, oxidative stress, and apoptosis, while the second one is characterized by the activation of the immune system that leads to neuroinflammation and further exacerbation of neuronal damage [14].

The brain damage usually is proportional to the length of the no-flow and low-flow periods, and involves mainly brain regions in the arterial-border zones and those with high metabolic consumption.

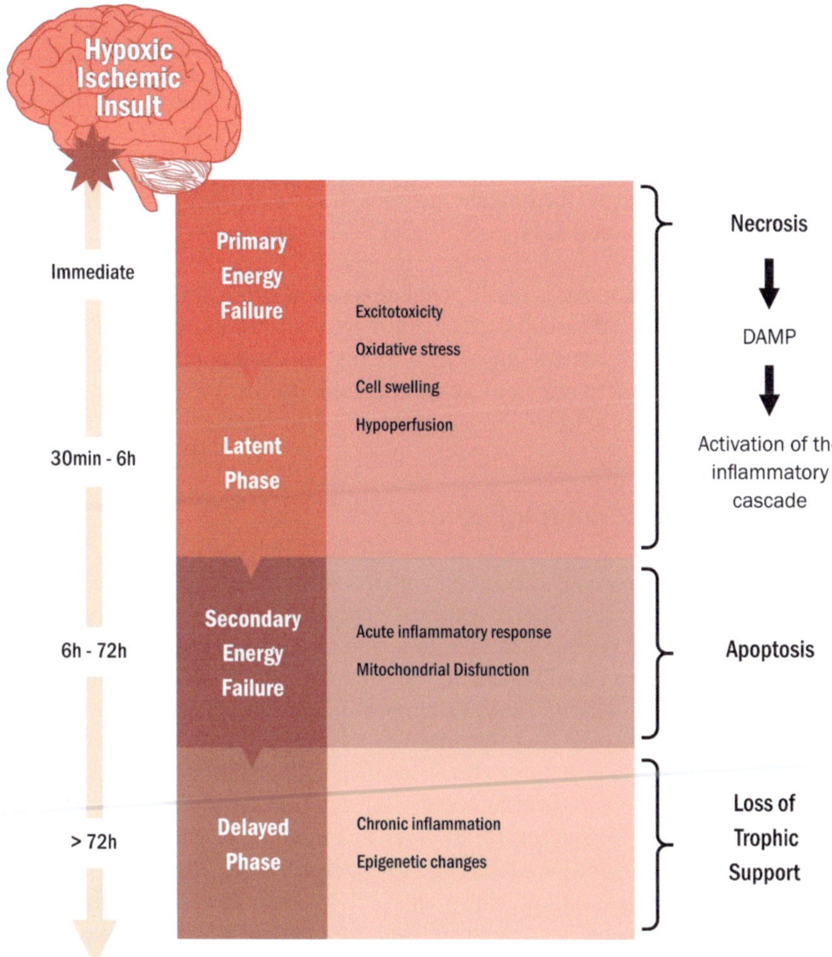

The regions in the arterial-border zones more affected are mainly three:

- The anterior border zone between the anterior (ACA) and middle cerebral artery (MCA)
- The posterior border zone between MCA and posterior cerebral artery
- The internal border zone between the superficial branches of the MCA and the deep branches of the MCA or ACA [10].

The deep white cerebral matter is particularly exposed to damage, not only because it lies in the internal border zones but also because of its vascular anatomy, consisting of widespread linear arterioles with not many anastomoses, which contribute to its sensibility to the hypoxic damage.

As for what concerns the areas with high metabolic consumption, the neurons more prone to be afflicted by hypoxic-ischemic damage are:

- CA1 pyramidal neurons of the hippocampus, leading to impairment in memory
- Purkinje cells of the cerebellum, with consequential truncal ataxia
- Pyramidal neurons in layers 3, 5, and 6 of the neocortex
- Basal ganglia neurons (the reticular neurons of the thalamus, the medium-sized neurons of the striatum) [21]

We specifically talk about these populations of neurons because it has been shown that glial cells and vascular cells in these areas are not as affected by hypoxia; a possible explanation for this impairment is that this sub-population of neurons expresses characteristic patterns of genes that code for early expressions of heat shock proteins [10].

10.5.2 Hypoxic-Ischemic Injury

Cardiac arrest leads to circulatory arrest with the sudden cessation of cerebral oxygen delivery (CDO2), resulting in neuronal hypoxia. The sudden reduction of O_2 availability leads to a decline and then to a stop of adenosine triphosphate (ATP) synthesis. The absence of ATP leads to a dysfunction of all those ATP-dependent ionic pump channels, altering the physiological ionic environment of the intracellular and extracellular space [14]. Specifically, potassium (K+) leaks in the extracellular environment while sodium (Na+) accumulates inside the cell leading to cytotoxic edema and to membrane depolarization. This depolarization causes the opening of N-methyl-D-aspartate (NMDA) channels with a sudden high increase of the intracellular concentration of Ca++, and hyper-activation of all those systems Ca++-dependent, such as the calpain system [22]. The calpain system is involved in signal transduction pathways, apoptosis, and the remodeling of cytoskeletal and membrane structures. The cytoskeletal ineffective remodeling leads to cytoskeletal damage and to the inability to maintain cell structure and function [23]. On the other hand, the consequent depolarization and the NMDA channels activity cause a continuous release of glutamate, excitatory neurotransmitter, increasing metabolic expenditure and causing the excitotoxic activation of glutamate receptors. This activation leads to the up-regulation of early genes, some of them with apparently protective function against free radical damage (such as Bcl-2 in the non-vulnerable areas of Hippocampus), but most of them involved in the synthesis of heat-shock protein and in inducing the excitotoxic activation of enzymes (such as lipases, nucleases, and proteases) involved in the neuronal tissue breakdown.

The increase of the intracellular Ca++ concentration causes a transient mitochondrial swelling, with polyribosome disaggregation and abnormal Golgi complexes ultimately leading to mitochondrial damage [10]. The mitochondrial dysfunction increases the inability of the system to buffer the calcium loads, worsens the ATP depletion, and is responsible for the release of free radical species and the production of nitric oxide (NO) and peroxynitrate (NO_3^-), the major mediator of NO damage. This process worsens the cytoskeletal damage of the neuron.

The decrease in nutrient availability reduces cellular functions deeply affecting protein synthesis. The reduction of protein synthesis starts relatively early in the process of ischemia and, in cells not permanently damaged, is restored to normality in about 12–48 h (depending on the animal model studied).

The reduction of the ATP synthesis causes a shift from aerobic metabolism to an anaerobic one, with the production of lactic acid that dissociates and produces hydrogen ions (H^+) cerebral lactate accumulation and metabolic acidosis [24]. The process involves initially the extracellular environment, and in a second moment (minutes later) the intracellular one, and leads to acidosis with pH values that can reach up to 6.1–6.5 (tolerable by the neurons for just about 10–12 min in rat models) [25]. The metabolic acidosis starts as a local problem, leading to cell damage and edema, and eventually becomes generalized with an imbalance between lactate production and removal.

During the first phase of circulatory arrest, there is an initial compensative cerebral vasodilatation, an attempt of the system to improve the oxygen delivery to the brain; this compensatory mechanism backfires shortly after, in fact the blood stasis that we have during the arrest leads to a fall in blood-viscosity, which lowers resistance in low resistance regions, such as capillary and veins, to buffer the pressure of adjacent high resistance regions [10].

10.5.3 Secondary Injury

Secondary injury mechanisms take place immediately after the return of spontaneous circulation (ROSC). If it is true that with the reperfusion of the brain, we witness the resumption of metabolic activity in those neurons that were not irreversibly damaged, it does not mean that neurological damage stops.

As soon as we have reperfusion, we witness a brief hyperemia of about 15 min, followed by a protracted period of global hypoperfusion that lasts up to 24 h [10]. This event is also called the no-reflow phenomenon, and it is responsible for diffuse secondary neurological damage, due to circulatory impairment with the reduction of blood flow that can decrease up to 50% of the normal blood flow level [14].

As we said before, initially during the cardiac arrest the increase of CO_2 levels and compensatory mechanisms induce cerebral vasodilatation, with blood stasis and, due to the ions and inorganic electrolytic disorders mentioned above, with the shift of water from the high pressure vascular lumen to the extravascular compartment, with subsequent brain edema and compression of the vascular district with low pressure, such as capillary and vein. We witness vascular spasms in big arterial branches. Still, the primary damage is due to microvascular impairment, where even brief periods of stasis have proved in animal models to induce brain damage up to 50% of the cerebral mass [26]. The compression of these low-pressure vascular districts causes a reduction in the caliber of the lumen, and blood flow reduction/obstruction, thus provoking a deterioration of the edema for further extravasation of water and other solutes [10]. On the other hand, we see blood cells sludging against each other, activating the coagulation cascade and causing micro-thrombosis and disseminated intravascular coagulation (CID), inducing eventually secondary hypoxia damage. It has to be mentioned also that during this no-reflow phenomenon, we observe an increase in the blood-brain barrier (BBB) permeability [26]. Whether this phenomenon is pathological or starts with reparative means the result is that the BBB becomes porous and permeable to substances normally poorly permeant such as sucrose; extravasation of water through these pores causes perivascular edema worsening the cerebrovascular resistance and the extraction of O_2. The damaged capillaries could also cause microhemorrhages [10].

10.5.4 Reperfusion Injury

Following the first phase of damage caused by the above mechanisms, there is a local activation of the inflammatory cascade that becomes systemic as soon as we have a resumption of the circulation.

During the hypoxic insult, we witness the activation of sensor proteins like AMP-activated protein kinase (AMPK), which in turn activates a pathway involving HMGB1 and S100A8/A9 proteins which signal through toll and RAGE receptors, ultimately leading to the activation of physiologically responsive transcription factors [27]. These factors, including HIF-1α and NF-kβ, are involved in the cell survival and necrosis processes, and in inflammatory response modulation. The cell death leads to the release of DAMPs, which in turn activates through pattern recognition receptors (PRRs), the nearby microglia, and macrophages with the production of chemokines and cytokines (TNF-alpha, IL1, IL6) [16].

Microglia, like macrophages, can be activated in two conformations:

- *M1*, promoted by pro-inflammatory cytokines and expressing CD68 and CD86, with pro-inflammatory function (expressed by the production of pro-inflammatory cytokines and other cytotoxic molecules including ROS, NO, and prostanoids) and enhanced phagocytic activity.
- *M2*, promoted by IL4, IL10, and TGF-beta, expressing CD206, anginase1, and Yml, with anti-inflammatory activity; this particular microglial function seems to be explicated by the phagocytosis of infiltrating neutrophils and the ingestion of dying neurons, a process known as phagoptosis [27].

Resident microglia are activated within minutes of hypoxia and start to proliferate and differentiate into M1 or M2 types. It then promotes the migration of resident microglia from other brain areas and the recruitment of peripheral immune cells like neutrophils, macrophages, and T lymphocytes, which contribute to the secondary damage [28].

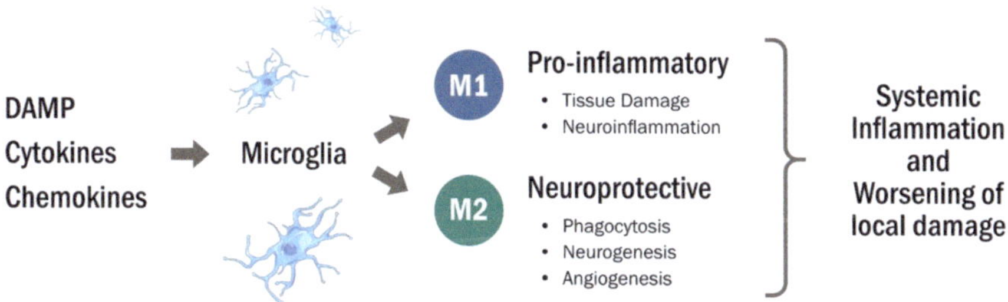

Neutrophils are the first non-resident immune cells to be enrolled. Within a few hours after ischemia onset, the neutrophils, after being exposed to pro-inflammatory cytokines, start to express cellular adhesion molecules (CAMs) like intercellular adhesion molecule 1 (ICAM-1). This molecule, as in any inflammatory response, is involved in the adhesion of the neutrophils to the endothelial membrane [29]. The adhesion to the membrane is facilitated by the degradation performed by free radicals and lytic enzymes of the glycoproteins, proteoglycans, and glycosaminoglycans blocks composing the glycocalyx [16]. The glycocalyx extends from the endothelial surface in the vascular lumen, is negatively charged, and serves as a first line of defense against macromolecules and circulating immune cells. The erosion of glycocalyx unleashes hyaluronic acid, syndecan-1, and heparan sulfate, uncovering P-selectin molecules and other adhesion factors that facilitate the recruitment, activation, and margination of leukocytes [30]. After the adhesion of the neutrophils to the endothelial surface, the neutrophils start rolling on it, and this process triggers the exocytosis of vesicles containing CD11b/CD18, an integrin complex that reinforces the cellular adhesion to the endothelium. The neutrophils then start secreting secondary granules containing matrix metalloproteases (MMPs) and other lytic enzymes such as IV-hyaluronidases and heparinases that deteriorate collagen (type IV and I), extracellular matrix, and the proteins forming the tight junctions (e-cadherin, claudins, occludins), thus facilitating the neutrophil margination but also leading the BBB, increasing its permeability and inducing cerebral edema [31].

The secretion of lytic enzymes also causes the loss of alpha6beta4, an integrin that conveys the adhesion of the astrocytic endfeet to the basal lamina, causing the detachment of the astrocytes from it and opening de facto a breach in the BBB [32].

Once activated and in situ neutrophils start causing direct damage (release of ROS, etc...) enhancing the inflammatory response by producing pro-inflammatory cytokines, and recruiting other leukocytes through the production of chemokines like IL8, CCL2, and CCL3 that attract monocytes and lymphocytes to the ischemic area, increasing the inflammatory damage to the tissues [20].

The breach in the BBB created by the neutrophils during their migration toward the areas of lesions permits the entry of the said leukocytes and also complement proteins, worsening the cellular edema and furthering the extrinsic microvascular collapse, oligemia, and finally secondary tissue ischemia.

Neutrophils also release azurophilic granules, which contain myeloperoxidase (MPO), defensins, cathepsins, and elastase that contribute to the BBB damage.

MPO produces HOCl that activates platelets and promotes the release of degradative enzymes and neutrophil extracellular traps (NETs), like decondensed chromatin and HGMB1, that exercise a pro-coagulant effect [20].

Some neutrophils, which express high levels of ICAM1 and ROS-generating abilities, undergo reverse migration going back into the vascular department and spreading inflammatory injury to distant locations, with particular tropism for lung tissue.

10.5.5 Clinical Manifestations

Clinically, these pathophysiological processes can manifest themselves as cognitive dysfunctions, cerebral edema, seizures, coma, stroke, and brain death [11].

10.6 Lung Damage

10.6.1 No-Flow Phase

During the no-flow phase of cardiac arrest, the lung, just as all the other organs, is subjected to hypoxia. Hypoxia induces on the lung tissue, aside from the switch to an anaerobic metabolisms from an aerobic one with consequent production of lactic acid and proinflammatory insult, a process of vascular remodeling involving monocytes, fibrocytes, and the resident vascular cells that ultimately leads to persistent vasoconstriction [11].

The impaired CO_2 clearance leads to an accumulation of CO_2 and consequent hypercapnia. Hypercapnia leads to the upregulation of genes such as miR-183, which in turn downregulates TCA enzymes causing mitochondrial dysfunction, which subsequently inhibits proliferation of the alveolar epithelial. It also causes a reduction in the macrophages activity of phagocytosis, and impairs alveolar epithelial cell migration in response to NF-Kbeta [11].

In the early phase of cardiac arrest, there is a first brief period of respiratory acidosis, followed by another brief phase of respiratory alkalosis (due to the mechanical ventilation), and lastly a phase of metabolic acidosis due to the impaired production and removal of lactate [33].

Acidosis in the lung causes a reduction in the ability of the lung epithelium to prevent/clear lung edema. In fact, the clearance of lung edema appears correlated to the expression on the lung epithelium of the ionic pump Na^+/K^+ATPase. During cardiac arrest, due to the low availability of ATP, the pump function is already undermined, and thus, activity is reduced [34]. The subset of acidosis activates AMP kinase (AMPK), which in turn activates the protein kinase C-Zeta (PKC-Zeta) that phosphorylates the alpha1 subunit of the Na^+/K^+ATPase pump, causing its endocytosis from the cell plasma membrane with consequent ionic imbalance between the extracellular and intracellular space.

Alkalosis, on the other hand, induces and amplifies the activation of the inflammatory cascade, and in the lung causes an increase in the mechanical power [11].

10.6.2 Low-Flow Phase

During the low-flow phase with the CPR maneuvers, the damage is primarily of an iatrogenic nature. Cardiopulmonary resuscitation induces mechanical trauma to the rib cage and to the lung; rib fractures and lung contusions are frequent consequences of CPR. On the other hand, iatrogenic trauma is frequently also associated with mechanical ventilation [35].

Mechanical ventilation itself with its set parameters can induce atelectrauma, volutrauma, and barotrauma (especially the latter has been correlated with hippocampal neuron apoptosis and consequent irreversible brain damage); it can also, as a positive pressure imposed to the thoracic system, easily increases the intrathoracic pressure, disturbing the lymphatic return outflow and thus inducing/worsening the pulmonary edema and affecting the gasses exchanges [36].

Mechanical ventilation often causes hyperventilation and subsequent hypocapnia. Hypocapnia increases the demand of metabolic energy and O_2. In a situation with low ATP production/availability, this leads to a sympathetic-like activation meant to counterweight the energy demands, which further increases the need for oxygen and the metabolic demand. This response, paired up with the cardiac damage and post-arrest cardiac pump failure, and with the increase in the diastolic cardiac pressure due to the inability of the myocardium in a low pH situation to relax, is accountable for the impaired cardiac function with increased cardiac pressure and worsening of the hyperventilation/hypocapnia.

It is not infrequent also the use of high concentration of O_2, during mechanical ventilation which leads to hyperoxia. Hyperoxia in the lung induces the transcription of p53 with consequent activation of miR34a which leads to abnormal cell proliferation, apoptosis, and impaired alveolarization [11].

Hyperoxia leads to overproduction of ROS and consequent saturation of the intrinsic antioxidant mechanisms of the lung, exposing its tissue to oxidative cellular injury, leading to activation of pro-apoptotic and proinflammatory factors like cyclooxygenase-2 (COX2), toll-like receptor 4 (TLR4), and caspase-3 protein, ultimately causing apoptosis and necrosis [37]. These damages are also carried out on the alveolar-capillary barrier inducing hemorrhagic pulmonary edema. Hyperoxia inhibits hypoxic pulmonary vasoconstriction and undermines the adsorption of atelectasis.

10.6.3 ROSC and Post-resuscitation Phase

After ROSC, we have a condition of metabolic acidosis due to the high production of lactate induced by the aforementioned mechanisms with all its described implications. What still needs to be mentioned is the high production of catecholamines induced by, among other mechanisms, acidosis itself, hypoxia, and high lactate levels [33]. These conditions induce a steady and increasing production of catecholamine. Whether of endogenous production or exogenous administration, catecholamines induce an increase in the oxygen consumption and in the metabolic needs of the organism. The response of the organism to catecholamine is deeply affected by the persistence of high levels of the same through time (which leads to downregulation and desensitization of adrenoreceptors and subsequent increase in the production of the same), but also by acidosis. Acidosis deeply reduces the sensitivity of the organism to catecholamine [38]. Through time, the clearance of lactate and the compensatory mechanisms mitigate the acidosis, suddenly improving the efficacy of catecholamines on target districts, causing a sudden toxicity of the molecules.

All the above cascades and pathways of damage added to the ischemic and reperfusion insult which the lung, just like all the other organs, undergoes lead to the activation of a systemic inflammatory response, the main responsible of damage in the post-resuscitation phase [11].

10.6.4 Inflammatory Mechanisms

The lung district filtrates the entire cardiac output and thus all the cells contained in it, even the quote from the thoracic duct. Neutrophils are physiologically bigger if compared to the diameter of the small alveolar capillaries, to the point that peripherally they have to deform to pass the narrow vases. This increases remarkably the time that they take to pass through the respiratory system and makes the lungs an indirect pool of reserve of neutrophils.

In certain conditions, the reticuloendothelial cells through the process of efferocytosis seem to be able to deprime activated neutrophils and to release or remove them from the circulation [39].

During inflammation, the production of cytokines and ROS causes the expression of iCAM and exposure of p-selectin, respectively, on neutrophils and endothelial cells promoting the neutrophils' adhesion to the endothelial surface and thus slowing their pace [40]. This process leads also to the activation and priming of the neutrophils, increasing the expression on their surface of toll-like receptors (TLRs) and making them more reactive to alarmins and more prone to react to damage insults. The neutrophil activation causes a reduction in their ability to deform and pass through the small blood vessels and thus lengthens their time of transit in the lungs, where they are removed from circulation and retained.

The neutrophils activated in the CNS that underwent reverse endothelial transmigration, highly activated, are filtered through the lung small blood vessels, where they migrate to the interstitial space and with their release of their granules cause damage to the lung tissue. The damaged lung tissue is unable to deprime neutrophils, and the constant release of ROS and pro-inflammatory cytokines ulteriorly aliments the inflammatory process [41]; it has also been suggested that the damaged lung could also perform a pro-inflammatory function directly, serving as a priming site, and not only indirectly by not explicating its depriming function [42].

The amplification of the inflammatory response in the lung tissue with the recruitment of other leukocytes and the increase in the capillary permeability and endothelial activation causes pulmonary edema, negatively affecting the gas exchanges with downsides on all the other organ's O_2 delivery and CO_2 washout.

The resident megakaryocytes (responsible for a good amount of the platelets produced) are likely to be affected by this inflammatory damage, with probably qualitative and quantitative changes in the platelets' functions [43].

As mentioned before, the lung has an intrinsic antioxidant defense system. It comprises superoxide dismutases (SOD) and catalase present in peroxisomes. Usually, the oxidative phosphorylation converts O_2 into H_2O, producing just a small amount of superoxide radical (O_2^-). This radical is converted to H_2O_2 by SOD and subsequently converted to water by catalase.

In the lung, we have an extracellular form of SOD (EC-SOD) encoded by the gene sod-3, with the function of stabilizing the extracellular matrix and inhibiting both inflammation and fibrosis under stress conditions. It plays a key role in protecting the lung against the damage caused by the highly reactive HOCl molecule generated by MPO released by the neutrophils.

In post-cardiac arrest systemic inflammation, this intrinsic mechanism of defense may be saturated and not completely effective in protecting the lung from damage induced by neutrophil toxicity and gut-associated xanthine oxidase activity, and an eventual ineffective response could lead to immediate damage or to a milieu of chronic inflammation [16].

10.6.5 Clinical Manifestations

In conclusion, clinically all these mechanisms of damage can result in *lung injury* (related to RCP, mechanical ventilation, and ischemia-reperfusion damage), neurogenic pulmonary edema, ARDS, and pneumonia.

Neurogenic pulmonary edema is a secondary damage induced by the effects of the inflammatory cascade on certain areas of the brain. As mentioned before, some of the districts more vulnerable to ischemic/inflammatory damage of the brain are the posterior hypothalamus, caudal ventrolateral medulla, nucleus tractus solitarius, and area postrema. It has been proposed that the inflammatory cascade activated in these regions during brain suffering may be responsible for neurogenic pulmonary edema (NPE) by driving sympathetically mediated surges in catecholamines. This sympathetic response causes pulmonary venoconstriction, increases the pulmonary capillary pressure, and raises the pulmonary vascular permeability, thus causing NPE.

Pulmonary edema may also be cardiogenic [44].

While for what concerns *ARDS*, two possible mechanisms have been proposed to explain its pathogenesis: one sees as leading actor an indirect activation of neutrophils with progressive inflammatory alveolar infiltrates, while the other proposes as the main culprit the direct damage of the epithelial barrier with endothelial cells activation induced by the ischemic reperfusion injury. Regardless of the ischemic or immune nature behind the beginning of the process, the consequence is the recruitment of leukocytes, thanks to the production of cytokines and chemokines and expression of CAMs, which, after transmigrating through the endothelium and epithelium, are sequestrated in the alveolar space where they release proinflammatory and cytotoxic mediators, causing ARDS [16]. Pneumonia may be related to aspiration during cardiac arrest or could be a consequence of therapeutic hypothermia, or could be a sovrainfection of the aforementioned lung complications [11].

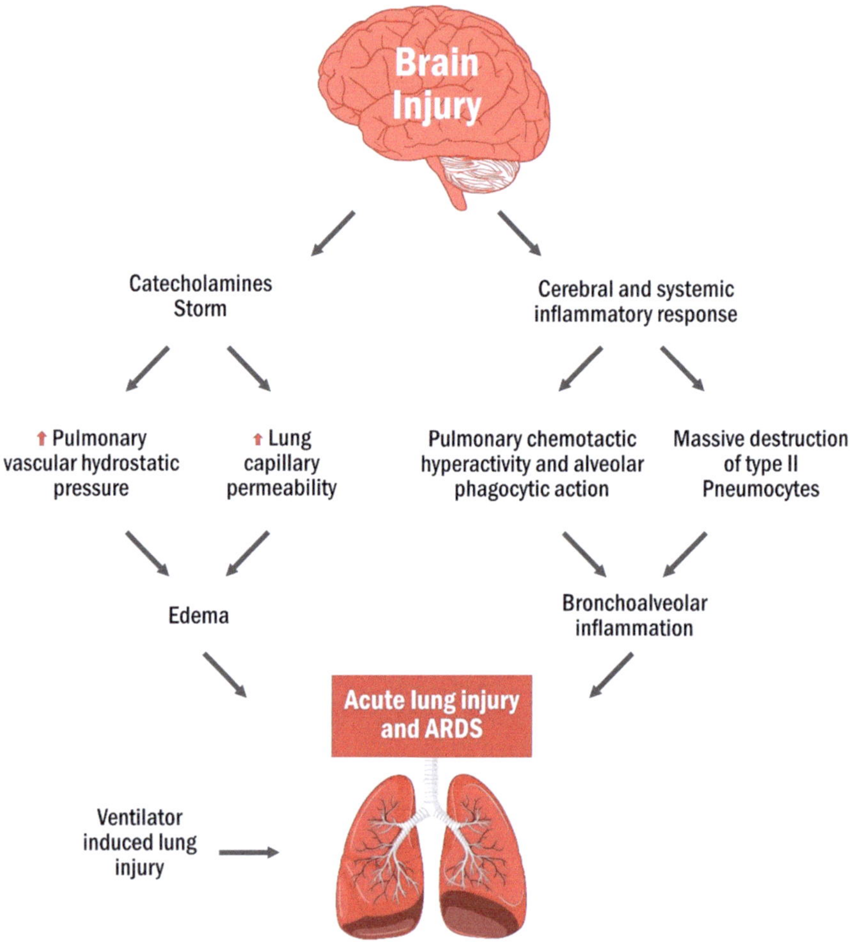

10.7 Gut Damage

Cardiac arrest induces non-occlusive mesenteric ischemia with subsequent endotoxemia. The gut in general is sensitive to ischemic damage, but the colon seems particularly prone to vasospasm and thus affected by hypoperfusion/hypotension states. The ischemic damage promotes the infiltration of the intestinal wall by hemorrhagic and inflammatory compounds, affecting its role of barrier against the enteric bacteria [45].

On the other hand, the high levels of DAMPS alone released during cardiac arrest even without mesenteric sufference seem to be able to induce an inflammatory response and infiltration in the intestinal wall.

The undermining of the intestinal wall favors the transmigration of enteric bacteria, pathogen-associated molecular patterns (PAMPs) like LPS, in the portal circulation where they cause a massive inflammatory cascade activation [46]. Apparently, even without bacteriemia, systemic immune activation can be witnessed. In fact, the lymphatic system associated with the gut alone can release proinflammatory factors in response to mesenteric injury, subsequently conveyed by the thoracic duct to the lung [16].

10.8 Myocardium Damage

During ischemia process caused by cardiac arrest, there is a blood supply restriction, with impaired oxygen and metabolic substrate supply. Simultaneously, there is a missing removal of waste metabolites. This phenomenon is at first balanced by a reduction in the systemic metabolic rate, but prolonged deprivation of blood flow leads inevitably to cell damage [9].

Oxygen deprivation leads to the shift from aerobic to anaerobic metabolism, due to an impairment in oxidative phosphorylation, developing a tissue acidotic status [47]. While performing CPR, we can witness an increased peripheral oxygen extraction, which is manifested by a decrease in ScvO2 levels [8].

Moreover, patients surviving after cardiac arrest often experience an ensemble of metabolic and respiratory disorders. More specifically, after the tissue's reperfusion process, there is a disproportion between lactate production and removal, leading to lactate acidosis. These acid-base imbalances lead inevitably to cell damage and dysfunction, with a depletion of cell's energy stores resulting in dysregulation of membrane ion pumps and, consequently, electrolyte and water imbalances. The result of all these processes is represented by mitochondrial damage, changes in gene expression, and production of ROS [7]. Acute lactic acidosis depresses left ventricular contractility, triggers the release of endogenous catecholamine, and decreases the responsiveness of the left ventricle to catecholamine [11].

Tissue damage caused by systemic I/R injury following cardiac arrest triggers a generalized activation of inflammatory and coagulation patterns which contribute to further damage and subsequent organ failure. This process has a similar profile to that observed in sepsis [8]. It involves innate and adaptive immunological response as well as complement system cascade. Indeed, innate immune cells are prevalent in the initial phase of reperfusion and are activated by DAMPS (damage-associated molecular patterns), produced by cell damage. Subsequently, T lymphocytes, as part of the adaptive immune system, are activated and further generate tissue injury.

Finally, complement activation amplifies local inflammation and differentiates healthy from injured tissue [7].

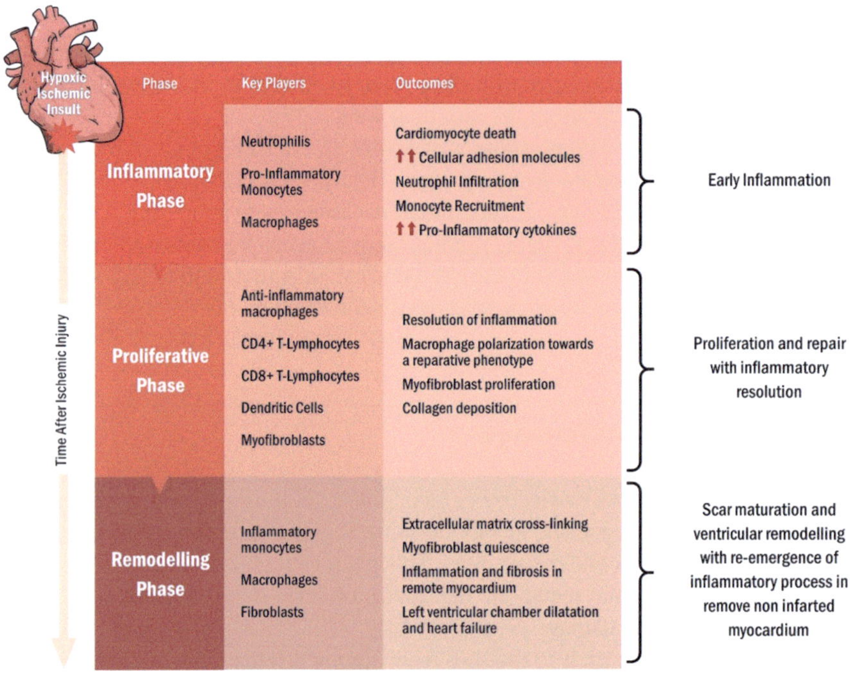

For what concerns heart involvement, according to recent studies, myocardial chronic low-grade inflammation is associated with some forms of heart disease, including cardiac injury due to ischemia/reperfusion process. This process involves complex and heterogeneous signaling patterns that promote disease progression. Among the main myocardial inflammatory pathways described may be reported [48]:

- Activation of Phospholipase A2: I/R cardiac injury may cause activation of this molecule, with an elevation in arachidonic acid levels and consensual increase in the production of eicosanoids, prostaglandins, and leukotrienes.
- ROS production, followed by release of proteases and DAMP2 (see below).
- TLRs/NLRs recognition of PAMPs/DAMPs: TLRs (Toll-like receptors) and NLRs (nucleotide oligomerization domain-like receptors) are found in immune cells as well as in endothelial cells and cardiomyocytes. Those receptors may be activated by damage-associated molecular patterns (DAMPs), leading to nuclear

translocation of NF-kB and subsequent release of cytokines (TNF-α, IL-1α, and IL-1β) and expression of adhesion molecules.

- Protease-activated receptors (PARs): These are a group of receptors found in endothelial cells, cardiac fibroblasts, and cardiomyocytes which seem to induce fibroblasts proliferation and hypertrophy.
- Mitogen-activated protein kinase (MAPK), phosphoinositide 3-kinase (PI3K), Akt pathway, Janus kinase (JAK)/ signal transducers and activator of transcription (STAT).
- Caspase 1 (interleukin-converting enzyme): The activation of this molecule is triggered by the inflammasome, a multiprotein complex, and leads to the release of IL-1beta.

The final effect of these molecular pathways is myocardial inflammation. This inflammatory state leads to matrix degradation, fibrosis, and collagen deposition inducing extracellular matrix remodeling, angiogenesis, and progressive loss of cardiomyocytes. This process induces the formation of a scar and is responsible for functional loss. This adverse ventricular remodeling induces LV dilatation, LV wall thinning, and systolic/diastolic dysfunction, ultimately leading to heart failure [48].

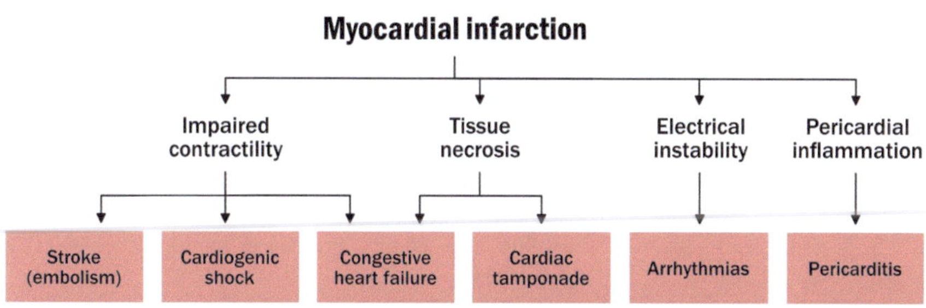

Aside from the aforementioned PCAS presentation, clinically all these damages can present themselves as acute myocardial infarction, dilatative, hypertrophic or restrictive cardiomyopathy, arrhythmias, and cardiovascular collapse.

10.9 Conclusions

In conclusion, inflammation plays a crucial role in the pathophysiology of cardiac arrest aftermath.

The study of inflammation in cardiac arrest is a rapidly evolving field. Future research should focus on elucidating the detailed mechanisms of the inflammatory response, identifying novel inflammatory markers, and developing effective anti-inflammatory therapies. The use of advanced technologies could provide new insights into the complex and dynamic nature of the inflammatory response following cardiac arrest. Moreover, the development of novel anti-inflammatory therapies, such as cytokine inhibitors and immune cell modulators, could provide new therapeutic options to improve the outcome for patients after cardiac arrest.

References

1. Perman SM, et al. 2023 American Heart Association focused update on adult advanced cardiovascular life support: an update to the American Heart Association guidelines for cardiopulmonary resuscitation and emergency cardiovascular care. Circulation. 2024;149(5):e254–73.
2. Andersen LW, Holmberg MJ, Berg KM, Donnino MW, Granfeldt A. In-hospital cardiac arrest. JAMA. 2019;321:1200.
3. Virani SS, et al. Heart disease and stroke statistics—2020 update: a report from the American Heart Association. Circulation. 2020;141(9):e139–596.
4. Chan PS, McNally B, Tang F, Kellermann A. Recent trends in survival from out-of-hospital cardiac arrest in the United States. Circulation. 2014;130:1876–82.
5. Chang W-T, et al. Postresuscitation myocardial dysfunction: correlated factors and prognostic implications. Intensive Care Med. 2006;33:88–95.
6. Wada T, et al. Disseminated intravascular coagulation with the fibrinolytic phenotype predicts the outcome of patients with out-of-hospital cardiac arrest. Thromb J. 2016;14:43.
7. Lazzarin T, et al. Post-cardiac arrest: mechanisms, management, and future perspectives. J Clin Med. 2022;12:259.
8. Nolan JP, et al. Post-cardiac arrest syndrome: epidemiology, pathophysiology, treatment, and prognostication. Resuscitation. 2008;79:350–79.
9. Mongardon N, et al. Postcardiac arrest syndrome: from immediate resuscitation to long-term outcome. Ann Intensive Care. 2011;1(1):45.
10. Busl KM, Greer DM. Hypoxic-ischemic brain injury: pathophysiology, neuropathology and mechanisms. NeuroRehabilitation. 2010;26. Preprint at https://doi.org/10.3233/NRE-2010-0531.
11. Robba C, et al. Pathophysiology and clinical consequences of arterial blood gases and pH after cardiac arrest. Intensive Care Med Exp. 2020;8. Preprint at https://doi.org/10.1186/s40635-020-00307-1.
12. Adrie C, et al. Coagulopathy after successful cardiopulmonary resuscitation following cardiac arrest. J Am Coll Cardiol. 2005;46:21–8.
13. Ruiz-Bailén M, et al. Reversible myocardial dysfunction after cardiopulmonary resuscitation. Resuscitation. 2005;66:175–81.
14. Sekhon MS, Ainslie PN, Griesdale DE. Clinical pathophysiology of hypoxic ischemic brain injury after cardiac arrest: a 'two-hit' model. Crit Care. 2017;21. Preprint at https://doi.org/10.1186/s13054-017-1670-9.
15. Battaglini D, et al. Brain-heart interaction after acute ischemic stroke. Crit Care. 2020;24. Preprint at https://doi.org/10.1186/s13054-020-02885-8.
16. Mai N, Miller-Rhodes K, Knowlden S, Halterman MW. The post-cardiac arrest syndrome: a case for lung–brain coupling and opportunities for neuroprotection. J Cereb Blood Flow Metab. 2019;39. Preprint at https://doi.org/10.1177/0271678X19835552.
17. Eltzschig HK, Eckle T. Ischemia and reperfusion—from mechanism to translation. Nat Med. 2011;17:1391–401.
18. Schneider A, Albertsmeier M, Böttiger BW, Teschendorf P. Post-resuscitation syndrome. Role of inflammation after cardiac arrest. Anaesthesist. 2012;61(5):424–36.
19. Sugita A, et al. Systemic impact on secondary brain aggravation due to ischemia/reperfusion injury in post-cardiac arrest syndrome: a prospective observational study using high-mobility group box 1 protein. Crit Care. 2017;21:247.

20. Xiang Y, et al. Inflammatory mechanisms involved in brain injury following cardiac arrest and cardiopulmonary resuscitation. Biomed Rep. 2016;5. Preprint at https://doi.org/10.3892/br.2016.677.
21. Baron J-C, Yamauchi H, Fujioka M, Endres M. Selective neuronal loss in ischemic stroke and cerebrovascular disease. J Cereb Blood Flow Metab. 2014;34:2–18.
22. Xiong W, Hoesch R, Geocadin R. Post-cardiac arrest encephalopathy. Semin Neurol. 2011;31:216–25.
23. Shi Y, et al. Rapid endothelial cytoskeletal reorganization enables early blood–brain barrier disruption and long-term ischaemic reperfusion brain injury. Nat Commun. 2016;7:10523.
24. Hossmann K-A, Lechtape-Grüter H, Hossmann V. The role of cerebral blood flow for the recovery of the brain after prolonged ischemia. Z Neurol. 1973;204:281–99.
25. Hoxworth JM, Xu K, Zhou Y, Lust WD, LaManna JC. Cerebral metabolic profile, selective neuron loss, and survival of acute and chronic hyperglycemic rats following cardiac arrest and resuscitation. Brain Res. 1999;821:467–79.
26. Ginsberg MD, Myers RE. The topography of impaired micro vascular perfusion in the primate brain following total circulatory arrest. Neurology. 1972;22:998.
27. Benakis C, Garcia-Bonilla L, Iadecola C, Anrather J. The role of microglia and myeloid immune cells in acute cerebral ischemia. Front Cell Neurosci. 2015;8:461.
28. Yenari MA, Kauppinen TM, Swanson RA. Microglial activation in stroke: therapeutic targets. Neurotherapeutics. 2010;7:378–91.
29. Price CJS, et al. Cerebral neutrophil recruitment, histology, and outcome in acute ischemic stroke. Stroke. 2004;35:1659–64.
30. Zhu J, et al. Glycocalyx degradation leads to blood–brain barrier dysfunction and brain edema after asphyxia cardiac arrest in rats. J Cereb Blood Flow Metab. 2018;38:1979–92.
31. Yenari MA, Xu L, Tang XN, Qiao Y, Giffard RG. Microglia potentiate damage to blood–brain barrier constituents. Stroke. 2006;37:1087–93.
32. Wagner S, Tagaya M, Koziol JA, Quaranta V, del Zoppo GJ. Rapid disruption of an astrocyte interaction with the extracellular matrix mediated by integrin $\alpha_6\beta_4$ during focal cerebral ischemia/reperfusion. Stroke. 1997;28:858–65.
33. Phypers B, Pierce JT. Lactate physiology in health and disease. Cont Educ Anaesth Crit Care Pain. 2006;6:128–32.
34. Michiels C. Physiological and pathological responses to hypoxia. Am J Pathol. 2004;164:1875–82.
35. Kim MJ, et al. Chest injury following cardiopulmonary resuscitation: a prospective computed tomography evaluation. Resuscitation. 2013;84:361–4.
36. Hedenstierna G, Lattuada M. Lymphatics and lymph in acute lung injury. Curr Opin Crit Care. 2008;14:31–6.
37. Hu G, Malik AB, Minshall RD. Toll-like receptor 4 mediates neutrophil sequestration and lung injury induced by endotoxin and hyperinflation*. Crit Care Med. 2010;38:194–201.
38. Mauch J, Ringer S, Spielmann N, Weiss M. Impact of catecholamines in cardiac arrest due to acute asphyxia—a study in piglets. Pediatr Anesth. 2014;24:933–9.
39. Robb CT, Regan KH, Dorward DA, Rossi AG. Key mechanisms governing resolution of lung inflammation. Semin Immunopathol. 2016;38:425–48.
40. Reitsma S, Slaaf DW, Vink H, van Zandvoort MAMJ, oude Egbrink MGA. The endothelial glycocalyx: composition, functions, and visualization. Pflugers Arch. 2007;454:345–59.
41. Singh NRP, et al. Acute lung injury results from failure of neutrophil de-priming: a new hypothesis. Eur J Clin Investig. 2012;42:1342–9.
42. Summers C, et al. Pulmonary retention of primed neutrophils: a novel protective host response, which is impaired in the acute respiratory distress syndrome. Thorax. 2014;69:623–9.
43. Lefrançais E, et al. The lung is a site of platelet biogenesis and a reservoir for haematopoietic progenitors. Nature. 2017;544:105–9.
44. Verein M, et al. Dynamics of extravascular pulmonary water and intracranial pressure in patients with ischemic stroke. Semin Cardiothorac Vasc Anesth. 2010;14:226–30.

45. Katsoulis IE, et al. Extensive colonic necrosis following cardiac arrest and successful cardiopulmonary resuscitation: report of a case and literature review. World J Emerg Surg. 2012;7:35.
46. Wang F, Li Q, Wang C, Tang C, Li J. Dynamic alteration of the colonic microbiota in intestinal ischemia-reperfusion injury. PLoS One. 2012;7:e42027.
47. Binks A, Nolan JP. Post-cardiac arrest syndrome. Minerva Anestesiol. 2010;76:362–8.
48. Ahn J, Kim J. Mechanisms and consequences of inflammatory signaling in the myocardium. Curr Hypertens Rep. 2012;14(6):510–6.

Part III

The Kidneys

Molecular Mechanisms of Kidney Crosstalk with Distant Organs

11

E. Sturdà, F. La Fergola, and M. Fiorentino

11.1 Introduction

Acute and chronic renal impairment are serious complications characterized by increasing prevalence and incidence worldwide. The accumulation of uremic toxins and the persistent chronic inflammation contribute to the onset of secondary injury in several organs. Similarly, an acute impairment of kidney function (acute kidney injury, AKI) may be typically associated with a multiorgan dysfunction syndrome leading to high morbidity and mortality among critically ill patients. Most studies focusing on organ crosstalk and multiorgan failure have highlighted the pathophysiological role of several proinflammatory and proapoptotic pathways, together with oxidative stress and the generation of reactive oxygen species (ROS) [1]. Leukocyte activation, the production of systemic cytokines and chemokines, and cell death regulation are potentially significant pathways involved in multiorgan dysfunction syndrome. Although the knowledge of the crosstalk between the kidney and other organs is still not entirely defined, a number of new molecular pathways and important mediators were discovered in recent years, leading to new potential therapeutic targets. In this chapter, we summarize the main underlying molecular mechanisms of organ crosstalk occurring during acute and chronic kidney diseases, focusing on the stunning interplay between kidneys and liver, heart, lung, and brain impairments.

E. Sturdà · F. La Fergola · M. Fiorentino (✉)
Department of Precision and Regenerative Medicine and Ionian Area (DiMePRE-J), Nephrology, Dialysis and Transplantation Unit, University of Bari Aldo Moro, Bari, Italy
e-mail: marco.fiorentino@uniba.it

D. Battaglini et al. (eds.), *Organ System Crosstalk in Critical Illness*,
https://doi.org/10.1007/978-3-032-01024-7_11

11.2 Kidney-Heart Crosstalk

Concurrent heart and kidney failure has a complex pathophysiology, referred to as cardiorenal syndrome (CRS). Distinct CRS subtypes that more precisely characterize the initiating event and potential factors sustaining acute or chronic end-organ failure have been defined [2, 3].

Cardiovascular dysfunction is a common cause of death in AKI patients, and several mechanisms have been proposed to define this crosstalk (Fig. 11.1). Specific cardiac alterations have been reported in this setting; during ischemic-reperfusion injury (IRI), left ventricular (LV) dilatation is described, as well as a decrease in fractional shortening, relaxation duration, and left ventricular end diastolic and end systolic diameter [4]. On the other hand, in certain situations, ischemic preconditioning of the kidney can result in protection for distant organs, limiting the permanent heart damage caused by chronic coronary artery closure [5]. It is commonly recognized that azotemia and water retention can cause heart failure in the setting of renal failure; however, the exact mechanism of heart injury during AKI remains unknown. Cardiac apoptosis and inflammatory response with neutrophil infiltration are known mechanisms linked to cardiac defects following AKI. During IRI-induced AKI, leukocyte activation and trafficking are crucial factors in inducing cardiac damage [6]. Following adhesion and chemotaxis,

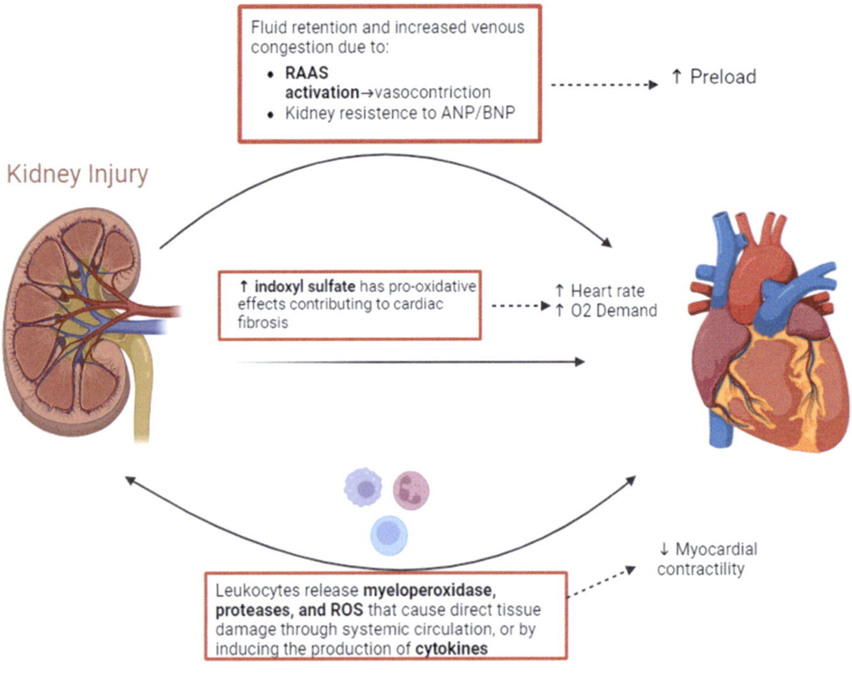

Fig. 11.1 Kidney-heart crosstalk. Legend: ANP atrial natriuretic peptide, BNP brain natriuretic peptide, RAS renin-angiotensin system, ROS reactive oxygen species

neutrophils are able to release specific substances such as myeloperoxidase, proteases, and ROS, leading to direct tissue damage or to an indirect one induced by cytokine production, which are essential in the pathophysiology of heart failure [7, 8]. Leukocyte infiltration and myocyte death are caused by both systemic and cardiac tumor necrosis factor-α (TNF-α), interleukin-1 (IL-1), and the increased mRNA expression of markers of endothelial dysfunction (ICAM-1) during AKI [4]. These studies pointout a potentially crucial function of the kidneys in preserving cardiac homeostasis and the balance of specific serum cytokines. Moreover, myocardial dysfunction can be avoided by blocking adhesion molecule receptors, using enteracept, a TNF-α receptor antagonist, or using anti-TNF-α antibodies [4]. Transgenic animals models have shown that deadly heart failure can result from cardiac myocyte apoptosis alone, indicating that this process plays a significant role in the pathogenesis of myocardial infarction [9].

Patients with CKD have significant rates of morbidity and mortality due to uremic cardiomyopathy. Urinary excretion of indoxyl sulfate (IS) and markers of oxidative stress in cardiac tissue have been shown to be linearly correlated [10]. Upon treatment with IS, cardiomyocytes exhibited elevated ROS generation and enhanced NOX2/NOX4 expression [11]. TNF-α, IL-6, and IL-1β are pro-inflammatory cytokines that have been linked to elevated levels of circulating IS. Conversely, the most prevalent arrhythmia in CKD patients is atrial fibrillation, linked to a higher risk of stroke, thromboembolism, and cardiovascular death. In addition, IS accumulation has been shown to contribute to cardiac fibrosis in both in vitro and in vivo studies, as this process may alter the normal electrical connection of heart tissue to enhance the vulnerability to arrhythmias [12].

Maladaptive inflammatory response and the persistence of hemodynamic-induced kidney dysfunction represent the milestones in the heart-kidney crosstalk, resulting in changes in cardiac output, extracellular volume, and renal sodium management. The activation of the sympathetic nervous system (SNS), the release of natriuretic peptides, and the activation of renin-angiotensin system have a pivotal role in this setting. Additionally, changes in the ratio of nitric oxide to ROS, inflammatory mediators, and SNS-induced cardiomyocyte hypertrophy, apoptosis, and infarction can all be linked to the pathophysiology of CRS [13]. These variables work together to change the left ventricle's structure, which accelerates the development of renal damage [3].

11.3 Kidney-Lung Crosstalk

Both preclinical and clinical studies have shown that lung impairment is a significant complication occurring during AKI course (Fig. 11.2). Acute lung injury (ALI) and AKI together account for almost 80% of the deaths of critically ill patients [1, 14]. Renal hemodynamics and function may typically deteriorate in the context of ALI, increasing the risk of AKI. In addition, ischemic AKI in rats induces profound alterations in the epithelial salt and water transporters at pulmonary level (ENaC, Na, K-ATPase, and aquaporin-5), resulting in their downregulation and the

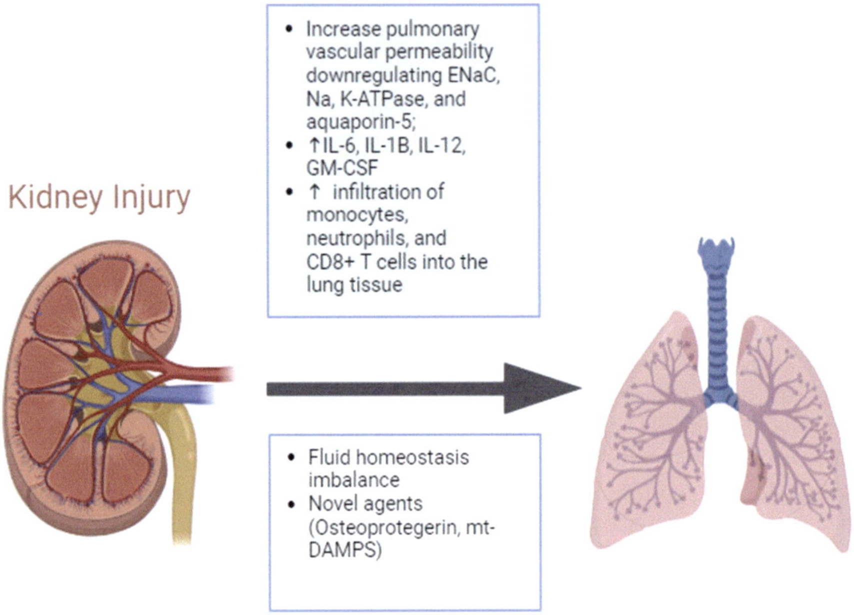

Fig. 11.2 Kidney-lung crosstalk. Legend: ENaC epithelial sodium channel, GM-CSF granulocyte-macrophage colony-stimulating factor, IL-6 interleukin 6, MT-DAMPS mitochondrial damage-associated molecular patterns

consequent reduced clearance of alveolar fluid [15]. In this context, the increased pulmonary vascular permeability with interstitial edema and alveolar hemorrhage, along with endothelial dysfunction and inflammatory cell infiltration, may result in lung impairment and respiratory failure [16]. Lung injury was well described in several murine models of kidney ischemia–reperfusion injury (IRI), reporting specific IRI-induced alterations in the lung transcriptome and involving an early activation of proinflammatory and proapoptotic pathways. Hassoun et al. identified 29 genes associated with inflammation and 66 genes related to apoptosis that are significantly activated in the lung during IRI-induced AKI [17].

The kidney-lung crosstalk is well recognized and described in the clinical setting, as several clinical epidemiological investigations have demonstrated that the most frequent complication occurring in the context of acute respiratory distress syndrome (ARDS) is renal dysfunction, encompassing hematuria, proteinuria, and worsening of renal function. ARSD is a well-known independent risk factor for AKI, as the incidence rate of AKI is significantly higher in patients with severe respiratory distress [15]. Moreover, AKI may have an impact on respiratory recovery, as patients with AKI needed more time to wean-off mechanical breathing and extend invasive intermittent mechanical ventilation (IMV) [18].

The development and aggravation of AKI are mostly attributed to inflammation and endothelial dysfunction, which affect multiple organ dysfunction. Lung neutrophil infiltration during AKI is indicative of lung injury, and neutrophils are important pathogenic mediators of ALI [16, 19]; the rapid activation of transcription factors, such as nuclear factor-kB (NF-kB) and activator protein-1 (AP-1) in the lung, the expression of lung tumor necrosis factor alpha (TNF-α), intercellular adhesion molecule-1 (ICAM-1), and the accumulation of pulmonary neutrophils after injury are additional characteristics of this early inflammatory response [18].

Cytokines are important mediators of inflammatory damage, and they are crucially involved in the onset and progression of both AKI and ALI [18, 20]. Conversely, IL-6 deficiency decreased lung neutrophil infiltration, myeloperoxidase activity, and the production of the chemokines MIP-2 (macrophage-inflammatory protein 2) and KC (chemokine CXCL-1), with consequent reduction in capillary leak in a mouse model [21]. Increased levels of IL-6, IL-1b, IL-12 (p40), and granulocyte macrophage colony-stimulating factor (GM-CSF) have been reported in AKI-related lung injury; by contrast, IL-10 inhibited the production and activity of multiple proinflammatory cytokines, which in turn decreased lung injury during AKI [22]. A systemic inflammatory response syndrome (SIRS) is characterized by a cytokine storm, in which elevated levels of circulating cytokines and chemokines are involved in the pathophysiology of multiorgan injury. SIRS can lead to lung and kidney inflammation, cell apoptosis, endothelial dysfunction, increased vascular permeability, oxidative stress, and worsening of pulmonary edema [23]. Among these proinflammatory molecules, IL-6 is reported as an important mediator of kidney-lung crosstalk; in this scenario, a decrease in IL-6 prevented ALI by reducing capillary leakage and pneumonia [24]. Moreover, immune cells are typical mediators of kidney-lung communication. In the context of AKI, monocyte and neutrophil infiltration at lung level is well described, leading to tissue damage and respiratory failure [25].

The decreased pulmonary fluid clearance capacity consequent to the downregulation of the expression of several transporters associated with the presence of oliguria or anuria in the context of renal failure increased the risk of respiratory failure due to fluid overload [26, 27]. Similarly, protein-bound uremic toxin indoxyl sulfate (IS) may induce IL-6 production, worsening therefore the risk of pulmunary edema due to overwhelming inflammation [28]. Additionally, the reduction of vital capacity and maximal breathing capacity was described in the context of uremic toxins accumulation during AKI [27]. Both hypoxemia and hypercapnia can reduce renal blood flow, either directly or indirectly, leading to renal dysfunction [25, 29].

Cell metabolism alterations at the lung level during AKI have not been fully investigated. The importance of metabolic alteration and mitochondrial damage associated molecular patterns (mt-DAMPs) in the kidney-lung crosstalk was recently described in a mouse model of IRI, where the authors demonstrated that fatty acid oxidation pathway was significantly altered at lung level, in line with a systemic mitochondrial dysfunction, and correlated with the extracellular accumulation of mtDAMPs and mitochondrial DNA (mtDNA) [30].

In a recent preclinical study with bilateral renal IRI, lung inflammation was reported, as evidenced by thicker alveolar walls and immune cell accumulation. In addition, osteopontin generated by damaged kidney tubular cells may have an impact on lung cells during the development of both AKI and ALI by doing single-cell RNA sequencing of the kidneys and lungs of these animals, followed by ligand-receptor pairing analysis [14].

11.4 Kidney-Brain Crosstalk

Ischemic AKI has a more noticeable impact on the brain and neurological dysfunction. Patients with AKI typically experience uremic encephalopathy, characterized by fatigue, apathy, clumsiness, and poor focus, leading to delirium, confusion, and coma. In a 10-year follow-up study including 2155 patients who had experienced their first acute stroke, about 27% of patients experienced AKI episodes after the stroke, and the 10-year mortality rate for AKI patients was dramatically high (75.9%) [31]. The bidirectional interplay between the kidney and the brain has been reported widely; AKI was also more likely to develop in patients with advanced age, chronic kidney disease, significant neurological impairments, and cardiac abnormalities [32]. On the other hand, encephalopathy and mental illnesses such as insomnia, epilepsy, coma, and chorea are at high risk for developing both acute and chronic kidney dysfunction [1].

The brain plays a crucial role in regulating specific kidney functions, as for instance salt and water reabsorption. Peritubular arginine vasopressin (AVP), secreted by the paraventricular and supra spinal nuclei of the hypothalamus, acts on distal convoluted tubules and gathers duct epithelial cells to increase water absorption [33]. In addition, renal vasoconstriction following the activation of sympathetic nervous system may modulate and alter the glomerular filtration rate [34]. AKI-induced brain injury is caused by a variety of factors, including aberrant cytokine/chemokine release during ischemic AKI and circulating uremic toxins (Fig. 11.3). Significant inflammatory alterations characterized by elevated levels of the soluble inflammatory proteins CXC (CXCL-1) and granulocyte colony-stimulating factor (G-CSF) have been reported at cerebral cortex and hippocampus after ischemic AKI [34]. Increases in KC and G-CSF are thought to have a pivotal role in drawing neutrophils to the areas of neuronal injury [34]. In this setting, the hyperproduction of these proinflammatory substances and their accumulation at the brain level due to an altered blood–brain barrier has a pivotal role in the onset of brain dysfunction [33]. Several preclinical studies have demonstrated a strong correlation between kidney and brain injury. In a mouse model of IRI, neuronal pyknosis and microgliosis at the brain level and altered permeability of the blood-brain barrier were reported in the context of renal dysfunction as compared to a sham group [35]. Furthermore, the upregulation of proinflammatory chemokines in the cerebral cortex and hippocampus, such as keratinocyte-derived chemoattractant and G-CSF, as well as the expression of glial fibrillary acidic protein in astrocytes located in the cortex and corpus callosum, has been documented [36]. Toll-like receptor 4 (TLR4) was markedly elevated in the striatum and hippocampal regions in a preclinical IRI model, indicating the critical role of TLR4 in neuroinflammation [37]. Additionally, a lower dopamine turnover was reported in the striatum, mesencephalon, and hypothalamus. In addition, ischemic AKI can cause changes in the balance of sodium and

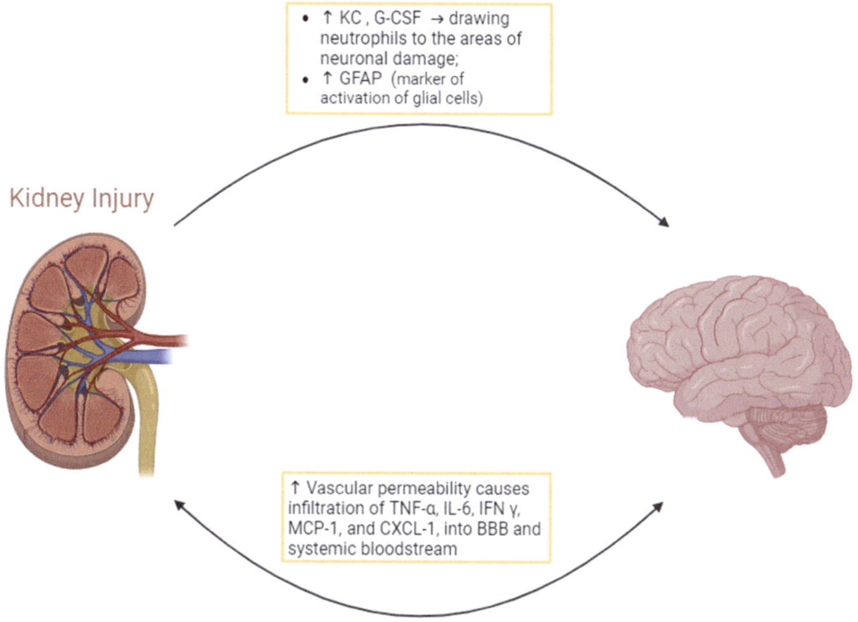

Fig. 11.3 Kidney-brain crosstalk. Legend: BBB blood-brain barrier, KC keratinocyte chemoattractant, G-CSF granulocyte colony-stimulating factor, GFAP glial fibrillary acidic protein, TNF-α tumor necrosis factor alpha, IL-6 interleukin 6, IFN-γ interferon-gamma, MCP-1 monocyte chemoattractant protein-1, CXCL-1 chemokine ligand 1

water, as well as electrolytes. It can also cause an immediate build-up of uremic toxins, such as guanidine molecules, potentially leading to uremic encephalopathy, impairment of the neurological system, peripheral vascular disease, myocardial infarction, and stroke [38].

11.5 Kidney-Liver Crosstalk

Kidney and liver play a key role in the elimination of harmful metabolic products and exogenous medications. There is a correlation between the degree of renal injury and the severity of liver damage and hepatocyte death. Ischemic AKI is characterized by elevated levels of malondialdehyde and serum alanine transaminase (ALT) and changes in liver architecture [39]. The development of hepatorenal syndrome (HRS), in which dysregulation of vasoactive mediators results in acute kidney dysfunction and systemic volume overload, is a significant cause of end-organ dysfunction in kidney-liver crosstalk (Fig. 11.4). A 40% chance of developing type 1-HRS (characterized by acute worsening of kidney function) within 5 years has been reported in a 10-year follow-up study [40]; similarly, a significant proportion of hospitalized patients with acute decompensated cirrhosis (up to 53%) was described in another prospective observational study [41].

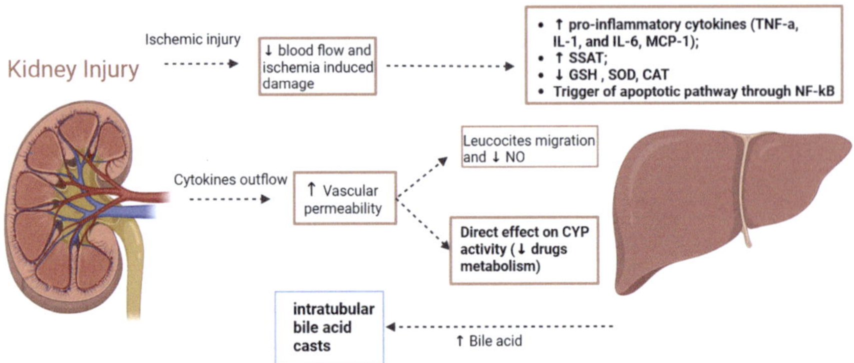

Fig. 11.4 Kidney-liver crosstalk. Legend: CAT catalase, CYP GSH glutathione, IL-1 interleukin 1, IL-6 interleukin 6, NF-kB nuclear factor kappa-light-chain-enhancer of activated B cells, NO nitric oxide, SOD Superoxide dismutase, SSAT spermine/spermidine-N1-acetyl transferase, TNF-α tumor necrosis factor alpha

Patients with cirrhosis who develop AKI have a lower 90-day survival rate, often reported at around 20% [42]. The relationship between kidney and liver dysfunction is bidirectional, as AKI episodes may also affect liver structure and function, which is linked to a high in-hospital mortality rate [43]. Increased vascular permeability and leukocyte infiltration at the liver level occur during AKI conditions, in addition to a profound dysregulation of oxidative stress, inflammation and apoptotic pathways, and hepatic tissue damage [39]. Furthermore, drug metabolism at the hepatic level may be altered and reduced when AKI occurs [36]. These findings point out the strong crosslink between the liver and the kidney; in addition, the reduced expression of drug transporters in the liver and the gut, including MDR1a, MRP2, and OATP3, as well as the expression level of CYP3A11 enzyme, may be connected to this process [44].

Acute kidney dysfunction is caused by renal blood flow being effectively reduced by hepatic failure. A splanchnic arterial vasodilation with consequent decrease of effective arterial blood volume and an increase of intrahepatic vascular resistance has been described in cirrhosis. In this scenario, systemic vasoconstrictor pathways including the sympathetic nervous system and arginine vasopressin (AVP) are activated [45]. A key component of HRS is the development of cirrhotic cardiomyopathy, which triggers the release of vasodilatory mediators (including nitric oxide, prostacyclin, and endothelin) leading to splanchnic dilation. Experimental models inhibiting nitric oxide synthases have been demonstrated to reduce AKI as a result of acute liver failure (ALF) [46]. Hemodynamic alterations during ALF include RAS hyperactivation, with consequent worsening of kidney function and avid salt absorption, leading to fluid retention and ascites [47]. This harmful reaction is controlled by the simultaneous impairment of cardiac, sympathomimetic, and splanchnic regulation, which highlights the intricate organ interaction.

Bile acid accumulation with evidence of intratubular casts has been described during ALF with consequent tubular damage; serum bilirubin concentrations above 10 mg/dL are linked to a worse prognosis in patients with AKI-HRS [48].

Almost half of patients with AKI-HRS experience systemic hyperinflammation. AKI-induced liver injury may be influenced by pro-inflammatory cytokines and ROS. The stimulation of pro-inflammatory cytokines, adhesion molecule expression, neutrophil infiltration, and the generation of cytokines, including TNF-α, IL-1, and IL-6, are the hallmarks of the acute inflammatory response [38]. Increases in serum chemokines and cytokines, such as MCP-1, TNF-α, and IL-6, increase the likelihood of tubular damage associated with tissue infiltration by neutrophils and macrophages. As a result, tubular cells in patients with AKI-HRS express more caspase-3 and TLR4, leading to hepatic cell apoptosis. On the other hand, cytokines including IL-6 and IL-17 are also responsible for AKI-induced liver injury. Administration of neutralizing antibodies against TNF-α, IL-17a, or IL-6 may protect against hepatic and small intestinal injury in wild-type mice with ischemia or non-ischemic AKI [49]. AKI raises IL-6 levels in the blood and kidney, and IL-6 stimulates Kupffer cells in the liver to release IL-10 [50]. Myeloperoxidase (MPO) activity is dramatically increased by a factor of 10 when renal ischemia-reperfusion occurs due to increased levels of hepatic TNF-α, which is mostly produced in liver Kupffer cells [38].

Oxidative stress may play a critical role in liver damage during AKI. Serteser et al. observed that hepatic glutathione (GSH) levels in the liver decreased along with hepatic superoxide dismutase (SOD) and catalase (CAT) activity [38]. Similarly, the rate-limiting enzyme of polyamine metabolism, spermine/spermidine-N1-acetyl transferase (SSAT), was upregulated in the liver 6 hours after kidney IRI or bilateral nephrectomy, leading to an increase in the production of reactive oxygen intermediates. In addition, the administration of GSH was found to significantly reduce liver injury during kidney IRI. Following AKI, Fadillioglu et al. identified elevated levels of protein carbonyl and malondialdehyde (MDA), two important markers of oxidative stress, in liver tissue [51].

Finally, cellular apoptosis is typically implicated in this kidney-liver crosstalk [52]. Although the regulation of the apoptotic machinery in liver cells is likely multifaceted, several evidence suggest that the Fas/FasL and perforin systems induce an immune-mediated route [53]. Dysregulated apoptosis can alter hepatocyte integrity, provoke hepatic inflammation, and set off harmful signaling cascades, mainly related to the release of pro-inflammatory cytokines [54]. These cytokines then trigger the apoptotic pathway through NF-kB, exacerbating liver injury [55]. Furthermore, oxidative stress and ROS directly cause hepatic apoptosis in the liver during renal IRI.

11.6 Conclusions

AKI is typically linked to distant organ dysfunction and represents a major risk factor for mortality among critically ill patients. The underlying mechanisms of organ crosstalk and AKI-induced multiorgan dysfunction have been discussed and reviewed, including oxidative stress, the role of uremic toxins, hemodynamic alterations, inflammation, immunological responses, and nervous system modulation. Further improvements in the understanding of these mechanisms and the consequent discovery of new potential therapeutic targets for novel treatment approaches are pivotal to improve clinical outcomes for critically ill patients.

References

1. Li X, Yuan F, Zhou L. Organ crosstalk in acute kidney injury: evidence and mechanisms. J Clin Med. 2022;11(22):6637.
2. Kociol R, Rogers J, Shaw A. Organ cross talk in the critically ill: the heart and kidney. Blood Purif. 2009;27(4):311–20.
3. Tsagalis G, Zerefos S, Zerefos N. Cardiorenal syndrome at different stages of chronic kidney disease. Int J Artif Organs. 2007;30(7):564–76.
4. Kelly KJ. Distant effects of experimental renal ischemia/reperfusion injury. J Am Soc Nephrol. 2003;14(6):1549–58.
5. Singh D, Chopra K. Evidence of the role of angiotensin AT(1) receptors in remote renal preconditioning of myocardium. Methods Find Exp Clin Pharmacol. 2004;26(2):117–22.
6. Forman MB, Virmani R, Puett DW. Mechanisms and therapy of myocardial reperfusion injury. Circulation. 1990;81(3 Suppl):Iv69–78.
7. Kapadia SR. Cytokines and heart failure. Cardiol Rev. 1999;7(4):196–206.
8. Morawietz H, Bornstein SR. Leptin, endothelin, NADPH oxidase, and heart failure. Hypertension. 2006;47(5):e20; author reply e-1.
9. MacLellan WR. Advances in the molecular mechanisms of heart failure. Curr Opin Cardiol. 2000;15(3):128–35.
10. Fujii H, Nishijima F, Goto S, Sugano M, Yamato H, Kitazawa R, et al. Oral charcoal adsorbent (AST-120) prevents progression of cardiac damage in chronic kidney disease through suppression of oxidative stress. Nephrol Dial Transplant. 2009;24(7):2089–95.
11. Gao H, Liu S. Role of uremic toxin indoxyl sulfate in the progression of cardiovascular disease. Life Sci. 2017;185:23–9.
12. Di Lullo L, Ronco C, Cozzolino M, Russo D, Russo L, Di Iorio B, et al. Nonvitamin K-dependent oral anticoagulants (NOACs) in chronic kidney disease patients with atrial fibrillation. Thromb Res. 2017;155:38–47.
13. Bongartz LG, Cramer MJ, Doevendans PA, Joles JA, Braam B. The severe cardiorenal syndrome: 'Guyton revisited'. Eur Heart J. 2005;26(1):11–7.
14. Khamissi FZ, Ning L, Kefaloyianni E, Dun H, Arthanarisami A, Keller A, et al. Identification of kidney injury released circulating osteopontin as causal agent of respiratory failure. Sci Adv. 2022;8(8):eabm5900.
15. Deng J, Hu X, Yuen PS, Star RA. Alpha-melanocyte-stimulating hormone inhibits lung injury after renal ischemia/reperfusion. Am J Respir Crit Care Med. 2004;169(6):749–56.
16. Kuiper JW, Groeneveld AB, Slutsky AS, Plötz FB. Mechanical ventilation and acute renal failure. Crit Care Med. 2005;33(6):1408–15.
17. Hassoun HT, Grigoryev DN, Lie ML, Liu M, Cheadle C, Tuder RM, et al. Ischemic acute kidney injury induces a distant organ functional and genomic response distinguishable from bilateral nephrectomy. Am J Physiol Renal Physiol. 2007;293(1):F30–40.

18. Klein CL, Hoke TS, Fang WF, Altmann CJ, Douglas IS, Faubel S. Interleukin-6 mediates lung injury following ischemic acute kidney injury or bilateral nephrectomy. Kidney Int. 2008;74(7):901–9.
19. Kramer AA, Postler G, Salhab KF, Mendez C, Carey LC, Rabb H. Renal ischemia/reperfusion leads to macrophage-mediated increase in pulmonary vascular permeability. Kidney Int. 1999;55(6):2362–7.
20. Grigoryev DN, Liu M, Hassoun HT, Cheadle C, Barnes KC, Rabb H. The local and systemic inflammatory transcriptome after acute kidney injury. J Am Soc Nephrol. 2008;19(3):547–58.
21. Ahuja N, Andres-Hernando A, Altmann C, Bhargava R, Bacalja J, Webb RG, et al. Circulating IL-6 mediates lung injury via CXCL1 production after acute kidney injury in mice. Am J Physiol Renal Physiol. 2012;303(6):F864–72.
22. Hoke TS, Douglas IS, Klein CL, He Z, Fang W, Thurman JM, et al. Acute renal failure after bilateral nephrectomy is associated with cytokine-mediated pulmonary injury. J Am Soc Nephrol. 2007;18(1):155–64.
23. Herrlich A. Interorgan crosstalk mechanisms in disease: the case of acute kidney injury-induced remote lung injury. FEBS Lett. 2022;596(5):620–37.
24. Bhargava R, Janssen W, Altmann C, Andrés-Hernando A, Okamura K, Vandivier RW, et al. Intratracheal IL-6 protects against lung inflammation in direct, but not indirect, causes of acute lung injury in mice. PLoS One. 2013;8(5):e61405.
25. Teixeira JP, Ambruso S, Griffin BR, Faubel S. Pulmonary consequences of acute kidney injury. Semin Nephrol. 2019;39(1):3–16.
26. Rabb H, Wang Z, Nemoto T, Hotchkiss J, Yokota N, Soleimani M. Acute renal failure leads to dysregulation of lung salt and water channels. Kidney Int. 2003;63(2):600–6.
27. Yabuuchi N, Sagata M, Saigo C, Yoneda G, Yamamoto Y, Nomura Y, et al. Indoxyl sulfate as a mediator involved in dysregulation of pulmonary aquaporin-5 in acute lung injury caused by acute kidney injury. Int J Mol Sci. 2016;18(1):11.
28. Adelibieke Y, Yisireyili M, Ng HY, Saito S, Nishijima F, Niwa T. Indoxyl sulfate induces IL-6 expression in vascular endothelial and smooth muscle cells through OAT3-mediated uptake and activation of AhR/NF-κB pathway. Nephron Exp Nephrol. 2014;128(1–2):1–8.
29. Hemlin M, Ljungman S, Carlson J, Maljukanovic S, Mobini R, Bech-Hanssen O, et al. The effects of hypoxia and hypercapnia on renal and heart function, haemodynamics and plasma hormone levels in stable COPD patients. Clin Respir J. 2007;1(2):80–90.
30. Hepokoski M, Wang J, Li K, Li Y, Gupta P, Mai T, et al. Altered lung metabolism and mitochondrial DAMPs in lung injury due to acute kidney injury. Am J Physiol Lung Cell Mol Physiol. 2021;320(5):L821–l31.
31. Tsagalis G, Akrivos T, Alevizaki M, Manios E, Theodorakis M, Laggouranis A, et al. Long-term prognosis of acute kidney injury after first acute stroke. Clin J Am Soc Nephrol. 2009;4(3):616–22.
32. MacWalter RS, Wong SY, Wong KY, Stewart G, Fraser CG, Fraser HW, et al. Does renal dysfunction predict mortality after acute stroke? A 7-year follow-up study. Stroke. 2002;33(6):1630–5.
33. Nongnuch A, Panorchan K, Davenport A. Brain-kidney crosstalk. Crit Care. 2014;18(3):225.
34. Sehara Y, Hayashi T, Deguchi K, Zhang H, Tsuchiya A, Yamashita T, et al. Decreased focal inflammatory response by G-CSF may improve stroke outcome after transient middle cerebral artery occlusion in rats. J Neurosci Res. 2007;85(10):2167–74.
35. Liu M, Liang Y, Chigurupati S, Lathia JD, Pletnikov M, Sun Z, et al. Acute kidney injury leads to inflammation and functional changes in the brain. J Am Soc Nephrol. 2008;19(7):1360–70.
36. Doi K, Rabb H. Impact of acute kidney injury on distant organ function: recent findings and potential therapeutic targets. Kidney Int. 2016;89(3):555–64.
37. Salama M, Farrag SM, Abulasrar S, Amin MM, Ali AA, Sheashaa H, et al. Up-regulation of TLR-4 in the brain after ischemic kidney-induced encephalopathy in the rat. CNS Neurol Disord Drug Targets. 2013;12(5):583–6.

38. Serteser M, Koken T, Kahraman A, Yilmaz K, Akbulut G, Dilek ON. Changes in hepatic TNF-alpha levels, antioxidant status, and oxidation products after renal ischemia/reperfusion injury in mice. J Surg Res. 2002;107(2):234–40.
39. Golab F, Kadkhodaee M, Zahmatkesh M, Hedayati M, Arab H, Schuster R, et al. Ischemic and non-ischemic acute kidney injury cause hepatic damage. Kidney Int. 2009;75(8):783–92.
40. Ginès A, Escorsell A, Ginès P, Saló J, Jiménez W, Inglada L, et al. Incidence, predictive factors, and prognosis of the hepatorenal syndrome in cirrhosis with ascites. Gastroenterology. 1993;105(1):229–36.
41. Huelin P, Piano S, Solà E, Stanco M, Solé C, Moreira R, et al. Validation of a staging system for acute kidney injury in patients with cirrhosis and association with acute-on-chronic liver failure. Clin Gastroenterol Hepatol. 2017;15(3):438–45.e5.
42. Salerno F, Cazzaniga M, Merli M, Spinzi G, Saibeni S, Salmi A, et al. Diagnosis, treatment and survival of patients with hepatorenal syndrome: a survey on daily medical practice. J Hepatol. 2011;55(6):1241–8.
43. Lee SA, Cozzi M, Bush EL, Rabb H. Distant organ dysfunction in acute kidney injury: a review. Am J Kidney Dis. 2018;72(6):846–56.
44. Sukkummee W, Jittisak P, Wonganan P, Wittayalertpanya S, Chariyavilaskul P, Leelahavanichkul A. The prominent impairment of liver/intestinal cytochrome P450 and intestinal drug transporters in sepsis-induced acute kidney injury over acute and chronic renal ischemia, a mouse model comparison. Ren Fail. 2019;41(1):314–25.
45. Simonetto DA, Gines P, Kamath PS. Hepatorenal syndrome: pathophysiology, diagnosis, and management. BMJ. 2020;370:m2687.
46. Dagher L, Moore K. The hepatorenal syndrome. Gut. 2001;49(5):729–37.
47. Islas-Carbajal MC, Covarrubias A, Grijalva G, Alvarez-Rodríguez A, Armendáriz-Borunda J, Rincón-Sánchez AR. Nitric oxide synthases inhibition results in renal failure improvement in cirrhotic rats. Liver Int. 2005;25(1):131–40.
48. Barreto R, Fagundes C, Guevara M, Solà E, Pereira G, Rodríguez E, et al. Type-1 hepatorenal syndrome associated with infections in cirrhosis: natural history, outcome of kidney function, and survival. Hepatology. 2014;59(4):1505–13.
49. Park SW, Chen SW, Kim M, Brown KM, Kolls JK, D'Agati VD, et al. Cytokines induce small intestine and liver injury after renal ischemia or nephrectomy. Lab Investig. 2011;91(1):63–84.
50. Daemen MA, van de Ven MW, Heineman E, Buurman WA. Involvement of endogenous interleukin-10 and tumor necrosis factor-alpha in renal ischemia-reperfusion injury. Transplantation. 1999;67(6):792–800.
51. Fadillioglu E, Kurcer Z, Parlakpinar H, Iraz M, Gursul C. Melatonin treatment against remote organ injury induced by renal ischemia reperfusion injury in diabetes mellitus. Arch Pharm Res. 2008;31(6):705–12.
52. Yoon JH, Gores GJ. Death receptor-mediated apoptosis and the liver. J Hepatol. 2002;37(3):400–10.
53. Canbay A, Friedman S, Gores GJ. Apoptosis: the nexus of liver injury and fibrosis. Hepatology. 2004;39(2):273–8.
54. Faouzi S, Burckhardt BE, Hanson JC, Campe CB, Schrum LW, Rippe RA, et al. Anti-Fas induces hepatic chemokines and promotes inflammation by an NF-kappa B-independent, caspase-3-dependent pathway. J Biol Chem. 2001;276(52):49077–82.
55. Paik YH, Schwabe RF, Bataller R, Russo MP, Jobin C, Brenner DA. Toll-like receptor 4 mediates inflammatory signaling by bacterial lipopolysaccharide in human hepatic stellate cells. Hepatology. 2003;37(5):1043–55.

Brain–Kidney Crosstalk in Acute Brain Injury: Understanding Polyuria and Augmented Renal Clearance from Pathophysiology to Clinical Practice

12

Daniel Agustin Godoy, Silvia De Rosa, Sergio Lassola, Denise Battaglini, and Juan Antonio Llompart-Pou

12.1 Introduction

Acute brain injury (ABI) remains a critical challenge in clinical management, necessitating careful attention to secondary insults to prevent exacerbation of primary injuries and facilitate recovery. Among these complications, polyuria—a condition characterized by excessive urine output—poses unique diagnostic and therapeutic challenges [1]. While polyuria is often viewed because of central diabetes insipidus (DI), cerebral salt-wasting syndrome (CSWS), or osmotic diuresis, emerging evidence suggests that it may also act as a marker of renal dysfunction [2]. The brain

D. A. Godoy
Unidad de Cuidados Neurointensivos, Sanatorio Pasteur, Human Resources and Planning (Government of Catamarca), Catamarca, Argentina

S. De Rosa (✉)
Centre for Medical Sciences-CISMed, University of Trento, Trento, Italy
e-mail: silvia.derosa@unitn.it

S. Lassola
Anesthesia and Intensive Care, Santa Chiara Hospital, APSS Trento, Trento, Italy
e-mail: sergio.lassola@apss.tn.it

D. Battaglini
Department of Surgical Sciences and Integrated Diagnostics, University of Genoa, Genoa, Italy

J. A. Llompart-Pou
Servei de Medicina Intensiva. Hospital Universitari Son Espases. Institut d'Investigació Sanitària Illes Balears (IdISBa), Palma, Spain
e-mail: juanantonio.llompart@ssib.es

D. Battaglini et al. (eds.), *Organ System Crosstalk in Critical Illness*,
https://doi.org/10.1007/978-3-032-01024-7_12

and kidneys share intricate physiological connections, and dysfunction in one organ can precipitate complications in the other—a phenomenon often referred to as the brain-kidney axis [3]. In ABI patients, polyuria can result from multiple mechanisms, and it can co-exist with augmented renal clearance (ARC), a phenomenon of increased renal excretion of circulating solutes, mostly defined by creatinine clearance (CrCl) >130mL/min/1.73 m^2 [4]. Persistent polyuria, if left unchecked, can lead to hypovolemia, electrolyte disturbances, and impaired renal perfusion, creating a vicious cycle that exacerbates both cerebral and renal functions [3]. Early recognition of this phenomenon is crucial, as timely intervention can often reverse the underlying pathology and prevent progression to established renal injury [5].

Despite its importance, the lack of a standardized definition complicates the assessment of polyuria prevalence and management strategies in ABI patients [6, 7].

Polyuria, as a secondary insult, can trigger detrimental mechanisms through multiple pathways. It can induce hypovolemia and arterial hypotension while also dysregulating sodium, water, osmolarity, and acid-base balance [8]. These disturbances contribute to systemic and intracranial pathophysiological changes, particularly affecting cerebral blood volume and flow, potentially resulting in lethal consequences such as increased intracranial pressure (ICP) and tissue hypoxia [6–8].

This scoping review aims to enhance understanding of polyuria in acute brain injury (ABI) by exploring it as both a symptom and a potential marker of renal injury. It highlights key pathophysiological mechanisms and stresses the importance of early recognition through clinical assessment, laboratory parameters, and neuroimaging. To facilitate systematic evaluation and timely intervention, we propose the mnemonic "VIDEOS." By addressing these critical aspects, this review seeks to improve diagnostic approaches and clinical management for ABI patients, providing a foundation for future research and enhanced patient care.

12.2 Definition of Polyuria and Augmented Renal Clearance in Acute Brain Injury

Polyuria, characterized by excessive urine output, has been variably defined in the literature [9, 10]. Common thresholds include urine volume exceeding 3000 mL per day, diuresis surpassing 150 mL/h, diuresis greater than 3 mL/kg/h, diuresis exceeding 50 mL/kg/day, or diuresis exceeding 10 mL/min [11–14]. However, for the purpose of this chapter, a pragmatic definition of polyuria as urine output exceeding 3 liters per day is adopted, offering a clear and clinically relevant threshold for identifying this condition in ABI patients [15]. Polyuria in ABI often coexists with ARC, a state of increased renal elimination of solutes characterized by CrCl exceeding 130 mL/min/1.73 m^2. ARC is frequently observed in critically ill patients, driven by hyperdynamic circulation, elevated cardiac output, sympathetic nervous system activation, and increased levels of atrial natriuretic peptide (ANP) [16]. These changes are exacerbated by aggressive fluid resuscitation, osmotherapy, and vasopressor use. Both polyuria and ARC contribute to fluid-electrolyte imbalances, subtherapeutic drug levels, and increased risk of acute kidney injury (AKI) [17].

12.2.1 Evaluation of Polyuria in the Clinical Setting

The diagnostic approach to polyuric states requires the simultaneous analysis of brain damage through physical examination, neuroimaging, and laboratory parameters [8, 11–14, 18]. Table 12.1 outlines the key steps in this diagnostic process. Additionally, urine examination is crucial for assessing volume, sediment, electrolyte concentration, urea, creatinine, glucose, ketone bodies, pH, density, and osmolarity [8, 11–14, 18].

However, challenges exist as measurements of urinary and plasma chemistry should ideally precede the administration of fluids or influencing agents [8, 11, 18, 19]. Obtaining urinary osmolarity directly with an osmometer is optimal but not always feasible in intensive care units (ICUs) worldwide; calculation is an alternative with some limitations [20].

In evaluating polyuria, urinary osmolarity (Osmu) plays a critical role. Two primary formulas are commonly used for its calculation:

1. *Formula 1 (Density-Based Calculation)* [21]*:*

   This method calculates Osmu by referencing urine density (UD) against water density.

   $$\text{Osmu}\left(\text{mOsm}/\text{kg}\right)=\left(\text{UD - 1000}\right)\times 35\text{Osmu}\left(\text{mOsm}/\text{kg}\right)=\left(\text{UD -1000}\right)\times 35$$

   Example: If UD = 1010 → Osmu = (1010 − 1000) × 35 = 350 mOsm/kg

   Limitations: Adjustments are required for glycosuria (subtract 0.004 per g/dL) and proteinuria (subtract 0.003 per g/dL). Additionally, this formula may not be reliable in patients under therapies involving mannitol, piperacillin, carbenicillin, or carbapenems.
2. *Formula 2 (Electrolyte-Based Calculation)* [22]*:*

   This method calculates Osmu based on urinary sodium (Na^+), potassium (K^+), and urea concentrations.

Table 12.1 Diagnostic approach to polyuria in acute brain injury: sequential steps in clinical evaluation

7 Steps	
1. Clinical assessment and neuroimaging	Detect signs of brain damage using physical examination and neuroimaging (CT/MRI)
2. Blood tests	Evaluate renal function, acid-base status, glucose, electrolytes, hemogram, and proteinogram
3. Diagnostic imaging	Assess renal structures using ultrasound or abdominal CT
4. Urinalysis	Analyze volume, sediment, electrolytes, urea, creatinine, glucose, ketones, pH, density, and osmolarity
5. Timing considerations	Measurements of urine and plasma chemistry should ideally precede fluid administration or pharmacological intervention
6. Integration of findings	Classify polyuric states into aqueous, osmotic, or mixed categories
7. Clinical decision-making	Guide treatment and ongoing monitoring based on findings

$$\text{Osmu}\left(\text{mOsm}/\text{kg}\right)=\left(\text{Nau}++\text{Ku}+\right)\times 2+\left(\text{Ureau}5.6\right)\text{Osmu}$$
$$\left(\text{mOsm}/\text{kg}\right)=\left(\text{Nau}++\text{Ku}+\right)\times 2+\left(5.6\text{Ureau}\right)$$

Limitations: This formula requires precise measurements of urinary electrolytes and urea, which may not always be readily available. It is also more complex and less practical in certain clinical scenarios.

Both formulas have their strengths and limitations, and their applicability depends on clinical and laboratory conditions. Accurate calculation of urinary osmolarity is crucial for the classification and management of polyuria in ABI patients.

12.2.2 Classification and Pathophysiology of Polyuric States

Polyuric states encompass a spectrum of conditions characterized by excessive urine production, each driven by distinct underlying causes and pathophysiological mechanisms [8, 11, 12, 19]. These conditions can be broadly categorized based on their cause-effect relationship into two primary groups:

1. *Adequate Polyuria* [8, 11, 12]:
   I. *Characteristics:* Result from increased fluid intake, often seen in clinical scenarios like aggressive fluid resuscitation or excessive voluntary water consumption.
   II. *Pathophysiology:* A balance exists between water intake and excretion, resulting in dilutional effects and increased urine output.
   III. *Clinical Features:* Low urinary osmolarity (Osmu < 150 mOsm/kg) and relatively normal urinary density (UD < 1010).
   IV. *Common Causes:* Excessive hydration, fluid resuscitation in critical care, or psychogenic polydipsia.
2. *Inadequate Polyuria*
   I. *Characteristics:* Arise from disturbances in water and solute balance, typically caused by impaired water reabsorption or increased solute excretion.
   II. *Pathophysiology:* Disruption in the regulatory mechanisms of antidiuretic hormone (ADH) secretion, renal tubular reabsorption, or solute clearance.
   III. *Clinical Features:* Abnormal urinary osmolarity and density depending on the underlying cause.
   IV. *Common Causes:* Central diabetes insipidus (ADH deficiency), nephrogenic diabetes insipidus (renal ADH resistance), diuretic use, hypernatremia correction, and cerebral salt-wasting syndrome CSWS.

This classification provides a functional distinction between polyuria driven by external fluid intake and those resulting from internal regulatory failures. It serves as a foundation for further diagnostic refinement using parameters such as urinary osmolarity and density, ultimately guiding targeted interventions for managing polyuria in ABI patients.

Polyuric states can also be categorized based on urinary osmolarity (Osmu) and urinary density (UD), allowing for a more systematic approach to diagnosis and management. These classifications provide insights into the underlying mechanisms and guide targeted interventions [8, 11, 12, 19]:

1. *Aqueous Polyuria*

Diabetes insipidus (DI) constitutes the most relevant entity within this group of polyuria and is the only one associated with ABI [8, 11, 13, 14, 18, 23, 24]. In its *central* form, DI results from alteration in the synthesis or release of ADH (vasopressin), leading to a partial or complete deficiency of the hormone [8, 11–14, 18, 23, 24]. Common causes of central DI include non-adenomatous pituitary tumors, severe traumatic brain injury (TBI), aneurysmal subarachnoid hemorrhage (SAH), and autoimmune diseases [8, 11–14, 18, 23, 24]. DI prevalence in ABI patients remains uncertain, but studies indicate its association with increased mortality and poor outcomes, particularly in severe TBI cases [25]. DI typically follows a transient course, with an onset within 48 hours of ABI and resolution within 3–5 days [8, 12–14, 23, 24, 26, 27]. This early pattern was found in aneurysmal SAH patients, who developed polyuria >6 L/24 h in 66% of the cases in which polyuria slightly preceded cerebral vasospasm [28]. Transient forms of DI have also been linked to sedative agents used in neurocritical care [29–31].

Nephrogenic DI occurs when the distal and collecting tubules fail to respond to ADH despite normal concentrations [13, 14, 32]. Common causes in neurocritical care patients include previous lithium intake, hypercalcemia/calciuria, persistent hypokalemia, propofol use, and intrinsic renal pathologies [13, 14, 29, 30, 32].

The diagnosis of DI relies on specific criteria, including excessive daily diuresis (>6–7 L), low urine osmolality (Osmu < 300 mmol/kg), low urine density (<1.005), high serum osmolality (>305 mmol/kg), and hypernatremia. Differential diagnosis between central and nephrogenic DI is based on clinical history, triggering etiologies, and specific diagnostic tests [8, 11, 12, 14, 29, 30, 32]. Hypernatremia worsens the prognosis and constitutes a risk factor for mortality [17, 33, 34].

The differential diagnosis between central and nephrogenic DI is primarily based on the analysis of the clinical history and triggering etiologies. Determining plasmatic vasopressin (ADH) levels presents methodological difficulties that have not yet been resolved, preventing its routine use [8, 11–14, 18, 23, 24, 32]. The water deprivation test is not widely applicable in critically ill patients. Positive results (decrease in urine volume, elevation of urine density, and urine osmolarity) during the deprivation test indicate central DI, while no response suggests nephrogenic DI [8, 11–14, 18, 23, 24, 32]. Recent advancements in copeptin analysis offer promising diagnostic potential, particularly in differentiating central and nephrogenic DI and predicting outcomes in TBI patients [13, 35–37]. However, routine clinical use remains limited pending further validation [37].

2. *Osmotic Polyuria*

From the pathophysiological perspective, the driving force is a solute with the capacity to simultaneously drag water with it [8, 11, 12]. Osmotic polyuria is then characterized by Osmu >300 mOsm/kg and UD >1015 [8, 11, 12]. The anatomical substrate primarily involves the renal tubules, compromised in their capacity to reabsorb solutes either by structural damage, drugs, solute hyperflux, or hemodynamic reasons. However, for practical purposes, we will identify them according to the solute excreted in osmotic polyuria, categorizing them as electrolytes or non-electrolytes polyuria [8, 9].

12.2.2.1 Electrolytes-Related Polyuria

In electrolytes-related polyuria, it is essential to carefully analyze the clinical picture, the daily excretion of each electrolyte, their total urinary elimination (TUE), urinary pH, and the determination of the remaining anion or urinary gap (UFA) [9]. Here, we will consider the most prevalent and relevant electrolyte polyuria types in ABI patients.

Sodium Chloride This is the most prevalent form [8, 9, 11, 12]. In this type, the electrolyte TUE exceeds 600 mEq/L, while the UFA ranges between 50 and 70 [8, 9]. Relevant etiologies include: (a) isotonic (fluid resuscitation) or hypertonic (intracranial hypertension control osmotherapy, hypernatremia correction) sodium chloride infusion commonly used in neurocritical care units [8, 9, 11, 12, 37]; (b) diuretics (furosemide) [9, 26]; (c) CSWS [38–41]; (d) adrenal insufficiency [42, 43]; (d) salt-losing nephropathies [9, 26]; (e) recovery phase of acute renal injury [9, 26]; (f) use of catecholamines, which generate natriuresis by multiple mechanisms, including: an increase in venous tone and ventricular filling pressure causing the release of natriuretic peptide; and hemodynamic effects such as inotropic and renal arteriolar vasodilatation with increased renal blood flow and inhibition of tubular sodium reabsorption and aldosterone (dopamine) secretion [40–42, 44].

Within this category, the role of CSW deserves further consideration. Its diagnosis has been controversial over the years due to the similarities with the syndrome of inappropriate antidiuretic hormone (SIADH), which shares several serum and urinary laboratory criteria. Indeed, ADH studies may not be helpful in CSW; decreased vascular volume resulting from high natriuresis and negative sodium balance triggers (appropriate) ADH secretion [38]. However, Lannou et al. have recently shown that in 60 patients with TBI, the decreased vascular volume resulting from a negative sodium balance was a major precipitating factor of hyponatremia. Predisposing factors for enhanced urinary sodium excretion were high sodium intake, high fractional excretion of urate, and augmented renal clearance over the first 7 days after ICU admission [45]. In a sample of 67 consecutive aneurysmal SAH patients, Igarashi et al. found that negative sodium and water balance and increased urine volume were predictors of symptomatic cerebral vasospasm, confirming a strong relationship of vasospasm with CSWS [46].

Sodium Bicarbonate To diagnose this type of polyuria, it is key to analyze the acid-base status, the UFA, and the urinary pH [9]. UFA levels >70 mEq/L may be caused by either chloride or bicarbonate [9]. To differentiate between them, it is necessary to measure the urinary pH. A urinary pH >7.5 indicates loss of bicarbonate. Possible causes include: (a) bicarbonate administration; (b) renal tubular acidosis; (c) tumor lysis syndrome; (d) acetazolamide administration.

Calcium The driving forces of polyuria have different mechanisms that potentiate each other. Hypercalciuria, as mentioned above, can cause aqueous polyuria secondary to the development of nephrogenic or osmotic DI, in which case the mandatory companion is sodium [9, 32]. The incidence of this type of polyuria is low, but it should be considered especially in patients with onco-hematologic disease, either due to the prolonged use of corticosteroids, furosemide, or during chemotherapy (tumor lysis syndrome) [47].

12.2.2.2 Non-electrolyte Polyuria

This type of polyuria is characterized by the excretion of osmotic molecules that carry water, generating hypertonic urine [8, 9, 11, 12]. The TUE of electrolytes does not exceed 600 mEq/L, and there is a marked simultaneous increase in the glomerular filtration rate of the solute involved and plasma osmolarity [26, 27]. The most frequent solutes are:

Glucose Glycemia levels >180–200 mg/dL generate polyuria by exceeding the maximum glucose absorption capacity at the level of the proximal convoluted tubules. Among its causes, we find diabetic ketoacidosis, response to ABI (stress hyperglycemia), and excessive glucose intake (parenteral feeding) [8, 9, 11, 12].

Urea Up to 12–20 grams of urea are eliminated daily through urine. In this setting, certain conditions are necessary to trigger polyuria: (a) presence of hyperazotemia, hypercatabolism, and acute renal injury (tubular necrosis, rhabdomyolysis, sepsis); or (b) urinary tract obstruction by ureteral stones or tumors, which when relieved produce an increase in urea tubular flow [9].

Others This group usually corresponds with adverse effects of drugs such as mannitol, commonly used in neurocritical care worldwide, that can cause polyuria and frequent hypotension (compromising cerebral perfusion pressure) especially with rapid infusions (<5 min). Briefly, mannitol increases the tonicity of the plasma. Since mannitol cannot cross the intact blood-brain barrier, the increased tonicity from the mannitol draws water out of the brain parenchyma and into the intravascular space. The water then travels with the mannitol to the kidneys, where it gets excreted in the urine [48].

Other drugs in this group are glycerol, diuretics, and aminoglycosides [9, 49].

12.2.2.3 Mixed Polyuria

Mixed polyuria exhibits characteristics of both aqueous and osmotic polyuria. Urinary osmolarity typically ranges between 150 and 300 mOsm/kg. Common causes include high sodium load, chronic renal failure, infiltrative renal pathology, prolonged urinary tract obstruction, or partial central DI [9, 11, 12, 18].

12.3 Integrative Algorithm and Insights from Evidence on Polyuria in Acute Brain Injury

Figure 12.1 shows an integrative algorithm encompassing the comprehensive, practical, and straightforward approach through the analysis of different clinical and biochemical parameters and the underlying conditions of the polyuric states. Figure 12.2 shows the mnemonic for easy recall *"VIDEOS,"* which summarizes the main features to consider when evaluating this sign that should not be overlooked in ABI patients.

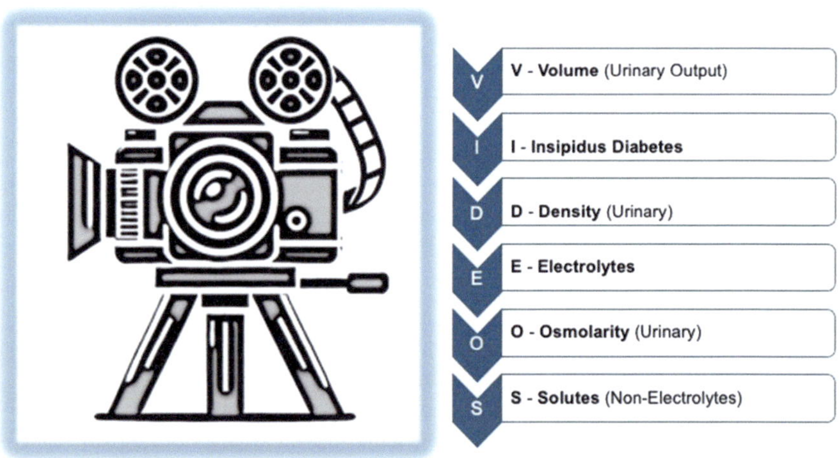

Fig. 12.1 Integrative algorithm encompassing the practical diagnostic approach using the analysis of clinical and biochemical parameters and the underlying conditions of the polyuric states
Osmolarityu urinary osmolarity, densityu urinary density, ml milliliters, L liters, mOsm miliosmoles, Na+ sodium, ADH antidiuretic hormone, TUE total urinary electrolytes, mEq miliequivalents, NaCl sodium chloride, CSWS cerebral salt wasting syndrome, UFA urinary electrolytes gap, Ca++ calcium, pHu urinary pH, DKA diabetic ketoacidosis, ATN acute tubular necrosis
Normal daily urinary electrolyte excretion [11, 30]

Na^+: 40–250 mEq/L
Cl^-: 110–250 mEq/L
HCO_3^-: 0–0.1 mEq/L
Ca++: <4 mg/kg
pH: 4.6–7.5
Urinary electrolytes gap (UFA): (Na+u + K+u) − Cl-u
Total urinary electrolytes (TUE): 2 × (Na+u + K+U) × Urinary volume

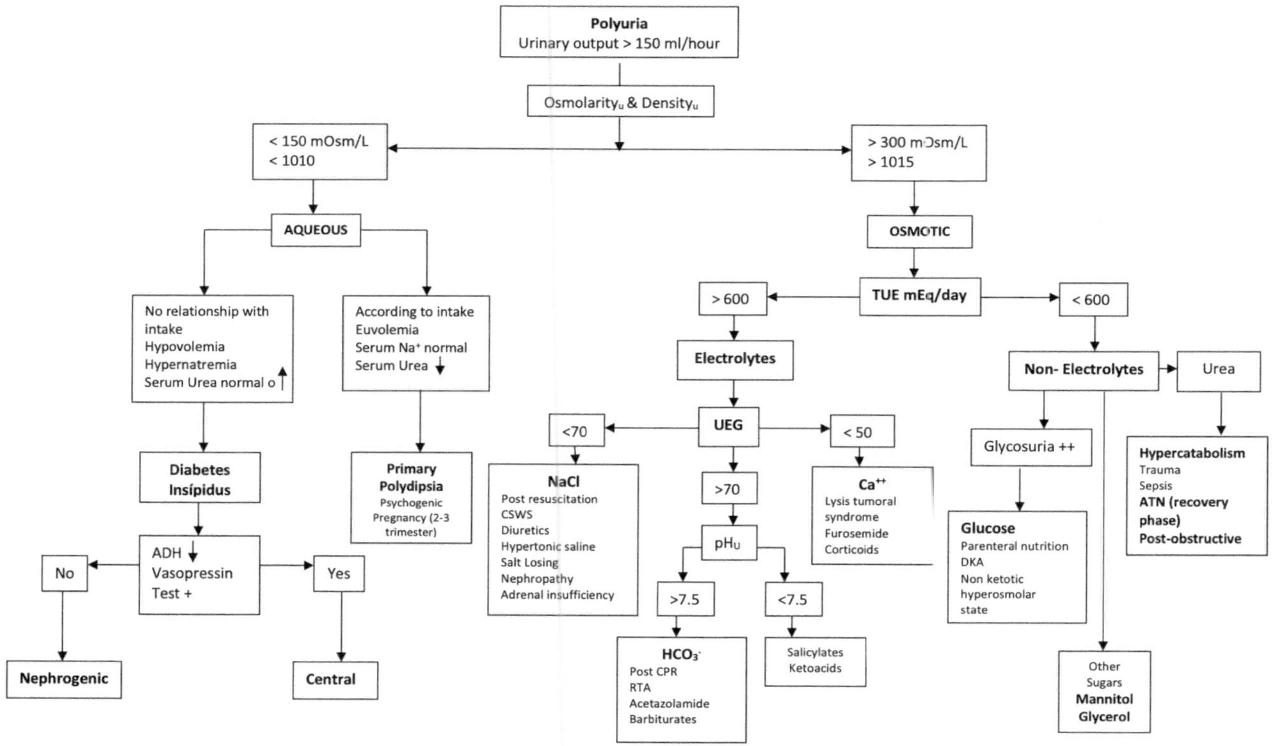

Fig. 12.2 The easy-to-remember acronym "VIDEOS" summarizes the key features to consider when evaluating polyuria in patients with acute brain injury

Observational studies have progressively shaped our understanding of polyuria in patients with acute brain injury (ABI), revealing its multifaceted nature and clinical impact. Early evidence from Gipstein and Boyle [50] highlighted the complications of hypernatremia resulting from prolonged mannitol-induced diuresis. This observation underscored the importance of cautious monitoring during osmotherapy to prevent severe electrolyte imbalances. Similarly, Manninen et al. investigated the effects of high-dose mannitol on serum and urinary electrolytes, demonstrating significant alterations that can further compromise cerebral perfusion if not carefully managed [51]. As research evolved, Chesnut et al. [6]. emphasized the role of secondary brain injuries, including fluid and electrolyte disturbances, in determining clinical outcomes after ABI. Thus, polyuria was recognized as more than just a symptom, framing it as a secondary insult that can exacerbate hypovolemia, hypotension, and cerebral edema. Later, Oster et al. [9] explored osmotic diuresis in ABI patients, stressing the diagnostic value of urinary osmolarity in differentiating underlying causes of polyuria. Their findings reinforced the importance of tailored therapeutic interventions based on precise biochemical markers.

In the 2000s, Aiyagari et al. [52] examined hypernatremia in neurocritical care settings, identifying a direct correlation between extreme sodium levels and adverse neurological outcomes. These findings were echoed by Tisdall et al. [53] and Bradshaw [54], who highlighted frequent sodium disturbances following brain injury and their implications for cerebral perfusion and overall prognosis. In a parallel investigation, Vedantam et al. [34]. demonstrated a strong association between the severity of hypernatremia and mortality rates in ABI patients, emphasizing the need for early recognition and intervention. Further insights emerged from Gempeler et al. [25], who documented a high incidence of diabetes insipidus in patients with severe ABI, linking this condition to increased mortality and prolonged ICU stays. Building on this, Christ-Crain et al. [55] proposed an integrated diagnostic and therapeutic approach, combining clinical assessment, neuroimaging, and biochemical analysis to improve the management of polyuria in neurocritical care settings.

Collectively, these studies chart an evolution in understanding polyuria in ABI, from initial observations of electrolyte imbalances caused by therapeutic interventions to the recognition of polyuria as a secondary insult with direct prognostic consequences. The evidence underscores the necessity for vigilant monitoring, standardized diagnostic frameworks, and tailored interventions to minimize complications and improve outcomes in ABI patients.

12.4 Conclusions

This scoping review provides a comprehensive overview of polyuria in ABI, highlighting its complex pathophysiology, diverse etiologies, and significant impact on patient outcomes. Polyuria remains an under-recognized yet critical secondary complication in ABI, with potential consequences including hypovolemia, electrolyte imbalances, and impaired cerebral perfusion. Despite advances in diagnostic tools and a growing body of evidence, inconsistencies in definitions and variability in clinical approaches continue to pose challenges for effective management. The introduction of practical tools, such as the "VIDEOS" mnemonic and diagnostic algorithms, offers clinicians actionable strategies to identify and address polyuria promptly. In conclusion, addressing polyuria in ABI requires a multidisciplinary approach, combining precise diagnostics, proactive monitoring, and evidence-based therapeutic strategies. By improving our understanding and management of polyuria, we can significantly enhance the prognosis and quality of care for ABI patients. Future research should focus on validating diagnostic algorithms and mnemonics like "VIDEOS" in diverse clinical settings and exploring the long-term outcomes of patients with polyuria post-ABI.

References

1. Stocchetti N, Carbonara M, Citerio G, Ercole A, Skrifvars MB, Smielewski P, et al. Severe traumatic brain injury: targeted management in the intensive care unit. Lancet Neurol. 2017;16(6):452–64.
2. Loh T, Lee W, Goh Y, Seow W. Combined central diabetes insipidus and cerebral salt wasting after craniotomy. Crit Care. 2000;4(Suppl 1):P178.
3. De Rosa S, Battaglini D, Robba C. Kidney dysfunction after acute brain injury. Nephrol Dial Transplant. 2024;39(2):170–3.
4. Cook AM, Hatton-Kolpek J. Augmented renal clearance. Pharmacotherapy. 2019;39(3):346–54.
5. Miller PD, Krebs RA, Neal BJ, McIntyre DO. Polyuric prerenal failure. Arch Intern Med. 1980;140(7):907–9.
6. Chesnut RM, Marshall LF, Klauber MR, Blunt BA, Baldwin N, Eisenberg HM, et al. The role of secondary brain injury in determining outcome from severe head injury. J Trauma. 1993;34(2):216–22.
7. McHugh GS, Engel DC, Butcher I, Steyerberg EW, Lu J, Mushkudiani N, et al. Prognostic value of secondary insults in traumatic brain injury: results from the IMPACT study. J Neurotrauma. 2007;24(2):287–93.
8. Godoy DA, Álvare E, Campi V, Soler C, Masotti L, Di Napoli M. Enfoque práctico para el diagnóstico y tratamiento de los estados poliúricos en pacientes con injuria cerebral aguda. Rev méd Chile. 2013;141(5):616–25.
9. Oster JR, Singer I, Thatte L, Grant-Taylor I, Diego JM. The polyuria of solute diuresis. Arch Intern Med. 1997;157(7):721–9.
10. Jakes AD, Bhandari S. Investigating polyuria. BMJ. 2013;347(dec02 1):f6772.
11. Bhasin B, Velez JCQ. Evaluation of polyuria: the roles of solute loading and water diuresis. Am J Kidney Dis. 2016;67(3):507–11.
12. Lithgow K, Corenblum B. Polyuria: a pathophysiologic approach. Can J Gen Int Med [Internet]. 2017 [citato 9 gennaio 2025];12(2). Disponibile su: http://www.cjgim.ca/index.php/csim/article/view/245.
13. Refardt J. Diagnosis and differential diagnosis of diabetes insipidus: update. Best Pract Res Clin Endocrinol Metab. 2020;34(5):101398.
14. Christ-Crain M, Winzeler B, Refardt J. Diagnosis and management of diabetes insipidus for the internist: an update. J Intern Med. 2021;290(1):73–87.
15. Ramírez-Guerrero G, Müller-Ortiz H, Pedreros-Rosales C. Polyuria in adults. A diagnostic approach based on pathophysiology. Rev Clin Esp (Barc). 2022;222(5):301–8.
16. Udy A, Boots R, Senthuran S, Stuart J, Deans R, Lassig-Smith M, et al. Augmented creatinine clearance in traumatic brain injury. Anesth Analg. 2010;111(6):1505–10.

17. Chand R, Chand R, Goldfarb DS. Hypernatremia in the intensive care unit. Curr Opin Nephrol Hypertens. 2022;31(2):199–204.
18. Robertson GL. Differential diagnosis of polyuria. Annu Rev Med. 1988;39(1):425–42.
19. Edoute Y, Davids MR, Johnston C, Halperin ML. An integrative physiological approach to polyuria and hyponatraemia: a «double-take» on the diagnosis and therapy in a patient with schizophrenia. QJM. 2003;96(7):531–40.
20. Heavens KR, Kenefick RW, Caruso EM, Spitz MG, Cheuvront SN. Validation of equations used to predict plasma osmolality in a healthy adult cohort. Am J Clin Nutr. 2014;100(5):1252–6.
21. Vidal-Mayo JDJ, Olivas-Martínez A, Pérez-Díaz I, López-Navarro JM, Sánchez-Landa E, Carrillo-Maravilla E, et al. Calculated versus measured urine osmolarity: accuracy of estimated urine density. Rev Invest Clin. 2018;70(6):1225.
22. Nguyen MK, Kurtz I. Derivation of a new formula for calculating urinary electrolyte-free water clearance based on the Edelman equation. Am J Physiol Renal Physiol. 2005;288(1):F1–7.
23. Tomkins M, Lawless S, Martin-Grace J, Sherlock M, Thompson CJ. Diagnosis and management of central diabetes insipidus in adults. J Clin Endocrinol Metabol. 2022;107(10):2701–15.
24. De Vries F, Lobatto DJ, Verstegen MJT, Van Furth WR, Pereira AM, Biermasz NR. Postoperative diabetes insipidus: how to define and grade this complication? Pituitary. 2021;24(2):284–91.
25. Gempeler A, Orrego-González E, Hernandez-Casanas A, Castro AM, Aristizabal-Mayor JD, Mejia-Mantilla JH. Incidence and effect of diabetes insipidus in the acute care of patients with severe traumatic brain injury. Neurocrit Care. 2020;33(3):718–24.
26. Kazda A, Jabor A, Zámečník M, Mašek K. Monitoring acid-base and electrolyte disturbances in intensive care. In: Advances in clinical chemistry [Internet]. Elsevier; 1989 [citato 9 gennaio 2025]. p. 201–268. Disponibile su: https://linkinghub.elsevier.com/retrieve/pii/S0065242308601845.
27. Halperin ML, Bohn D. Clinical approach to disorders of salt and water balance. Crit Care Clin. 2002;18(2):249–72.
28. Brown RJ, Epling BP, Staff I, Fortunato G, Grady JJ, McCullough LD. Polyuria and cerebral vasospasm after aneurysmal subarachnoid hemorrhage. BMC Neurol. 2015;15(1):201.
29. Kraus MB, Leuzinger K, Reynolds E, Gallo De Moraes A, Smith J, Sharpe EE, et al. Diabetes insipidus related to sedation in the intensive care unit: a review of the literature. J Crit Care. 2023;75:154233.
30. Van Decar LM, Reynolds EG, Sharpe EE, Harbell MW, Kosiorek HE, Kraus MB. Perioperative diabetes insipidus caused by anesthetic medications: a review of the literature. Anesth Analg. 2022;134(1):82–9.
31. Herity LB, Baker C, Kim C, Lowe DK, Cahoon WD. Delayed onset of central diabetes insipidus with ketamine sedation: a report of 2 cases. J Pharm Pract. 2021;34(2):314–8.
32. Vaz De Castro PAS, Bitencourt L, De Oliveira Campos JL, Fischer BL, Soares De Brito SBC, Soares BS, et al. Nephrogenic diabetes insipidus: a comprehensive overview. J Pediatr Endocrinol Metab. 2022;35(4):421–34.
33. Hoffman H, Jalal MS, Chin LS. Effect of hypernatremia on outcomes after severe traumatic brain injury: a nationwide inpatient sample analysis. World Neurosurg. 2018;118:e880–6.
34. Vedantam A, Robertson CS, Gopinath SP. Morbidity and mortality associated with hypernatremia in patients with severe traumatic brain injury. Neurosurg Focus. 2017;43(5):E2.
35. Winzeler B, Zweifel C, Nigro N, Arici B, Bally M, Schuetz P, et al. Postoperative copeptin concentration predicts diabetes insipidus after pituitary surgery. J Clin Endocrinol Metabol. 2015;100(6):2275–82.
36. Berton AM, Gatti F, Penner F, Varaldo E, Prencipe N, Rumbolo F, et al. Early copeptin determination allows prompt diagnosis of post-neurosurgical central diabetes insipidus. Neuroendocrinology. 2020;110(6):525–34.
37. Jeon JP, Kim S, Kim TY, Han SW, Lim SH, Youn DH, et al. Association between copeptin and six-month neurologic outcomes in patients with moderate traumatic brain injury. Front Neurol. 2022;12:749110.

38. Froelich M, Ni Q, Wess C, Ougorets I, Härtl R. Continuous hypertonic saline therapy and the occurrence of complications in neurocritically ill patients*. Crit Care Med. 2009;37(4):1433–41.
39. Singh R, Watchorn JC, Zarbock A, Forni LG. Prognostic biomarkers and AKI: potential to enhance the identification of post-operative patients at risk of loss of renal function. Res Rep Urol. 2024;16:65–78.
40. Harrigan MR. Cerebral salt wasting syndrome: a review. Neurosurgery. 1996;38(1):152–60.
41. Epstein FH, Levin ER, Gardner DG, Samson WK. Natriuretic peptides. N Engl J Med. 1998;339(5):321–8.
42. Hannon MJ, Sherlock M, Thompson CJ. Pituitary dysfunction following traumatic brain injury or subarachnoid haemorrhage – In "Endocrine Management in the Intensive Care Unit". Best Pract Res Clin Endocrinol Metab. 2011;25(5):783–98.
43. Mahajan C, Prabhakar H, Bilotta F. Endocrine dysfunction after traumatic brain injury: an ignored clinical syndrome? Neurocrit Care. 2023;39(3):714–23.
44. Singh S, Bohn D, Carlotti APCP, Cusimano M, Rutka JT, Halperin ML. Cerebral salt wasting: truths, fallacies, theories, and challenges. Crit Care Med. 2002;30(11):2575–9.
45. Lannou A, Carrie C, Rubin S, Cane G, Cottenceau V, Petit L, et al. Salt wasting syndrome in brain trauma patients: a pathophysiologic approach using sodium balance and urinary biochemical analysis. BMC Neurol. 2020;20(1):190.
46. Igarashi Y, Norii T, Sung-Ho K, Nagata S, Yoshino Y, Hamaguchi T, et al. Airway obstruction time and outcomes in patients with foreign body airway obstruction: multicenter observational choking investigation. Acute Med Surg. 2022;9(1):e741.
47. Hori D, Kobayashi R, Suzuki D, Kodama K, Yanagi M, Matsushima S, et al. A survey of hypercalciuria during chemotherapy in acute lymphoblastic leukemia. Pediatr Int. 2021;63(8):923–8.
48. Tenny S, Patel R, Thorell W. Mannitol. In: StatPearls [Internet]. Treasure Island: StatPearls Publishing; 2025. [citato 9 gennaio 2025]. Disponibile su: http://www.ncbi.nlm.nih.gov/books/NBK470392/.
49. Freeman N, Welbourne J. Osmotherapy: science and evidence-based practice. BJA Educ. 2018;18(9):284–90.
50. Gipstein RM, Boyle JD. HYPERNATREMIA COMPLICATING PROLONGED MANNITOL DIURESIS. N Engl J Med. 1965;272:1116–7.
51. Manninen PH, Lam AM, Gelb AW, Brown SC. The effect of high-dose mannitol on serum and urine electrolytes and osmolality in neurosurgical patients. Can J Anaesth. 1987;34(5):442–6.
52. Aiyagari V, Deibert E, Diringer MN. Hypernatremia in the neurologic intensive care unit: how high is too high? J Crit Care. 2006;21(2):163–72.
53. Tisdall M, Crocker M, Watkiss J, Smith M. Disturbances of sodium in critically ill adult neurologic patients: a clinical review. J Neurosurg Anesthesiol. 2006;18(1):57–63.
54. Bradshaw K, Smith M. Disorders of sodium balance after brain injury. Contin Educ Anaesth Crit Care Pain. 2008;8(4):129–33.
55. Christ-Crain M. EJE AWARD 2019: new diagnostic approaches for patients with polyuria polydipsia syndrome. Eur J Endocrinol. 2019;181(1):R11–21.

Kidney-Gut Crosstalk in Acute Kidney Injury

13

Ilaria Godi, Andrea Ballin, and Silvia De Rosa

Abbreviations

AKI	acute kidney injury
I/R	ischemia reperfusion
SCFA	short-chain fatty acids
TMAO	trimethylamine-N-oxide

13.1 Introduction

The microbiome is the collection of microorganisms, including bacteria, viruses, fungi, and other microbes, that live within and on the human body. These microorganisms are found in various body parts, such as the skin, mouth, gut, and reproductive organs.

The human microbiome is crucial in maintaining our overall health and well-being. It performs essential functions such as aiding digestion, synthesizing vitamins, regulating the immune system, and protecting against harmful pathogens. The composition and diversity of the microbiome can vary from person to person and even within different parts of an individual's body.

Acute kidney injury (AKI) is a severe complication of critical illness. AKI is a complex and multifactorial process, but our understanding of its pathogenesis still

I. Godi · A. Ballin
Anesthesiology and Intensive Care Medicine, University Hospital of Padua, Padua, Italy

S. De Rosa (✉)
Centre for Medical Sciences-CISMed, University of Trento, Trento, Italy

D. Battaglini et al. (eds.), *Organ System Crosstalk in Critical Illness*,
https://doi.org/10.1007/978-3-032-01024-7_13

needs to be completed. One of the merging pathophysiologic themes is the role of the gut microbiome in AKI. During critical illness, several factors can disrupt the average balance of the microbiome. These include broad-spectrum antibiotics, diet changes, gut environment alterations, and invasive medical procedures. These disruptions can lead to a condition known as dysbiosis. Recent research has focused on understanding the relationship between the microbiome and AKI to develop strategies for prevention and treatment. However, it is essential to note that microbiome research in critical illness still evolves, and many questions remain unanswered. This chapter reviews the current literature on the complex interactions between the microbiome, host immune system, and AKI.

13.2 The Intestinal Barrier and Gut Microbiome

A healthy gut contains the largest absorptive surface in the body, the vast majority of the body's immune cells, and at least one thousand genera of microbes, forming three barriers, including physical, immune, and biological barriers [1], as shown in Fig. 13.1.

1. Physical barrier: refers to intestinal epithelial cells, whose apical tight junctions serve two main functions.
    - Tight junctions regulate the permeability of solutes between adjacent cells.
    - Tight junctions maintain the polarity of intestinal epithelial cells, controlling the diffusion of lipids and proteins from the intestinal lumen to the basolateral lamina propria.
2. Immune barrier: refers to intestinal cells able to activate the immune response.
    - Dendritic cells in the lamina propria recruit regulatory T cells via non-classical autophagy pathways to activate adaptive immune response.
    - Epithelial cells release cytokines to control pro-inflammatory response.
    - Innate lymphoid cells in the gut epithelium produce or activate cytokines related to adaptive or innate immune response.
    - Paneth cells secrete antimicrobial proteins and IgA to protect the mucosal surface and favor host-microbiota mutualism.
3. Biological barrier: refers to bacterial and fungal symbionts, which colonize the gut (gut microbiome).
    - Anaerobic symbionts secrete antimicrobial proteins via Paneth cells to defend against pathogens.
    - Commensal bacteria break down indigestible carbohydrates into short-chain fatty acids (SCFAs), used as an energy source by epithelial cells, contributing to restoring tight junctions.
    - Gut microbiome synthesizes K and B vitamins.

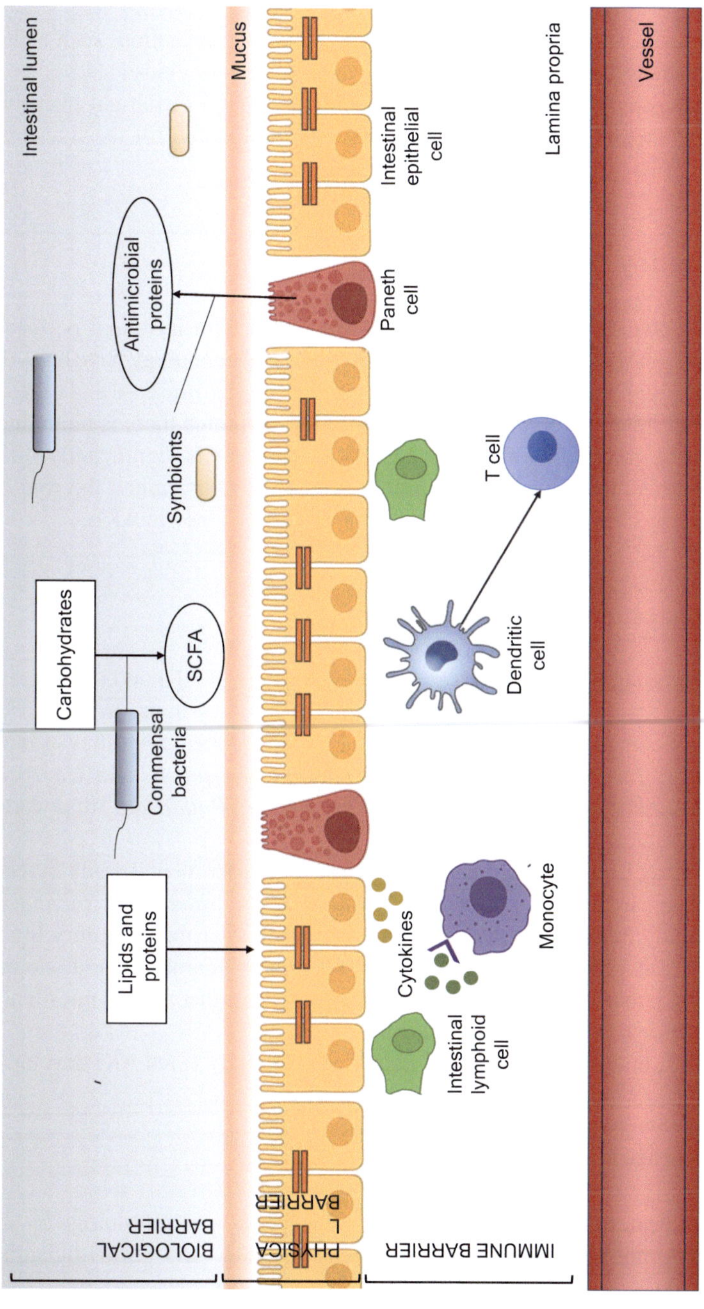

Fig. 13.1 Gut microbiome and intestinal barriers (physical, immune, and biological barriers). SCFA short-chain fatty acid

- Symbionts compete with pathological bacteria to inhibit colonization (colonization resistance).

Many factors may influence the gut microbiome's composition, such as human genetics, diet and lifestyle, circadian cycle, and use of antibiotics [1].

It is increasingly clear that an imbalance or disruption of the gut microbiome, known as dysbiosis, is associated with disease development in the intestine and other organs [1].

13.3 Kidney-Gut Crosstalk in AKI

It is well known that kidney diseases are associated with intestinal permeability disorder and gut dysfunction. More recent advances in technology have helped clarify the role of gut microbiome in the pathogenesis of kidney disease and explore the kidney-gut crosstalk in chronic kidney disease [2]. Although there is mounting evidence that the microbiota signature in various diseases is significantly different from that in healthy controls, only limited studies have examined the role of the microbiome and the crosstalk between the gut and the kidney in AKI.

13.3.1 Microbiome Composition and AKI

Microbiome composition has a role in the development of AKI and its progression. Experimental studies on ischemia/reperfusion (I/R) kidney injury in mice revealed that different composition of intestinal flora leads to different severities of injury: a prevalence of *Prevotella copri*, *Faecalibacterium prausnitzii*, and *Coprococcus eutactus* was associated with no or mild injury, whereas *Rothia* and *Staphylococcus* positively correlated with severe injury [3].

On the other hand, AKI induces dysbiosis: in an experimental study by Nakade et al., there were increased numbers of *Lactobacillus*, *Clostridium*, and *Ruminococcus* and decreased numbers of *Bifidobacterium* and TM7 after the I/R injury [4]. Yang et al. colonized germ-free mice with post-I/R injury microbiota and showed an increased AKI severity in recipient mice, demonstrating that altered intestinal flora negatively affects post-AKI outcome [5].

In humans, alteration of intestinal flora appears rapidly when AKI develops [6].

13.3.2 Metabolites and AKI

Evidence indicates that the gut microbiota influences human physiology by signaling through metabolic products such as SCFAs and trimethylamine-N-oxide (TMAO).

SCFAs are produced due to saccharolytic fermentation of dietary fibers by gut microbiota. The most abundant SCFAs are acetate, propionate, and butyrate.

Locally, SCFAs are energy sources for colonocytes; SCFAs not metabolized by the colonocytes are transported into the portal circulation, inducing systemic effects. So far, researchers have found that SCFAs may mediate renin secretion by binding G protein-coupled receptor 41 and olfactory receptor 78 expressed in the kidneys [7]. In murine models, treatment with SCFAs reduced renal inflammation and oxidative damage after ischemia-reperfusion, contrast-induced, or gentamycin-induced kidney injury, most likely via epigenetic modification [8–10]. Another mechanism by which SCFAs regulate systemic functions is by inhibiting histone deacetylase activity [8, 11]. Al-Harbi et al. demonstrated that acetate ameliorated sepsis-induced AKI and restored oxidant-antioxidant balance by attenuating histone deacetylase activity in T cells [12]. Thus, evidence shows that SCFAs have the reno-protective effect, but conversely, alteration of gut microbiota and, consequently elevated SCFAs levels are responsible for dysregulated T-cell responses and tissue inflammation in the renal system [13].

TMAO is derived from a diet containing choline, lecithin, betaine, and carnitine through gut flora digestion. It has been shown that the serum level of TMAO can promote inflammatory activation of vascular endothelial cells and platelet aggregation, leading to atherosclerosis and cardiovascular events. More recently, gut microbiota-derived TMAO has been demonstrated to contribute to renal interstitial fibrosis in a mouse model of a high-choline diet [14]. A recent study confirms the contribution of TMAO to renal interstitial inflammation by activation of the inflammatory pathway favoring the release of cytokines and oxidative stress, which ultimately aggravates kidney injury [15].

13.3.3 Immune System Interaction and AKI

A series of investigations have demonstrated a key role of T-cells in the pathogenesis of AKI and repair [16]. Dysregulation in gut microbiota-immune system interactions leads to imbalances in T-cell sub-populations.

The role of microbiota-induced immune modulation in AKI was first studied by Jang et al., which investigated differences in microbial status and their effects on kidney lymphocyte trafficking, cytokines, function, and structure in normal kidneys and after AKI [17]. Abundant T-cells, especially natural killer T-cells with lower expression of anti-inflammatory cytokines, were found in germ-free mice kidneys in the absence of kidney disease. T-cells trafficking increased after I/R AKI in germ-free mice, with more severe renal structural injury and functional decline, suggesting a reno-protective effect of microbiota by influencing the phenotype of renal lymphocytes and the expression of cytokines. Conventionalizing germ-free mice with stools from control mice limited the extent of renal injury, modulating the outcome of I/R AKI.

Gut-derived SCFAs modulate T-cell function via histone deacetylase activity in T-cells during sepsis-induced AKI, suggesting an important role for SCFA signaling in AKI [12]. Recently, it appeared that microbiota-derived T-helper 17 cells can be recruited to inflamed kidneys via the chemokine axis, a new pathological mechanism in autoimmune kidney disease [18].

Depletion of microbiota limits T helper cell response while amplifying functions of T regulatory cells and macrophages [5].

Monocytes/macrophages play another critical role in initiating and progressing of inflammatory diseases, such as AKI. Inflammation causes monocytes to migrate and infiltrate into organs, where they differentiate into pathogen-killing or tissue-repair phenotypes. Thus, Emal et al. investigated the effect of gut microbiota depletion with broad-spectrum antibiotics on the maturation status of renal resident macrophages and bone marrow monocytes in AKI [19]. This investigation showed microbiota depletion was protective against I/R AKI, affecting macrophage/monocyte maturation status, release of chemokines, and migration capacity. The protective effect and macrophage alterations were reversed after reintroduction of microbiota after fecal transplantation.

13.3.4 Effect of AKI on Gastrointestinal Tract

Kidney clearance deficiency leads to the accumulation of metabolic waste products and urea in plasma. Uremic toxins and metabolites mediated the intestinal epithelial colonic barrier by increasing colonic wall thickness and accumulation of mononuclear leucocytes in lamina propria and by depletion of transcellular and intracellular components of colonic epithelial tight junctions [20, 21]. Uremic toxins are predominantly excreted through the kidneys and partly through the colon. However, deterioration of kidney function shifts the primary site of excretion from the kidneys to the colon. The sustained presence of uremic toxins in the colon leads to gut dysbiosis by proliferation of urease-producing bacteria. Barrios et al. showed an association between three metabolic uremic products (indoxyl-sulfate, p-cresyl-sulfate, and phenylacetylglutamate) and gut flora composition [6]. Together with uremic toxins, the altered serum levels of amino acids (elevated levels of acetylcarnitine, a drop of other three amino acids, and altered balance of D-/L- serine) were associated with some bacterial clades in experimental studies [3, 4]. The shift in microbiota composition enhances gut ammonia production, thus raising the physiological pH of the intestinal lumen and leading to mucosal irritation and damage of the epithelial colonic barrier [22]. This results in increased intestinal permeability, commonly called "leaky gut."

Consequently, endotoxins and bacterial products translocate into circulation and induce both local (via Paneth cells and interleukin 17) and systemic inflammation, further exacerbating the deterioration of kidney function [23, 24].

Thus, microbiota contribute substantially to producing harmful uremic solutes, but conversely, growth without microbiota has harmful effects on renal damage progression [25].

13.3.5 Therapeutic Potentials

As the gut plays a vital role in the progression of inflammation and AKI, efforts to modulate the gut microbiome and barrier function to improve outcomes make great sense. However, one must bear in mind that human data are still evolving in this therapeutic area. The strategies which were most studied are set out in the following.

- A prebiotic is "a selectively fermented ingredient that results in specific changes in the composition and/or activity of the gastrointestinal microbiota, thus conferring benefits upon host health" [26]. The beneficial effects of many prebiotics have been demonstrated in different settings, including chronic kidney disease. In the field of AKI, the effects of prebiotics are unclear, and it is expected to be clarified by an ongoing study focusing on prebiotics and probiotics in septic AKI patients (registered in clinicaltrials.gov as NCT 03877081).
- Probiotics are "the preparation of inanimate microorganisms and/or their components that confers a health benefit on the host" [26]. Several probiotics, including *Lactobacillus*, *Bifidobacterium* species, and microbial cocktails, show beneficial effects in attenuating AKI severity [27, 28].
- Synbiotic is a supplemental treatment combining probiotics and prebiotics. Even though the idea of getting the synergistic effect from the two therapies sounds promising, there are limited and inconclusive studies in chronic kidney disease. As for AKI, the evidence still needs to be included.
- Postbiotic describes nonviable bacteria or metabolic byproducts from probiotic microorganisms, such as vitamins, SCFAs, and enzymes, which may positively affect gut microbiota and the host. It has been shown in animal experiments that therapy with microbiota-derived SCFAs protects against AKI, mainly through the reduction of local and systemic inflammation and oxidative stress [8–10, 12]. Furthermore, the possible underlying mechanism was proposed to boost mitochondrial biogenesis via epigenetic modification and nuclear factor kappa-light chain-enhancer of activated B cells [9, 10].
- Oral adsorbent of uremic toxins, like AST-120, is a new strategy to remove protein-bound uremic toxins with great affinity. A study by Fujii et al. shows a reduction of toxin levels and limitation of renal expression of mRNAs of injury-related markers in a murine model of AKI treated with AST-150 [29].
- Selective decontamination of the digestive tract uses non-absorbable microbials, which are applied in the oropharynx and the gastrointestinal tract to prevent secondary colonization and overgrowth of potential bacterial pathogens while preserving the anaerobic microbiota. A comprehensive systematic review and meta-analysis suggested that selective decontamination of the digestive tract can decrease mortality in critically ill patients [30]. However, randomized controlled trials are still needed in the AKI context.
- Gut-microbiota depletion following administration of broad-spectrum antibiotics also demonstrates protective effects against AKI [19]. Moreover, long-term use of rifaximin is associated with decreased AKI incidence and hepatorenal syndrome in a population of cirrhotic patients [31]. The discordant results still

need a valid explanation. Some authors suggest that antibiotics may protect against AKI independent of gut microbiota depletion or that antibiotic treatment may preferentially deplete pro-injurious bacteria but not the protective ones [32].
- Fecal microbiota transplantation is a method to restore the microbial community by introducing a healthy donor's local gut microbes to a dysbiotic gut via either capsules or colonoscopy. Despite the protective effect of fecal microbial transplantation shown in mice, information about its benefit on kidney disease in humans is still insufficient.

13.4 Conclusions

Intestinal dysbiosis, altered mucosal immune responses, and loss of barrier integrity are emerging factors responsible for injury or inflammation in AKI. At the same time, AKI induces microbiota alteration in the gastrointestinal system, favoring a vicious cycle of injury and inflammation (Fig. 13.2). Despite advances in our understanding of kidney-gut crosstalk, insight into the complex interplay between the gut microbiome with its metabolites and immunity in the pathogenesis of AKI is rather primitive. In theory, rational therapies aimed at restoring gut integrity, the microbiome, and the homeostatic balance between the two systems represent an exciting avenue in the battle against AKI in critical patients.

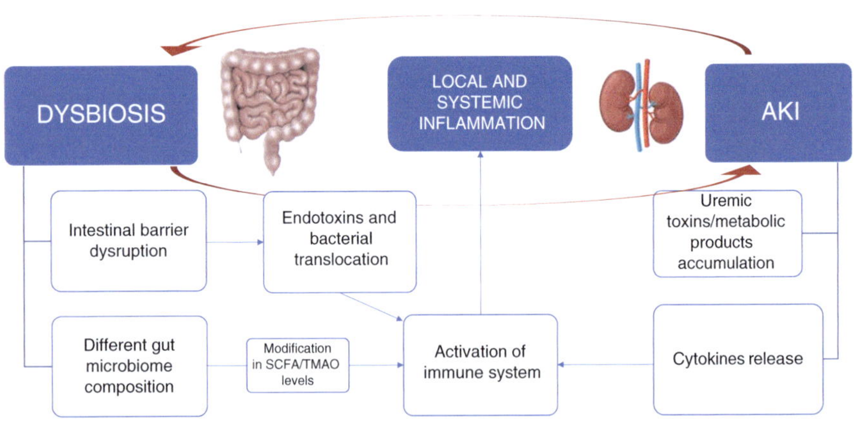

Fig. 13.2 Gut-kidney crosstalk. The combined effect of intestinal barrier disruption, a shift in the composition, and virulence of intestinal microbes may lead to the point where cascading inflammation drives AKI. During AKI, the clearance of inflammatory mediators is decreased, and metabolic products accumulate that can increase systemic inflammation. This feeds a continuous cycle of local and systemic inflammation

References

1. Gilbert JA, Blaser MJ, Caporaso JG, Jansson JK, Lynch SV, Knight R. Current understanding of the human microbiome. Nat Med. 2018;24(4):392–400.
2. Chen YY, Chen DQ, Chen L, Liu JR, Vaziri ND, Guo Y, et al. Microbiome–metabolome reveals the contribution of gut–kidney axis on kidney disease. J Transl Med. 2019;17(1):5.
3. Andrianova NV, Popkov VA, Klimenko NS, Tyakht AV, Baydakova GV, Frolova OY, et al. Microbiome-metabolome signature of acute kidney injury. Meta. 2020;10(4):142.
4. Nakade Y, Iwata Y, Furuichi K, Mita M, Hamase K, Konno R, et al. Gut microbiota–derived D-serine protects against acute kidney injury. JCI Insight. 2018;3(20):e97957.
5. Yang J, Kim CJ, Go YS, Lee HY, Kim MG, Oh SW, et al. Intestinal microbiota control acute kidney injury severity by immune modulation. Kidney Int. 2020;98(4):932–46.
6. Barrios C, Beaumont M, Pallister T, Villar J, Goodrich JK, Clark A, et al. Gut-microbiota-metabolite axis in early renal function decline. Remuzzi G, editor. PLoS One. 2015;10(8):e0134311.
7. Pluznick JL, Protzko RJ, Gevorgyan II, Peterlin Z, Sipos A, Han J, et al. Olfactory receptor responding to gut microbiota-derived signals plays a role in renin secretion and blood pressure regulation. Proc Natl Acad Sci. 2013;110(11):4410–5.
8. Sun X, Zhang B, Hong X, Zhang X, Kong X. Histone deacetylase inhibitor, sodium butyrate, attenuates gentamicin-induced nephrotoxicity by increasing prohibitin protein expression in rats. Eur J Pharmacol. 2013;707(1–3):147–54.
9. Andrade-Oliveira V, Amano MT, Correa-Costa M, Castoldi A, Felizardo RJF, De Almeida DC, et al. Gut bacteria products prevent AKI induced by ischemia-reperfusion. J Am Soc Nephrol. 2015;26(8):1877–88.
10. Machado RA, Constantino LDS, Tomasi CD, Rojas HA, Vuolo FS, Vitto MF, et al. Sodium butyrate decreases the activation of NF- B reducing inflammation and oxidative damage in the kidney of rats subjected to contrast-induced nephropathy. Nephrol Dial Transplant. 2012;27(8):3136–40.
11. Yanda MK, Liu Q, Cebotaru V, Guggino WB, Cebotaru L. Histone deacetyl inhibition reduces cysts by decreasing cAMP and Ca^{2+} in knock-out mouse models of polycystic kidney disease. J Biol Chem. 2017;292(43):17897–908.
12. Al-Harbi NO, Nadeem A, Ahmad SF, Alotaibi MR, AlAsmari AF, Alanazi WA, et al. Short chain fatty acid, acetate ameliorates sepsis-induced acute kidney injury by inhibition of NADPH oxidase signaling in T cells. Int Immunopharmacol. 2018;58:24–31.
13. Park J, Goergen CJ, HogenEsch H, Kim CH. Chronically elevated levels of short-chain fatty acids induce T cell–mediated ureteritis and hydronephrosis. J Immunol. 2016;196(5):2388–400.
14. Sun G, Yin Z, Liu N, Bian X, Yu R, Su X, et al. Gut microbial metabolite TMAO contributes to renal dysfunction in a mouse model of diet-induced obesity. Biochem Biophys Res Commun. 2017;493(2):964–70.
15. Lai Y, Tang H, Zhang X, Zhou Z, Zhou M, Hu Z, et al. Trimethylamine-N-oxide aggravates kidney injury via activation of p38/MAPK signaling and upregulation of HuR. Kidney Blood Press Res. 2022;47(1):61–71.
16. Gong J, Noel S, Pluznick JL, Hamad ARA, Rabb H. Gut microbiota-kidney cross-talk in acute kidney injury. Semin Nephrol. 2019;39(1):107–16.
17. Jang HR, Gandolfo MT, Ko GJ, Satpute S, Racusen L, Rabb H. Early exposure to germs modifies kidney damage and inflammation after experimental ischemia-reperfusion injury. Am J Physiol Renal Physiol. 2009;297(5):F1457–65.
18. Krebs CF, Paust HJ, Krohn S, Koyro T, Brix SR, Riedel JH, et al. Autoimmune renal disease is exacerbated by S1P-receptor-1-dependent intestinal Th17 cell migration to the kidney. Immunity. 2016;45(5):1078–92.
19. Emal D, Rampanelli E, Stroo I, Butter LM, Teske GJ, Claessen N, et al. Depletion of gut microbiota protects against renal ischemia-reperfusion injury. J Am Soc Nephrol. 2017;28(5):1450–61.

20. Vaziri ND, Yuan J, Rahimi A, Ni Z, Said H, Subramanian VS. Disintegration of colonic epithelial tight junction in uremia: a likely cause of CKD-associated inflammation. Nephrol Dial Transplant. 2012;27(7):2686–93.
21. Vaziri ND, Yuan J, Norris K. Role of urea in intestinal barrier dysfunction and disruption of epithelial tight junction in chronic kidney disease. Am J Nephrol. 2013;37(1):1–6.
22. Ichii O, Otsuka-Kanazawa S, Nakamura T, Ueno M, Kon Y, Chen W, et al. Podocyte injury caused by indoxyl sulfate, a uremic toxin and aryl-hydrocarbon receptor ligand. Rastaldi MP, editor. PLoS One. 2014;9(9):e108448.
23. Park SW, Kim M, Kim JY, Ham A, Brown KM, Mori-Akiyama Y, et al. Paneth cell–mediated multiorgan dysfunction after acute kidney injury. J Immunol. 2012;189(11):5421–33.
24. Li J, Moturi KR, Wang L, Zhang K, Yu C. Gut derived-endotoxin contributes to inflammation in severe ischemic acute kidney injury. BMC Nephrol. 2019;20(1):16.
25. Mishima E, Fukuda S, Mukawa C, Yuri A, Kanemitsu Y, Matsumoto Y, et al. Evaluation of the impact of gut microbiota on uremic solute accumulation by a CE-TOFMS–based metabolomics approach. Kidney Int. 2017;92(3):634–45.
26. Davani-Davari D, Negahdaripour M, Karimzadeh I, Seifan M, Mohkam M, Masoumi S, et al. Prebiotics: definition, types, sources, mechanisms, and clinical applications. Foods. 2019;8(3):92.
27. Lee T, Park D, Kim Y, Lee I, Kim S, Oh C, et al. Lactobacillus salivarius BP121 prevents cisplatin-induced acute kidney injury by inhibition of uremic toxins such as indoxyl sulfate and p-cresol sulfate via alleviating dysbiosis. Int J Mol Med [Internet]. 2020 [cited 2023 Sep 5]; Available from: http://www.spandidos-publications.com/10.3892/ijmm.2020.4495.
28. Yang J, Ji GE, Park MS, Seong YJ, Go YS, Lee HY, et al. Probiotics partially attenuate the severity of acute kidney injury through an immunomodulatory effect. Kidney Res Clin Pract. 2021;40(4):620–33.
29. Fujii H, Yonekura Y, Yamashita Y, Kono K, Nakai K, Goto S, et al. Anti-oxidative effect of AST-120 on kidney injury after myocardial infarction: effect of AST-120 on kidney injury. Br J Pharmacol. 2016;173(8):1302–13.
30. Price R, MacLennan G, Glen J, on behalf of the SuDDICU collaboration. Selective digestive or oropharyngeal decontamination and topical oropharyngeal chlorhexidine for prevention of death in general intensive care: systematic review and network meta-analysis. BMJ. 2014;348(2):g2197.
31. Dong T, Aronsohn A, Gautham Reddy K, Te HS. Rifaximin decreases the incidence and severity of acute kidney injury and hepatorenal syndrome in cirrhosis. Dig Dis Sci. 2016;61(12):3621–6.
32. Chou YT, Kan WC, Shiao CC. Acute kidney injury and gut dysbiosis: a narrative review focus on pathophysiology and treatment. Int J Mol Sci. 2022;23(7):3658.

Myokine-Mediated Muscle-Kidney Crosstalk 14

Paolo Formenti and Michele Umbrello

14.1 Introduction

Myokines are defined as cytokines and other peptides that are produced, expressed, and released by muscle fibers in response to muscular contractions, and exert either autocrine, paracrine, or endocrine effects [87]. Myokines mediate communication between muscle and other organs — brain, adipose tissue, bone, liver, gut, pancreas, the vascular bed, and skin — as well as within the muscle itself [6]. They affect lipid and glucose metabolism, insulin sensitivity, bone formation, endothelial function, and skin structure [28]. As biomarkers, they can be useful for monitoring the type and amount of exercise required as a therapeutic form in cancer, diabetes, or neurodegenerative diseases [23], while the identification of new myokines and their specific roles might lead to novel therapeutic targets. There is an emerging understanding of skeletal muscle as a secretory organ, and of myokines as mediators of muscular status [86], which have already been shown to be involved in tissue regeneration and repair, maintenance of healthy functioning, and immunomodulation. Different muscle fiber types release different clusters of myokines during contraction. Some myokines exert their effects within the muscle itself and are involved in muscle hypertrophy and myogenesis, and in the mediation of fat oxidation [100]. Studies in the past few years have suggested the existence of yet unidentified factors, secreted from muscle cells, which may influence cancer cell growth and pancreas function [26, 88]. Because many muscle-derived proteins depend on contraction, physical

P. Formenti
SC Anestesia, Rianimazione e Terapia Intensiva, ASST Nord Milano, Ospedale Bassini, Cinisello Balsamo, Italy

M. Umbrello (✉)
SC Anestesia e Rianimazione II, ASST Santi Paolo e Carlo – Polo Universitario, Ospedale San Carlo Borromeo, Milan, Italy
e-mail: michele.umbrello@asst-santipaolocarlo.it

D. Battaglini et al. (eds.), *Organ System Crosstalk in Critical Illness*,
https://doi.org/10.1007/978-3-032-01024-7_14

inactivity likely alters the myokine response. This may help explain the association between sedentary behavior and many chronic diseases [20]. In fact, when muscles contract, they produce hormone-like chemical messengers such as myokines allowing muscles to communicate with many other tissues [3]. This represents a new way of looking at muscle as one of the most active endocrine organs in our body. The research-based benefits offered by myokines are described in Table 14.1. Accumulating evidence suggests muscle–kidney crosstalk mediated by mitochondrial RNA. These RNAs appear to be secreted by muscle via exosomes [130]. In this framework, the catabolic influence on skeletal muscle results in a maladaptive behavior of several factors associated with the acceleration of organ dysfunction. Low muscle mass seems to be associated with an increased prevalence of chronic kidney disease (CKD) [51, 61]. Intensive care unit patients skeletal muscle wasting due to critical illness itself, and this has important clinical implications, hindering rehabilitation and increasing both morbidity and mortality [74, 111]. Intensive care unit-acquired weakness (ICUAW) brings about skeletal muscle wasting due to critical illness and has important consequences, possibly due to the effect of organ-organ (specifically, muscle-organ) crosstalk [41, 63]. Thus, myokines may become new targets for the diagnosis and treatment of different conditions. In this chapter,

Table 14.1 The research-based benefits offered by myokines

Research-based benefits	Research-based mechanism
Building of muscle tissue mass	Downregulation of myostatin and upregulation of decorin, a myokine associated with gene expression that promotes muscle growth
Decreased fat	Including visceral (organ), intramuscular (within muscle), and subcutaneous (under the skin)
Increased resting energy expenditure	A number of myokines are able to modulate adipose tissue metabolism and thermogenic activity, liver endogenous glucose production, and β-cell insulin secretion
Prevention of bone mineral density loss	Myostatin is involved in osteoclast formation and bone destruction; transforming growth factor-β, follistatin, insulin-like growth factor-I, fibroblast growth factor-2, osteoglycin, FAM5C, irisin, interleukin (IL)-6, leukemia inhibitory factor, IL-7, IL-15, monocyte chemoattractant protein-1, ciliary neurotrophic factor, osteonectin, and matrix metalloproteinase 2 also affect bone cells in various manners
Improved insulin sensitivity	Increased cellular glucose uptake
Decreased chronic, systemic inflammation	Exercise-induced interleukin-6 myokine (IL-6) increases circulating levels of potent anti-inflammatory hormones, such as IL-1RA and IL-10
Inhibition of mammary cancer cell growth	SPARC and OSM myokines have an anti-tumorigenic effect
Benefits on learning and memory	Upregulated the expression of the brain-derived neurotrophic factor (BDNF) myokine, which has been identified as a key factor in controlling body mass and energy homeostasis, as well as cognitive function

we will focus on principal myokines related to muscle mass disruption and the evidence of their kidney crosstalk mediation.

14.2 Muscle Myokines

The myokine network described above can be considered as the conceptual framework for analyzing and understanding the crosstalk between muscles and a variety of other distant organs. At present, more than 600 myokines have been described [39]. The vast majority still require functional analysis. Among the hundreds of recognized myokines which have been identified, the vast majority was shown to be regulated at the mRNA or secretory level by differentiation, contraction, or other stimuli. Many of them most likely act in a complex autocrine fashion, which is very difficult to analyze. Moreover, many of these myokines have been described only in cell-culture models. Their relevance for in vivo crosstalk remains to be validated. For instance, less than 30 myokines were analyzed on the ex vivo human skeletal muscle biopsies taken before and after acute exercise and exercise training, showing how some of them could play a role in the communication between skeletal muscle and other organs [19]. Figure 14.1 summarizes the main characteristics of the most important muscles' myokine.

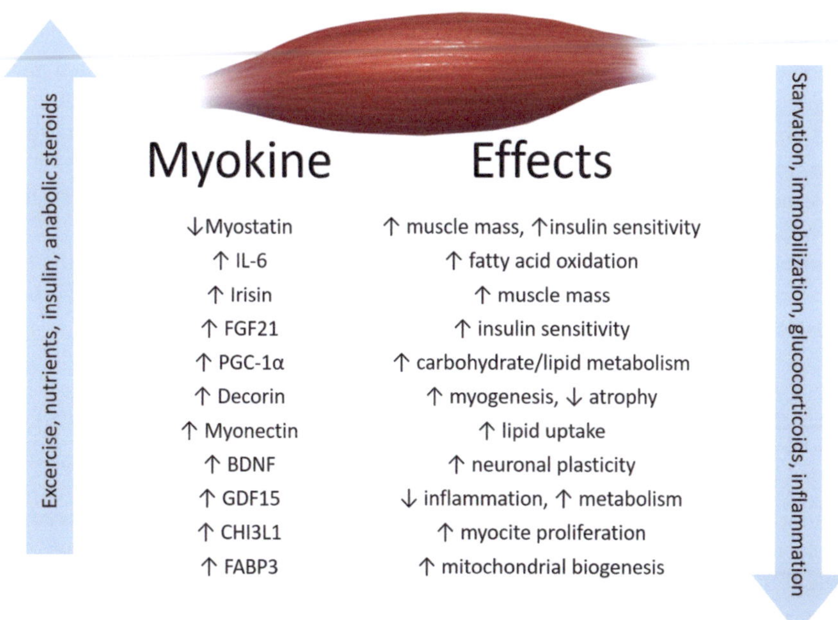

Fig. 14.1 Main characteristics of the most important muscle myokines

14.2.1 Myostatin

Myostatin is a protein synthesized and secreted by the skeletal muscle, which negatively regulates muscle mass [3]. In addition, myostatin seems to have an important role in the crosstalk between skeletal muscle and adipose tissue and is involved in insulin sensitivity. In fact, both aerobic and resistance exercise attenuate myostatin expression, and myostatin inactivation potentiates the beneficial effects of endurance exercise on metabolism [33].

14.2.2 Interleukins

A systemic cytokine response is secreted in response to muscle activity [31]. Among these, IL-6 was identified as a myokine based on the observation that it exponentially increased in proportion to the amount of muscle mass engaged in the exercise [88]. Following exercise, the basal plasma IL-6 concentration may increase up to 100-fold. The exercise-induced increase of plasma IL-6 occurs in an exponential manner, and the peak IL-6 level is reached at the end of the exercise or shortly thereafter. It is the combination of mode, intensity, and duration of the exercise that determines the magnitude of the exercise-induced increase of plasma IL-6 [88]. Moreover, its increment is followed by a cascade that includes the increment in IL-1 and the anti-inflammatory cytokine IL-10 [9, 16]. It was initially hypothesized that the exercise-induced IL-6 response was related to muscle damage, since its increment was studied in the pro-inflammatory context of sepsis [43]. IL-6 has also been reported to directly affect myofibrils by activating many signaling pathways involved in muscle protein degradation or promoting muscle atrophy-related gene expression [125]. Then, chronic muscle injury is characteristic of fatty infiltration and fibrosis. Many myokines have been proven to regulate adipose or cell proliferation. Interleukin-15 stimulates fat oxidation, glucose uptake, mitochondrial biogenesis, and myogenesis in skeletal muscle and adipose tissue [79]. Recent observation screened the potential role of IL-15 in regulating the fatty infiltration in muscle injury [54], supporting the potential role of this myokine as a modulator of the fate of adipogenicity progenitors in injured muscle and as a novel therapy for chronic muscle injury.

14.2.3 Fibronectin Type III Domain-Containing Protein 5 (FNDC5) or Irisin

Irisin (fibronectin type III domain-containing protein 5 or FNDC5) is produced by skeletal muscles after physical exercise. It was originally described as a molecule able to promote energy expenditure in white adipose tissue [14]. Recently, it has been shown that the myokine irisin affects skeletal metabolism in vivo [92]. An experimental study showed how mice treated with a micro-dose of irisin displayed improved cortical bone mass, geometry, and strength, resembling the effect of physical activity in developing an efficient load-bearing skeleton [128]. Additional studies highlighted the autocrine effect of irisin on skeletal muscle, showing how irisin is increased by physical activity and how it is strictly correlated with adipose thermogenesis [70]. Research regarding irisin receptor is still controversial. Experimental studies showed how it increases both osteocytes survival and production of sclerostin, a local modulator of bone remodeling, demonstrating that αV integrin receptors may act as the receptors of irisin to mediate signal transfer into cells [58]. Few papers showed that irisin injections can impact skeletal remodeling by improving cortical bone mineral density and strength in mice [24]. Other studies focused on kidney effects, showing how irisin could reduce renal tubular cell injury by inhibiting the TGF-β type 1 receptor [89]. However, the receptor repertoire of irisin needs to be further elucidated in the future to clarify the mechanisms underlying irisin effects.

14.2.4 Fibroblast Growth Factor 21 (FGF21)

FGF is a superfamily of polypeptides released into the blood circulation, acting as hormones that regulate important metabolic pathways [104]. Striated muscles have been found to be an important source of FGF21 [107]. When FGF binds to its receptors, it mediates intracellular signaling through different paths, which include mitogen-activated protein kinase (MAPK) signaling, phosphatidylinositol 3-kinase (PI3K)/serine-threonine protein kinase signaling pathway, signal transducer and activator of transcription signaling pathway, and phosphoinositide phospholipase C signaling pathway [104]. As a regulatory metabolic molecule, FGF21 plays an important role in maintaining metabolic homeostasis [113]. One study showed that FGF21 inhibited glucolipid-induced islet cell apoptosis, promoted beta cell survival and function, and increased the number of insulin-positive islets, contributing to the maintenance of glucose homeostasis and prevention of hyperglycemia [82]. Conversely, the absence of FGF21 resulted in insulin resistance and islet dysfunction [44]. Recent studies confirmed that the expression of FGF21 in skeletal muscles is upregulated upon activation of the phosphatidylinositol 3-kinase/Akt signaling pathway, which is induced by exercise and muscle contraction [56]. Acute exercise increases FGF21 concentrations in both serum and metabolic organs. Moreover, in animal model, it was shown to increase the expression of FGF21 in skeletal muscle, complemented by the phosphorylation of Akt [106]. Finally, few studies have confirmed that FGF21 plays an important role in the progression of kidney disease [96].

14.2.5 Peroxisome Proliferator-Activated Receptor Gamma 1-Alpha Coactivator (PGC-1 Alpha)

PGC-1 alpha seems to be correlated with muscle hypertrophy by stimulating the macrophages. M1 macrophages, once stimulated, release IL-6, insulin growth factor type 1 (IGF-1), and vascular endothelial growth factor (VEGF). M2 macrophages stimulate satellite cells for proliferation and growth by acting as anti-inflammatory, while M1 stimulates blood vessels and produces pro-inflammatory cytokines [91]. In particular, it stimulates mitochondrial biogenesis and promotes the remodeling of muscle tissue to a fiber-type composition that is metabolically more oxidative and less glycolytic in nature, and it participates in the regulation of both carbohydrate and lipid metabolism [68]. It has recently been proposed as a new target against oxidative stress, mitochondrial dysfunction, and cellular senescence in kidney cells [32].

14.2.6 Decorin

Decorin seems to play a role in muscle growth. Few papers investigated this myokine, showing how it is secreted from myotubules in response to exercise, and it is involved in the regulation of muscle hypertrophy playing a role in exercise-related restructuring processes of skeletal muscle [55]. In particular, its overexpression stimulates the pro-myogenic factor Mighty (which is negatively regulated by myostatin) and reduce muscle-specific ubiquitin ligases atrogin1 and MuRF1, which are involved in atrophic pathways.

14.2.7 Myonectin

Myonectin is expressed and secreted by the muscle tissue. Circulating levels of myonectin were tightly regulated by the metabolic state as fasting suppressed it, while refeeding dramatically increased its mRNA and serum levels [99]. Myonectin stimulates the lipid uptake capacity of adipose tissue and liver by upregulating proteins involved in lipid uptake, reducing circulating free fatty acids levels without significantly affecting the lipolysis and glucose homeostasis of adipose cells [37]. Therefore, myonectin may act as a nutrition-sensing factor that can timely transmit information about the nutritional status of the body to various tissues. Few studies have explored the potential mechanism through which myonectin acts in renal disease.

14.2.8 Brain-Derived Neurotrophic Factor (BDNF)

BDNF is produced by contracting muscle, enhancing the oxidation of fat. It plays an important role in neuronal survival and growth, supplies as a neurotransmitter modulator, and takes part in neuronal plasticity [13]. It is widely expressed in the central nervous system, gut, and other tissues. BDNF and insulin-like growth factor-1 have similar downstream signaling mechanisms that increase the expression of pro-survival genes [47]. Decreased levels of BDNF are associated with neurodegenerative diseases with neuronal loss, such as Parkinson's disease, Alzheimer's disease, multiple sclerosis, and Huntington's disease [8]. BDNF has also been identified as a key component of the hypothalamic pathway that controls body mass and energy homeostasis [90].

14.2.9 Growth Differentiation Factor 15 (GDF15)

GDF15 is a stress-inducing hormone and is released by cells, such as vascular smooth muscle cells, heart and endothelial cells, macrophages, and fat cells in response to external stimuli resulting from various stress states, such as obesity, insulin resistance, heart failure, and cancer [27]. GDF-15 acts through a recently identified receptor called glial-derived neurotrophic factor (GDNF) receptor alpha-like (GFRAL) which signals through the rearranged during transfection (RET) tyrosine kinase receptor [121]. The effects of GDF-15 are pleiotropic and include appetite regulation and actions on metabolism, pregnancy, cell survival, immune response, and inflammation. GDF-15 also plays different roles in the pathophysiology of cardiovascular disease, autoimmunity, cancer-associated anorexia/cachexia, and diabetes [49]. Exercise is a key factor causing increased GDF15 levels in the blood circulation as shown by experimental and clinical observations [60]. GDF15 plays a role also in metabolic diseases. For instance, it was associated with faster deterioration of renal function and was found to be a predictor of all-cause and cardiovascular mortality [48] and morbidity in patients with chronic kidney disease [76]. It has been investigated also in lung-related diseases, showing how in patients with COPD high levels of GDF15 were independently associated with a higher yearly rate of exacerbations, higher mortality, and increased decline in both FEV1 and FVC [115].

14.2.10 Chitinase-3-Like Protein 1 (CHI3L1/YKL-40)

CHI3L1/YKL-40 is one of the several myokine non-enzymatic chitinase-like proteins (CLPs) [129]. Its stimulation is induced by acute exercise activating myocyte proliferation, which is important for the restructuring of skeletal muscle in response to exercise training [40]. After secretion into the blood stream, CHI3L1 can move to target organs to promote cell proliferation, differentiation, and anti-apoptosis [29]. Recent evidence has implicated YKL-40 in patients with inflammatory diseases [108] and cardio-metabolic disorders [29], making it potentially useful to evaluate disease severity, prognosis, and survival. YKL-40 may also act as a potential serological marker for the diagnosis of asthma, assessment of severity, indicator of the disease state, and differential diagnosis [52]. The level of YKL-40 was found to be increased in the early stage of kidney disease and was correlated with its progression [64]. Finally, YKL-40 may have a potential role in neurodegenerative disease [25].

14.2.11 Fatty Acid-Binding Protein 3 (FABP3)

Fatty acids function both as an energy source and as metabolic signaling molecules and affect many vital processes [103]. This complexity, combined with the chemical characteristics of lipids, presents many challenges in their trafficking, compartmentalization, and specific target engagement properties within and between cells [36]. At least nine FABPs have been identified to date, which exhibit unique patterns of tissue expression. FABP3 is the most widely distributed, mainly in muscle, kidney, lung, brain, and ovary tissues. Its concentrations were determined for tissues from Sprague-Dawley rats and found to occur at highest concentrations in cardiac muscle and in skeletal muscles containing an abundance of type I fibers, such as the soleus muscle [66]. Studies have revealed that FABP3 is also involved in the progression of many diseases such as cardiac hypertrophy and cardiac insufficiency [133]. Moreover, the downregulation of FABP3 expression can lead to changes in mitochondrial morphology, decrease intracellular ATP synthesis, increase mitochondrial ROS production, and ultimately induce apoptosis [132]. Unfortunately, few studies have explored the involvement of FABP3 in kidney disease.

14.3 Muscle-Kidney Crosstalk

Chronic kidney disease, also known as chronic renal disease or CKD, is a condition characterized by a gradual loss of kidney function over time. It includes conditions that damage the kidneys and decrease their ability to maintain a healthy status. CKD is associated with complications such as chronic inflammation, oxidative stress, early vascular aging, and cellular senescence leading to a dysregulated ageing process [18]. Chronic renal failure is independently associated with cardiovascular mortality by its cause mortality and by its progression to end-stage kidney failure [109]. Furthermore, glucose metabolism, metabolic acidosis, microinflammation, and altered cellular protein turnover are all affected by renal insufficiency. Moreover, patients with CKD exhibit a catabolic state, which is known to be associated with protein wasting and with multiple metabolic imbalances due, in part, to elevated uremic toxins [42]. It is reasonable that catabolic conditions associated with CKD would affect skeletal muscle mass. While low muscle mass was not predictive of incident CKD or CKD progression, low muscle mass was independently associated with increased risk of mortality in CKD patients [21]. Within this perspective, bone and skeletal muscles may be negatively affected by CKD in terms of function and activity, contributing to increased morbidity and mortality. Indeed, both organs are anatomically and physiologically coupled, and together regulate functional and metabolic mechanisms. Recent research clarifies how the crosstalk between the skeleton and muscle contraction occurs through the interaction of myokines and osteokines [65].

A third player in this biochemical crosstalk is adipose tissue and the secretion of adipokines. The detection of bone and muscle-derived cytokine secretion following physical exercise has strengthened the idea of cross communication between these organs. Basically, myokines, osteokines, and adipokines exert a local and systemic autocrine and paracrine effect to regulate muscle, bone, and fat metabolism [59]. Several myokines exert anabolic/catabolic effects on bone; the osteokines seem to be able to induce muscle anabolism and catabolism, while adipokines modulate muscle and bone metabolism. Thus, physical activity plays an important role in the balance between all these cytokines. In fact, aging, and the subsequent reduction in physical activity, determines adipocyte hypertrophy and increments the immunological cells releasing the pro-inflammatory adipokines which induces chronic low-grade inflammation. Conversely, muscle-bone-fat crosstalk can induce stimulation of bioactive cytokines after muscular exercises, leading to an increase in muscle anabolism, bone formation, mitochondrial biogenesis, glucose utilization, and fatty acid oxidation [84]. Advanced stages of CKD are often associated with a sedentary lifestyle [5, 53, 98]. Conversely, it has been demonstrated how a highly physical activity reduced up to 25% all-cause of mortality [62] with a beneficial impact on bone mass, through promotion of bone formation and inhibition of bone resorption, and an increased muscle mass [2].

14.4 Main Myokines Implicated in Muscle-Kidney Crosstalk

Several myokines such as irisin, myostatin, IL-15, IL-6, MG53, FGF21, FABP3 exert favorable physiological and metabolic effects in skeletal muscle and bone and are associated with modifications during kidney disease. Irisin plays a role in diet-induced insulin resistance by raising the total energy expenditure, which leads to protein-energy waste and resultant greater mortality in chronic renal failure [123]. The exact mechanisms responsible for deregulation of energy expenditure in chronic renal failure patients are not fully understood. Some authors showed how the resting irisin levels were significantly decreased in chronic kidney disease patients and were inversely correlated with the levels of blood urea nitrogen and creatinine [119]. Other findings suggest that irisin may be involved in the regulation of biochemical factor levels in CKD patients through the progression kidney disease as it was significantly decreased with the progression of CKD from stage 2 to stage 4 [94]. Irisin concentration was found to be lower in type 2 diabetes mellitus compared to non-diabetic individuals. Wang et al. showed that irisin was found to be significantly lower in patients with microalbuminuria and macroalbuminuria, and their serum level further decreased with the increase in proteinuria and decrease in the glomerular filtration rate [116]. Moreover, irisin was shown to be increased in diabetic nephropathy patients, and it was negatively correlated with GFR [71]. Experimental studies suggest a potential renal protective effect of exercise mediated by the irisin pathway. The use of an irisin receptor blocker decreased the positive effects of aerobic physical exercise in reducing albuminuria, glomerular hypertrophy, and inflammation in the kidney of rats compared to sedentary diabetic rats [35]. The existing literature also suggests a possible link between irisin and ischemia-reperfusion, involving mechanisms similar to those associated with exercise [117]. In mice with ischemia-reperfusion-induced acute kidney injury, irisin could protect renal mitochondrial function and reduce oxidative stress and inflammation [126]. Moreover, it has been suggested that myokine-mediated muscle-kidney crosstalk can suppress metabolic reprogramming and fibrogenesis during kidney disease. The induction of irisin improved kidney energy metabolism and prevented kidney damage in mice [89]. Specifically, metabolomics analysis reveals increased ATP production and improved energy metabolism in injured kidneys, identifying irisin as a serum factor that mediates these metabolic effects during progressive kidney injury by inhibiting TGF-β type 1 receptor. Regarding its potential role in to reno-protective effects, irisin could reduce vascular calcification in chronic kidney disease by maintaining mitochondrial function or inhibiting pyroptosis [83]. These studies suggest that irisin could be used as a potential target for kidney therapy in the future. Contrasting results prevented an understanding of the effects of exercise on bone-muscle biomarkers in CKD. For instance, irisin was unaffected by resistance exercise in hemodialysis patients [75], while myostatin levels were shown to decrease following aerobic and resistive training [46, 93] but were found to be higher following months of exercise training CKD patients [131].

A recent systematic review investigated the effects of physical activity in CKD patients and reported beneficial effects of resistance exercise on bone health [17]. Age-related decline of renal function may reflect multicellular dysfunction that leads to reduced capability of the kidney to repair or regenerate in response to stress. A novel finding showed links between Mitsugumin 53 (MG53) and the control of intracellular calcium signaling to modulation of inflammatory activation associated with kidney injury and fibrosis. In fact, renal proximal tubular epithelia contain MG53 protein, and a compromised function to repair renal injury could be an intrinsic mechanism that contributes to reduced kidney function. A loss of the crosstalk from muscle to kidney may constitute an extrinsic mechanism leading to the increased vulnerability of the kidney to function properly during aging. MG53 was previously identified as a key component of cell membrane repair, which plays a vital role in protection against kidney injury [69]. These findings represent a novel concept that engineering of macrophages with tailored secretion of MG53 can enhance renal protection using inflammation and fibrotic remodeling associated with CKD.

Metabolic disorders often present in CKD have been proposed to contribute to the elevation of FGF21 levels in CKD, as it increases from the early stage and predicts renal progression in diabetes and all-cause mortality [96]. Although high FGF21 levels may be advantageous for surviving CKD, excess FGF21 may also have adverse effects. FGF21 was found to be negatively correlated with GFR. The benefits of FGF21 in combination with other treatments for kidney disease have been investigated. For instance, fenofibrate, a commonly used lipid-lowering drug used to treat hyperlipidemia, could play a renal protective role directly through FGF21. This has been investigated in experimental and human studies. It prevents type 1 diabetes-induced pathological and functional abnormalities of the heart by increasing FGF21 that may upregulate Sirt1-mediated autophagy [127] and plays a renal protective role by promoting the expression of FGF21 and thereby activating the Akt2/GSK-3β/Fyn/Nrf2 antioxidant and AMPK pathway [22]. Similarly, in humans, long-term fenofibrate treatment could increase serum FGF21 levels over 5 years in patients with type 2 diabetes [80]. One study explored therapeutic effect and mechanism of combined use of FGF21 and Insulin on diabetic nephropathy [72]. The combination of FGF21 with insulin exhibits reciprocal sensitization on glucose and lipid metabolism in mice with type 2 diabetes. Compared with insulin or FGF21 alone, FGF21 combined with insulin can further improve blood glucose levels and renal pathological changes, oxidative stress, and AGEs caused by high glucose. Finally, the combination of low-dose radiation with FGF21 significantly reduced diabetes-induced renal fibrosis, inflammation, and oxidative damage [101]. These findings seem to suggest that FGF21 is closely related to the progression of nephropathy and can be used as a therapeutic target.

FABP3 is located in the renal mesangial and distal tubular cells and has been shown to be a sensitive marker of renal injury, potentially a mediator in the pathogenesis of CKD. Current studies suggest that FABP3 may be an important predictor of kidney disease even if is still not completely understood whether it tends to increase in a compensatory manner in response to kidney injury or whether it is also of non-muscular origin. Experimentally, it has been shown to be associated with MCP-1 expression and lymphocytes renal infiltration, significantly increased in the kidneys of diabetic eNOS knockout mice [81]. Similarly, in human observations, it was found to be significantly increased in the urine [77] and independently and significantly correlated with GFR stages of diabetic patients [124]. These findings suggest that FABP3 levels in the blood and urine are significantly increased in kidney disease and may play an adverse role in the progression of kidney disease. Research data showed that local activation of IL-6 trans-signaling pathway is implicated in renal autoimmune and inflammatory diseases. Kidney resident cells can secrete IL-6, but only podocyte expresses IL-6R [78]. This is upregulated by proinflammatory factors and high glucose level. Some authors showed that the progression of diabetic nephropathy may be attenuated by blocking IL-6 and its downstream mediators such as IL-6R and gp130 [57]. This myokine seems to be implicated in some autoimmune nephropathies such as IgA nephropathy in which immune complex and complement component can stimulate mesangial cell to secrete IL-6 and ensue its proliferation and inflammatory cell recruitment [105], or in lupus nephritis, in which it was found increased [45, 50]. Higher IL-6 levels act as a trigger for the progression of CKD and its related complications. Since CKD is caused by the increased generation of oxidative stress from chronic inflammation and its impaired renal function reduce its clearance, an elevated plasma IL-6 level is commonly observed in these patients [85]. Its role in the progression of renal disease is probably also associated with the chronic vascular disease as IL6 initiates the endothelial injury mainly via reducing endothelial nitric oxide synthase and adiponectin (an anti-atherogenic adipokine) expression [15]. Recently, IL-15 has been implicated in fibrosis protection in several organs by regulating collagen synthesis of myofibroblasts and through the modulation of inflammation [30]. In the tubulo-interstitial and glomerular kidney diseases, it has been reported that IL-15 and the IL-15 receptor are constitutively expressed in normal tubular epithelial cells. IL-15 decreases the induction of a nephrogenic chemokine, MCP-1, that attracts leukocytes into the kidney [102].

Data suggest that decorin exerts beneficial effects on tubulointerstitial fibrosis, primarily by influencing the expression of a key cyclin-dependent kinase inhibitor and by limiting the degree of apoptosis, mononuclear cell infiltration, tubular atrophy, and expression of TGF-beta1 [97]. A new approach for treating renal insufficiency with gene therapy has been investigated in animal models. The authors implanted decorin-expressing fibroblasts within the renal tissue of rats with renal failure to neutralize TGF-β1 activity, showing how it can alleviate fibrosis and delay the progression of renal failure [67]. Similarly, decorin may have a protective effect on acute ischemia-reperfusion injury in the rat kidney model by reducing TGF-β1 level as an initiator of fibrotic and apoptotic activity [1]. Few studies have investigated the plasma concentrations of myostatin in CKD patients. Although it has been shown how its level is increased in chronic disease and in dialysis-patients [7], its role is still debated. The application of a specific antibody that neutralizes myostatin demonstrated inconsistent results, with some that suggest the possibility to reduce the risk of falls or physical dependency in older weak faller [11], and others that suggest a dose-dependent increase in appendicular lean body mass and decrease in fat mass [122]. The main myokines implicated in a muscle-kidney crosstalk are reported in Table 14.2.

14.5 Any Role for Myokines in the Critical Care Setting?

A pathological crosstalk may be responsible for multiple organ dysfunction syndrome in critically ill patients admitted to the intensive care unit (ICU) [4]. Moreover, multiple organ failure may occur in a serial sequence, such as during cardiogenic shock which may lead to ischemic hepatitis, or in parallel, such as during septic shock where sepsis leads to acute respiratory distress syndrome, acute kidney injury, and neurological impairment [10]. Hypoperfusion, triggering interactions between immune cells of the human body, pathogen, and damage-associated molecular patterns released from the pathogen, is the likely factors behind this complicated pathophysiologic process. All these may be considered as distant organ crosstalk effects of various cytokines released due to critical event. Many pathophysiological factors are linked with the high risk of developing clinically significant muscle weakness in the patients ICU (ICUAW) [34]. This relatively new entity has recently

Table 14.2 Main myokines implicated in muscle-kidney crosstalk

Myokine	Role and mechanism
Irisin	Reduced resting levels in CKD, reduced levels with progression of CKD stage: less protection of the kidneys against I-R damage
FGF21	Increased levels in CKD and negative association with GFR
FABP3	Blood levels correlated with the stage of diabetic nephropathy
Decorin	Reduced in CKD with less protection against tubulointerstitial fibrosis
Myostatin	Increased in end-stage renal disease

been advocated as one of the causes associated with the increased risk of death and prolonged dependency on mechanical ventilation and other intensive care complications [112]. Frequently, critically ill patients are prone to develop a catabolic state as a consequence of a number of factors which include immobilization and hormonal changes [38, 110]. This sarcopenia-induced status alters the secretions of myokines leading to a multisystemic dysfunction. The isolated secretion of myokines in the critically ill patient has previously been reported in this context; however, there is no research focused on this specific topic. More detailed investigations regarding myokine secretion and their local or systemic effects in the critically ill patient, especially in early stages of disease, is a potentially promising novel approach yet to be developed. Few is known about serum/plasma concentrations of these proteins or affected metabolites and their association with the outcome of critical illness.

Sepsis remains one of the major complications in the ICU [95], and recent research focused on its pathogenesis, which includes ferroptosis, an iron-dependent programmed cell death inside the mitochondria. In this contest, irisin, which improves mitochondrial function, has been proposed as a target of treatment. It has been showed how serum irisin levels are decreased and negatively correlated with disease severity in patients with sepsis, and how irisin treatment suppresses ferroptosis and restores mitochondrial function in experimental sepsis [118]. In particular, in mice subjected to cecal ligation and puncture (CLP), exogenous irisin administration suppressed ferroptosis, inhibited inflammatory response, decreased reactive oxygen species (ROS) production, restored abnormal mitochondrial morphology, and increased mtDNA copy number and adenosine triphosphate (ATP) content. The effect of irisin on ferroptosis was confirmed in LPS-treated hepatocytes and CLP-induced septic mice. Inhibition of glutathione peroxidase 4 (GPX4), a central regulator of ferroptosis, reduced irisin's protective effects in LPS-treated hepatocytes and CLP-induced septic mice, while blocking the irisin receptor with RGD peptide or Echistain decreased irisin-induced GPX4 expression. Very recently, observations suggest how the expression of the FNDC5/irisin was affected by critical illness and associated with clinical outcomes, with limited effects of interventions that attenuate muscle wasting or weakness [111]. Similarly, in an exploratory study, the serum levels of IL-8, IL-15, and tumor necrosis factor-α (TNF-α) among patients receiving mechanical ventilation were investigated together with their association to outcomes of patient delirium, muscle strength, activities of daily living, duration of mechanical ventilation, and length of ICU stay [120]. The results showed how IL-8, IL-15, and TNF-α were highly variable and consistently elevated, and almost 30% were positive for significant muscle weakness at discharge from ICU. Repeated values of mean post-activity IL-8 serum values were significantly associated only with ADL following ICU discharge. Patients with heart failure (HF) manifest the highest-risk, most complex, and most resource-intensive disease states in ICU [73]. Incidence of cardiac cachexia in HF is accompanied by crossover changes in the spectrum of the myokines. Elevated serum concentrations of myostatin and IL-6 were found, whereas isirin, FGF-21, and myonectin were significantly decreased [12]. The serum levels of decorin, BDNF, and GDF-11 were variable and exhibited a strong relation to the age of the HF patients rather than severity of contractility dysfunction and sarcopenia [114]. Finally, myokines influence not only skeletal muscles but also the myocardium and adipose tissue and ensure their autocrine metabolic regulation of energy homeostasis, hypertrophy, reparation, and adaptation of skeletal muscles to physical exercise.

14.6 Conclusions

Skeletal muscle can produce hundreds of different myokines, with only approximately less than 5% having a defined biological function. The number of kidney-derived factors, which may alter skeletal muscle mass and function, is currently unknown. Some of them are upregulated in CKD promoting skeletal muscle atrophy, while others may improve renal functioning. Any knowledge on the mechanistic role so far is dependent on preclinical animal models and the methodological concerns regarding the accuracy of measurements need to be carefully considered in future research. Thus, their roles on kidney function require further systematic research, including any antiatrophic effects, and human clinical pharmacological interventions. Finally, numerous key questions remain unanswered. Among these, further research should investigate if there is any connection between renal disease and sarcopenia, if one condition come first or metabolically influence the other, if the loss of muscle only related to comparable changes in bone over the course of CKD progression, and if other tissues are involved in the observed deleterious changes to bone and muscle in CKD. Similar questions should be addressed in the critical care setting.

References

1. Alan C, Kocoglu H, Altintas R, Alici B, Resit Ersay A. Protective effect of decorin on acute ischaemia-reperfusion injury in the rat kidney. Arch Med Sci. 2011;7(2):211–6. https://doi.org/10.5114/aoms.2011.22069.
2. Alghadir AH, Gabr SA, Al-Eisa ES, Alghadir MH. Correlation between bone mineral density and serum trace elements in response to supervised aerobic training in older adults. Clin Interv Aging. 2016;11:265–73. https://doi.org/10.2147/CIA.S100566.
3. Argilés JM, Orpí M, Busquets S, López-Soriano FJ. Myostatin: more than just a regulator of muscle mass. Drug Discov Today. 2012;17(13–14):702–9. https://doi.org/10.1016/j.drudis.2012.02.001.
4. Armutcu F. Organ crosstalk: the potent roles of inflammation and fibrotic changes in the course of organ interactions. Inflamm Res. 2019;68(10):825–39. https://doi.org/10.1007/s00011-019-01271-7.
5. Avesani CM, Trolonge S, Deléaval P, Baria F, Mafra D, Faxén-Irving G, Chauveau P, Teta D, Kamimura MA, Cuppari L, Chan M, Heimbürger O, Fouque D. Physical activity and energy expenditure in haemodialysis patients: an international survey. Nephrol Dial Transplant. 2012;27(6):2430–4. https://doi.org/10.1093/ndt/gfr692.
6. Barbalho SM, Prado Neto EV, De Alvares GR, Bechara MD, Baisi Chagas EF, Audi M, Guissoni Campos LM, Landgraf Guiger E, Buchaim RL, Buchaim DV, Cressoni Araujo

A. Myokines: a descriptive review. J Sports Med Phys Fitness. 2020;60(12):1583–90. https://doi.org/10.23736/S0022-4707.20.10884-3.
7. Bataille S, Chauveau P, Fouque D, Aparicio M, Koppe L. Myostatin and muscle atrophy during chronic kidney disease. Nephrol Dial Transplant. 2021;36(11):1986–93. https://doi.org/10.1093/ndt/gfaa129.
8. Bathina S, Das UN. Brain-derived neurotrophic factor and its clinical implications. Arch Med Sci. 2015;11(6):1164–78. https://doi.org/10.5114/aoms.2015.56342.
9. Batista ML, Rosa JC, Lopes RD, Lira FS, Martins E, Yamashita AS, Brum PC, Lancha AH, Lopes AC, Seelaender M. Exercise training changes IL-10/TNF-α ratio in the skeletal muscle of post-MI rats. Cytokine. 2010;49(1):102–8. https://doi.org/10.1016/j.cyto.2009.10.007.
10. Bauer M, Coldewey SM, Leitner M, Löffler B, Weis S, Wetzker R. Deterioration of organ function as a Hallmark in sepsis: the cellular perspective. Front Immunol. 2018;9:1460. https://doi.org/10.3389/fimmu.2018.01460.
11. Becker C, Lord SR, Studenski SA, Warden SJ, Fielding RA, Recknor CP, Hochberg MC, Ferrari SL, Blain H, Binder EF, Rolland Y, Poiraudeau S, Benson CT, Myers SL, Hu L, Ahmad QI, Pacuch KR, Gomez EV, Benichou O, STEADY Group. Myostatin antibody (LY2495655) in older weak fallers: a proof-of-concept, randomised, phase 2 trial. Lancet Diabetes Endocrinol. 2015;3(12):948–57. https://doi.org/10.1016/S2213-8587(15)00298-3.
12. Berezin AE, Berezin AA, Lichtenauer M. Myokines and heart failure: challenging role in adverse cardiac remodeling, myopathy, and clinical outcomes. Dis Markers. 2021;2021:e6644631. https://doi.org/10.1155/2021/6644631.
13. Binder DK, Scharfman HE. Brain-derived neurotrophic factor. Growth Factors. 2004;22(3):123–31. https://doi.org/10.1080/08977190410001723308.
14. Boström P, Wu J, Jedrychowski MP, Korde A, Ye L, Lo JC, Rasbach KA, Boström EA, Choi JH, Long JZ, Kajimura S, Zingaretti MC, Vind BF, Tu H, Cinti S, Højlund K, Gygi SP, Spiegelman BM. A PGC1-α-dependent myokine that drives brown-fat-like development of white fat and thermogenesis. Nature. 2012;481(7382):463–8. https://doi.org/10.1038/nature10777.
15. Bruun JM, Lihn AS, Verdich C, Pedersen SB, Toubro S, Astrup A, Richelsen B. Regulation of adiponectin by adipose tissue-derived cytokines: in vivo and in vitro investigations in humans. Am J Physiol Endocrinol Metab. 2003;285(3):E527–33. https://doi.org/10.1152/ajpendo.00110.2003.
16. Cannon JG, Fielding RA, Fiatarone MA, Orencole SF, Dinarello CA, Evans WJ. Increased interleukin 1 beta in human skeletal muscle after exercise. Am J Phys. 1989;257(2 Pt 2):R451–5. https://doi.org/10.1152/ajpregu.1989.257.2.R451.
17. Cardoso DF, Marques EA, Leal DV, Ferreira A, Baker LA, Smith AC, Viana JL. Impact of physical activity and exercise on bone health in patients with chronic kidney disease: a systematic review of observational and experimental studies. BMC Nephrol. 2020;21(1):334. https://doi.org/10.1186/s12882-020-01999-z.
18. Carney EF. The impact of chronic kidney disease on global health. Nat Rev Nephrol. 2020;16(5):251. https://doi.org/10.1038/s41581-020-0268-7.
19. Catoire M, Mensink M, Kalkhoven E, Schrauwen P, Kersten S. Identification of human exercise-induced myokines using secretome analysis. Physiol Genomics. 2014;46(7):256–67. https://doi.org/10.1152/physiolgenomics.00174.2013.
20. Chen W, Wang L, You W, Shan T. Myokines mediate the cross talk between skeletal muscle and other organs. J Cell Physiol. 2021;236(4):2393–412. https://doi.org/10.1002/jcp.30033.
21. Cheng T-C, Huang S-H, Kao C-L, Hsu P-C. Muscle wasting in chronic kidney disease: mechanism and clinical implications-a narrative review. Int J Mol Sci. 2022;23(11):6047. https://doi.org/10.3390/ijms23116047.
22. Cheng Y, Zhang X, Ma F, Sun W, Wang W, Yu J, Shi Y, Cai L, Xu Z. The role of Akt2 in the protective effect of fenofibrate against diabetic nephropathy. Int J Biol Sci. 2020;16(4):553–67. https://doi.org/10.7150/ijbs.40643.

23. Coelho-Junior HJ, Picca A, Calvani R, Uchida MC, Marzetti E. If my muscle could talk: myokines as a biomarker of frailty. Exp Gerontol. 2019;127:110715. https://doi.org/10.1016/j.exger.2019.110715.
24. Colaianni G, Cuscito C, Mongelli T, Pignataro P, Buccoliero C, Liu P, Lu P, Sartini L, Di Comite M, Mori G, Di Benedetto A, Brunetti G, Yuen T, Sun L, Reseland JE, Colucci S, New MI, Zaidi M, Cinti S, Grano M. The myokine irisin increases cortical bone mass. Proc Natl Acad Sci USA. 2015;112(39):12157–62. https://doi.org/10.1073/pnas.1516622112.
25. Connolly K, Lehoux M, O'Rourke R, Assetta B, Erdemir GA, Elias JA, Lee CG, Huang Y-WA. Potential role of chitinase-3-like protein 1 (CHI3L1/YKL-40) in neurodegeneration and Alzheimer's disease. Alzheimers Dement. 2023;19(1):9–24. https://doi.org/10.1002/alz.12612.
26. de Oliveira dos Santos AR, de Oliveira Zanuso B, Miola VFB, Barbalho SM, Santos Bueno PC, Flato UAP, Detregiachi CRP, Buchaim DV, Buchaim RL, Tofano RJ, Mendes CG, Tofano VAC, dos Santos Haber JF. Adipokines, myokines, and hepatokines: crosstalk and metabolic repercussions. Int J Mol Sci. 2021;22(5):2639. https://doi.org/10.3390/ijms22052639.
27. De Paepe B. The cytokine growth differentiation factor-15 and skeletal muscle health: portrait of an emerging widely applicable disease biomarker. Int J Mol Sci. 2022;23(21):13180. https://doi.org/10.3390/ijms232113180.
28. Delezie J, Handschin C. Endocrine crosstalk between skeletal muscle and the brain. Front Neurol. 2018;9:698. https://doi.org/10.3389/fneur.2018.00698.
29. Deng Y, Li G, Chang D, Su X. YKL-40 as a novel biomarker in cardio-metabolic disorders and inflammatory diseases. Clin Chim Acta. 2020;511:40–6. https://doi.org/10.1016/j.cca.2020.09.035.
30. Devocelle A, Lecru L, Ferlicot S, Bessede T, Candelier J-J, Giron-Michel J, François H. IL-15 prevents renal fibrosis by inhibiting collagen synthesis: a new pathway in chronic kidney disease? Int J Mol Sci. 2021;22(21):11698. https://doi.org/10.3390/ijms222111698.
31. Docherty S, Harley R, McAuley JJ, Crowe LAN, Pedret C, Kirwan PD, Siebert S, Millar NL. The effect of exercise on cytokines: implications for musculoskeletal health: a narrative review. BMC Sports Sci Med Rehabil. 2022;14(1):5. https://doi.org/10.1186/s13102-022-00397-2.
32. Donate-Correa J, Martín-Carro B, Cannata-Andía JB, Mora-Fernández C, Navarro-González JF. Klotho, oxidative stress, and mitochondrial damage in kidney disease. Antioxidants (Basel). 2023;12(2):239. https://doi.org/10.3390/antiox12020239.
33. Elliott B, Renshaw D, Getting S, Mackenzie R. The central role of myostatin in skeletal muscle and whole body homeostasis. Acta Physiol (Oxf). 2012;205(3):324–40. https://doi.org/10.1111/j.1748-1716.2012.02423.x.
34. Formenti P, Umbrello M, Coppola S, Froio S, Chiumello D. Clinical review: peripheral muscular ultrasound in the ICU. Ann Intensive Care. 2019;9(1):57. https://doi.org/10.1186/s13613-019-0531-x.
35. Formigari GP, Dátilo MN, Vareda B, Bonfante ILP, Cavaglieri CR, Lopes de Faria JM, Lopes de Faria JB. Renal protection induced by physical exercise may be mediated by the irisin/AMPK axis in diabetic nephropathy. Sci Rep. 2022;12:9062. https://doi.org/10.1038/s41598-022-13054-y.
36. Furuhashi M, Hotamisligil GS. Fatty acid-binding proteins: role in metabolic diseases and potential as drug targets. Nat Rev Drug Discov. 2008;7(6):489–503. https://doi.org/10.1038/nrd2589.
37. Gamas L, Matafome P, Seiça R. Irisin and myonectin regulation in the insulin resistant muscle: implications to adipose tissue: muscle crosstalk. J Diabetes Res. 2015;2015:359159. https://doi.org/10.1155/2015/359159.
38. Gao Y, Arfat Y, Wang H, Goswami N. Muscle atrophy induced by mechanical unloading: mechanisms and potential countermeasures. Front Physiol. 2018;9:235. https://doi.org/10.3389/fphys.2018.00235.

39. Görgens SW, Eckardt K, Jensen J, Drevon CA, Eckel J. Exercise and regulation of adipokine and myokine production. Prog Mol Biol Transl Sci. 2015;135:313–36. https://doi.org/10.1016/bs.pmbts.2015.07.002.
40. Görgens SW, Hjorth M, Eckardt K, Wichert S, Norheim F, Holen T, Lee S, Langleite T, Birkeland KI, Stadheim HK, Kolnes KJ, Tangen DS, Kolnes AJ, Jensen J, Drevon CA, Eckel J. The exercise-regulated myokine chitinase-3-like protein 1 stimulates human myocyte proliferation. Acta Physiol (Oxf). 2016;216(3):330–45. https://doi.org/10.1111/apha.12579.
41. Grunow JJ, Reiher K, Carbon NM, Engelhardt LJ, Mai K, Koch S, Schefold JC, Z'Graggen W, Schaller SJ, Fielitz J, Spranger J, Weber-Carstens S, Wollersheim T. Muscular myostatin gene expression and plasma concentrations are decreased in critically ill patients. Crit Care. 2022;26(1):237. https://doi.org/10.1186/s13054-022-04101-1.
42. Gulcicek S, Seyahi N. Factors associated with sarcopenia in patients with chronic kidney disease: a cross-sectional single-center study. Med Sci Monit. 2023;29:e939457-1–e939457-12. https://doi.org/10.12659/MSM.939457.
43. Haddad F, Zaldivar F, Cooper DM, Adams GR. IL-6-induced skeletal muscle atrophy. J Appl Physiol (1985). 2005;98(3):911–7. https://doi.org/10.1152/japplphysiol.01026.2004.
44. Hale C, Chen MM, Stanislaus S, Chinookoswong N, Hager T, Wang M, Véniant MM, Xu J. Lack of overt FGF21 resistance in two mouse models of obesity and insulin resistance. Endocrinology. 2012;153(1):69–80. https://doi.org/10.1210/en.2010-1262.
45. Herrera-Esparza R, Barbosa-Cisneros O, Villalobos-Hurtado R, Avalos-Díaz E. Renal expression of IL-6 and TNFalpha genes in lupus nephritis. Lupus. 1998;7(3):154–8. https://doi.org/10.1191/096120398678919949.
46. Hittel DS, Axelson M, Sarna N, Shearer J, Huffman KM, Kraus WE. Myostatin decreases with aerobic exercise and associates with insulin resistance. Med Sci Sports Exerc. 2010;42(11):2023–9. https://doi.org/10.1249/MSS.0b013e3181e0b9a8.
47. Huang EJ, Reichardt LF. Neurotrophins: roles in neuronal development and function. Annu Rev Neurosci. 2001;24:677–736. https://doi.org/10.1146/annurev.neuro.24.1.677.
48. Husebø GR, Grønseth R, Lerner L, Gyuris J, Hardie JA, Bakke PS, Eagan TM. Growth differentiation factor-15 is a predictor of important disease outcomes in patients with COPD. Eur Respir J. 2017;49(3):1601298. https://doi.org/10.1183/13993003.01298-2016.
49. Iglesias P, Silvestre RA, Díez JJ. Growth differentiation factor 15 (GDF-15) in endocrinology. Endocrine. 2023. https://doi.org/10.1007/s12020-023-03377-9.
50. Iwano M, Dohi K, Hirata E, Kurumatani N, Horii Y, Shiiki H, Fukatsu A, Matsuda T, Hirano T, Kishimoto T. Urinary levels of IL-6 in patients with active lupus nephritis. Clin Nephrol. 1993;40(1):16–21.
51. Jenkin KA, Perry BD. Skeletal muscle and kidney crosstalk in chronic kidney disease. Cell Physiol Biochem. 2022;56(5):587–601. https://doi.org/10.33594/000000578.
52. Jin Y, Song J, Xu F, Zhang D, He J, Zheng J, Zhang Y, Li J, Guo Y, Xu M, Yu X, Liu Y, Liu Q, Yan J. Association between YKL-40 and asthma: a systematic meta-analysis. Sleep Breath. 2022;26(3):1011–22. https://doi.org/10.1007/s11325-021-02495-w.
53. Johansen KL, Chertow GM, Ng AV, Mulligan K, Carey S, Schoenfeld PY, Kent-Braun JA. Physical activity levels in patients on hemodialysis and healthy sedentary controls. Kidney Int. 2000;57(6):2564–70. https://doi.org/10.1046/j.1523-1755.2000.00116.x.
54. Kang X, Yang M-Y, Shi Y-X, Xie M-M, Zhu M, Zheng X-L, Zhang C-K, Ge Z-L, Bian X-T, Lv J-T, Wang Y-J, Zhou B-H, Tang K-L. Interleukin-15 facilitates muscle regeneration through modulation of fibro/adipogenic progenitors. Cell Commun Signal. 2018;16(1):42. https://doi.org/10.1186/s12964-018-0251-0.
55. Kanzleiter T, Rath M, Görgens SW, Jensen J, Tangen DS, Kolnes AJ, Kolnes KJ, Lee S, Eckel J, Schürmann A, Eckardt K. The myokine decorin is regulated by contraction and involved in muscle hypertrophy. Biochem Biophys Res Commun. 2014;450(2):1089–94. https://doi.org/10.1016/j.bbrc.2014.06.123.
56. Keipert S, Ost M, Johann K, Imber F, Jastroch M, van Schothorst EM, Keijer J, Klaus S. Skeletal muscle mitochondrial uncoupling drives endocrine cross-talk through the induc-

tion of FGF21 as a myokine. Am J Physiol Endocrinol Metab. 2014;306(5):E469–82. https://doi.org/10.1152/ajpendo.00330.2013.

57. Kim DI, Park SH. Sequential signaling cascade of IL-6 and PGC-1α is involved in high glucose-induced podocyte loss and growth arrest. Biochem Biophys Res Commun. 2013;435(4):702–7. https://doi.org/10.1016/j.bbrc.2013.05.046.
58. Kim H, Wrann CD, Jedrychowski M, Vidoni S, Kitase Y, Nagano K, Zhou C, Chou J, Parkman V-JA, Novick SJ, Strutzenberg TS, Pascal BD, Le PT, Brooks DJ, Roche AM, Gerber KK, Mattheis L, Chen W, Tu H, Bouxsein ML, Griffin PR, Baron R, Rosen CJ, Bonewald LF, Spiegelman BM. Irisin mediates effects on bone and fat via αV integrin receptors. Cell. 2018;175(7):1756–1768.e17. https://doi.org/10.1016/j.cell.2018.10.025.
59. Kirk B, Feehan J, Lombardi G, Duque G. Muscle, bone, and fat crosstalk: the biological role of myokines, osteokines, and adipokines. Curr Osteoporos Rep. 2020;18(4):388–400. https://doi.org/10.1007/s11914-020-00599-y.
60. Klein AB, Nicolaisen TS, Ørtenblad N, Gejl KD, Jensen R, Fritzen AM, Larsen EL, Karstoft K, Poulsen HE, Morville T, Sahl RE, Helge JW, Lund J, Falk S, Lyngbæk M, Ellingsgaard H, Pedersen BK, Lu W, Finan B, Jørgensen SB, Seeley RJ, Kleinert M, Kiens B, Richter EA, Clemmensen C. Pharmacological but not physiological GDF15 suppresses feeding and the motivation to exercise. Nat Commun. 2021;12:1041. https://doi.org/10.1038/s41467-021-21309-x.
61. Kruse NT, Buzkova P, Barzilay JI, Valderrabano RJ, Robbins JA, Fink HA, Jalal DI. Association of skeletal muscle mass, kidney disease and mortality in older men and women: the cardiovascular health study. Aging. 2020;12(21):21023–36. https://doi.org/10.18632/aging.202135.
62. Kuo C-P, Tsai M-T, Lee K-H, Lin Y-P, Huang S-S, Huang C-C, Tseng W-C, Tarng D-C. Dose-response effects of physical activity on all-cause mortality and major cardiorenal outcomes in chronic kidney disease. Eur J Prev Cardiol. 2022;29(3):452–61. https://doi.org/10.1093/eurjpc/zwaa162.
63. Latronico N, Herridge M, Hopkins RO, Angus D, Hart N, Hermans G, Iwashyna T, Arabi Y, Citerio G, Ely EW, Hall J, Mehta S, Puntillo K, Van den Hoeven J, Wunsch H, Cook D, Dos Santos C, Rubenfeld G, Vincent J-L, Van den Berghe G, Azoulay E, Needham DM. The ICM research agenda on intensive care unit-acquired weakness. Intensive Care Med. 2017;43(9):1270–81. https://doi.org/10.1007/s00134-017-4757-5.
64. Laucyte-Cibulskiene A, Ward LJ, Ebert T, Tosti G, Tucci C, Hernandez L, Kautzky-Willer A, Herrero M-T, Norris CM, Pilote L, Söderberg M, Brismar TB, Ripsweden J, Stenvinkel P, Raparelli V, Kublickiene K. Role of GDF-15, YKL-40 and MMP 9 in patients with end-stage kidney disease: focus on sex-specific associations with vascular outcomes and all-cause mortality. Biol Sex Differ. 2021;12:50. https://doi.org/10.1186/s13293-021-00393-0.
65. Leal DV, Ferreira A, Watson EL, Wilund KR, Viana JL. Muscle-bone crosstalk in chronic kidney disease: the potential modulatory effects of exercise. Calcif Tissue Int. 2021;108(4):461–75. https://doi.org/10.1007/s00223-020-00782-4.
66. Li B, Syed MH, Khan H, Singh KK, Qadura M. The role of fatty acid binding protein 3 in cardiovascular diseases. Biomedicine. 2022;10(9):2283. https://doi.org/10.3390/biomedicines10092283.
67. Li R, Wang Q-F, Li W-W, Niu X-C. Effect of treating renal failure with decorin gene therapy. Eur Rev Med Pharmacol Sci. 2018;22(8):2483–9. https://doi.org/10.26355/eurrev_201804_14843.
68. Liang H, Ward WF. PGC-1alpha: a key regulator of energy metabolism. Adv Physiol Educ. 2006;30(4):145–51. https://doi.org/10.1152/advan.00052.2006.
69. Liu C, Hu Y, Han Y, Wang Y, Zhang Y, Zhang X, He D, Ren H, Liu Y, Wang H, Tan T, Lin P, Li H, Rovin BH, Ma J, Zeng C. MG53 protects against contrast-induced acute kidney injury by reducing cell membrane damage and apoptosis. Acta Pharmacol Sin. 2020;41(11):1457–64. https://doi.org/10.1038/s41401-020-0420-8.
70. Ma C, Ding H, Deng Y, Liu H, Xiong X, Yang Y. Irisin: a new code uncover the relationship of skeletal muscle and cardiovascular health during exercise. Front Physiol. 2021;12:620608. https://doi.org/10.3389/fphys.2021.620608.

71. Mageswari R, Sridhar MG, Nandeesha H, Parameshwaran S, Vinod KV. Irisin and visfatin predicts severity of diabetic nephropathy. Indian J Clin Biochem. 2019;34(3):342–6. https://doi.org/10.1007/s12291-018-0749-7.
72. Meng F, Cao Y, Khoso MH, Kang K, Ren G, Xiao W, Li D. Therapeutic effect and mechanism of combined use of FGF21 and insulin on diabetic nephropathy. Arch Biochem Biophys. 2021;713:109063. https://doi.org/10.1016/j.abb.2021.109063.
73. Metkus TS, Lindsley J, Fair L, Riley S, Berry S, Sahetya S, Hsu S, Gilotra NA. Quality of heart failure care in the intensive care unit. J Card Fail. 2021;27(10):1111–25. https://doi.org/10.1016/j.cardfail.2021.08.001.
74. Moisey LL, Mourtzakis M, Cotton BA, Premji T, Heyland DK, Wade CE, Bulger E, Kozar RA, for the Nutrition and Rehabilitation Investigators Consortium (NUTRIC). Skeletal muscle predicts ventilator-free days, ICU-free days, and mortality in elderly ICU patients. Crit Care. 2013;17(5):R206. https://doi.org/10.1186/cc12901.
75. Moraes C, Leal VO, Marinho SM, Barroso SG, Rocha GS, Boaventura GT, Mafra D. Resistance exercise training does not affect plasma irisin levels of hemodialysis patients. Horm Metab Res. 2013;45(12):900–4. https://doi.org/10.1055/s-0033-1354402.
76. Nair V, Robinson-Cohen C, Smith MR, Bellovich KA, Bhat ZY, Bobadilla M, Brosius F, de Boer IH, Essioux L, Formentini I, Gadegbeku CA, Gipson D, Hawkins J, Himmelfarb J, Kestenbaum B, Kretzler M, Magnone MC, Perumal K, Steigerwalt S, Ju W, Bansal N. Growth differentiation factor-15 and risk of CKD progression. J Am Soc Nephrol. 2017;28(7):2233–40. https://doi.org/10.1681/ASN.2016080919.
77. Nauta FL, Boertien WE, Bakker SJL, van Goor H, van Oeveren W, de Jong PE, Bilo H, Gansevoort RT. Glomerular and tubular damage markers are elevated in patients with diabetes. Diabetes Care. 2011;34(4):975–81. https://doi.org/10.2337/dc10-1545.
78. Nechemia-Arbely Y, Barkan D, Pizov G, Shriki A, Rose-John S, Galun E, Axelrod JH. IL-6/IL-6R axis plays a critical role in acute kidney injury. J Am Soc Nephrol. 2008;19(6):1106–15. https://doi.org/10.1681/ASN.2007070744.
79. Nielsen AR, Mounier R, Plomgaard P, Mortensen OH, Penkowa M, Speerschneider T, Pilegaard H, Pedersen BK. Expression of interleukin-15 in human skeletal muscle—effect of exercise and muscle fibre type composition. J Physiol. 2007;584(Pt 1):305–12. https://doi.org/10.1113/jphysiol.2007.139618.
80. Ong KL, Rye K-A, O'Connell R, Jenkins AJ, Brown C, Xu A, Sullivan DR, Barter PJ, Keech AC, FIELD study investigators. Long-term fenofibrate therapy increases fibroblast growth factor 21 and retinol-binding protein 4 in subjects with type 2 diabetes. J Clin Endocrinol Metab. 2012;97(12):4701–8. https://doi.org/10.1210/jc.2012-2267.
81. Ozawa S, Ueda S, Li Y, Mori K, Asanuma K, Yanagita M, Nakagawa T. Fatty acid binding protein 3 as a potential mediator for diabetic nephropathy in eNOS deficient mouse. Biochem Biophys Res Commun. 2014;454(4):531–6. https://doi.org/10.1016/j.bbrc.2014.10.121.
82. Pan Y, Wang B, Zheng J, Xiong R, Fan Z, Ye Y, Zhang S, Li Q, Gong F, Wu C, Lin Z, Li X, Pan X. Pancreatic fibroblast growth factor 21 protects against type 2 diabetes in mice by promoting insulin expression and secretion in a PI3K/Akt signaling-dependent manner. J Cell Mol Med. 2019;23(2):1059–71. https://doi.org/10.1111/jcmm.14007.
83. Pang Q, Wang P, Pan Y, Dong X, Zhou T, Song X, Zhang A. Irisin protects against vascular calcification by activating autophagy and inhibiting NLRP3-mediated vascular smooth muscle cell pyroptosis in chronic kidney disease. Cell Death Dis. 2022;13(3):283. https://doi.org/10.1038/s41419-022-04735-7.
84. Peake JM, Della Gatta P, Suzuki K, Nieman DC. Cytokine expression and secretion by skeletal muscle cells: regulatory mechanisms and exercise effects. Exerc Immunol Rev. 2015;21:8–25.
85. Pecoits-Filho R, Heimbürger O, Bárány P, Suliman M, Fehrman-Ekholm I, Lindholm B, Stenvinkel P. Associations between circulating inflammatory markers and residual renal function in CRF patients. Am J Kidney Dis. 2003;41(6):1212–8. https://doi.org/10.1016/s0272-6386(03)00353-6.

86. Pedersen BK. Muscle as a secretory organ. Compr Physiol. 2013;3(3):1337–62. https://doi.org/10.1002/cphy.c120033.
87. Pedersen BK, Åkerström TCA, Nielsen AR, Fischer CP. Role of myokines in exercise and metabolism. J Appl Physiol. 2007;103(3):1093–8. https://doi.org/10.1152/japplphysiol.00080.2007.
88. Pedersen BK, Febbraio MA. Muscle as an endocrine organ: focus on muscle-derived interleukin-6. Physiol Rev. 2008;88(4):1379–406. https://doi.org/10.1152/physrev.90100.2007.
89. Peng H, Wang Q, Lou T, Qin J, Jung S, Shetty V, Li F, Wang Y, Feng X-H, Mitch WE, Graham BH, Hu Z. Myokine mediated muscle-kidney crosstalk suppresses metabolic reprogramming and fibrosis in damaged kidneys. Nat Commun. 2017;8(1):1493. https://doi.org/10.1038/s41467-017-01646-6.
90. Podyma B, Parekh K, Güler AD, Deppmann CD. Metabolic homeostasis via BDNF and its receptors. Trends Endocrinol Metab. 2021;32(7):488–99. https://doi.org/10.1016/j.tem.2021.04.005.
91. Puigserver P, Spiegelman BM. Peroxisome proliferator-activated receptor-gamma coactivator 1 alpha (PGC-1 alpha): transcriptional coactivator and metabolic regulator. Endocr Rev. 2003;24(1):78–90. https://doi.org/10.1210/er.2002-0012.
92. Reza MM, Subramaniyam N, Sim CM, Ge X, Sathiakumar D, McFarlane C, Sharma M, Kambadur R. Irisin is a pro-myogenic factor that induces skeletal muscle hypertrophy and rescues denervation-induced atrophy. Nat Commun. 2017;8(1):1104. https://doi.org/10.1038/s41467-017-01131-0.
93. Ryan AS, Ivey FM, Prior S, Li G, Hafer-Macko C. Skeletal muscle hypertrophy and muscle myostatin reduction after resistive training in stroke survivors. Stroke. 2011;42(2):416–20. https://doi.org/10.1161/STROKEAHA.110.602441.
94. Sadeghi Shad J, Akbari R, Qujeq D, Hajian-Tilaki K. Measurement of serum irisin in the different stages of chronic kidney disease. Caspian J Intern Med. 2019;10(3):314–9. https://doi.org/10.22088/cjim.10.3.314.
95. Sakr Y, Jaschinski U, Wittebole X, Szakmany T, Lipman J, Ñamendys-Silva SA, Martin-Loeches I, Leone M, Lupu M-N, Vincent J-L. Sepsis in intensive care unit patients: worldwide data from the intensive care over nations audit. Open Forum Infect Dis. 2018;5(12):ofy313. https://doi.org/10.1093/ofid/ofy313.
96. Salgado JV, Goes MA, Salgado Filho N. FGF21 and chronic kidney disease. Metabolism. 2021;118:154738. https://doi.org/10.1016/j.metabol.2021.154738.
97. Schaefer L, Macakova K, Raslik I, Micegova M, Gröne H-J, Schönherr E, Robenek H, Echtermeyer FG, Grässel S, Bruckner P, Schaefer RM, Iozzo RV, Kresse H. Absence of decorin adversely influences tubulointerstitial fibrosis of the obstructed kidney by enhanced apoptosis and increased inflammatory reaction. Am J Pathol. 2002;160(3):1181–91. https://doi.org/10.1016/S0002-9440(10)64937-1.
98. Segura-Ortí E, Gordon PL, Doyle JW, Johansen KL. Correlates of physical functioning and performance across the spectrum of kidney function. Clin Nurs Res. 2018;27(5):579–96. https://doi.org/10.1177/1054773816689282.
99. Seldin MM, Wong GW. Regulation of tissue crosstalk by skeletal muscle-derived myonectin and other myokines. Adipocytes. 2012;1(4):200–2. https://doi.org/10.4161/adip.20877.
100. Severinsen MCK, Pedersen BK. Muscle-organ crosstalk: the emerging roles of myokines. Endocr Rev. 2020;41(4):594–609. https://doi.org/10.1210/endrev/bnaa016.
101. Shao M, Yu L, Zhang F, Lu X, Li X, Cheng P, Lin X, He L, Jin S, Tan Y, Yang H, Zhang C, Cai L. Additive protection by LDR and FGF21 treatment against diabetic nephropathy in type 2 diabetes model. Am J Physiol Endocrinol Metab. 2015;309(1):E45–54. https://doi.org/10.1152/ajpendo.00026.2015.
102. Shinozaki M, Hirahashi J, Lebedeva T, Liew FY, Salant DJ, Maron R, Kelley VR. IL-15, a survival factor for kidney epithelial cells, counteracts apoptosis and inflammation during nephritis. J Clin Invest. 2002;109(7):951–60. https://doi.org/10.1172/JCI14574.

103. Smathers RL, Petersen DR. The human fatty acid-binding protein family: evolutionary divergences and functions. Hum Genomics. 2011;5(3):170–91. https://doi.org/10.1186/1479-7364-5-3-170.
104. Staiger H, Keuper M, Berti L, Hrabe de Angelis M, Häring H-U. Fibroblast growth factor 21-metabolic role in mice and men. Endocr Rev. 2017;38(5):468–88. https://doi.org/10.1210/er.2017-00016.
105. Tamouza H, Chemouny JM, Raskova Kafkova L, Berthelot L, Flamant M, Demion M, Mesnard L, Paubelle E, Walker F, Julian BA, Tissandié E, Tiwari MK, Camara NOS, Vrtovsnik F, Benhamou M, Novak J, Monteiro RC, Moura IC. The IgA1 immune complex-mediated activation of the MAPK/ERK kinase pathway in mesangial cells is associated with glomerular damage in IgA nephropathy. Kidney Int. 2012;82(12):1284–96. https://doi.org/10.1038/ki.2012.192.
106. Tanimura Y, Aoi W, Takanami Y, Kawai Y, Mizushima K, Naito Y, Yoshikawa T. Acute exercise increases fibroblast growth factor 21 in metabolic organs and circulation. Physiol Rep. 2016;4(12):e12828. https://doi.org/10.14814/phy2.12828.
107. Tezze C, Romanello V, Sandri M. FGF21 as modulator of metabolism in health and disease. Front Physiol. 2019;10:419. https://doi.org/10.3389/fphys.2019.00419.
108. Tizaoui K, Yang JW, Lee KH, Kim JH, Kim M, Yoon S, Jung Y, Park JB, An K, Choi H, Song D, Jung H, Ahn S, Yuh T, Choi HM, Ahn JH, Kim Y, Jee S, Lee H, Jin S, Kang J-G, Koo B, Lee JY, Min KM, Yoo W, Rhyu HJ, Yoon Y, Lee MH, Kim SE, Hwang J, Koyanagi A, Jacob L, Park S, Shin JI, Smith L. The role of YKL-40 in the pathogenesis of autoimmune diseases: a comprehensive review. Int J Biol Sci. 2022;18(9):3731–46. https://doi.org/10.7150/ijbs.67587.
109. Tonelli M, Wiebe N, Culleton B, House A, Rabbat C, Fok M, McAlister F, Garg AX. Chronic kidney disease and mortality risk: a systematic review. J Am Soc Nephrol. 2006;17(7):2034–47. https://doi.org/10.1681/ASN.2005101085.
110. Van den Berghe G. On the neuroendocrinopathy of critical illness. Perspectives for feeding and novel treatments. Am J Respir Crit Care Med. 2016;194(11):1337–48. https://doi.org/10.1164/rccm.201607-1516CI.
111. Vanhorebeek I, Gunst J, Casaer MP, Derese I, Derde S, Pauwels L, Segers J, Hermans G, Gosselink R, Van den Berghe G. Skeletal muscle myokine expression in critical illness, association with outcome and impact of therapeutic interventions. J Endocr Soc. 2023;7(3):bvad001. https://doi.org/10.1210/jendso/bvad001.
112. Vanhorebeek I, Latronico N, Van den Berghe G. ICU-acquired weakness. Intensive Care Med. 2020;46(4):637–53. https://doi.org/10.1007/s00134-020-05944-4.
113. Velingkar A, Vuree S, Prabhakar PK, Kalashikam RR, Banerjee A, Kondeti S. Fibroblast growth factor 21 as a potential master regulator in metabolic disorders. Am J Physiol Endocrinol Metab. 2023;324(5):E409–24. https://doi.org/10.1152/ajpendo.00244.2022.
114. Vu TT, Marquez J, Le LT, Nguyen ATT, Kim HK, Han J. The role of decorin in cardiovascular diseases: more than just a decoration. Free Radic Res. 2018;52(11–12):1210–9. https://doi.org/10.1080/10715762.2018.1516285.
115. Wan Y, Fu J. GDF15 as a key disease target and biomarker: linking chronic lung diseases and ageing. Mol Cell Biochem. 2023:1–14. https://doi.org/10.1007/s11010-023-04743-x.
116. Wang R, Liu H. Association between serum irisin and diabetic nephropathy in patients with type 2 diabetes mellitus: a meta-analysis. Horm Metab Res. 2021;53(5):293–300. https://doi.org/10.1055/a-1475-4444.
117. Wang Y, Liu H, Sun N, Li J, Peng X, Jia Y, Karch J, Yu B, Wehrens XHT, Tian J. Irisin: a promising target for ischemia-reperfusion injury therapy. Oxidative Med Cell Longev. 2021;2021:5391706. https://doi.org/10.1155/2021/5391706.
118. Wei S, Bi J, Yang L, Zhang J, Wan Y, Chen X, Wang Y, Wu Z, Lv Y, Wu R. Serum irisin levels are decreased in patients with sepsis, and exogenous irisin suppresses ferroptosis in the liver of septic mice. Clin Transl Med. 2020;10(5):e173. https://doi.org/10.1002/ctm2.173.
119. Wen M-S, Wang C-Y, Lin S-L, Hung K-C. Decrease in irisin in patients with chronic kidney disease. PLoS One. 2013;8(5):e64025. https://doi.org/10.1371/journal.pone.0064025.

120. Winkelman C, Johnson KD, Gordon N. Associations between muscle-related cytokines and selected patient outcomes in the ICU. Biol Res Nurs. 2015;17(2):125–34. https://doi.org/10.1177/1099800414532709.
121. Wischhusen J, Melero I, Fridman WH. Growth/differentiation factor-15 (GDF-15): from biomarker to novel targetable immune checkpoint. Front Immunol. 2020;11:951. https://doi.org/10.3389/fimmu.2020.00951.
122. Woodhouse L, Gandhi R, Warden SJ, Poiraudeau S, Myers SL, Benson CT, Hu L, Ahmad QI, Linnemeier P, Gomez EV, Benichou O, Study Investigators. A phase 2 randomized study investigating the efficacy and safety of myostatin antibody LY2495655 versus placebo in patients undergoing elective Total hip arthroplasty. J Frailty Aging. 2016;5(1):62–70. https://doi.org/10.14283/jfa.2016.81.
123. Yano N, Zhao YT, Zhao TC. The physiological role of irisin in the regulation of muscle glucose homeostasis. Endocrine. 2021;2(3):266–83. https://doi.org/10.3390/endocrines2030025.
124. Yu T-H, Hsuan C-F, Wu C-C, Hung W-C, Lee T-L, Tsai I-T, Wei C-T, Houng J-Y, Chung F-M, Lee Y-J, Lu Y-C. Association of plasma fatty acid-binding protein 3 with estimated glomerular filtration rate in patients with type 2 diabetes mellitus. Int J Med Sci. 2022;19(1):82–8. https://doi.org/10.7150/ijms.66876.
125. Zanders L, Kny M, Hahn A, Schmidt S, Wundersitz S, Todiras M, Lahmann I, Bandyopadhyay A, Wollersheim T, Kaderali L, Luft FC, Birchmeier C, Weber-Carstens S, Fielitz J. Sepsis induces interleukin 6, gp130/JAK2/STAT3, and muscle wasting. J Cachexia Sarcopenia Muscle. 2022;13(1):713–27. https://doi.org/10.1002/jcsm.12867.
126. Zhang J, Bi J, Ren Y, Du Z, Li T, Wang T, Zhang L, Wang M, Wei S, Lv Y, Wu R. Involvement of GPX4 in irisin's protection against ischemia reperfusion-induced acute kidney injury. J Cell Physiol. 2021;236(2):931–45. https://doi.org/10.1002/jcp.29903.
127. Zhang J, Cheng Y, Gu J, Wang S, Zhou S, Wang Y, Tan Y, Feng W, Fu Y, Mellen N, Cheng R, Ma J, Zhang C, Li Z, Cai L. Fenofibrate increases cardiac autophagy via FGF21/SIRT1 and prevents fibrosis and inflammation in the hearts of Type 1 diabetic mice. Clin Sci (Lond). 2016;130(8):625–41. https://doi.org/10.1042/CS20150623.
128. Zhang Y, Li R, Meng Y, Li S, Donelan W, Zhao Y, Qi L, Zhang M, Wang X, Cui T, Yang L-J, Tang D. Irisin stimulates browning of white adipocytes through mitogen-activated protein kinase p38 MAP kinase and ERK MAP kinase signaling. Diabetes. 2014;63(2):514–25. https://doi.org/10.2337/db13-1106.
129. Zhao T, Su Z, Li Y, Zhang X, You Q. Chitinase-3 like-protein-1 function and its role in diseases. Signal Transduct Target Ther. 2020;5(1):201. https://doi.org/10.1038/s41392-020-00303-7.
130. Zhou S, Cheing GLY, Cheung AKK. Role of exosomes and exosomal microRNA in muscle-kidney crosstalk in chronic kidney disease. Front Cell Dev Biol. 2022;10:951837. https://doi.org/10.3389/fcell.2022.951837.
131. Zhou Y, Hellberg M, Hellmark T, Höglund P, Clyne N. Muscle mass and plasma myostatin after exercise training: a substudy of Renal Exercise (RENEXC)-a randomized controlled trial. Nephrol Dial Transplant. 2021;36(1):95–103. https://doi.org/10.1093/ndt/gfz210.
132. Zhu C, Hu DL, Liu YQ, Zhang QJ, Chen FK, Kong XQ, Cao KJ, Zhang JS, Qian LM. Fabp3 inhibits proliferation and promotes apoptosis of embryonic myocardial cells. Cell Biochem Biophys. 2011;60(3):259–66. https://doi.org/10.1007/s12013-010-9148-2.
133. Zhuang L, Mao Y, Liu Z, Li C, Jin Q, Lu L, Tao R, Yan X, Chen K. FABP3 deficiency exacerbates metabolic derangement in cardiac hypertrophy and heart failure via PPARα pathway. Front Cardiovasc Med. 2021;8:722908. https://doi.org/10.3389/fcvm.2021.722908.

Renal Disease and Neural Circuits: Brain-Kidney Crosstalk

15

Lilia Rizo-Topete, Gonzalo Ramírez-Guerrero, and Cristian Pedreros-Rosales

15.1 Introduction

The kidneys and brain maintain a dynamic interplay, where disruptions in renal function can lead to neurological complications and vice versa. The brain-kidney axis involves complex interactions between the autonomic nervous system, inflammatory mediators, and the hypothalamic-pituitary-adrenal (HPA) axis. In critical care settings, AKI frequently coexists with ABI, exacerbating systemic and organ-specific damage. Despite growing recognition of this interplay, the underlying mechanisms remain incompletely understood, necessitating further research into the neurophysiological and molecular links between these organ systems.

15.2 Epidemiology of Neurological Disorders in Patients with Impaired Kidney Function

Epidemiological evidence indicates a strong correlation between reduced renal function and an elevated risk of cerebrovascular disease. Specifically, an estimated glomerular filtration rate (eGFR) below 60 mL/min/1.73 m^2 has been associated

L. Rizo-Topete (✉)
Department of Nephrology, Hospital Universitario "José Eleuterio González", Universidad Autónoma de Nuevo León, Monterrey, Nuevo León un, Mexico

G. Ramírez-Guerrero
Nephrology Service, Hospital Las Higueras, Talcahuano, Chile

C. Pedreros-Rosales
Nephrology Service, Hospital Las Higueras, Talcahuano, Chile

Departamento de Medicina Interna, Facultad de Medicina, Universidad de Concepción, Concepción, Chile

D. Battaglini et al. (eds.), *Organ System Crosstalk in Critical Illness*,
https://doi.org/10.1007/978-3-032-01024-7_15

with a higher likelihood of both ischemic and hemorrhagic strokes, whether fatal or non-fatal, in the general population. Notably, this risk increases progressively as eGFR declines and is further exacerbated in the presence of albuminuria [1, 2].

Moreover, chronic kidney disease (CKD) has been linked to an increased prevalence of cognitive impairment, particularly affecting executive functions. The prevalence of cognitive dysfunction among CKD patients ranges from 30% to 60%, with a reported 11% rise in cognitive impairment for every 10 mL/min/1.73 m^2 reduction in eGFR [3–5]. Some studies suggest that hemodialysis may temporarily enhance cognitive performance, possibly due to the clearance of uremic toxins [6].

In addition to cerebrovascular and cognitive consequences, declining eGFR has been associated with movement disorders, particularly Parkinson's disease. Independent risk factors for Parkinson's include both reduced eGFR and proteinuria, with an adjusted hazard ratio (HR) of 1.74 (95% CI: 1.32–1.63) for individuals with an eGFR below 30 mL/min/1.73 m^2. This relationship is likely driven by shared pathophysiological mechanisms, including oxidative stress, accumulation of protein-bound uremic toxins, and hypertension [7–10].

Beyond CKD, AKI is a significant concern in neurocritical patients. Non-neurological complications, including AKI, are independent predictors of worse clinical outcomes, increasing morbidity, mortality, and the risk of prolonged hospitalization [11–13]. AKI is highly prevalent in neurocritical care, with an incidence ranging from 8% to 43%, depending on the definitions used and the specific neurological condition. Reported AKI rates in neurocritical patients vary by pathology, with 9.2% in traumatic brain injury (TBI), 14.5–20.9% in acute ischemic stroke (AIS), 19–59.8% in intracerebral hemorrhage (ICH), and 12–43.3% in subarachnoid hemorrhage (SAH). Furthermore, severe AKI (KDIGO stage 3), requiring renal replacement therapy (RRT), occurs in 3–12% of neurocritical patients, significantly worsening prognosis [11, 13–23].

The brain-kidney connection plays a pivotal role in AKI development among neurocritical patients. AKI is not merely a localized renal disorder but a systemic condition that influences and is influenced by the central nervous system. The presence of AKI in neurocritical patients has far-reaching clinical consequences. It increases the risk of cerebral edema, prolonged mechanical ventilation, and in-hospital mortality [13]. In one cohort study, AKI was identified as an independent predictor of mortality, with a 40% death rate among AKI patients compared to 14.5% in those without AKI [11, 13].

Understanding the intricate brain-kidney connection is essential, as it highlights the bidirectional impact of renal dysfunction on neurological outcomes and vice versa. A comprehensive, multidisciplinary approach that acknowledges this interplay is crucial to improving renal and neurological prognoses in critically ill patients.

15.3 The Kidney and the Brain Interactions

15.3.1 Neural Regulation of Renal Function

The autonomic nervous system (ANS) plays a pivotal role in kidney homeostasis. Sympathetic overactivation, commonly observed in AKI and CKD, contributes to hypertension, endothelial dysfunction, and progression of renal injury. Renal afferent nerves relay information to central autonomic centers, modulating renal blood flow and sodium handling. Dysregulation of this neural feedback loop can promote maladaptive responses, exacerbating renal and cerebrovascular pathology.

ABI can disrupt the blood-brain barrier, leading to metabolic and inflammatory disorders that can worsen AKI. Conversely, AKI can exacerbate intracranial hypertension and cerebral edema [12]. Systemic inflammation after ABI can cause functional alterations and apoptosis in renal tubular cells, potentially leading to subclinical AKI [24]. AKI can also cause an increase in proinflammatory cytokines that reduce cerebral blood flow and contribute to brain edema [25, 26] (Fig. 15.1).

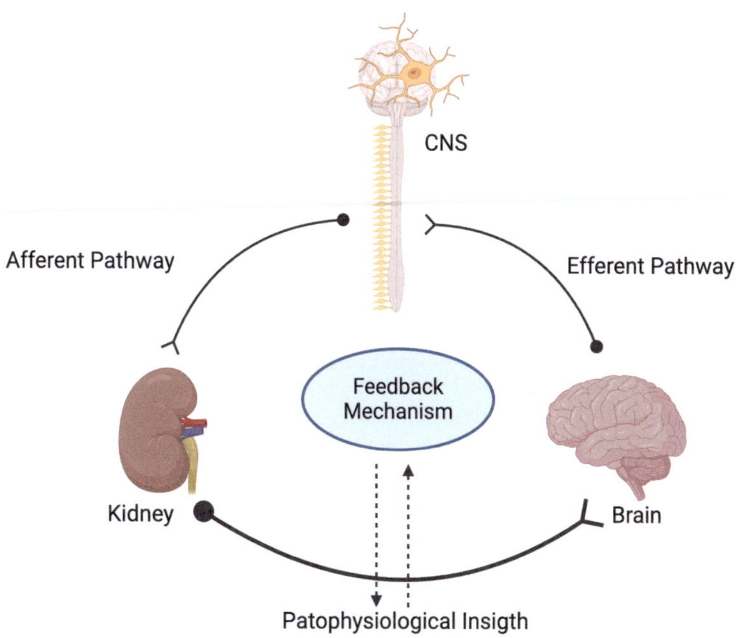

Fig. 15.1 Flowchart of brain-kidney crosstalk

15.4 Efferent Pathways (Brain to Kidney)

Sympathetic Nervous System Efferent fibers originating from the intermediolateral cell column of the spinal cord (T10–L2 levels) project to the kidneys, where the release of norepinephrine affects renal blood vessels, tubular cells, and juxtaglomerular apparatus, influencing renal blood flow, sodium reabsorption, and renin release.

Parasympathetic Nervous System Although less prominent, the parasympathetic innervation via the vagus nerve modulates certain aspects of renal function.

15.5 Afferent Pathways (Kidney to Brain)

Sensory Afferent Nerves Renal sensory nerves transmit information from mechanoreceptors and chemoreceptors in the kidneys to the CNS via the dorsal root ganglia and spinal cord. These signals inform the brain about renal status, contributing to reflex regulation of renal function and blood pressure.

Feedback Mechanisms CNS adjusts renal function based on afferent input, maintaining homeostasis. Dysregulation in these pathways can lead to conditions such as hypertension, acute kidney injury, or contribute to neurogenic inflammation.

15.6 Neuroinflammation and Blood-Brain Barrier Disruption in Kidney Disease

Systemic inflammation and uremic toxins in CKD and AKI contribute to blood-brain barrier (BBB) disruption, facilitating neuroinflammation and cognitive dysfunction. Elevated levels of proinflammatory cytokines, such as IL-6 and TNF-α, have been implicated in both renal and neural injury. Moreover, oxidative stress and endothelial dysfunction further potentiate the neurovascular damage observed in patients with kidney disease [27–33].

15.7 Brain Injury-Induced Renal Dysfunction

Acute neurological insults, including ischemic stroke, TBI, and SAH, often precipitate renal dysfunction. Mechanisms include sympathetic nervous system overactivation, release of damage-associated molecular patterns (DAMPs), and dysregulation of fluid balance. Understanding these pathways is essential for preventing secondary organ dysfunction in neurocritical care. Recent studies have highlighted the incidence of AKI in neurocritical patients and its association with worse clinical outcomes, emphasizing the need for vigilant monitoring and early intervention in this population [11–13].

A common example is stroke, a major neurological disorder and leading cause of disability and death, which often inflicts damage to the kidneys. Changes in GFR, urine output, and biomarkers such as creatinine and albuminuria can occur. In 2018, the incidence rates reported were 9.61% and 11.6%, respectively, for AKI following stroke [20, 34, 35].

15.8 Neuroinflammation and Blood-Brain Barrier Disruption in Kidney Disease

The interplay between kidney dysfunction and neurological impairment is increasingly recognized as a crucial determinant of clinical outcomes. AKI and CKD are both associated with systemic inflammation, oxidative stress, and neuroinflammatory processes that lead to blood-brain barrier (BBB) disruption and neuronal injury. This bidirectional relationship, commonly referred to as the brain-kidney axis, has been extensively investigated in both clinical and preclinical studies [11, 12, 26].

15.9 Molecular Mechanisms of Neuroinflammation in Kidney Disease

At the molecular level, AKI triggers a systemic inflammatory cascade characterized by elevated levels of proinflammatory cytokines, oxidative stress mediators, and endothelial dysfunction. Experimental models have demonstrated that AKI leads to increased serum concentrations of tumor necrosis factor-alpha (TNF-α), interleukin-6 (IL-6), interleukin-1β (IL-1β), and monocyte chemoattractant protein-1 (MCP-1), which contribute to both systemic and central nervous system (CNS) inflammation. These cytokines enhance microglial activation, disrupt astrocytic function, and compromise BBB integrity, leading to increased permeability and neuronal damage [11, 12, 26].

Murine models of ischemia-reperfusion injury (IRI)-induced AKI have shown significant upregulation of matrix metalloproteinase-9 (MMP-9), an enzyme responsible for the degradation of tight junction proteins within the BBB. Increased MMP-9 activity leads to vascular leakage, infiltration of peripheral immune cells into the brain parenchyma, and heightened neuroinflammation [25, 36–40]. Additionally, aquaporin-4 (AQP4), a key regulator of water transport in the brain, is upregulated following AKI, exacerbating vasogenic cerebral edema [41].

Beyond AKI, CKD-related uremic toxins, such as indoxyl sulfate, p-cresyl sulfate, and guanidino compounds, have been implicated in microglial activation and neuronal apoptosis. These toxins disrupt mitochondrial function, leading to excessive production of reactive oxygen species (ROS), which further damages endothelial cells and promotes neuroinflammation [27, 42].

15.10 Neurotransmitter Alterations and Cognitive Dysfunction

Kidney disease disrupts the delicate balance of neurotransmitter homeostasis, which plays a fundamental role in cognitive function and neuronal signaling. Animal models of AKI have shown altered expression of the sodium-independent cationic amino acid transporter (CAT1/SLC7A1), which regulates the influx of L-arginine and other amino acids essential for neurotransmitter synthesis. Dysregulation of this system leads to decreased levels of taurine, glycine, and creatine, all of which are critical for synaptic plasticity and neuronal metabolism [11, 12, 43].

Furthermore, AKI and CKD induce excessive glutamate accumulation, resulting in excitotoxicity—a key driver of neuronal death in neurodegenerative diseases. Experimental evidence suggests that metabolic acidosis secondary to kidney dysfunction impairs astrocytic glutamate uptake, leading to increased synaptic glutamate concentrations and overstimulation of N-methyl-D-aspartate receptors. This process contributes to neuronal calcium overload, oxidative stress, and ultimately, cell death [44, 45].

Neurotransmitter imbalances in kidney disease also extend to dopaminergic dysfunction. A rat model of AKI demonstrated reduced dopamine turnover in the striatum, mesencephalon, and hypothalamus, correlating with impaired motor function and cognitive deficits. This finding aligns with clinical observations showing a higher prevalence of Parkinson's disease in patients with advanced CKD [46, 47].

15.11 Murine Studies on the Brain-Kidney Axis

Rodent models have provided compelling evidence of the direct effects of kidney disease on brain structure and function. Studies using bilateral renal ischemia-reperfusion injury (IRI) models have consistently shown increased BBB permeability, neuronal apoptosis, and neuroinflammation. Notably, microglial activation in the hippocampus and prefrontal cortex has been observed within 24 hours of AKI onset, suggesting that kidney injury rapidly triggers a neuroinflammatory response [25].

In addition, a study using Evans blue dye extravasation to assess BBB integrity found significant leakage in AKI mice, indicating loss of endothelial tight junction integrity. This breakdown of the BBB facilitates the entry of systemic inflammatory mediators and circulating uremic toxins into the CNS, exacerbating neuronal injury [25].

15.12 Causes of Neuroinflammation and BBB Disruption in Kidney Disease

Several factors contribute to neuroinflammation and BBB dysfunction in the context of kidney disease, including [11, 12]:

1. Systemic Inflammation—AKI induces a cytokine storm that exacerbates neuroinflammation and endothelial dysfunction.
2. Oxidative Stress—Increased production of reactive oxygen species damages neurons and disrupts BBB integrity.
3. Uremic Toxins—Indoxyl sulfate, p-cresyl sulfate, and advanced glycation end-products (AGEs) promote neuroinflammation and neurodegeneration.
4. Sympathetic Overactivation—AKI triggers excessive sympathetic nervous system activation, leading to hypertension, cerebrovascular dysregulation, and neuronal injury.
5. Dysregulated Autoregulation—The brain and kidney share similar vascular autoregulatory mechanisms; dysfunction in one organ often leads to parallel impairments in the other.

15.13 Polyuric Syndromes and Augmented Renal Clearance in Brain-Kidney Connection

15.13.1 Polyuria and the Brain-Kidney Crosstalk

Polyuria is a frequent manifestation of brain-kidney crosstalk, reflecting the intricate interplay between the central nervous system and renal function, particularly in critically ill patients. In neurocritical conditions such as TBI, SAH, and AIS, disturbances in autonomic regulation, inflammatory signaling, and neurohormonal control profoundly impact renal function, leading to excessive urine output [48, 49].

15.13.2 Epidemiology of Polyuria in Neurocritical Patients

Polyuria is highly prevalent in neurocritical care settings, with a reported incidence of 50% in patients with acute neurological injury, according to a retrospective cohort study by Ramírez-Guerrero et al. [49]. The prevalence varies depending on the underlying neurological disorder, with higher rates in patients with TBI and SAH, where increased sympathetic activation and augmented renal clearance (ARC) play a key role. Polyuria was particularly frequent in patients with an ARTIC score ≥ 6, a validated tool for predicting ARC, suggesting that younger neurocritical patients with preserved renal reserve are at increased risk of excessive urine output. Additionally, hypernatremia was observed in 40.9% of patients, while hyponatremia occurred in 16.9%, emphasizing the clinical significance of fluid and electrolyte management in neurocritical care [48].

The study also highlighted that polyuria correlates with a lower incidence of AKI and reduced short-term mortality, possibly due to enhanced renal clearance in these patients. However, the long-term impact of persistent polyuria on cerebral perfusion, neurological recovery, and overall patient prognosis remains an area of active investigation [48].

15.13.3 Pathophysiology of Polyuria in Brain-Kidney Crosstalk

One of the key mechanisms underlying polyuria in brain-injured patients is the dysregulation of the hypothalamic-pituitary axis, which disrupts antidiuretic hormone (ADH) secretion. This imbalance can manifest as central diabetes insipidus (CDI), characterized by inadequate ADH release and subsequent failure of the kidneys to concentrate urine, resulting in profound water loss and hypernatremia [49]. Additionally, excessive sympathetic nervous system activation in response to neurological injury can lead to augmented renal clearance (ARC), further exacerbating polyuria by increasing GFR and renal blood flow [48].

Another contributor to polyuria within the brain-kidney axis is osmotic diuresis, which occurs due to increased solute excretion, particularly in states of uremic toxin accumulation, hypernatremia, or mannitol administration for cerebral edema management. The excessive renal elimination of osmotically active substances results in high urine output, perpetuating intravascular volume depletion and worsening neurological outcomes by compromising cerebral perfusion [48, 49].

15.13.4 Augmented Renal Clearance and the Brain-Kidney Crosstalk

Augmented renal clearance (ARC) represents a key component of the brain-kidney connection, particularly in neurocritical patients. This phenomenon, characterized by supraphysiologic renal filtration rates exceeding 130 mL/min/1.73 m^2, is frequently observed in patients with acute brain injuries. The pathophysiology of ARC is multifactorial, involving hyperdynamic circulation, increased cardiac output, systemic inflammatory response syndrome (SIRS), and neurohormonal activation. The sympathetic nervous system plays a pivotal role, as acute neurological injury induces excessive sympathetic drive, leading to vasodilation of renal afferent arterioles and enhanced glomerular filtration. Furthermore, neuroendocrine alterations, including increased levels of natriuretic peptides and suppressed arginine vasopressin (AVP), contribute to excessive diuresis and renal hyperfiltration. While ARC has been associated with reduced rates of AKI and lower mortality, its presence complicates pharmacokinetic dosing, leading to subtherapeutic antibiotic and antiepileptic drug levels, thereby influencing clinical outcomes. Recognizing ARC as part of the brain-kidney axis is essential for optimizing treatment strategies in neurocritical care [48].

15.14 Therapeutic Implications and RRT Management

Targeting brain-kidney crosstalk offers a promising avenue for therapeutic intervention. Strategies such as autonomic modulation, anti-inflammatory treatments, and endothelial protection may mitigate the deleterious effects of AKI and ABI. Continuous renal replacement therapy (CRRT) has evolved significantly, providing not only renal support but also aiding in the management of fluid balance and removal of inflammatory mediators in critically ill patients.

These patients are at risk for cerebral edema, elevated intracranial pressure, and cerebral ischemia due to breakdown of the blood-brain barrier and disrupted cerebral blood flow. These issues can be worsened by conventional hemodialysis, hence the preference for CRRT.

CRRT includes several modalities: continuous slow ultrafiltration (SCUF), continuous venovenous hemofiltration (CVVH), continuous venovenous hemodialysis (CVVHD), and continuous venovenous hemodiafiltration (CVVHDF) [12]. CVVH is often favored for ABI patients because it provides better hemodynamic stability and reduces the risk of cerebral edema [11, 26]. This is based on convection, which is more efficient at clearing larger molecular weight substances like cytokines. At the same time, CVVHD relies on diffusion and is better at clearing smaller substances [11, 26].

Optimal control of variables such as the timing of initiation, prescribed dose, composition of replacement fluid, and anticoagulation is important for neurocritical patients with AKI [11, 12]. The Kidney Disease Improving Global Outcomes (KDIGO) group recommends an effluent flow of 20–25 ml/kg/h, but a dose of 30–35 ml/kg/h is suggested to account for circuit pauses [12]. The delivered dose is affected by blood flow, treatment time, circuit preservation via anticoagulation, and the location of replacement fluid [12, 26, 50].

Anticoagulation is crucial for CRRT to prevent circuit clotting, but it needs careful consideration in ABI patients due to the risk of bleeding [12, 34]. Regional citrate anticoagulation (RCA) is recommended over other methods, especially in patients with a high bleeding risk [11, 12]. Citrate chelates divalent ions, inhibiting the coagulation cascade. Trisodium citrate is commonly used, and the objective is to achieve an ionic calcium concentration <0.4 mmol/L15. However, citrate can cause acid-base and electrolyte imbalances [11, 12].

The composition of replacement fluid is important to avoid complications. Acetate-free solutions are recommended for rapid control of metabolic acidosis. Sodium balance is critical in neurocritical patients, and supraphysiologic sodium concentrations may be used to prevent increases in intracranial pressure, although commercial replacement solutions are lower in sodium [11]. In patients with hyponatremia, the increase in serum sodium should be gradual [11, 12]. The calcium concentration in the replacement solution is also important, especially when using RCA [12].

There is no consensus on the optimal timing to initiate CRRT, especially in ABI patients. Some studies suggest early initiation to ameliorate the osmotic effect of cytokines, but more research is needed.

15.15 Conclusion

The interplay between the kidneys and brain is a critical yet understudied aspect of critical illness. Disruptions in this axis contribute to poor clinical outcomes in patients with AKI, CKD, and neurological disorders. A deeper understanding of brain-kidney interactions is essential for advancing neuroprotective and renoprotective strategies in critically ill patients.

In conclusion, there is a delicate balance required when managing patients with both ABI and AKI. CVVH is the preferred CRRT modality due to its hemodynamic stability and benefits in mitigating cerebral edema. However, individualized therapy with careful consideration of timing, dose, fluid composition, and anticoagulation is essential for optimizing patient outcome.

Future research should focus on elucidating the precise molecular interactions between renal and neural circuits to develop targeted therapies.

References

1. Holzmann MJ, Aastveit A, Hammar N, et al. Renal dysfunction increases the risk of ischemic and hemorrhagic stroke in the general population. Ann Med. 2012;44:607–15.
2. Masson P, Webster AC, Hong M, et al. Chronic kidney disease and the risk of stroke: a systematic review and meta-analysis. Nephrol Dial Transplant. 2015;30:1162–9.
3. Bugnicourt JM, Godefroy O, Chillon JM, et al. Cognitive disorders and dementia in CKD: the neglected kidney-brain axis. J Am Soc Nephrol. 2013;24:353–63.
4. Puy L, Bugnicourt JM, Liabeuf S, et al. Cognitive impairments and dysexecutive behavioral disorders in chronic kidney disease. J Neuropsychiatry Clin Neurosci. 2018;30:310–7.
5. Kurella Tamura M, Wadley V, Yaffe K, et al. Kidney function and cognitive impairment in US adults: the Reasons for Geographic and Racial Differences in Stroke (REGARDS) Study. Am J Kidney Dis. 2008;52:227–34.
6. Schneider SM, Malecki AK, Muller K, et al. Effect of a single dialysis session on cognitive function in CKD5D patients: a prospective clinical study. Nephrol Dial Transplant. 2015;30:1551–9.
7. Nam GE, Kim NH, Han K, et al. Chronic renal dysfunction, proteinuria, and risk of Parkinson's disease in the elderly. Mov Disord. 2019;34:1184–91.
8. Wang IK, Lin CL, Wu YY, et al. Increased risk of Parkinson's disease in patients with end-stage renal disease: a retrospective cohort study. Neuroepidemiology. 2014;42:204–10.
9. Rojas A, Lindner C, Schneider I, Gonzalez I, Uribarri J. The RAGE axis: a relevant inflammatory hub in human diseases. Biomolecules. 2024;14:412.
10. Meléndez-Flores JD, Estrada-Bellmann I. Linking chronic kidney disease and Parkinson's disease: a literature review. Metab Brain Dis. 2021;36:1–12.
11. Ramírez-Guerrero G, Baghetti-Hernández R, Ronco C. Acute kidney injury at the neurocritical care unit. Neurocrit Care. 2022;36(2):640–9. https://doi.org/10.1007/s12028-021-01345-7.
12. Husain-Syed F, Takeuchi T, Neyra JA, et al. Acute kidney injury in neurocritical care. Crit Care. 2023;27(1):341. https://doi.org/10.1186/s13054-023-04632-1.
13. Ramírez-Guerrero G, Lucero C, Villagrán-Cortés F, et al. Acute kidney injury in neurocritical patients: a retrospective cohort study. Int Urol Nephrol. 2023;55(7):1875–83. https://doi.org/10.1007/s11255-023-03502-7.
14. Tsagalis G. Renal dysfunction in acute stroke: an independent predictor of long-term all combined vascular events and overall mortality. Nephrol Dial Transplant. 2009;24(1):194–200.

15. Corral L. Impact of non-neurological complications in severe traumatic brain injury outcome. Crit Care. 2012;16(2):R44.
16. Zacharia BE. Renal dysfunction as an independent predictor of outcome after aneurysmal subarachnoid hemorrhage: a single-center cohort study. Stroke. 2009;40(7):2375–81.
17. Moore EM, Bellomo R, Nichol A, Harley N, Macisaac C, Cooper DJ. The incidence of acute kidney injury in patients with traumatic brain injury. Ren Fail. 2010;32(9):1060–5.
18. Covic A, Schiller A, Mardare NG, et al. The impact of acute kidney injury on short-term survival in an Eastern European population with stroke. Nephrol Dial Transplant. 2008;23(7):2228–34.
19. Buttner S, Stadler A, Mayer C, et al. Incidence, risk factors, and outcome of acute kidney injury in neurocritical care. J Intensive Care Med. 2020;35(4):338–46.
20. Zorrilla-Vaca A, Ziai W, Sander E, Geocadin R, Thompson R, Rivera-lara L. Acute kidney injury following acute ischemic stroke and intracerebral hemorrhage: a meta-analysis of prevalence rate and mortality risk. Cerebrovasc Dis. 2017;45:1–9.
21. Tujjar O, Belloni I, Hougardy JM, et al. Acute kidney injury after subarachnoid hemorrhage. J Neurosurg Anesthesiol. 2017;29(2):140–9.
22. Wang D, Guo Y, Zhang Y, Li Z, Li A, Luo Y. Epidemiology of acute kidney injury in patients with stroke: a retrospective analysis from the neurology ICU. Intern Emerg Med. 2018;13(1):17–25.
23. Li N, Zhao WG, Zhang WF. Acute kidney injury in patients with severe traumatic brain injury: implementation of the acute kidney injury network stage system. Neurocrit Care. 2011;14:377–81.
24. Civiletti F, Assenzio B, Mazzeo AT, et al. Acute tubular injury is associated with severe traumatic brain injury: in vitro study on human tubular epithelial cells. Sci Rep. 2019;9(1):6090.
25. Liu M, Liang Y, Chigurupati S, et al. Acute kidney injury leads to inflammation and functional changes in the brain. J Am Soc Nephrol. 2008;19(7):1360–70.
26. Ramírez-Guerrero G, Reis T, Husain-Syed F, Zanella M, Ronco C. Oliguria, acute kidney injury, and principles of blood purification. In: Mahanna Gabrielli E, et al., editors. Textbook of neurointensive care: volume 1. Cham: Springer; 2024. https://doi.org/10.1007/978-3-031-62220-5_14.
27. Bobot M, Thomas L, Moyon, Fernandez S, McKay N, Balasse L, et al. Uremic toxic blood-brain barrier disruption mediated by AhR activation leads to cognitive impairment during experimental renal dysfunction. J Am Soc Nephrol. 2020;31(7):1509–21.
28. Bobot M, Guedj E, Ressenguier N, Faraut J, Garrigue P, Nail V, et al. Increased blood-brain barrier permeability and cognitive impairment in patients with end-stage kidney disease. Kidney Int Rep. 2024;9(10):2988–95.
29. Banks WA, Lynch JL, Price TO. Cytokines and the blood-brain barrier. In: Siegel A, Zalcmann SS, editors. The neuroimmunological basis of behavior and mental disorders. Boston: Springer, US. 2009; p. 3–17.
30. Disdier C, Chalansonnet M, Gagnaire F, et al. Brain inflammation, blood brain barrier dysfunction and neuronal synaptophysin decrease after inhalation exposure to titanium dioxide nano-aerosol in aging rats. Sci Rep. 2017;7(1):12196.
31. Koyama Y, Sun Y, Shimada S. Inflammation from peripheral organs to the brain: how does systemic inflammation cause neuroinflammation? Front Aging Neurosci. 2022;14:903455.
32. Dias-Carvalho A, Sa SI, Carvalho F, Fernandes E, Costa VM. Inflammation as common link to progressive neurological diseases. Arch Toxicol. 2024;98(1):95–119.
33. Xue Y, Zeng X, Tu WJ, Zhao J. Tumor necrosis factor-α: the next marker of stroke. Dis Markers. 2022;2022(27):2395269.
34. Chen X, Yang DX, Zhao H, et al. Stroke-induced renal dysfunction: underlying mechanisms and challenges of the brain-kidney axis. CNS Neurosci Ther. 2024;30(11):e70114.
35. Arnold J, Ng KP, Sims D, Gill P, Cockwell P, Ferro C. Incidence and impact on outcomes of acute kidney injury after a stroke: a systematic review and meta-analysis. BMC Nephrol. 2018;19:283.

36. Andres-Hernando A, Dursun B, Altmann C, et al. Cytokine production increases and cytokine clearance decreases in mice with bilateral nepherectomy. Nephrol Dial Transplant. 2012;27:4339–47.
37. Nongunch A, Panorchan K, Davenport A. Brain-kidney crosstalk. Crit Care. 2014;18:225.
38. Lu R, Kiernan MC, Murray A, Rosner MH, Ronco C. Kidney-brain crosstalk in the acute and chronic setting. Nat Rev Nephrol. 2015;11(12):707–19.
39. Tsao N, Hsu HP, Wu CM, Liu CC, Lei HY. Tumor necrosis factor-alpha causes an increase in blood-brain barrier permeability during sepsis. J Med Microbiol. 2001;50:812–21.
40. Trinh-Trang-Tan MM, Cartron JP, Bankir L. Molecular basis for the dialysis disequilibrium syndrome: altered aquaporin and urea transporter expression in the brain. Nephrol Dial Transplant. 2005;20:1984–8.
41. de Vries DK, Lindeman JH, Ringers J, et al. Donor brain death predisposes human kidney grafts to a proinflammatory reaction after transplantation. Am J Transplant. 2011;11:1064–70.
42. Adesso S, Magnus T, Cuzzocrea S, Campolo M, Rissiek B, Paciello O, et al. Indoxyl sulfate affects glial function, increasing oxidative stress and neuroinflammation in chronic kidney disease: interaction between astrocytes and microglia. Front Pharmacol. 2017;8:370.
43. O'Kane RL, Vina JR, Simpson I, Zaragoza R, Mokashi A, Hawkins RA. Cationic amino acid transport across the blood-brain barrier is mediated exclusively by system y+. Am J Physiol Endocrinol Metab. 2006;291:412–9.
44. Zaganas I, Pajecka K, Wender C, Schousboe A, Waagepetersen HS, Plaitakis A. The effect of pH and ADP on ammonia affinity for human glutamate dehydrogenases. Metab Brain Dis. 2013;28(2):127–31.
45. Rothman D, De Feyter HM, Maciejewski PK, Behar KL. Is there in vivo evidence for amino acid shuttles carrying ammonia from neurons to astrocytes? Neurochem Res. 2012;37(11):2597–612.
46. Adachi N, Lei B, Deshpande G, Seyfried FJ, Shimizu I, Nagaro T, Arai T. Uraemia suppresses central dopaminergic metabolism and impairs motor activity in rats. Intensive Care Med. 2001;27(10):1655–60.
47. Tevzadze G, Barbakadze T, Kvergelidze E, Zhuravliova E, Shanshiashvili L, Mikeladze D. Gut neurotoxin p-cresol induces brain-derived neurothrophic factor secretion and increases the expression of neurofilament subunits in PC- 12 cells. AIMS Neurosci. 2022;9(1):12–23.
48. Ramírez-Guerrero G, Vera-Calzaretta A, Torres V, et al. Augmented renal clearance in neurocritical care patients: a retrospective cohort study. J Transl Crit Care Med. 2024;6(2):e24–00002.
49. Ramírez-Guerrero G, Muller-Ortiz H, Pedreros-Rosales C. Polyuria in adults. A diagnostic approach base on pathophysiology. Rev Clin Esp. 2022;222(5):301–8.
50. Cruz-Llanos L, Molano A, Rizo-Topete L. Continuous renal replacement therapy in acute brain injury. Front Nephrol. 2022;2:853677.

Cardiorenal Syndromes: Role of Humoral Signaling 16

Marco Casarotti, Sonia Guarino, Francesco Cundari, and Sergio Lassola

16.1 Introduction

Cardiorenal syndrome (CRS) defines a spectrum of disorders in which cardiac and renal dysfunction are intricately linked, with impairment in one organ leading to adverse effects on the other [1]. This bidirectional relationship is increasingly recognized as a critical area in cardiovascular and renal medicine due to its high prevalence and significant impact on patient outcomes [2]. The concept of CRS emerged as researchers began to identify distinct patterns in how heart failure and kidney disease interact, leading to various types of syndromes based on the initial organ affected and the acute or chronic nature of the dysfunction [1]. The heart-kidney connection holds profound implications for understanding the disease mechanisms underlying CRS [3]. Cardiac and renal systems are closely interconnected through hemodynamic, neurohormonal, and inflammatory pathways, each capable of triggering a cascade that exacerbates dysfunction in the other organ. For instance, decreased cardiac output in heart failure can reduce renal perfusion, while renal dysfunction can lead to volume overload and electrolyte disturbances, further straining cardiac function [4]. The objectives of this chapter are to provide a comprehensive overview of the classification, pathophysiology, and clinical implications of

M. Casarotti · S. Lassola (✉)
Department of Anesthesia and Intensive Care, Santa Chiara Hospital, Trento, Italy
e-mail: sergio.lassola@apss.tn.it

S. Guarino
Department of Morphology, Surgery and Experimental Medicine, Section of Anesthesia and Intensive Care, Sant'Anna Hospital, University of Ferrara, Ferrara, Italy

F. Cundari
Department of Surgical, Medical, Molecular Pathology and Critical Care Medicine, University of Pisa, Pisa, Italy
e-mail: f.cundari@studenti.unipi.it

D. Battaglini et al. (eds.), *Organ System Crosstalk in Critical Illness*,
https://doi.org/10.1007/978-3-032-01024-7_16

CRS. We will delve into the five major types of CRS as categorized by the Acute Dialysis Quality Initiative consensus, examining how different patterns of organ injury can guide diagnosis and treatment strategies. Furthermore, we will explore the role of humoral signaling—specifically, how biochemical signals between the heart and kidneys contribute to the progression of CRS. Through this discussion, we aim to shed light on the importance of targeting these pathways to mitigate disease progression and improve clinical outcomes.

16.2 Pathophysiological Interactions

Cardiorenal syndrome (CRS) represents a complex pathological interaction between the heart and kidneys, where dysfunction in one organ can lead to deterioration in the other [1].

This interdependence is mediated by hemodynamic and neurohormonal pathways. For example, reduced cardiac function decreases renal perfusion, activating compensatory mechanisms in the kidneys that, over time, worsen cardiac dysfunction [5]. Conversely, renal impairment can exacerbate heart failure through volume overload and electrolyte imbalances [5].

This bidirectional relationship is integral to understanding the dynamics of CRS [6]. CRS is perpetuated by a series of feedback loops that accelerate the progressive decline of both organs. One of the main mechanisms is the activation of the renin-angiotensin-aldosterone system (RAAS) and the sympathetic nervous system (SNS) [7]. RAAS activation promotes sodium and water retention and vasoconstriction, increasing blood pressure and cardiac workload. Simultaneously, SNS activation raises myocardial oxygen demand and reduces renal perfusion, further straining both organs [7].

These interconnected pathways create self-reinforcing loops that worsen the patient's overall condition [8]. Humoral factors, including pro-inflammatory cytokines (such as TNF-alpha and IL-6), uremic toxins, and natriuretic peptides, play a critical role in the progression of CRS [9]. Inflammatory cytokines drive fibrosis in both the heart and kidneys, exacerbating the loss of function in each organ. Additionally, factors like fibroblast growth factor 23 (FGF23), released by compromised kidneys, can lead to cardiac hypertrophy and remodeling, worsening heart failure [10]. Although initially protective, natriuretic peptides may lose effectiveness due to receptor downregulation, contributing to fluid overload [11]. The complex interactions of these humoral signals highlight the progressive nature of CRS [6]. The intertwined networks of humoral and neurohormonal signals, coupled with self-sustaining feedback mechanisms, underscore the chronic and progressive nature of CRS. Breaking these pathological cycles remains a key goal in improving therapeutic outcomes and reducing the high mortality rates associated with this syndrome [1, 6].

16.3 Overview of Cardiorenal Syndromes

The first formal attempt to define cardiorenal syndrome (CRS) came from the National Heart, Lung, and Blood Institute Working Group in 2004 [3]. Their cardio-centric definition emphasized the increase in circulatory and non-circulatory compartment volumes due to kidney failure, which worsens heart failure and decreases sensitivity to decongestive therapies [12]. The most widely used classification of CRS originates from the Acute Dialysis Quality Initiative consensus outlined in 2008 [13]. This classification divides CRS into two main groups based on the primary affected organ, or "primum movens": types 1 (acute) and 2 (chronic) for heart-initiated dysfunction, and types 3 (acute) and 4 (chronic) for kidney-initiated dysfunction. A fifth category includes systemic processes that result in dysfunction in both organs [13]. As illustrated in Table 16.1, each type of CRS is associated with specific initiating organs, key characteristics, and representative examples.

Table 16.1 Classification and characteristics of cardiorenal syndromes (CRS)

CRS type	Initiating organ	Description	Examples
Type 1—acute cardiorenal syndrome	Heart	Acute cardiac event leads to kidney failure, often due to reduced cardiac output, volume overload, and RAAS activation	Acute coronary syndrome resulting in cardiogenic shock; heart failure with acute kidney injury (AKI)
Type 2—chronic cardiorenal syndrome	Heart	Persistent cardiac dysfunction gradually impairs kidney function over time, often involving chronic inflammation and fibrosis	Chronic heart failure (HF), heart failure with preserved ejection fraction (HFpEF), atrial fibrillation (AF), and ischemic heart disease
Type 3—acute renocardiac syndrome	Kidney	Acute kidney injury (AKI) results in cardiac impairment, primarily due to volume overload, hyperuremia, electrolyte imbalances, and RAAS activation	AKI leading to fluid overload, left ventricular heart failure (LVHF), or pulmonary edema; increased risk of heart failure by 58%
Type 4—chronic renocardiac syndrome	Kidney	Chronic kidney disease (CKD) contributes to progressive cardiac dysfunction, often due to RAAS activation, fluid retention, and systemic conditions	CKD-associated cardiomyopathy, left ventricular hypertrophy, and congestive heart failure (CHF) in end-stage renal disease (ESRD)
Type 5—secondary cardiorenal syndrome	Systemic processes	Systemic diseases simultaneously affect both heart and kidney function, typically through inflammation, RAAS activation, and oxidative stress	Sepsis, vasculitis, diabetes, amyloidosis, cirrhosis, systemic inflammation, and hypertension

Note. *CRS* cardiorenal syndrome, *AKI* acute kidney injury, *RAAS* renin–angiotensin–aldosterone system, *HF* heart failure, *HFpEF* heart failure with preserved ejection fraction, AF atrial fibrillation, *LVHF* left ventricular heart failure, *CKD* chronic kidney disease, *CHF* congestive heart failure, *ESRD* end-stage renal disease

CRS, by nature, is an evolving entity. This evolution can often blur the lines between different phenotypes, making it challenging to pinpoint the initial organ of injury. The primary utility of this classification lies in identifying the main source of dysfunction, as targeted treatment could potentially halt or even reverse secondary damage. Alternative classifications, based on clinical manifestations rather than the primary affected organ, have also been proposed but are less frequently used. Type 1 CRS is defined as a rapid decline in cardiac function that induces AKI, according to the KDIGO 2012 guidelines (increase in sCr by $\geq$0.3 mg/dl within 48 hours; or increase in sCr to $\geq$1.5 times baseline within the prior 7 days; or urine volume $\leq$0.5 ml/kg/h for 6 hours) [14]. This form affects roughly one in four individuals with acute decompensated heart failure. Acute heart failure decreases cardiac output and increases central venous pressure (CVP), causing volume overload, sluggish intravascular flow, and reduced glomerular filtration rate (GFR) [15]. These conditions activate the RAAS cascade, leading to vasoconstriction of renal efferent arterioles to restore GFR while promoting salt reabsorption in the proximal tubule, exacerbating volume overload. Angiotensin II also boosts endothelin-1 production, stimulating aldosterone-driven salt reabsorption in the distal tubules [16]. This peptide acts as a potent pro-inflammatory and pro-fibrotic agent, contributing to pathological changes and generating oxidative stress in a vicious cycle [17]. Type 2 CRS is a persistent cardiac dysfunction that gradually leads to CKD, likely due to chronic inflammation and fibrosis that result in cellular damage [3]. Older theories suggested that reduced renal perfusion was the main cause, but recent findings underscore the critical role of IL-6 and TNF-α in promoting inflammatory cell accumulation in the renal interstitium and mesangial cell death, along with oxidative stress [13]. Common conditions associated with type 2 CRS include HFpEF, congenital heart diseases, atrial fibrillation, and ischemic heart disease. Studies have shown improved cardiac function with erythropoiesis-stimulating agents in this context [13]. Type 3 CRS results in a gradual decline in kidney function due to AKI, ischemia, or glomerulonephritis, leading to acute cardiac impairment, with a 58% increased risk of heart failure [3]. Misregulated RAAS activation causes sodium and water retention, fluid overload, and eventual left ventricular heart failure and pulmonary edema. This also heightens the risk of sudden death from electrolyte imbalances [5]. Type 4 CRS is characterized by cardiac dysfunction because of CKD. Renal impairment is an independent risk factor for cardiovascular disease: about 40% of end-stage renal disease (ESRD) patients also have ischemic coronary disease, and 40% of these patients develop chronic heart failure [3, 13]. Fluid retention in CKD is mediated by vasoconstriction, oxidative stress, RAAS activation, and sodium and water reabsorption, which inhibit endothelial proliferation, impair wound healing, and increase renal damage, perpetuating a vicious cycle [18]. Recent research highlights fibroblast growth factor 23 (FGF23), involved in vitamin D and phosphorus metabolism, as a cardiovascular risk marker in CKD and ESRD, with elevated levels linked to left ventricular hypertrophy and mortality [19]. CKD patients often have other systemic conditions, like diabetes, obesity, and dyslipidemia, which further compromise heart function [20]. Type 5 CRS can be divided into four stages: hyperacute (0–72 hours from diagnosis), acute (3–7 days), subacute (7–30 days), and chronic (>30 days) [3]. Systemic diseases that affect both heart and kidney functions are generally complement-mediated, inducing cytokine and RAAS activation, which leads to organ damage through oxidative stress, increased vascular resistance, and eventual ischemia [21]. In intensive care, sepsis and septic shock are classic examples, increasing prostacyclin and thromboxane levels, along with TNF and IL-1, leading to endothelial dysfunction, impaired autoregulation, and, in some cases, disseminated intravascular coagulation (DIC) [22]. The organ interactions mentioned above are mediated by humoral signaling proteins, which sometimes serve as biomarkers of disease.

16.4 Role of Humoral Signaling

The term "organ crosstalk" refers to the complex interactions between organs mediated by biochemical signals [23]. While these interactions can have protective effects, they may also contribute to damage, as seen in acute kidney injury (AKI), where renal damage triggers pathological responses in other organs, including the heart, lungs, and brain [23, 24]. Cardiorenal syndrome is a key example, where alterations in renal function impair cardiac function and vice versa, creating a self-perpetuating cycle of deterioration [1, 13]. Initially, the mechanisms of cardiorenal damage, known as cardio-renal connectors, were thought to be solely the result of hemodynamic changes [25]. However, evidence now indicates that cardio-renal connectors such as the renin-angiotensin-aldosterone system (RAAS), sympathetic nervous system (SNS), and inflammatory mediators like TNF-alpha and IL-6 play crucial roles in this process. These biochemical signals can worsen both cardiac and renal function through mechanisms such as oxidative stress, vasoconstriction, and fibrosis. Natriuretic peptides, particularly BNP and NT-proBNP, are essential indicators of fluid overload and cardiac stress, while fibroblast growth factor 23 (FGF23) contributes to cardiac remodeling [11]. As summarized in Table 16.2, each of these biomarkers plays a distinct role in the progression of CRS, providing valuable insights for diagnosis, prognosis, and therapeutic monitoring. Understanding these biomarkers aids in guiding clinical decisions, ultimately improving the management of CRS.

However, evidence shows that patients with heart failure without significant hemodynamic changes may experience a more rapid decline in glomerular filtration rate (GFR) than expected [26]. This observation suggests that factors beyond hemodynamics play a role [26]. Currently, the renin-angiotensin-aldosterone system (RAAS), the sympathetic nervous system (SNS), and inflammatory responses are recognized as central contributors [27]. Venous congestion, a primary trigger for renal dysfunction, leads to increased renal venous pressure, causing vasoconstriction and reduced GFR [28]. This cycle of volume overload is perpetuated by RAAS, leading to sodium and water retention, elevated central venous pressure, and renal vein pressure [29]. As summarized in Table 16.3, multiple mechanisms contribute to the deterioration of both cardiac and renal function in CRS. These mechanisms include RAAS activation, sympathetic dysregulation, inflammatory responses, and

Table 16.2 Key biomarkers in cardiorenal syndrome (CRS)

Biomarker	Source	Role in CRS	Clinical relevance
BNP	Cardiac ventricles	Indicates cardiac stress and fluid overload	Diagnostic tool in heart failure; elevated in CRS
NT-proBNP	Cardiac ventricles	Inactive precursor of BNP; reflects cardiac stress	Useful in diagnosis and monitoring of heart failure
FGF23	Compromised kidneys	Promotes cardiac hypertrophy and remodeling	Elevated levels linked to poor cardiovascular outcomes
TNF-alpha	Immune cells in kidneys	Promotes inflammation and fibrosis in kidneys and heart	Indicator of inflammatory response; worsens CRS
IL-6	Immune cells	Contributes to inflammation and kidney fibrosis	Associated with worsening renal and cardiac outcomes
Endothelin-1	Vascular endothelium	Increases vasoconstriction and sodium reabsorption	Marker of endothelial dysfunction in heart failure
CD40	Renal proximal tubules	Activates inflammatory signaling and TNF-alpha production	Potential target for reducing renal inflammation

Note. *BNP* B-type natriuretic peptide, *NT-proBNP* N-terminal prohormone of BNP, *FGF23* fibroblast growth factor 23, *TNF-alpha* tumor necrosis factor-alpha, *IL-6* interleukin 6, *CD40* cluster of differentiation 40

oxidative stress. Together, they create a vicious cycle of cellular and functional damage across both organs.

16.5 Natriuretic Peptides

Natriuretic peptides are a group of hormones vital for cardiovascular regulation, particularly in managing blood volume and vascular tone [11]. The primary types include atrial natriuretic peptide (ANP), B-type natriuretic peptide (BNP), and C-type natriuretic peptide (CNP) [11]. ANP is mainly secreted by the atria in response to increased blood volume, BNP by the ventricles due to ventricular stretch and pressure overload, and CNP in lower quantities by endothelial cells, impacting local vascular functions [6, 30]. These peptides exert their effects by binding to natriuretic peptide receptors (NPR-A, NPR-B, and NPR-C), activating the intracellular messenger cyclic guanosine monophosphate (cGMP) [31]. This cascade results in vasodilation, increased glomerular filtration rate (GFR), and inhibition of the renin-angiotensin-aldosterone system (RAAS) [11]. Through NPR-A, ANP and BNP induce vasodilation and natriuresis, lowering blood pressure and volume. CNP, acting mainly on NPR-B, supports vascular relaxation. NPR-C, a clearance receptor, regulates circulating levels of natriuretic peptides through degradation mechanisms [11]. The principal role of ANP and BNP is in fluid and electrolyte homeostasis. In response to increased cardiac chamber pressures, such as in heart failure, ANP and BNP are released to promote natriuresis (sodium excretion) and diuresis (water excretion), enhancing GFR and reducing both preload and afterload

Table 16.3 Mechanisms of organ crosstalk in cardiorenal syndrome (CRS)

Mechanism	Description	Impact on organs
Venous congestion	Increased renal venous pressure due to volume overload	Leads to vasoconstriction, reduced GFR, and kidney damage
RAAS activation	Triggered by venous congestion, increasing aldosterone and promoting fibrosis	Causes fibrosis in both heart and kidneys, oxidative stress
SNS activation	Upregulated in heart failure, contributing to renal vasoconstriction and reduced GFR	Fuels RAAS, sodium reabsorption, and raises blood pressure
Inflammatory responses	Inflammatory signals from kidneys activate cytokines, chemokines, and cell adhesion molecules	Leads to neutrophil migration, endothelial dysfunction
Reactive oxygen species (ROS)	Oxidative stress caused by RAAS and mitochondrial dysfunction	Promotes inflammation and fibrosis in heart and kidneys
CD40 activation in renal cells	Proximal tubular cells activate CD40, producing TNF-alpha and recruiting immune cells	Increases inflammation and tubular damage in kidneys
Systemic effects on other organs	Venous congestion and reduced intestinal perfusion allow endotoxins into the bloodstream	Leads to chronic inflammation; affects heart, lungs, brain
Cardiomyocyte apoptosis	Caused by humoral signaling and oxidative stress, leading to cellular death in heart muscle cells	Contributes to cardiac dysfunction in type 3 CRS

Note. *GFR* glomerular filtration rate, *RAAS* renin-angiotensin-aldosterone system, *SNS* sympathetic nervous system, *ROS* reactive oxygen species, *CD40* cluster of differentiation 40, *TNF-alpha* tumor necrosis factor-alpha

on the heart [11, 32]. Additionally, these peptides inhibit aldosterone, thereby preventing further sodium and water retention, and counterbalance the RAAS and sympathetic nervous system, which are typically upregulated in heart failure and CRS [1]. Natriuretic peptides, particularly BNP and its precursor NT-proBNP, hold significant clinical importance in CRS, where both cardiac and renal dysfunction coexist. High levels of BNP or NT-proBNP serve as biomarkers for diagnosing heart failure and gauging its severity [33]. In CRS, elevated natriuretic peptides reflect cardiac stress and fluid overload. However, interpreting these markers in patients with chronic kidney disease (CKD) can be complex due to reduced renal clearance, which keeps BNP levels elevated even in stable states [34]. Despite this, these markers remain critical in differentiating dyspnea related to heart failure from other causes. Furthermore, interventions targeting natriuretic peptide pathways, such as neprilysin inhibitors, show promise in heart failure treatment by enhancing these peptides' beneficial effects [35]. Natriuretic peptides play an essential role in managing cardiovascular and renal homeostasis through vasodilation, natriuresis, and RAAS inhibition [36]. Their ability to mitigate fluid overload makes them invaluable in heart failure and CRS management, providing crucial insights for diagnostics and therapeutics in complex clinical conditions like CRS [37].

16.6 Conclusion

This chapter highlights the complex interplay between the heart and kidneys in cardiorenal CRS, emphasizing the critical role of humoral signaling in the disease's progression. CRS is a multifaceted disorder, where dysfunction in one organ induces impairment in the other through hemodynamic, neurohormonal, and inflammatory mechanisms. The classification into five types of CRS provides a structured approach for identifying and managing the primary source of dysfunction, which is essential for developing targeted treatments. Key contributors to CRS include the RAAS, SNS, inflammatory cytokines, and natriuretic peptides. Each of these mechanisms can sustain a vicious cycle, leading to progressive decline in both heart and kidney function. Biomarkers such as BNP, NT-proBNP, and FGF23 serve as valuable tools for diagnosis, risk stratification, and treatment guidance. Understanding these humoral signals enables clinicians to better assess disease severity and monitor therapeutic efficacy. The findings presented in this chapter underscore the importance of a multidisciplinary approach to CRS, addressing both cardiac and renal contributions to disease progression. Future research should focus on identifying novel therapeutic targets within the humoral signaling pathways, with the aim of interrupting the pathological cycle between the heart and kidneys, thereby improving patient outcomes and reducing morbidity and mortality associated with CRS. Understanding how microbial and immune mediators orchestrate systemic inflammation provides the foundation for interpreting organ crosstalk mechanisms. These principles are further expanded in Chaps. 23 and 24, which explore the systemic and imaging perspectives of organ interaction.

References

1. Rangaswami J, Bhalla V, Blair JEA, Chang TI, Costa S, Lentine KL, et al. Cardiorenal Syndrome: Classification, Pathophysiology, Diagnosis, and Treatment Strategies: A Scientific Statement From the American Heart Association. Circulation. 2019:139. https://doi.org/10.1161/CIR.0000000000000664.
2. Marassi M, Fadini GP. The cardio-renal-metabolic connection: a review of the evidence. Cardiovasc Diabetol. 2023;22:195. https://doi.org/10.1186/s12933-023-01937-x.
3. Prastaro M, Nardi E, Paolillo S, Santoro C, Parlati ALM, Gargiulo P, et al. Cardiorenal syndrome: Pathophysiology as a key to the therapeutic approach in an under-diagnosed disease. J Clin Ultrasound. 2022;50:1110–24. https://doi.org/10.1002/jcu.23265.
4. Raina R, Nair N, Chakraborty R, Nemer L, Dasgupta R, Varian K. An Update on the Pathophysiology and Treatment of Cardiorenal Syndrome. Cardiol Res. 2020;11:76–88. https://doi.org/10.14740/cr955
5. Mann DL, Felker GM. Mechanisms and Models in Heart Failure: A Translational Approach. Circulation Research. 2021;128:1435–50. https://doi.org/10.1161/CIRCRESAHA.121.318158.
6. Cicoira M, Anker SD, Ronco C. Cardio-renal cachexia syndromes (CRCS): pathophysiological foundations of a vicious pathological circle. J Cachexia Sarcopenia Muscle 2011;2:135–142. https://doi.org/https://doi.org/10.1007/s13539-011-0038-2.

7. Kanugula AK, Kaur J, Batra J, Ankireddypalli AR, Velagapudi R. Renin-Angiotensin System: Updated Understanding and Role in Physiological and Pathophysiological States. Cureus. 2023;15:e40725. https://doi.org/10.7759/cureus.40725.
8. Xu G, Law JA. Loops, crosstalk, and compartmentalization: it takes many layers to regulate DNA methylation. Current Opinion in Genetics & Development. 2024;84:102147. https://doi.org/10.1016/j.gde.2023.102147.
9. Megha KB, Joseph X, Akhil V, Mohanan PV. Cascade of immune mechanism and consequences of inflammatory disorders. Phytomedicine. 2021;91:153712. https://doi.org/10.1016/j.phymed.2021.153712.
10. Li H, Chen C, Wang DW. Inflammatory Cytokines, Immune Cells, and Organ Interactions in Heart Failure. Front Physiol. 2021;12:695047. https://doi.org/10.3389/fphys.2021.695047.
11. Volpe M, Rubattu S, Burnett J. Natriuretic peptides in cardiovascular diseases: current use and perspectives. European Heart Journal. 2014;35:419–25. https://doi.org/10.1093/eurheartj/eht466.
12. Núñez J, De La Espriella R, Rossignol P, Voors AA, Mullens W, Metra M, et al. Congestion in heart failure: a circulating biomarker-based perspective. A review from the Biomarkers Working Group of the Heart Failure Association, European Society of Cardiology. European J of Heart Fail 2022;24:1751–1766. https://doi.org/10.1002/ejhf.2664.
13. Ronco C, McCullough P, Anker SD, Anand I, Aspromonte N, Bagshaw SM, et al. Cardio-renal syndromes: report from the consensus conference of the Acute Dialysis Quality Initiative. European Heart Journal. 2010;31:703–11. https://doi.org/10.1093/eurheartj/ehp507.
14. Fu K, Hu Y, Zhang H, Wang C, Lin Z, Lu H, et al. Insights of Worsening Renal Function in Type 1 Cardiorenal Syndrome: From the Pathogenesis. Biomarkers to Treatment. Front Cardiovasc Med. 2021;8:760152. https://doi.org/10.3389/fcvm.2021.760152.
15. Pang PS, Levy P. Pathophysiology of Volume Overload in Acute Heart Failure Syndromes. Congestive Heart Failure. 2010;16 https://doi.org/10.1111/j.1751-7133.2010.00167.x.
16. Ruan Y, Yu Y, Wu M, Jiang Y, Qiu Y, Ruan S. The renin-angiotensin-aldosterone system: An old tree sprouts new shoots. Cellular Signalling. 2024;124:111426. https://doi.org/10.1016/j.cellsig.2024.111426.
17. Antar SA, Ashour NA, Marawan ME, Al-Karmalawy AA. Fibrosis: Types, Effects, Markers, Mechanisms for Disease Progression, and Its Relation with Oxidative Stress, Immunity, and Inflammation. IJMS. 2023;24:4004. https://doi.org/10.3390/ijms24044004.
18. Jia G, Aroor AR, Hill MA, Sowers JR. Role of Renin-Angiotensin-Aldosterone System Activation in Promoting Cardiovascular Fibrosis and Stiffness. Hypertension. 2018;72:537–48. https://doi.org/10.1161/HYPERTENSIONAHA.118.11065.
19. Latic N, Erben RG. FGF23 and Vitamin D Metabolism. JBMR Plus. 2021;5:e10558. https://doi.org/10.1002/jbm4.10558.
20. Jankowski J, Floege J, Fliser D, Böhm M, Marx N. Cardiovascular Disease in Chronic Kidney Disease: Pathophysiological Insights and Therapeutic Options. Circulation. 2021;143:1157–72. https://doi.org/10.1161/CIRCULATIONAHA.120.050686.
21. Schefold JC, Filippatos G, Hasenfuss G, Anker SD, Von Haehling S. Heart failure and kidney dysfunction: epidemiology, mechanisms and management. Nat Rev Nephrol. 2016;12:610–23. https://doi.org/10.1038/nrneph.2016.113.
22. Iba T, Helms J, Connors JM, Levy JH. The pathophysiology, diagnosis, and management of sepsis-associated disseminated intravascular coagulation. J Intensive Care. 2023;11:24. https://doi.org/10.1186/s40560-023-00672-5.
23. Virzì G, Day S, de Cal M, Vescovo G, Ronco C. Heart-kidney crosstalk and role of humoral signaling in critical illness. Crit Care. 2014;18:201. https://doi.org/10.1186/cc13177.
24. Colombo PC, Ganda A, Lin J, Onat D, Harxhi A, Iyasere JE, et al. Inflammatory activation: cardiac, renal, and cardio-renal interactions in patients with the cardiorenal syndrome. Heart Fail Rev. 2012;17:177–90. https://doi.org/10.1007/s10741-011-9261-3.
25. Junho CVC, Trentin-Sonoda M, Panico K, Dos Santos RSN, Abrahão MV, Vernier ICS, et al. Cardiorenal syndrome: long road between kidney and heart. Heart Fail Rev. 2022;27:2137–53. https://doi.org/10.1007/s10741-022-10218-w.

26. Beldhuis IE, Lam CSP, Testani JM, Voors AA, Van Spall HGC, Ter Maaten JM, et al. Evidence-Based Medical Therapy in Patients With Heart Failure With Reduced Ejection Fraction and Chronic Kidney Disease. Circulation. 2022;145:693–712. https://doi.org/10.1161/CIRCULATIONAHA.121.052792.
27. Kingma JG, Simard D, Rouleau JR, Drolet B, Simard C. The Physiopathology of Cardiorenal Syndrome: A Review of the Potential Contributions of Inflammation. J Cardiovasc Dev Dis. 2017;4:21. https://doi.org/10.3390/jcdd4040021.
28. Polsinelli VB, Marteau L, Shah SJ. The role of splanchnic congestion and the intestinal microenvironment in the pathogenesis of advanced heart failure. Curr Opin Support Palliat Care. 2019;13:24–30. https://doi.org/10.1097/SPC.0000000000000414.
29. Mullens W, Abrahams Z, Francis GS, Sokos G, Taylor DO, Starling RC, et al. Importance of venous congestion for worsening of renal function in advanced decompensated heart failure. J Am Coll Cardiol. 2009;53:589–96. https://doi.org/10.1016/j.jacc.2008.05.068.
30. Sarzani R, Allevi M, Di Pentima C, Schiavi P, Spannella F, Giulietti F. Role of Cardiac Natriuretic Peptides in Heart Str and Function. IJMS. 2022;23:14415. https://doi.org/10.3390/ijms232214415.
31. Della Corte V, Pacinella G, Todaro F, Pecoraro R, Tuttolomondo A. The Natriuretic Peptide System: A Single Entity. Pleiotropic Effects. IJMS. 2023;24:9642. https://doi.org/10.3390/ijms24119642.
32. Potter LR, Yoder AR, Flora DR, Antos LK, Dickey DM. Natriuretic peptides: their structures, receptors, physiologic functions and therapeutic applications. Handb Exp Pharmacol. 2009:341–66. https://doi.org/10.1007/978-3-540-68964-5_15.
33. Weber M. Role of B-type natriuretic peptide (BNP) and NT-proBNP in clinical routine. Heart. 2005;92:843–9. https://doi.org/10.1136/hrt.2005.071233.
34. Tagore R, Ling LH, Yang H, Daw H-Y, Chan Y-H, Sethi SK. Natriuretic peptides in chronic kidney disease. Clin J Am Soc Nephrol. 2008;3:1644–51. https://doi.org/10.2215/CJN.00850208.
35. Seliger S. The Cardiorenal Syndrome: Mechanistic Insights and Prognostication with Soluble Biomarkers. Curr Cardiol Rep. 2020;22:114. https://doi.org/10.1007/s11886-020-01360-8.
36. Nishikimi T, Maeda N, Matsuoka H. The role of natriuretic peptides in cardioprotection. Cardiovascular Research. 2006;69:318–28. https://doi.org/10.1016/j.cardiores.2005.10.001.
37. Ronco C, Kaushik M, Valle R, Aspromonte N, Peacock WF. Diagnosis and Management of Fluid Overload in Heart Failure and Cardio-Renal Syndrome: The "5B" Approach. Seminars in Nephrology. 2012;32:129–41. https://doi.org/10.1016/j.semnephrol.2011.11.016.

Part IV

The Liver

Liver-Kidney Crosstalk: Hepatorenal Syndrome

17

Kevin Roedl, Christian Schmidt-Lauber, Markus Haar, and Valentin Fuhrmann

17.1 Introduction

In patients with liver cirrhosis, acute kidney injury (AKI) is a common finding. Reports describe AKI rates of up to 50% in hospitalized patients with liver cirrhosis [1–5]. For patients in critical illness, AKI rates of up to 80% were described [5, 6]. Due to heterogeneity in the severity of illness, the clinical settings, the aetiology of AKI, and variations in definitions of AKI, the reported incidence rates show a considerable variance [7]. The occurrence of AKI in patients with liver cirrhosis is associated with increased morbidity and mortality [1, 3, 5]. Furthermore, an increased progression from AKI to chronic kidney disease (CKD) was observed [1–3, 5, 8, 9]. The prognostic importance of kidney function in liver disease is underlined by the inclusion of serum creatinine in commonly used scores such as the Model of End Stage Liver Disease (MELD) score or the CLIF-C Acute-on-Chronic Liver Failure (ACLF) score [10, 11]. In general, three main causes of AKI can be distinguished: (I) Renal hypoperfusion (pre-renal AKI), (II) intrinsic due to a structural kidney injury, and (III) post-renal injury due to urinary obstruction [12].

K. Roedl (✉) · M. Haar
Department of Intensive Care Medicine, University Medical Centre Hamburg-Eppendorf, Hamburg, Germany
e-mail: k.roedl@uke.de; m.haar@uke.de

C. Schmidt-Lauber
III. Department of Medicine, University Medical Center Hamburg-Eppendorf, Hamburg, Germany

Hamburg Center for Kidney Health (HCKH), University Medical Center Hamburg-Eppendorf, Hamburg, Germany
e-mail: c.schmidt-lauber@uke.de

V. Fuhrmann
Department of Medicine and Gastroenterology, Heilig Geist-Hospital, Cologne, Germany

D. Battaglini et al. (eds.), *Organ System Crosstalk in Critical Illness*,
https://doi.org/10.1007/978-3-032-01024-7_17

See also Table 17.1. Furthermore, in patients with liver cirrhosis, there is a unique cause of AKI that can be observed, which is mainly explained due to renal hypoperfusion which is the result of splanchnic vasodilatation and renal vasoconstriction, called hepatorenal syndrome (HRS) [2]. Renal hypoperfusion due to hypovolaemia accounts for approximately 50% of AKI cases in patients with liver cirrhosis, intrinsic causes (e.g. acute tubular necrosis) account for approximately 30%, and HRS accounts for approximately 15–20% [13]. Post-renal obstruction accounts for only <1% of AKI cases in patients with liver cirrhosis [13].

17.2 Diagnostic Criteria: Acute Kidney Injury and Hepatorenal Syndrome

The diagnostic criteria for AKI and HRS in patients with liver cirrhosis have changed several times during the last decade [2, 7]. Of interest, before 2012 criteria defining AKI, specifically in patients with liver cirrhosis, were absent. However, there was a definition of HRS defining it as a syndrome occurring in patients with cirrhosis and portal hypertension [14]. It was further characterized by impaired kidney function (serum creatinine >1.5 mg/dl) in the absence of an underlying kidney disease [14]. Furthermore, HRS was classified by the clinical course of the kidney function in HRS type-1 and HRS type-2. HRS type-1 was characterized by a rapid reduction in kidney function alongside with an increase in serum creatinine to levels >2.5 mg/dl in a period <2 weeks [14]. HRS type-2 was characterized by a chronic deterioration in kidney function [14].

Recently, the diagnostic criteria for AKI and HRS were revised. During a joint meeting of the Acute Disease Quality Initiative (ADQI) and International Club of

Table 17.1 Main causes of acute kidney injury

Pre-renal
Renal hypoperfusion due to
Hypovolaemia (low blood volume)
Low arterial perfusion
Venous congestion
Intrinsic
Structural kidney injury due to
Glomerulonephritis
Acute tubular necrosis (ATN)
Acute interstitial nephritis (AIN)
Vascular disease (such as thrombotic microangiopathies)
Post-renal
Urinary obstruction due to
Benign prostatic hyperplasia
Obstructed urinary catheter
Cancer (bladder, ureters or prostate)
Bladder or kidney stones

Ascites (ICA), the definition of kidney dysfunction in patients with cirrhosis was refined [15].

The new definition of AKI was harmonized with the Kidney Disease: Improving Global Outcomes (KDIGO) definition. Acute kidney injury in patients with liver cirrhosis was defined as an increase in serum creatinine of ≥0.3 mg/dl within 48 hours or ≥50% from baseline value known or presumed to have occurred within the prior 7 days and/or urine output ≤0.5 ml/kg for ≥6 hours [15]. Of note, the inclusion of the urine output criteria was considered important. Studies showed that urine output serves as a sensitive marker of AKI in patients with cirrhosis which was associated with worse outcomes [5]. The reference value of serum creatinine should be estimated from the values obtained within the last 3 months. However, in the case of no obtainable serum creatinine values within the last 3 months, it is recommended using the last 12 months as baseline period or if not applicable use the serum creatinine on admission [15].

Hepatorenal syndrome describes a specific phenotype of kidney dysfunction [7]. This form of kidney dysfunction is usually observed in patients with clinically significant ascites and liver cirrhosis. Furthermore, this can also be observed in the presence of tubular injury, proteinuria, and/or pre-existing chronic kidney disease. For HRS, the newly consented definition eliminated the threshold for serum creatinine (see above) with the intention to allow earlier diagnosis and treatment in patients with normal serum creatinine levels but reduced kidney function (e.g. older patients, sarcopenia, woman) [2, 15]. Additionally, the two forms of HRS (type 1 and type 2) were reclassified into an acute form, termed HRS-AKI, and a chronic form, HRS-CKD [15]. Till the last definition of HRS, there was a need to exclude the presence of parenchymal kidney disease by proteinuria >500 mg/day, microhaematuria >50 red cells/high-power field or abnormal renal findings on ultrasonography [16]. Although excluding this criterion makes the diagnosis of HRS easier, it is considered one of the major limitations of the definition. Especially, the worldwide increase in obesity has led to a marked increase in non-alcoholic steatohepatitis and a higher presence of underlying CKD due to arterial hypertension and diabetes mellitus [17]. However, the prognostic and therapeutic implications of HRS-AKI in patients with CKD have to be determined and will probably differ from patients who progress to HRS-CKD [2, 18, 19]. Further changes in the diagnostic criteria for HRS-AKI were proposed. Currently, it is recommended that HRS-AKI should be considered in patients with liver cirrhosis of any degree, presence of ascites, and AKI, where intravascular volume status is deemed adequate, unless there is strong evidence for an alternative explanation for AKI, such as sepsis or nephrotoxic exposure [15]. The intravascular volume status should be assessed in all patients with AKI using standard methods [20]. When indicated, volume resuscitation should be initiated within 24 hours, to prevent fluid overload and ensure timely initiation of vasoconstrictor therapy for HRS-AKI [7, 15]. Additionally, the routine administration of intravenous albumin for 48 hours is no longer required and is not considered for the diagnosis of HRS-AKI. The diagnosis of HRS-AKI will often co-exist with other common causes of AKI or pre-existing CKD. Treatment with vasopressors should be initiated if HRS-AKI is thought to be the primary cause of AKI. The

Table 17.2 Diagnostic criteria for HRS-AKI [15]

Cirrhosis with ascites
Increase in serum creatinine ≥0.3 mg/dl within 48 hours or ≥50% from baseline value known or presumed to have occurred within the prior 7 days and/or urinary output ≤0.5 ml/kg for ≥6 hours
Absence of improvement in serum creatinine and/or urine output within 24 hours following adequate volume resuscitation (when clinically indicated)
Absence of strong evidence for an alternative explanation as the primary cause of AKI

diagnosis of HRS-AKI should be made on the best available parameters and regularly re-evaluated, and if necessary, excluded in the further clinical course [7] (Table 17.2).

17.3 Pathophysiology

The current understanding of the pathophysiology of HRS-AKI is mostly based on observational studies in humans [21]. There is a lack of reproducible experimental models of HRS. Different mechanisms can contribute to the development of several phenotypes of AKI in patients with hepatic cirrhosis [7]. Background susceptibility to renal injury varies across individuals, according to non-modifiable and modifiable factors. These factors are usually liver, kidney, and cardiovascular related but may include comorbidities and other external factors [7]. The degree of liver, kidney, and cardiac derangement, together with concomitant precipitating events and exposures, may lead to a variety of clinical phenotypes of AKI [15]. The different phenotypes of AKI include the presence of functional changes, structural damage, or both [7, 15].

In patients with liver cirrhosis, the course of the disease is tightly intertwined with the development of portal hypertension, which plays an important role in further development of complications and pathophysiological changes in this patient cohort. The initial pathophysiological change leading to portal hypertension is the increased intrahepatic resistance, mainly due to the changes from normal liver tissue to liver fibrosis. The activation of vasodilators in the splanchnic circulation, primarily nitric oxide, results in progressive vasodilation, not only in the splanchnic region but also systemically. Intestinal dysbiosis, bacterial overgrowth, and changes in tight-junction proteins increase bacterial translocation, further contributing to this effect, leading to a reduction in effective arterial blood volume and, thereby, triggering the activation of neurohumoral systems, including the renin-angiotensin-aldosterone, sympathetic, and arginine-vasopressin systems. Consequently, sodium and water retention occur, leading to the formation of ascites [2, 22, 23].

Clinical and histopathological evidence suggests that uncompensated hyperdynamic circulation is a key feature of AKI-HRS [21]. Other factors contributing to the development of AKI-HRS include systemic inflammation, cirrhotic cardiomyopathy, and adrenal insufficiency.

17.3.1 Circulatory Dysfunction

Haemodynamic changes in patients with cirrhosis are associated with splanchnic dilatation, sodium retention, ascites development, and subsequent kidney dysfunction [24]. Cirrhosis increases intrahepatic vascular resistance, causing splanchnic vasodilation primarily due to an increased production of vasodilators, e.g. nitric oxide, carbon monoxide, prostacyclins, and endocannabinoids. Hence, arterial hypotension can frequently be observed as a consequence of decreased effective arterial blood volume (EABV) and arterial pressure. As liver disease progresses, a decline in cardiac output often precedes the onset of HRS, while peripheral vascular resistance remains unchanged, indicating a potential role of cirrhotic cardiomyopathy in this syndrome's pathogenesis [25]. In order to compensate for the reduced EABV, systemic vasoconstrictor pathways are activated. These mechanisms promote sodium retention, impair solute-free water excretion, and cause renal vasoconstriction, consequently, reducing renal blood flow. In earlier stages, normal glomerular filtration rate can be preserved due to the vasodilatory effects of renal prostaglandins (like prostaglandin I2 and E2) on afferent renal arterioles, allowing glomerular pressure to remain stable despite decreased renal blood flow (renal autoregulation). However, this balance is disrupted as liver disease progresses, leading to a reduction in glomerular filtration and the development of AKI. Elevated ammonia levels in cirrhosis affect the metabolism of arginine, an essential amino acid for nitric oxide synthesis [26], thereby impairing renal microcirculation leading to subsequent functional and ischaemic kidney injury.

17.3.2 Systemic Inflammation

HRS-AKI is closely related to systemic inflammatory response syndrome (SIRS) and specifically spontaneous bacterial peritonitis (SBP). SIRS is seen in nearly half of patients with AKI-HRS, even in the absence of infection [27]. Patients with AKI-HRS have elevated plasma levels of pro-inflammatory cytokines (such as interleukin-6, TNF-α, vascular cell adhesion protein-1, and interleukin-8) and higher urinary monocyte chemoattractant protein-1 compared to those with decompensated cirrhosis without AKI or AKI from pre-renal azotaemia [28]. Systemic inflammation represents the centre of the pathophysiology of patients with liver cirrhosis and acute-on-chronic liver failure (ACLF) as well as HRS-AKI [29]. Patients with ACLF exhibit significantly higher inflammatory blood markers (e.g. CRP, leukocytes, cytokines) [30]. ACLF is often triggered by infections or excessive alcohol consumption—including alcoholic hepatitis [31–33]. These are associated with a considerable systemic inflammatory reaction [31, 34]. Furthermore, there is an increased risk of bacterial infection in the context of gastrointestinal bleeding [35]. Bacterial translocation via the gastrointestinal tract with subsequent SBP plays a pivotal role in the development of ACLF and may also be of relevance in the pathophysiology of HRS-AKI [34]. In the case of a bacterial infection, the innate immune system is activated by recognizing foreign molecular signatures (pathogen-associated molecular pattern, PAMP) [36]. PAMPs are detected via pattern recognition receptors, which initiating systemic inflammation [36]. In addition to PAMPs, toxins and other virulence factors can serve as stimuli as well [37]. Importantly, the activation of pathogen defence via PAMPs also leads to local suppression of normal tissue functions, thus enabling damage to healthy tissue cells [37]. In sepsis, an excessive inflammatory reaction leads to tissue damage that releases cellular components (damage-associated molecular pattern, DAMP) [36]. These in turn lead to the activation of the same pattern recognition receptors that have already been activated by PAMPs and can thus contribute to the further maintenance of the inflammatory reaction [34, 36]. A pronounced systemic inflammatory reaction can lead to organ failure via several pathways or mechanisms [34]. In the splanchnic area, the systemic inflammatory reaction results in the stimulation and release of nitric oxide (NO), which leads to vasodilation in this vascular area [34, 37]. This subsequently leads to pooling of the circulating blood volume in the splanchnic area and thus to effective hypovolaemia with consecutive development of hypotension [37]. Counter-regulatory mechanisms include the activation of endogenous vasoconstrictors, although in this case, excessive vasoconstriction leads to the development of renal hypoperfusion. This can subsequently develop into AKI or HRS-AKI [38]. Tissue damage can occur as part of an excessive inflammatory reaction and contribute to further organ damage [34, 36]. Moreover, severe systemic inflammation can lead to mitochondrial dysfunction in peripheral tissues [34, 39]. The resulting reduced adenosine triphosphate production may contribute significantly to the development of organ failure [39].

17.3.3 Hepato-Adrenal Syndrome

Relative adrenal insufficiency (RAI) occurs in 24–47% of patients with decompensated cirrhosis and ascites, potentially contributing to the development of HRS [40–42]. Patients with relative adrenal insufficiency (RAI) have lower arterial pressure, elevated serum levels of renin and noradrenaline, and face a higher risk of developing AKI-HRS, sepsis, and short-term mortality compared to those with normal adrenal function [21]. The mechanisms behind hepato-adrenal syndrome are still unclear but may involve depletion of cortisol synthesis substrates and dysfunction of the hypothalamic-pituitary axis. Hydrocortisone treatment is used in the treatment of septic shock and RAI. However, to date it is unknown if glucocorticoid replacement in the absence of shock may be beneficial in the prevention and treatment of HRS.

17.3.4 Cholaemic (or Bile Cast) Nephropathy

Cholaemic nephropathy has been observed in patients with cirrhosis and elevated serum bilirubin levels, believed to result from the formation of obstructive intratubular bile acid casts and the direct toxic effects of bile acids on tubular cells.

Histopathologic studies have identified intratubular bile acid casts in 18–75% of patients with AKI-HRS [43, 44]. Cholaemic nephropathy is likely present in many patients with jaundice and AKI-HRS, potentially influencing both outcomes and treatment response. However, its prevalence is probably underestimated. Increased bilirubin levels have been associated with a lower rate of response to vasopressors [45, 46]. Therefore, targeting bile acids in patients with jaundice and AKI-HRS may theoretically be beneficial.

17.3.5 Intra-Abdominal Hypertension

Elevated intra-abdominal pressure (>12 mm Hg) is an underappreciated cause of AKI. It may play a role in the development of HRS in patients with refractory ascites, and paracentesis of ascites was shown to improve creatinine clearance in HRS as a result of reduced intra-abdominal pressure [47]. Careful monitoring of systemic haemodynamic parameters, along with guided plasma expansion, is essential to prevent the onset of post-paracentesis circulatory dysfunction [21]. Bedsides echocardiography, abdominal ultrasound can help identify if intra-abdominal hypertension is contributing to renal dysfunction.

17.3.6 Hepatorenal Reflex Hypothesis

A connection between the kidneys and the liver has been proposed, indicating that osmoreceptors, chemoreceptors, and baroreceptors in the liver directly influence kidney function via complex neural pathways [21, 48]. Experimental studies have supported this hypothesis by manipulating portal blood osmolality, composition, and pressure. These findings hold potential clinical significance; however, further research is needed to confirm their relevance in humans.

17.4 Prevention of AKI

The occurrence of acute kidney injury (AKI) is a frequent yet serious complication in patients with cirrhosis. As a result, it is crucial to identify and address factors that may lead to AKI, especially in individuals with ascites [2, 49].

Volume depletion, as one the reasons for AKI, should be prevented through the mindful use of diuretics, lactulose, and prevention of variceal haemorrhage [50]. Intravenous albumin infusions, administered at a dose of 4–6 g/l of ascites removed, have been shown to improve circulatory function and prevent AKI following large-volume paracentesis (>5 l) [51]. Additionally, albumin infusions have demonstrated the potential to reduce the incidence of AKI and lower mortality rates in patients with spontaneous bacterial peritonitis [52]. However, although albumin used in patients with cirrhosis and infection other than spontaneous bacterial peritonitis delayed the onset of renal failure, it did not improve renal function and led to an increased incidence of pulmonary oedema [52]. In addition, maintaining albumin levels of 3 g/dl did not improve outcomes and was associated with an increased incidence of pulmonary oedema [53]. Therefore, the use of albumin must be carefully monitored and frequently reassessed.

Certain medications, such as nonsteroidal anti-inflammatory drugs (NSAIDs), can have direct nephrotoxic effects by disrupting intrarenal blood flow. Other agents, including radiocontrast dye, aminoglycosides, vancomycin, and amphotericin B, can cause direct toxicity to the renal tubules, while drugs like beta-lactam antibiotics and proton pump inhibitors may lead to allergic interstitial injury [2, 7, 15]. Therefore, kidney function should be carefully monitored in patients with cirrhosis and ascites who are receiving these medications. Although data on the use of intravenous contrast in this population are limited, it is recommended to use it with caution [2, 7, 15].

17.5 Treatment/Management of HRS-AKI

Besides ruling out other causes of AKI, patients with liver cirrhosis presenting with elevated renal biomarkers and fulfilling the diagnosis of AKI should undergo a precise assessment of volume status [7, 20, 54, 55]. Therefore, a combined approach using different techniques including physical examination, ultrasound and static/dynamic measurements (when available) should be used [54].

17.5.1 Pharmacologic Treatment

Upon diagnosis of HRS-AKI, immediate initiation of vasoconstrictor therapy (first-line agent: terlipressin) in combination with 20–25% albumin should be established, as recommended by current guidelines [15]. However, it must be noted that this therapy has not universally been shown to improve long-term outcomes, and severe adverse events can occur.

Regarding the use of vasoconstrictive agents, currently, terlipressin—a vasopressin analogue—is the most common vasoconstrictor used worldwide for HRS-AKI [2]. Furthermore, its use is encouraged in current European and US guidelines as a first-line agent [15, 56, 57]. The treatment with terlipressin can be administered intravenously either as bolus or as a continuous infusion showing similar efficacy. However, it has been demonstrated that the cumulative daily dose required for effective treatment as well as the incidence of adverse events is lower with a continuous infusion [58]. The initial dose of terlipressin can be increased, maintained, or discontinued, according to the therapeutic response and is defined as change in the serum creatinine levels. Of interest, serum creatinine levels inversely correlate with increases in mean arterial pressure induced by vasoconstrictors [59]. Large randomized trials showed the short-term efficacy of terlipressin in patients with HRS-AKI [60]. However, the use of terlipressin was associated with serious adverse events, including respiratory failure due to pulmonary oedema [60]. If there is clinical evidence of intravascular volume overload, it is essential to withhold terlipressin and albumin [2]. Several meta-analyses and systematic reviews have shown that other vasopressors (i.e. norepinephrine) have comparative effects to terlipressin for reversal of HRS-AKI [2, 15], with the notable difference that norepinephrine requires continuous infusion and, usually, the placement of a central venous catheter [15]. If norepinephrine is already administered due to other reasons, terlipressin should be withheld. The combination of octreotide and midodrine has weak vasoconstrictive activity, and it was shown that the effect of reversing HRS-AKI was inferior compared to terlipressin [61]. Therefore, the use of octreotide and midodrine should be only temporarily and only if terlipressin is unavailable or contraindicated [2]. Patients receiving vasoconstrictors should be monitored for adverse events (mainly ischaemic) which are usually mitigated by drug discontinuation, lowering the dose, or in the case of terlipressin, changing from bolus dosing to continuous infusion [15]. However, vasoconstrictors in general have not shown to improve survival in HRS-AKI. Therefore, their use should be considered as bridge to transplantation [2]. Currently, guidelines recommend daily use of 20–25% albumin (20–40 g/day) during the treatment of HRS-AKI [15]. To date, the optimal dosing of albumin and length of administration are not well defined. Furthermore, cautious use of albumin is recommended, with discontinuation if there is evidence of pulmonary oedema [15].

17.5.2 Transjugular Intrahepatic Portosystemic Shunt

Advanced liver cirrhosis can result in portal hypertension. The presence of portal hypertension can lead to important clinical consequences like ascites and gastrointestinal varices [62, 63]. Transjugular intrahepatic portosystemic shunt (TIPS) placement represents a relevant therapeutic option in advanced liver cirrhosis [50]. The management of refractory ascites and variceal gastrointestinal bleeding is supported by the strongest evidence [50, 62, 63]. A meta-analysis demonstrated that TIPS improved kidney function and led to a potential survival benefit in patients with HRS-AKI but with a high incidence of hepatic encephalopathy [64]. Although TIPS could be a promising option in the treatment of HRS-AKI, there is currently insufficient evidence to recommend its routine use as treatment option.

17.5.3 Renal Replacement Therapy and Liver Support Therapy

In general, renal replacement therapy (RRT) and extracorporeal liver support in critically ill patients with liver cirrhosis have been regarded as bridge to liver transplantation [65]. Initiation of RRT in patients who are not candidates for liver transplantation represents a cohort with the highest observed mortality rates and is therefore controversial [66]. However, mortality for RRT in patients with HRS was comparable to RRT in patients without RRT and liver cirrhosis [67]. Where liver transplantation is not an option, discussion with the patient and/or caregivers regarding goals of therapy and long-term prognosis is imperative [7]. Currently, there is no consensus on whether or when RRT and/or liver support should be initiated in patients with cirrhosis and AKI [2]. Several RCTs have not shown a benefit of early initiation of RRT in the general ICU population. However, patients with liver cirrhosis were mainly excluded from these RCTs. Initiation of RRT and liver support in patients with cirrhosis should be individualized and based on underlying conditions, for instance, the presence of hyperkaliaemia, acidosis, fluid overload, uremic complications, and overall prognosis [2].

17.5.4 Liver Transplantation

Liver transplantation is the preferred treatment for patients with HRS-AKI. For those with end-stage kidney disease prior to liver transplantation, combined liver and kidney transplantation may be a viable therapeutic option, as the likelihood of kidney function recovery is lower in these patients as compared to those with a shorter duration of kidney impairment [2]. Predicting the duration as well as the severity of kidney dysfunction remains challenging. A kidney biopsy could aid in diagnosing, assessing the reversibility of kidney dysfunction, and determining the necessity of simultaneous liver and kidney transplantation [68]. Biomarkers that predict AKI recovery post-transplantation are needed to help guide the allocation of kidney grafts [69, 70]. However, in the Eurotransplant area in Europe, kidney transplantation is only possible with end-stage renal disease and therefore not with HRS-AKI.

17.6 Biomarkers

In the current guidelines of the Acute Disease Quality Initiative (ADQI) and International Club of Ascites (ICA) also biomarkers were described to aid timely detection and accurate differential diagnosis of the diagnosis [15]. The expert panel suggested the use of functional biomarkers (e.g. serum Creatinine, cystatin C) as well as damage-related kidney biomarkers (e.g. albuminuria, urine neutrophil gelatinase-associated lipocalin (uNGAL)). This should not only lead to a better differential diagnosis, it should also lead to a more individual approach regarding suitable specific therapeutic interventions [7]. Although newer damage biomarkers can help to identify AKI, their additional diagnostic benefit remains unknown. Especially, in the situation where standard biomarkers remain in normal levels (subclinical AKI), specific cut-offs for damage biomarkers have yet to be defined. It was shown that an uNGAL value of 220–250 µg/g can differentiate patients with acute tubular injury from other AKI phenotypes [71]. If these values are different, applying the new diagnostic criteria for HRS-AKI remains unknown. However, a change in biomarker is more relevant than an absolute cutoff, and persistent elevations in selected biomarkers (e.g. NGAL) can indicate irreversible injury. Some time will pass till novel biomarkers can replace serum creatinine in guideline-based evaluation and management of HRS-AKI.

17.7 Conclusion

In patients with liver cirrhosis, kidney injury is a common finding and its occurrence is associated with increased morbidity and mortality. Due to heterogeneity in the severity of illness, the clinical settings, the aetiology of AKI, and variations in definitions of AKI, the reported incidence rates show a considerable variance. However, the diagnostic criteria for AKI and HRS in patients with liver cirrhosis have changed several times during the last decade. Especially the last update of guidelines on diagnosis and definition leads to earlier diagnosis and treatment of HRS-AKI in patients with liver cirrhosis. Whether the change of diagnostic criteria will have an impact on the outcome remains to be observed. The development of urinary biomarkers and their inclusion in diagnostic or treatment algorithm could potentially improve the differential diagnosis and guide treatment in patients with HRS-AKI.

References

1. Tandon P, James MT, Abraldes JG, Karvellas CJ, Ye F, Pannu N. Relevance of new definitions to incidence and prognosis of acute kidney injury in hospitalized patients with cirrhosis: a retrospective population-based cohort study. PLoS One. 2016;11(8):e0160394.
2. Nadim MK, Garcia-Tsao G. Acute kidney injury in patients with cirrhosis. N Engl J Med. 2023;388(8):733–45.
3. Belcher JM, Garcia-Tsao G, Sanyal AJ, Bhogal H, Lim JK, Ansari N, et al. Association of AKI with mortality and complications in hospitalized patients with cirrhosis. Hepatology. 2013;57(2):753–62.
4. Desai AP, Knapp SM, Orman ES, Ghabril MS, Nephew LD, Anderson M, et al. Changing epidemiology and outcomes of acute kidney injury in hospitalized patients with cirrhosis - a US population-based study. J Hepatol. 2020;73(5):1092–9.
5. Amathieu R, Al-Khafaji A, Sileanu FE, Foldes E, DeSensi R, Hilmi I, et al. Significance of oliguria in critically ill patients with chronic liver disease. Hepatology. 2017;66(5):1592–600.
6. Staufer K, Roedl K, Kivaranovic D, Drolz A, Horvatits T, Rasoul-Rockenschaub S, et al. Renal replacement therapy in critically ill liver cirrhotic patients-outcome and clinical implications. Liver Int. 2017;37(6):843–50.
7. Nadim MK, Forni LG, Ostermann M. Hepatorenal syndrome in the intensive care unit. Intensive Care Med. 2024;50(6):978–81.
8. Wang PL, Silver SA, Djerboua M, Thanabalasingam S, Zarnke S, Flemming JA. Recovery from dialysis-treated acute kidney injury in patients with cirrhosis: a population-based study. Am J Kidney Dis. 2022;80(1):55–64.e1.
9. Nadim MK, Genyk YS, Tokin C, Fieber J, Ananthapanyasut W, Ye W, et al. Impact of the etiology of acute kidney injury on outcomes following liver transplantation: acute tubular necrosis versus hepatorenal syndrome. Liver Transpl. 2012;18(5):539–48.
10. Wiesner R, Edwards E, Freeman R, Harper A, Kim R, Kamath P, et al. Model for end-stage liver disease (MELD) and allocation of donor livers. Gastroenterology. 2003;124(1):91–6.

11. Jalan R, Saliba F, Pavesi M, Amoros A, Moreau R, Gines P, et al. Development and validation of a prognostic score to predict mortality in patients with acute-on-chronic liver failure. J Hepatol. 2014;61(5):1038–47.
12. Ronco C, Bellomo R, Kellum JA. Acute kidney injury. Lancet. 2019;394(10212):1949–64.
13. Garcia-Tsao G, Parikh CR, Viola A. Acute kidney injury in cirrhosis. Hepatology. 2008;48(6):2064–77.
14. Salerno F, Gerbes A, Gines P, Wong F, Arroyo V. Diagnosis, prevention and treatment of hepatorenal syndrome in cirrhosis. Gut. 2007;56(9):1310–8.
15. Nadim MK, Kellum JA, Forni L, Francoz C, Asrani SK, Ostermann M, et al. Acute kidney injury in patients with cirrhosis: Acute Disease Quality Initiative (ADQI) and International Club of Ascites (ICA) joint multidisciplinary consensus meeting. J Hepatol. 2024;81(1):163–83.
16. Salerno F, Gerbes A, Ginès P, Wong F, Arroyo V. Diagnosis, prevention and treatment of hepatorenal syndrome in cirrhosis. Gut. 2007;56(9):1310–8.
17. Calzadilla-Bertot L, Jeffrey GP, Jacques B, McCaughan G, Crawford M, Angus P, et al. Increasing incidence of nonalcoholic steatohepatitis as an indication for liver transplantation in Australia and New Zealand. Liver Transpl. 2019;25(1):25–34.
18. Nadim MK, Kellum JA, Davenport A, Wong F, Davis C, Pannu N, et al. Hepatorenal syndrome: the 8th International Consensus Conference of the Acute Dialysis Quality Initiative (ADQI) Group. Crit Care. 2012;16(1):R23.
19. Angeli P, Garcia-Tsao G, Nadim MK, Parikh CR. News in pathophysiology, definition and classification of hepatorenal syndrome: a step beyond the International Club of Ascites (ICA) consensus document. J Hepatol. 2019;71(4):811–22.
20. Durand F, Kellum JA, Nadim MK. Fluid resuscitation in patients with cirrhosis and sepsis: a multidisciplinary perspective. J Hepatol. 2023;79(1):240–6.
21. Simonetto DA, Gines P, Kamath PS. Hepatorenal syndrome: pathophysiology, diagnosis, and management. BMJ (Clinical research ed). 2020;370:m2687.
22. Traykova D, Schneider B, Chojkier M, Buck M. Blood microbiome quantity and the hyperdynamic circulation in decompensated cirrhotic patients. PLoS One. 2017;12(2):e0169310.
23. Wiest R, Das S, Cadelina G, Garcia-Tsao G, Milstien S, Groszmann RJ. Bacterial translocation in cirrhotic rats stimulates eNOS-derived NO production and impairs mesenteric vascular contractility. J Clin Invest. 1999;104(9):1223–33.
24. Schrier RW, Arroyo V, Bernardi M, Epstein M, Henriksen JH, Rodés J. Peripheral arterial vasodilation hypothesis: a proposal for the initiation of renal sodium and water retention in cirrhosis. Hepatology. 1988;8(5):1151–7.
25. Ruiz-del-Arbol L, Monescillo A, Arocena C, Valer P, Ginès P, Moreira V, et al. Circulatory function and hepatorenal syndrome in cirrhosis. Hepatology. 2005;42(2):439–47.
26. Varga ZV, Erdelyi K, Paloczi J, Cinar R, Zsengeller ZK, Jourdan T, et al. Disruption of renal arginine metabolism promotes kidney injury in hepatorenal syndrome in mice. Hepatology. 2018;68(4):1519–33.
27. Thabut D, Massard J, Gangloff A, Carbonell N, Francoz C, Nguyen-Khac E, et al. Model for end-stage liver disease score and systemic inflammatory response are major prognostic factors in patients with cirrhosis and acute functional renal failure. Hepatology. 2007;46(6):1872–82.
28. Solé C, Solà E, Huelin P, Carol M, Moreira R, Cereijo U, et al. Characterization of inflammatory response in hepatorenal syndrome: relationship with kidney outcome and survival. Liver Int. 2019;39(7):1246–55.
29. Bernardi M, Moreau R, Angeli P, Schnabl B, Arroyo V. Mechanisms of decompensation and organ failure in cirrhosis: from peripheral arterial vasodilation to systemic inflammation hypothesis. J Hepatol. 2015;63(5):1272–84.
30. Claria J, Stauber RE, Coenraad MJ, Moreau R, Jalan R, Pavesi M, et al. Systemic inflammation in decompensated cirrhosis: characterization and role in acute-on-chronic liver failure. Hepatology. 2016;64(4):1249–64.
31. Moreau R, Jalan R, Gines P, Pavesi M, Angeli P, Cordoba J, et al. Acute-on-chronic liver failure is a distinct syndrome that develops in patients with acute decompensation of cirrhosis. Gastroenterology. 2013;144(7):1426–37, 37 e1–9.

32. Fernandez J, Acevedo J, Wiest R, Gustot T, Amoros A, Deulofeu C, et al. Bacterial and fungal infections in acute-on-chronic liver failure: prevalence, characteristics and impact on prognosis. Gut. 2018;67(10):1870–80.
33. Lucey MR, Mathurin P, Morgan TR. Alcoholic hepatitis. N Engl J Med. 2009;360(26):2758–69.
34. Arroyo V, Moreau R, Jalan R. Acute-on-chronic liver failure. N Engl J Med. 2020;382(22):2137–45.
35. Thalheimer U, Triantos CK, Samonakis DN, Patch D, Burroughs AK. Infection, coagulation, and variceal bleeding in cirrhosis. Gut. 2005;54(4):556–63.
36. Angus DC, van der Poll T. Severe sepsis and septic shock. N Engl J Med. 2013;369(9):840–51.
37. Huebener P, Braun G, Fuhrmann V. [Acute-on-chronic liver failure: a diagnostic and therapeutic challenge for intensive care]. Medizinische Klinik, Intensivmedizin und Notfallmedizin. 2018;113(8):649–57.
38. Gines P, Schrier RW. Renal failure in cirrhosis. N Engl J Med. 2009;361(13):1279–90.
39. Moreau R, Claria J, Aguilar F, Fenaille F, Lozano JJ, Junot C, et al. Blood metabolomics uncovers inflammation-associated mitochondrial dysfunction as a potential mechanism underlying ACLF. J Hepatol. 2020;72(4):688–701.
40. Jang JY, Kim TY, Sohn JH, Lee TH, Jeong SW, Park EJ, et al. Relative adrenal insufficiency in chronic liver disease: its prevalence and effects on long-term mortality. Aliment Pharmacol Ther. 2014;40(7):819–26.
41. Singh RR, Walia R, Sachdeva N, Bhalla A, Singh A, Singh V. Relative adrenal insufficiency in cirrhotic patients with ascites (hepatoadrenal syndrome). Dig Liver Dis. 2018;50(11):1232–7.
42. Piano S, Favaretto E, Tonon M, Antonelli G, Brocca A, Sticca A, et al. Including relative adrenal insufficiency in definition and classification of acute-on-chronic liver failure. Clin Gastroenterol Hepatol. 2020;18(5):1188–96.e3.
43. Bräsen JH, Mederacke YS, Schmitz J, Diahovets K, Khalifa A, Hartleben B, et al. Cholemic nephropathy causes acute kidney injury and is accompanied by loss of aquaporin 2 in collecting ducts. Hepatology. 2019;69(5):2107–19.
44. van Slambrouck CM, Salem F, Meehan SM, Chang A. Bile cast nephropathy is a common pathologic finding for kidney injury associated with severe liver dysfunction. Kidney Int. 2013;84(1):192–7.
45. Nazar A, Pereira GH, Guevara M, Martín-Llahi M, Pepin MN, Marinelli M, et al. Predictors of response to therapy with terlipressin and albumin in patients with cirrhosis and type 1 hepatorenal syndrome. Hepatology. 2010;51(1):219–26.
46. Barreto R, Fagundes C, Guevara M, Solà E, Pereira G, Rodríguez E, et al. Type-1 hepatorenal syndrome associated with infections in cirrhosis: natural history, outcome of kidney function, and survival. Hepatology. 2014;59(4):1505–13.
47. Umgelter A, Reindl W, Wagner KS, Franzen M, Stock K, Schmid RM, et al. Effects of plasma expansion with albumin and paracentesis on haemodynamics and kidney function in critically ill cirrhotic patients with tense ascites and hepatorenal syndrome: a prospective uncontrolled trial. Crit Care. 2008;12(1):R4.
48. Lang F, Tschernko E, Schulze E, Ottl I, Ritter M, Völkl H, et al. Hepatorenal reflex regulating kidney function. Hepatology. 1991;14(4 Pt 1):590–4.
49. O'Leary JG, Levitsky J, Wong F, Nadim MK, Charlton M, Kim WR. Protecting the kidney in liver transplant candidates: practice-based recommendations from the American Society of Transplantation Liver and Intestine Community of Practice. Am J Transplant. 2016;16(9):2516–31.
50. de Franchis R, Bosch J, Garcia-Tsao G, Reiberger T, Ripoll C. Baveno VII - renewing consensus in portal hypertension. J Hepatol. 2022;76(4):959–74.
51. Bernardi M, Caraceni P, Navickis RJ, Wilkes MM. Albumin infusion in patients undergoing large-volume paracentesis: a meta-analysis of randomized trials. Hepatology. 2012;55(4):1172–81.
52. Sort P, Navasa M, Arroyo V, Aldeguer X, Planas R, Ruiz-del-Arbol L, et al. Effect of intravenous albumin on renal impairment and mortality in patients with cirrhosis and spontaneous bacterial peritonitis. N Engl J Med. 1999;341(6):403–9.

53. China L, Freemantle N, Forrest E, Kallis Y, Ryder SD, Wright G, et al. A randomized trial of albumin infusions in hospitalized patients with cirrhosis. N Engl J Med. 2021;384(9):808–17.
54. De Backer D, Aissaoui N, Cecconi M, Chew MS, Denault A, Hajjar L, et al. How can assessing hemodynamics help to assess volume status? Intensive Care Med. 2022;48(10):1482–94.
55. Nadim MK, Durand F, Kellum JA, Levitsky J, O'Leary JG, Karvellas CJ, et al. Management of the critically ill patient with cirrhosis: a multidisciplinary perspective. J Hepatol. 2016;64(3):717–35.
56. Biggins SW, Angeli P, Garcia-Tsao G, Ginès P, Ling SC, Nadim MK, et al. Diagnosis, evaluation, and management of ascites, spontaneous bacterial peritonitis and hepatorenal syndrome: 2021 practice guidance by the American Association for the Study of Liver Diseases. Hepatology. 2021;74(2):1014–48.
57. EASL Clinical Practice Guidelines for the management of patients with decompensated cirrhosis. J Hepatol. 2018;69(2):406–60.
58. Cavallin M, Piano S, Romano A, Fasolato S, Frigo AC, Benetti G, et al. Terlipressin given by continuous intravenous infusion versus intravenous boluses in the treatment of hepatorenal syndrome: a randomized controlled study. Hepatology. 2016;63(3):983–92.
59. Velez JC, Nietert PJ. Therapeutic response to vasoconstrictors in hepatorenal syndrome parallels increase in mean arterial pressure: a pooled analysis of clinical trials. Am J Kidney Dis. 2011;58(6):928–38.
60. Wong F, Pappas SC, Curry MP, Reddy KR, Rubin RA, Porayko MK, et al. Terlipressin plus albumin for the treatment of type 1 hepatorenal syndrome. N Engl J Med. 2021;384(9):818–28.
61. Cavallin M, Kamath PS, Merli M, Fasolato S, Toniutto P, Salerno F, et al. Terlipressin plus albumin versus midodrine and octreotide plus albumin in the treatment of hepatorenal syndrome: a randomized trial. Hepatology. 2015;62(2):567–74.
62. Garcia-Tsao G, Abraldes JG, Berzigotti A, Bosch J. Portal hypertensive bleeding in cirrhosis: risk stratification, diagnosis, and management: 2016 practice guidance by the American Association for the study of liver diseases. Hepatology. 2017;65(1):310–35.
63. Angeli P, Bernardi M, Villanueva C, Francoz C, Mookerjee RP, Trebicka J, et al. EASL Clinical Practice Guidelines for the management of patients with decompensated cirrhosis. J Hepatol. 2018;69(2):406–60.
64. Song T, Rössle M, He F, Liu F, Guo X, Qi X. Transjugular intrahepatic portosystemic shunt for hepatorenal syndrome: a systematic review and meta-analysis. Dig Liver Dis. 2018;50(4):323–30.
65. Fuhrmann V, Bauer M, Wilmer A. The persistent potential of extracorporeal therapies in liver failure. Intensive Care Med. 2020;46(3):528–30.
66. Martin-Llahi M, Guevara M, Torre A, Fagundes C, Restuccia T, Gilabert R, et al. Prognostic importance of the cause of renal failure in patients with cirrhosis. Gastroenterology. 2011;140(2):488–96 e4.
67. Allegretti AS, Parada XV, Eneanya ND, Gilligan H, Xu D, Zhao S, et al. Prognosis of patients with cirrhosis and AKI who initiate RRT. Clinical journal of the American Society of Nephrology: CJASN. 2018;13(1):16–25.
68. Pichler RH, Huskey J, Kowalewska J, Moiz A, Perkins J, Davis CL, et al. Kidney biopsies may help predict renal function after liver transplantation. Transplantation. 2016;100(10):2122–8.
69. Levitsky J, Asrani SK, Klintmalm G, Schiano T, Moss A, Chavin K, et al. Discovery and validation of a biomarker model (PRESERVE) predictive of renal outcomes after liver transplantation. Hepatology. 2020;71(5):1775–86.
70. Levitsky J, Asrani SK, Abecassis M, Ruiz R, Jennings LW, Klintmalm G. External validation of a pretransplant biomarker model (REVERSE) predictive of renal recovery after liver transplantation. Hepatology. 2019;70(4):1349–59.
71. Asrani SK, Shankar N, da Graca B, Nadim MK, Cardenas A. Role of novel kidney biomarkers in patients with cirrhosis and after liver transplantation. Liver Transpl. 2022;28(3):466–82.

Gut-Liver Crosstalk in Sepsis-Induced Liver Injury

18

Francesco Alessandri, Vlad Cristian Sanda, Giancarlo Ceccarelli, and Ricard Ferrer

18.1 Introduction

Sepsis is a multisystem condition with high mortality, which rises significantly—to between 54% and 68%—when liver dysfunction or failure occurs. During microbial infection, pathogen-associated molecular patterns (PAMPs), present in several microorganisms but absent in the host, alert the immune system to the presence of pathogens, thereby promoting immunity [1]. The gastrointestinal tract plays a crucial role in the pathophysiology of sepsis has been demonstrated, being the main source of lipopolysaccharides (LPS). Under normal conditions, the amount of LPS and other PAMPs is managed by the liver with its local immune cells. However, in pathological conditions such as sepsis or systemic inflammation, microcirculation

F. Alessandri (✉)
Intensive Care Unit, Department of General and Specialistic Surgery, "Sapienza" University of Rome, Rome, Italy

Azienda Ospedaliera-Universitaria Policlinico Umberto I, Rome, Italy
e-mail: francesco.alessandri@uniroma1.it

V. C. Sanda
Azienda Ospedaliera-Universitaria Policlinico Umberto I, Rome, Italy

G. Ceccarelli
Azienda Ospedaliera-Universitaria Policlinico Umberto I, Rome, Italy

Department of Public Health and Infectious Diseases, "Sapienza" University of Rome, Rome, Italy
e-mail: giancarlo.ceccarelli@uniroma1.it

R. Ferrer
Servicio de Medicina Intensiva, Hospital Universitario Vall d'Hebron, Barcelona, España; SODIR, Vall d'Hebron Institut de Recerca, Barcelona, España

Departamento de Medicina, Universitat Autònoma de Barcelona, Barcelona, Spain
e-mail: ricard.ferrer@vallhebron.cat

D. Battaglini et al. (eds.), *Organ System Crosstalk in Critical Illness*, https://doi.org/10.1007/978-3-032-01024-7_18

alterations impair liver function [2]. As the patient's condition deteriorates, intestinal LPS translocation and hepatic inflammation both intensify. The crosstalk between the gut and liver and vice versa is fundamental in limiting the inflammation in the liver and the homeostasis of the gut barrier [2, 3]. Liver damage during sepsis can range from active hepatocellular dysfunction to potentially fatal fulminant liver failure, causing severe systemic inflammation affecting other organs. Increased levels of inflammatory cytokines, along with issues in bacterial and bile acid excretion, are indicators of hepatic dysfunction and can lead to intestinal barrier disruption and gut microbiota dysbiosis [1, 4].

18.2 Gastrointestinal Microbiome

The human gut provides an ideal environment due to the abundance of available nutrients. These microorganisms are mainly represented by bacteria and live symbiotically with the host [5]. There are more than 100 bacterial species in the gut, the so-called microbiome, among which we find several bacterial types like *Bacteroides*, *Prevotella*, and *Ruminococcus*. The *Bacteroides* perform saccharolytic and proteolytic functions and synthetize biotin, riboflavin, pantothenate, and ascorbate. The *Prevotella* enterotype is known for its role in degrading mucin glycoproteins, synthesizing thiamine and folate. The *Ruminococcus* enterotype is involved in mucin degradation and sugar membrane transportation. Normally all individuals have different percentages of enterotypes [5, 6]. Despite the great variability among individuals, some microbial members serve as the "core microbiota," while others function as a "flexible pool." The "core microbiota" ensures stability, while the "flexible pool" aids in host adaptation [7]. The flexible pool is typically acquired from diet, water, and environmental factors. There are exchanges of genetic material between core and flexible pool species that help the host adapt to environmental or dietary changes. Structurally, the microbiota is organized into mucosa-associated microbiota and luminal microbiota. The former contributes more to host cell protection and gut barrier function than the luminal, due to direct interaction with gut-associated lymphoid tissues [8]. Considering the different anatomical characteristics of the gut also the microbiome distribution is variable [9]. In the duodenum where there is a high concentration of bile acids, pancreatic secretions, and a fast transit of food there is a low bacterial density, primarily Firmicutes and Actinobacteria. In the jejunum, there is a wide bacterial colonization primarily represented by Gram positive aerobes and facultative anaerobes like Lactobacilli, Enterococci, and Streptococci. Near the ileo-cecal valve, there is a large number of anaerobes and Gram-negative bacteria; in this zone, the population starts to be similar as the colon one. The colon is the section of the gastrointestinal tract that harbors the highest concentration of bacteria, predominantly anaerobic species such as *Bacteroides*, *Bifidobacterium*, *Streptococcus*, Enterobacteriaceae, *Clostridium*, *Lactobacillus*, and *Ruminococcus* [10]. The human gastrointestinal tract is responsible for the digestion of the food consumed through the diet. Almost all the nutrients are digested by the host enzymes; however, the microbiome contributes to approximately 10% to 30% of energy intake. Some dietary fibers, like lignin, non-starch polysaccharides, resistant starch, and some oligosaccharides resist host enzymes but not those of the microbiome. Bacteroidetes and Firmicutes have genes encoding for glycoside hydrolase that can digest these polysaccharides [11]. In the gut, there is a continuous fermentation process where all the aliments consumed with the diet are transformed with the microbiome enzymes releasing gases, small chain fatty acids (SCFAs) (acetate, propionate, butyrate, valerate, isovalerate, and hexanoate), organic acids (lactate and succinate), and alcohols (methanol and ethanol) [11]. SCFAs are influenced by food intake. Primary producers of these SCAFs include *Roseburia* spp., *Eubacterium rectale*, *Faecalibacterium prausnitzii*, and various *Clostridium* species. After their production, these fatty acids are absorbed in the colon and can contribute up to 10% of the human caloric requirement [12]. SCFAs not only provide caloric energy, each molecule serves distinct functions within the body: acetate is primarily used by peripheral tissue and it plays a role in lipogenesis and cholesterol biosynthesis in the liver; butyrate is predominantly consumed by the colon cells, and it also has an endocrine function as it stimulates the secretion of leptin and glucagon like peptide-1 [13]. Additionally, over 90% of propionic acid is metabolized by the liver, where it serves as a substrate for lipogenesis, gluconeogenesis and protein synthesis.

Microbiota is essential for the digestion of nutrients that would otherwise remain nonabsorbable, while also contributes to maintenance of a healthy intestinal barrier. This is achieved through its ongoing interaction with the gut immune system which encompasses gut-associated lymphoid and Peyer's patches [12, 13].

18.3 Physiological Interaction Between Gut and Liver

The gut-liver axis and the liver-gut represent the bidirectional connections between the gastrointestinal tract, specifically the gut, and the liver. Anatomically, this connection is made by the portal vein which drains blood from the gastrointestinal tract to the liver and by the bile duct, which delivers bile acids from the liver into the gut. In this context, the role of the microbiota, the immune response to the microbiota, and the liver function are crucial to understand the presentation of potential pathological issues of the liver itself or the gut, as this is a two-way interaction (Fig. 18.1) [14].

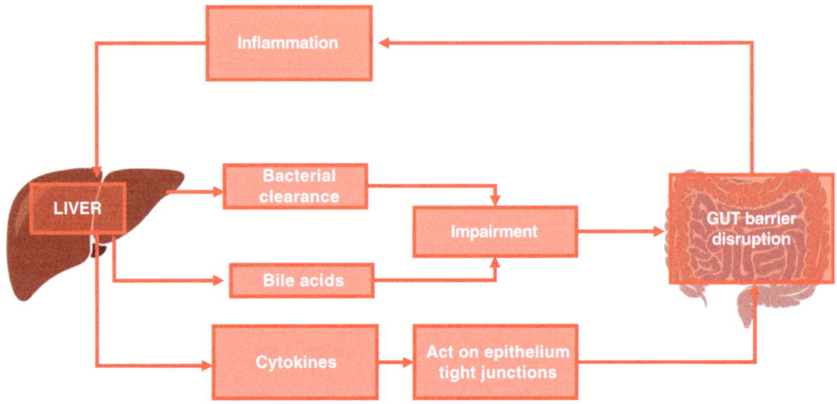

Fig. 18.1 Sepsis-induced liver injury on the gut

18.4 Gut-Liver Axis

When discussing the gut-liver axis, it is essential to consider the harmful effects of the microbiota. The LPS interacts with Toll-like receptors TLR, especially TLR 4, in both gut and liver cells (mostly in macrophages), leading to the production of inflammatory cytokines and inflammasomes. If the level of LPS exceeds the capacity of the liver to process it, the continued inflammatory stress may lead to liver diseases such as fibrosis. The amount of LPS that reaches the liver depends directly on the permeability of the intestinal barrier [15].

The intestinal barrier consists of a single epithelial layer that prevents LPS and other dangerous PAMPs from entering the bloodstream and throughout the portal system to reach the liver. The resistance of the barrier is maintained by tight junction proteins: intramembrane proteins [claudin, occludin, tricellulin, junctional adhesion molecule (JAM)] and intracellular connector proteins [zonula occludens (ZO), myosin light chain] link the tight junctions to the intracellular cytoskeleton [16, 17]. During sepsis, increased levels of cytokines can modulate intestinal permeability by regulating the expression of these proteins. The cytokines involved in the disequilibrium of the intestinal barrier are all the pro-inflammatory ones (TNF, IFNg, IL-6, and IL-1b), while IL-22 has a protective role in enhancing the barrier. The alteration of intestinal barrier function increases systemic inflammation through a positive feedback loop. Intestinal permeability and bacterial translocation are increased by cell apoptosis, reduction in villus height, and mucus layer thickness. It has been proven that the microbiota has a central role in maintaining the integrity of the barrier by producing SCFAs and improving the production of antimicrobial molecules by the gut-associated lymphoid tissue (GALT): Firmicutes and Bacteroidetes exert beneficial effects while Proteobacteria increase inflammation at the mucosal surface and impair the epithelial barrier in experimental models. It is clear how dysbiosis is a central issue in the permeability of the intestinal barrier. It has been proven that a high-fat diet may impair the epithelial barrier and increase endotoxemia. [16, 18]

Besides the direct influence through the increased concentration of LPS, the gut can influence the liver even with glucagon-like peptide-1 (GLP-1) and fibroblast growth factor 19 (FGF-19), secreted by the epithelial cells in the ileum and the colon. GLP-1 takes part in the control of glucose metabolism in the liver and in gastric emptying and satiety. FGF-19 participates in bile acid synthesis, lipid metabolism, and glucose liver metabolism. Its secretion is induced by bile acids representing a two-way interaction between gut and liver.

18.5 Liver-Gut Axis

In addition to the intestinal epithelial barrier, the liver is also an important line of defense against bacterial spread. Hepatocytes, B cells, and Kupffer cells can phagocytose pathogens that pass through the sinusoid cell layer. The intestine and local immune system work together to prevent intestinal bacteria from entering the portal vein [19]. Alterations in the reticulo-endothelial system, decreased complement production, and phagocytic activity of neutrophils impair the liver's ability to eliminate bacteria. Changes in the gut microbiota significantly impact the gut-liver axis. Intestinal dysbiosis directly aggravates the liver damage induced by sepsis, intensifying the systemic inflammatory response, altering intestinal microbial communities, causing hemodynamic instability and organ damage, and facilitating the translocation of bacteria and toxins [20].

In case of dysbiosis or another pathological problem that leads to increased translocation of LPS into the bloodstream, a gut-derived molecule can reduce inflammasome activation in the liver by binding LPS to macrophages. High-density lipoprotein 3, a gut-derived lipoprotein, can sequester LPS from the macrophages, disrupting the persistence of inflammatory stimuli [19].

Bile acids are synthesized in the liver by several enzymes from cholesterol. The primary bile acids, such as chenodeoxycholic acid (CDCA) and cholic acid (CA), are then bound to glycine to form acids such as taurocholic acid (TCA), taurochenodeoxycholic acid (TCDCA), glycocholic acid (GCA), and glycochenodeoxycholic acid (GCDCA) which are secreted, passing through the gallbladder, into the duodenum. In the gastrointestinal tract, bile acids have cleansing function, as they are amphipathic molecules that regulate the composition of the intestinal flora [21]. Bile acids have bactericidal properties and decrease intestinal permeability to endotoxins. The bactericidal qualities of bile are diminished by increased deconjugation of bile acids, which leads to the growth of bacteria that encourage further deconjugation of bile acids and, eventually, bacterial translocation and endotoxemia under homeostasis conditions [19].

About 95% of bile acids are reabsorbed by the distal ileum and return to liver by the portal circulation (enterohepatic cycle). The remaining bile acids are modified by the gut microbiome. Oxidation, deconjugation and epimerization are the main processes that transform bile acids into secondary products such as lithocholic acid (LCA) and deoxycholic acid (DCA) [21]. The bacteria mainly involved in these processes are *Bacteroides*, *Clostridium*, *Lactobacillus*, *Bifidobacterium*, and

Listeria. Most of these secondary bile acids are reabsorbed and transported to the liver, while a few unabsorbed are eliminated with feces. The absorption of bile acids in the distal ileum is a sodium-dependent system. Bile acids are key signaling molecules which have an indirect role in the homeostasis of gut microbiome; they alter signaling through receptors by metabolizing bile acids. Farnesoid X receptor (FXR) is a nuclear receptor involved in the reduction of inflammasome and cholestasis [13]. Another important receptor induced by bile acids is TGR-5, a G protein-coupled receptor expressed on many types of cells. Its effect is to induce secretion of GLP-1, insulin, improve peristalsis, reduce NF-κB, and regulate immunity and inflammation. There are other minor receptors of bile acids such as sphingosine-1-phosphate-receptor-2 (S1PR2), involved in inflammation and fibrosis. Other factors regulated by bile acids in the gut and the liver are vitamin D receptor (VDR), pregnane X receptor (PXR), and retinoic acid-related orphan receptor (ROR γt). During liver dysfunction, the increased bile acid levels activate inflammatory and oxidative stress and result in apoptosis, necrosis, fibrosis, and cirrhosis [22–24].

18.6 Therapeutic Implications

Sepsis-induced liver injury involves a complex interplay of inflammatory cascades, immune cell activation, and microcirculatory dysfunction. The liver, a central organ in immune regulation and host defense, is particularly vulnerable to the systemic inflammatory response triggered by sepsis. This response often leads to significant alterations in hepatic microcirculation, characterized by impaired sinusoidal perfusion, leukocyte adhesion, and increased vascular permeability. The inflammatory milieu of sepsis promotes the release of various mediators, including cytokines, chemokines, and reactive oxygen species, which contribute to endothelial dysfunction and disruption of the hepatic microvascular barrier. This disruption facilitates the extravasation of fluid and inflammatory cells into the liver parenchyma, worsening tissue edema and inflammation. Furthermore, activated neutrophils and other immune cells adhere to the sinusoidal endothelium, obstructing blood flow and further compromising oxygen delivery to hepatocytes. This impaired microcirculation contributes to hepatocellular hypoxia and subsequent necrosis, ultimately driving liver dysfunction and failure [25].

Table 18.1 Therapeutic strategies for sepsis via the gut-liver axis

Therapeutic target	Intervention strategies	Potential benefits
Restoring intestinal barrier integrity	Tight junction modulators, probiotics, prebiotics, fecal microbiota transplantation	Reduced bacterial translocation, decreased inflammation
Modulating the gut microbiome	Probiotics, prebiotics, antibiotics, fecal microbiota transplantation	Restoration of healthy gut microbiota, reduced production of harmful bacterial products
Targeting hepatic inflammation and immune cell activation	Anti-inflammatory agents, immunomodulators	Mitigation of liver inflammation and immune cell activation
Improving hepatic microcirculation	Vasodilators, fluid resuscitation, anti-thrombotic agents	Improved blood flow and oxygen delivery to hepatocytes

The interplay between the gut and the liver plays a crucial role in sepsis-induced liver injury. Increased intestinal permeability, a hallmark of sepsis, allows translocation of bacteria and their products into the portal circulation, exposing the liver to a significant inflammatory burden. This gut-derived inflammation further amplifies the hepatic inflammatory response and contributes to microcirculatory dysfunction. Therapeutic strategies targeting the hepatic microcirculation and gut-liver axis hold promise for mitigating sepsis-induced liver injury. These strategies include interventions aimed at restoring endothelial barrier function, reducing leukocyte adhesion, and improving sinusoidal perfusion [26]. Modulation of the gut microbiome and enhancement of intestinal barrier integrity may also prove beneficial in attenuating the inflammatory burden on the liver (Table 18.1).

Table 18.2 provides an in-depth overview of innovative therapeutic approaches for managing sepsis. These strategies target key pathological mechanisms, including epithelial barrier integrity, modulation of the gut microbiome, and systemic inflammation. Evidence from experimental models and clinical studies highlights their potential efficacy, while limitations and risks are also addressed. The table includes detailed mechanisms of action, supporting scientific evidence, and relevant references for further exploration.

Further research is needed to fully elucidate the complex mechanisms underlying sepsis-induced liver injury and to develop effective therapeutic interventions.

Table 18.2 Emerging therapies for sepsis via the gut-liver axis

Therapy	Mechanism of action	Scientific evidence	References
Epithelial barrier-targeting therapy	Regulation of claudin-2-dependent paracellular channels and tight junction (TJ) gating; inhibition of miR-155 to reduce inflammation	Claudin-2 regulation may have therapeutic potential for epithelial barrier failure inhibition of miR-155 alleviates inflammation and improves intestinal barrier function in sepsis-induced mice	[26, 27]
Probiotics	Live nonpathogenic microorganisms that keep the intestinal barrier, inhibit bacterial translocation, and prevent infections	A meta-analysis confirmed the efficacy of probiotics in preventing infections however, genomic studies in ICU patients linked probiotics to cases of bacteremia due to microbial transfer from the capsule to the bloodstream	[28, 29]
Prebiotics	Indigestible dietary components promote the growth of beneficial gut microbiota	Cellulose supplementation partially reduces systemic inflammation and improves survival in murine sepsis models	[30, 31]
Fecal microbiota transplantation (FMT)	Restores systemic immunity and enhances pathogen clearance; associated with the spread of butyrate-producing *Bacteroidetes*	FMT rescues mice from lethal sepsis caused by human pathogensdonor screening is crucial to prevent the transmission of harmful infections, and patient-specific benefits and risks need to be carefully evaluated	[32]
Absorbent materials	Remove enterogenic toxins and bacterial products to prevent their entry into systemic circulation and the liver	Cation-exchange resins effectively treat hyperkalemia and hyperphosphatemia Nonabsorbable nanoporous carbon reduces portal vein pressure and liver biomarkers in bile duct-ligated rats, decreasing endotoxin-induced Kupffer cell activation	[33–35]
HDL as a potential therapy	Neutralizes lipopolysaccharides (LPS) and accelerates their clearance via SR-BI receptors; apolipoproteins remove endotoxins	Studies show HDL reduces endotoxin-induced tissue damage in the lung, liver, and intestinelow HDL and Apo AI levels in severe sepsis patients are associated with increased mortality, prolonged ICU stay, and hospital-acquired infectionsreconstituted HDL improves survival in animal models	[36–44]

18.7 Conclusions

Sepsis even nowadays has a high impact on public health because of its high mortality, morbidity, and costs. It is a systemic condition that involves the GI tract and liver. During sepsis, the tight junctions and all the GI barrier complex are stressed and loosen, allowing pro-inflammatory products to enter the portal circulation.

Once in the portal vein, the PAMPs reach the liver, where inflammation is exacerbated by the local immune cells as Kupffer cells, macrophage, LSEC, and the circulating immune cells attracted by the pro-inflammatory cytokines. The net result is liver damage with the production of DAMPs and increased inflammation, leading to greater stress and higher permeability of the gastrointestinal barrier. Stopping this vicious cycle must be a primary goal for physicians. Unfortunately, the mechanisms that drive and maintain the hyperpermeability of the gastrointestinal barrier are still partially unknown.

Currently, there are some therapeutic proposals that aim to modulate the hyperpermeability of the gastrointestinal barrier in pathological conditions. One approach targets Claudin 2 due to its role in modulating paracellular permeability influencing tight junctions [26]. Another logical target is the gut microbiome. Recent evidence suggests that favoring the predominance of the "good" bacteria in the gut might have a protective role in sepsis. To enhance the presence of bacteria such as *Bacteroides*, we can use probiotics, or lately, a new strategy is fecal microbial transplantation. Other strategies involve the use of absorbent materials to prevent PAMPs from entering the portal bloodstream.

High-density lipoproteins may improve prognosis in septic patients because of their ability to bind LPS and induce its degradation through metabolic pathways that do not stimulate, or stimulate to a lesser extent, inflammasome activation [19].

The mechanisms underlying the entire crosstalk between gut and liver are still partially unknown. It is clear that this interaction plays an important role during sepsis, but further research is needed to fully understand the pathophysiology and identify potential interventions.

References

1. Yan J, Li S, Li S. The role of the liver in sepsis. Int Rev Immunol. 2014;33(6):498–510.
2. An L, Wirth U, Koch D, Schirren M, Drefs M, Koliogiannis D, Nieß H, Andrassy J, Guba M, Bazhin AV, Werner J, Kühn F. The role of gut-derived lipopolysaccharides and the intestinal barrier in fatty liver diseases. J Gastrointest Surg. 2022;26(3):671–83.
3. Rodrigues SG, van der Merwe S, Krag A, Wiest R. Gut-liver axis: pathophysiological concepts and medical perspective in chronic liver diseases. Semin Immunol. 2024;71:101859.
4. Sun J, Zhang J, Wang X, Ji F, Ronco C, Tian J, Yin Y. Gut-liver crosstalk in sepsis-induced liver injury. Crit Care. 2020;24(1):614.
5. Adak A, Khan MR. An insight into gut microbiota and its functionalities. Cell Mol Life Sci. 2019;76:473–93.
6. Konturek PC, Harsch IA, Konturek K, Schink M, Konturek T, Neurath MF, Zopf Y. Gut⁻liver axis: how do gut bacteria influence the liver? Med Sci (Basel). 2018;6(3):79.
7. McNally L, Brown SP. Microbiome: ecology of stable gut communities. Nat Microbiol. 2016;1:15016.
8. Brahe LK, Astrup A, Larsen LH. Can we prevent obesity-related metabolic diseases by dietary modulation of the gut microbiota? Adv Nutr. 2016;7(1):90–101.
9. Shapira M. Gut microbiotas and host evolution: scaling up symbiosis. Trends Ecol Evol. 2016;31(7):539–49.
10. Hollister EB, Gao C, Versalovic J. Compositional and functional features of the gastrointestinal microbiome and their effects on human health. Gastroenterology. 2014;146(6):1449–58.

11. Duncan SH, Belenguer A, Holtrop G, Johnstone AM, Flint HJ, Lobley GE. Reduced dietary intake of carbohydrates by obese subjects results in decreased concentrations of butyrate and butyrate-producing bacteria in feces. Appl Environ Microbiol. 2007;73(4):1073–8.
12. Donohoe DR, Garge N, Zhang X, Sun W, O'Connell TM, Bunger MK, Bultman SJ. The microbiome and butyrate regulate energy metabolism and autophagy in the mammalian colon. Cell Metab. 2011;13(5):517–26.
13. Nicholson JK, Holmes E, Kinross J, Burcelin R, Gibson G, Jia W, Pettersson S. Host-gut microbiota metabolic interactions. Science. 2012;336(6086):1262–7.
14. Brandl K, Kumar V, Eckmann L. Gut-liver axis at the frontier of host-microbial interactions. Am J Physiol Gastrointest Liver Physiol. 2017;312(5):G413–9.
15. Peterson LW, Artis D. Intestinal epithelial cells: regulators of barrier function and immune homeostasis. Nat Rev Immunol. 2014;14(3):141–53.
16. Tilg H, Adolph TE, Trauner M. Gut-liver axis: pathophysiological concepts and clinical implications. Cell Metab. 2022;34(11):1700–18.
17. Yan M, Man S, Sun B, Ma L, Guo L, Huang L, Gao W. Gut liver brain axis in diseases: the implications for therapeutic interventions. Signal Transduct Target Ther. 2023;8(1):443.
18. Dumitru A, Matei E, Cozaru GC, Chisoi A, Alexandrescu L, Popescu RC, Butcaru MP, Dumitru E, Rugină S, Tocia C. Endotoxin inflammatory action on cells by dysregulated-immunological-barrier-linked ROS-apoptosis mechanisms in gut-liver axis. Int J Mol Sci. 2024;25(5):2472.
19. Zhang X, Liu H, Hashimoto K, Yuan S, Zhang J. The gut-liver axis in sepsis: interaction mechanisms and therapeutic potential. Crit Care. 2022;26(1):213.
20. Albillos A, Lario M, Álvarez-Mon M. Cirrhosis-associated immune dysfunction: distinctive features and clinical relevance. J Hepatol. 2014;61(6):1385–96.
21. Dawson PA, Karpen SJ. Intestinal transport and metabolism of bile acids. J Lipid Res. 2015;56(6):1085–99.
22. Burg N, Salmon JE, Hla T. Sphingosine 1-phosphate receptor-targeted therapeutics in rheumatic diseases. Nat Rev Rheumatol. 2022;18:335–51.
23. Poland JC, Flynn CR. Bile acids, their receptors, and the gut microbiota. Physiology (Bethesda). 2021;36(4):235–45.
24. Carazo A, Mladěnka P, Pávek P. Marine ligands of the Pregnane X receptor (PXR): an overview. Mar Drugs. 2019;17(10):554.
25. Jaeschke H. Reactive oxygen and mechanisms of inflammatory liver injury: present concepts. J Gastroenterol Hepatol. 2011;26(Suppl 1):173–9.
26. Weber CR, Liang GH, Wang Y, Das S, Shen L, Yu AS, et al. Claudin-2-dependent paracellular channels are dynamically gated. elife. 2015;4:e9906.
27. Cao Y, Wang Z, Wang Z, Jiang X, Lu W. Inhibition of miR-155 alleviates sepsis-induced inflammation and intestinal barrier dysfunction by inactivating NF-κB signaling. Int Immunopharmacol. 2021;90:107218.
28. Manzanares W, Lemieux M, Langlois PL, Wischmeyer PE. Probiotic and synbiotic therapy in critical illness: a systematic review and meta-analysis. Crit Care. 2016;20:262.
29. Yelin I, Flett KB, Merakou C, Mehrotra P, Stam J, Snesrud E, et al. Genomic and epidemiological evidence of bacterial transmission from probiotic capsule to blood in ICU patients. Nat Med. 2019;25:1728–32.
30. Everard A, Lazarevic V, Derrien M, Girard M, Muccioli GG, Neyrinck AM, et al. Responses of gut microbiota and glucose and lipid metabolism to prebiotics in genetic obese and diet-induced leptin-resistant mice. Diabetes. 2011;60:2775–86.
31. Morowitz MJ, Di Caro V, Pang D, Cummings J, Firek B, Rogers MB, et al. Dietary supplementation with nonfermentable fiber alters the gut microbiota and confers protection in murine models of sepsis. Crit Care Med. 2017;45:e516–23.
32. Kim SM, DeFazio JR, Hyoju SK, Sangani K, Keskey R, Krezalek MA, et al. Fecal microbiota transplant rescues mice from human pathogen mediated sepsis by restoring systemic immunity. Nat Commun. 2020;11:2354.

33. Sterns RH, Grieff M, Bernstein PL. Treatment of hyperkalemia: something old, something new. Kidney Int. 2016;89:546–54.
34. Macnaughtan J, Soeda J, Mouralidarane A, Sandeman S, Howell C, Kozynchenko O, et al. PMO-127 biological effects of oral nanoporous carbon in bile duct ligated rats. Gut. 2012;61:A124.
35. Macnaughtan J, Soeda J, Mouralidarane A, Sandeman S, Howell C, Milkhalovsky S, et al. PMO-128 Effects of oral nanoporous carbon therapy in leptin null mice as a model of non-alcoholic steatohepatitis. Gut. 2012;61:A121–5.
36. Morin EE, Guo L, Schwendeman A, Li X. HDL in sepsis—risk factor and therapeutic approach. Front Pharmacol. 2015;6:244.
37. Flegel WA, Baumstark MW, Weinstock C, Berg A, Northoff H. Prevention of endotoxin-induced monokine release by human low- and high-density lipoproteins and by apolipoprotein A-I. Infect Immun. 1993;61:5140–6.
38. de Bont N, Netea MG, Demacker PN, Verschueren I, Kullberg BJ, van Dijk KW, et al. Apolipoprotein E knock-out mice are highly susceptible to endotoxemia and Klebsiella pneumoniae infection. J Lipid Res. 1999;40:680–5.
39. Van Oosten M, Rensen PCN, Van Amersfoort ES, Van Eck M, Van Dam A, Brevé JJP, et al. Apolipoprotein E protects against bacterial lipopolysaccharide-induced lethality. J Biol Chem. 2001;276:8820–4.
40. Berbee JF, van der Hoogt CC, Kleemann R, Schippers EF, Kitchens RL, van Dissel JT, et al. Apolipoprotein CI stimulates the response to lipopolysaccharide and reduces mortality in gram-negative sepsis. FASEB J. 2006;20:2162–4.
41. Thompson PA, Berbee JF, Rensen PC, Kitchens RL. Apolipoprotein A-II augments monocyte responses to LPS by suppressing the inhibitory activity of LPS-binding protein. Innate Immun. 2008;14:365–74.
42. Chien J, Jerng J, Yu C, Yang P. Low serum level of high-density lipoprotein cholesterol is a poor prognostic factor for severe sepsis. Crit Care Med. 2005;33:1688–93.
43. McDonald MC, Dhadly P, Cockerill GW, Cuzzocrea S, Mota-Filipe H, Hinds CJ, et al. Renstituted high-density lipoprotein attenuates organ injury and adhesion molecule expression in a rodent model of endotoxic shock. Shock. 2003;20:551–7.
44. Tanaka S, Genève C, Zappella N, Yong-Sang J, Planesse C, Louedec L, et al. Reconstituted high-density lipoprotein therapy improves survival in mouse models of sepsis. Anesthesiology. 2020;132:825–38.

Muscle-Liver Crosstalk and Sarcopenia 19

David Pérez-Torres and Isabel Canas-Pérez

The preservation of homeostatic equilibrium within skeletal muscle tissue necessitates intricate interplay among various organs, environmental stimuli, and nutritional inputs. Perturbations in the interorgan communication dynamics linking skeletal muscle tissue and the liver can yield noteworthy repercussions on the individual, exhibiting both advantageous and adverse outcomes. This chapter aims to delineate the principal modalities of inter-organ communication, explaining their intricate associations with sarcopenia.

19.1 The Skeletal Muscle as a Secretory Organ

Skeletal muscle cells are highly specialized in the conversion of chemical energy into mechanical energy, predominantly for locomotion, facilitated by the utilization of adenosine triphosphate (ATP) to generate force or execute work. In individuals with optimal physical conditioning, skeletal muscle typically comprises approximately 30–40% of total body weight [20]. An emerging body of evidence underscores the endocrine role of skeletal muscle tissue, positing it as a secretory organ [34]. These secreted molecules are collectively referred to as myokines when their release is contingent upon muscle contraction, or as exerkines when elicited in response to exercise stimuli. The repertoire of myokines encompasses a diverse array of molecules including metabolites, hormones, cytokines, proteins, and nucleic acids, which manifest physiological effects on distal organs such as the liver and adipose tissue. Importantly, alterations in physical activity, metabolic

D. Pérez-Torres (✉) · I. Canas-Pérez
Servicio de Medicina Intensiva, Hospital Universitario Río Hortega, Gerencia Regional de Salud de Castilla y León (SACYL), Valladolid, Spain
e-mail: dperezt@saludcastillayleon.es; icanasp@saludcastillayleon.es

D. Battaglini et al. (eds.), *Organ System Crosstalk in Critical Illness*,
https://doi.org/10.1007/978-3-032-01024-7_19

disturbances, and dietary modifications occurring in critical illness can markedly influence the profile of myokine secretion [46].

19.2 The Central Role of the Liver in Metabolism

The liver serves as the primary site for processing most nutrients absorbed in the gastrointestinal tract, including carbohydrates, lipids, and proteins.

With respect to carbohydrate metabolism, the liver assumes the pivotal role of converting sugars into glucose via gluconeogenesis, while concurrently acting as a reservoir for glucose, storing excess amounts as glycogen during postprandial intervals. Subsequently, during periods of heightened energy demand, the liver facilitates the release of stored glucose into the bloodstream to meet metabolic exigencies.

Additionally, the liver actively engages in lipid metabolism, predominantly through the oxidation of fatty acids, thereby furnishing energy substrates for various physiological processes. Hepatocytes orchestrate the synthesis of lipids from intermediary products of carbohydrate metabolism and participate in the biosynthesis of lipoproteins, cholesterol, and phospholipids.

Concerning protein metabolism, the liver demonstrates remarkable versatility, being proficient in the synthesis of non-essential amino acids and orchestrating the deamination of amino acids, thereby yielding by-products conducive to carbohydrate synthesis, particularly under conditions of severe energy deficit. Moreover, the liver serves as the primary site for the synthesis of a vast array of plasma proteins, with the notable exception of immunoglobulins. Importantly, the liver plays a pivotal role in the metabolism of ammonia, a by-product of protein catabolism, converting it into urea for subsequent excretion via the renal route.

Nowadays, the liver is acknowledged as an endocrine entity capable of secreting hepatokines, thereby facilitating bidirectional intercommunication with various tissues. Dysregulation in the signaling pathways mediated by specific hepatokines has been implicated in the pathogenesis of conditions including insulin resistance, obesity, and metabolic dysfunction-associated steatotic liver disease (MASLD) [15].

19.3 Proteins as a Linking Element Between the Skeletal Muscle and the Liver

Roughly three-quarters of the body's solid constituents are comprised of proteins, serving diverse roles including structural support, enzymatic catalysis, and facilitation of transport processes, alongside their involvement in nucleoprotein synthesis and mediation of muscle contraction. Despite their intrinsic energetic potential, proteins are not typically utilized as a primary substrate for energy production under basal physiological conditions, undergoing degradation solely in scenarios where carbohydrates and lipids are insufficiently available.

Upon ingestion, the process of protein digestion and subsequent absorption unfolds gradually over a span of approximately 2–3 hours, culminating in a modest elevation in circulating amino acid levels. Subsequently, these amino acids undergo rapid cellular uptake, with hepatocytes being the primary beneficiaries of this influx within the bloodstream.

In the absence of exogenous protein intake, a portion of the body's protein reservoir undergoes continual degradation, resulting in the liberation of amino acids, subsequent deamination, and oxidation, in a process that is collectively termed obligatory nitrogen losses. To mitigate this phenomenon, critically ill patients are advised to receive a protein intake of approximately 1.3 grams per kilogram of body weight per day, a recommendation advocated by the European Society for Clinical Nutrition and Metabolism (ESPEN) [42, 43]. Notably, some studies have demonstrated a correlation between adherence to such protein intake guidelines and improved survival outcomes among critically ill patients [51].

19.4 Hormonal Liver-Muscle Crosstalk

Several hormones exert significant effects on protein metabolism, with implications for both skeletal muscle and hepatic function.

Insulin facilitates the transportation of amino acids into cells, thereby stimulating protein synthesis. Additionally, it mitigates protein degradation and enhances cellular glucose availability, thereby exerting a protein-sparing effect. Insulin deficiency or resistance, as observed in critically ill patients, can severely limit protein synthesis.

Glucocorticoids promote protein degradation primarily through the ubiquitin-proteasome system and lysosomal autophagy pathways, leading to muscle atrophy. They also hinder the synthesis of new myofibrillar proteins by inhibiting translation initiation. Furthermore, glucocorticoids act antagonistically to hormones with anabolic properties, exacerbating protein and muscle mass loss [5]. The resultant increase in plasma amino acid concentration may stimulate the synthesis of hepatic and plasma proteins.

Growth hormone stimulates protein synthesis at the tissue level, although the precise mechanism remains incompletely understood. It is believed that growth hormone may facilitate DNA and RNA transcription and translation processes, thereby promoting protein synthesis.

Testosterone is known to promote protein deposition in body tissues, particularly in muscles [47]. The effect of testosterone appears to diminish over time compared to growth hormone. Despite its initial efficacy, testosterone's impact on protein metabolism may wane with prolonged exposure.

19.5 The Concept of Sarcopenia

Sarcopenia is a generalized, progressive disease of skeletal muscle characterized by a rapid loss of muscle mass and function. While it is commonly associated with aging (primary sarcopenia), it can also stem from other significant factors such as systemic diseases, physical inactivity, or malnutrition (secondary sarcopenia). Identifying sarcopenia in clinical practice can be challenging and typically necessitates the presence of low muscle strength, diminished muscle quality or quantity, and impaired physical performance. Given its association with adverse outcomes such as falls, functional decline, frailty, and mortality, some experts regard sarcopenia as an organ failure, specifically referring to it as muscle failure [7, 8, 41].

19.6 The Delicate Balance Between Muscle Tissue Synthesis and Degradation

Skeletal muscle exhibits remarkable plasticity, allowing its mass to dynamically fluctuate in response to various physiological and pathological conditions. In scenarios characterized by reduced muscular activity, such as during hospitalization, the rate of degradation of contractile proteins surpasses that of synthesis, leading to a net loss of muscle mass, a phenomenon commonly referred to as muscle wasting [3]. The findings from a recent meta-analysis underscore the severity of muscle loss among critically ill patients, with an estimated decline of nearly 2% of skeletal muscle mass per day within the initial week of intensive care unit (ICU) admission [9]. Paradoxically, proteolysis plays a crucial role in averting cellular damage and the progression of certain diseases.

The ubiquitin-proteasome system (UPS) serves as the principal proteolytic pathway accountable for the degradation of muscle proteins [18]. The pathogenesis of sarcopenia encompasses a multitude of molecular dysregulations that, cumulatively, promote the UPS activity. Regulation of this system is intricately governed by various signaling pathways, notably including Smad, nuclear factor kappa-light-chain-enhancer of activated B cells (NF-κB), and forkhead box protein O (FoxO).

Hypercatabolic states, fasting, or denervation provoke an escalation in the UPS activity. Moreover, the UPS can undergo rapid activation triggered by various signaling pathways, including transforming growth factor-beta (TGF-β) or the myostatin/activin system (via Smad), pro-inflammatory cytokines (via NF-κB), or glucocorticoids (via FoxO). Disturbances in insulin/insulin-like growth factor-1 (IGF-1) signaling or androgen deficiency downregulate the phosphoinositide 3-kinase (PI3K)/Akt pathway, consequently upregulating FoxO, thereby enhancing the UPS activity [10, 24].

Autophagy represents a pivotal pathway involved in protein degradation, facilitating the removal of redundant or damaged cellular constituents. Typically, under basal conditions in healthy individuals, autophagy exhibits minimal activity. However, in response to both endogenous and exogenous stressors, such as starvation or oxidative stress, autophagy is activated, thereby contributing to muscle wasting [18]. Depending on the nature of substrates transported into lysosomes, autophagy is categorized into macroautophagy, microautophagy, and chaperone-mediated autophagy [27]. The regulation of autophagy is intricate, with pathways such as AMP-activated protein kinase (AMPK)/mTOR and Akt/mTOR playing crucial roles [48]. While autophagy and the UPS were initially perceived as independent pathways, current evidence underscores the presence of crosstalk between them [31].

Autophagy plays a critical protective role against sarcopenia by regulating satellite cell regeneration, mitigating oxidative stress, and dampening inflammatory responses. Consequently, inhibition of autophagy is frequently observed in individuals with sarcopenia, and such inhibition appears to exacerbate the progression of sarcopenia development [48].

19.7 Muscle-Liver Crosstalk Via Myokines

The skeletal muscle communicates with various tissues and organs through the secretion of myokines. These molecules play a pivotal role in conveying crucial information regarding the metabolic state of skeletal muscle. Myokines have attracted considerable interest owing to their involvement in conditions such as insulin resistance, obesity, and other metabolic disorders. Below, we describe some of the most relevant ones.

19.7.1 Interleukin 6 (IL-6)

At the onset of the twenty-first century, it was revealed that muscle tissue releases factors into the bloodstream during contraction, thereby mediating some of the effects of physical activity on distant organs such as the liver or adipose tissue. Interleukin 6 (IL-6) emerged as the first molecule attributed to this behavior, thus earning the distinction of being the first described myokine [33, 36]. Despite its well-documented pro-inflammatory activity in syndromes prevalent in Intensive Care Medicine, such as sepsis or acute respiratory distress syndrome, IL-6 also assumes significant physiological and anti-inflammatory roles [23], particularly in its capacity as a myokine, wherein it inhibits the production of tumor necrosis factor (TNF) [35].

The expression of the IL-6 gene is swiftly activated during physical activity, a response that is further potentiated as muscle glycogen stores are depleted [21], thereby facilitating myogenic differentiation at the muscular level [12]. Metabolically, IL-6 promotes glucose uptake by muscle by facilitating GLUT4 transporter translocation [32] and stimulates hepatic glucose production by activating gluconeogenesis through induction of phosphoenolpyruvate carboxykinase (PEPCK) expression [1]. Additionally, IL-6 enhances fatty acid oxidation in skeletal muscle and adipose tissue by activating AMP-activated protein kinase (AMPK) [39]. Lastly, certain studies have indicated that IL-6 may interfere with insulin signaling and perturb glucose homeostasis via the JNK1, STAT3, and SOCS3 pathways [17, 40, 45].

19.7.2 Irisin

Muscular physical activity triggers the upregulation of the transcriptional coactivator PGC1α, which orchestrates a plethora of biological pathways crucial for energy metabolism and the beneficial outcomes associated with muscular exercise. These pathways include mitochondrial biogenesis, angiogenesis, and fiber-type switching [11]. Irisin, a hormone generated through the proteolysis of a type I membrane protein encoded by the Fndc5 gene, is activated by PGC1α [4]. Irisin exerts profound effects on hepatic metabolism, where it mitigates insulin resistance by suppressing gluconeogenesis and promoting glycogenesis through the PI3K/Akt/FoxO1 pathway in hepatocytes [37]. Furthermore, irisin demonstrates notable effects on adipose tissue by inducing the conversion of white adipocytes into beige cells, thereby enhancing energy expenditure and fostering weight loss [6].

19.7.3 Interleukin 15

Interleukin 15 (IL-15), a member of the IL-2 superfamily, stands out as one of the myokines released by skeletal muscle fibers in response to exercise, primarily exerting anabolic effects [28]. Among its diverse functions, IL-15 enhances glucose uptake in skeletal muscle by activating the JAK3/STAT3 pathway, thereby facilitating GLUT4 translocation. Moreover, it stimulates the activity of PGC1α, thereby promoting beneficial metabolic outcomes such as mitochondrial biogenesis and fatty acid oxidation in skeletal muscle [25]. Additionally, IL-15 plays a pivotal role in mediating crosstalk with adipose tissue, where it demonstrates the ability to reduce visceral fat without affecting lean body mass or perturbing signaling by other cytokines in animal models [38].

19.8 Liver-Muscle Crosstalk Via Hepatokines

The liver communicates with multiple organs through the production of hepatokines, which are essential for transmitting information about the liver's metabolic status. Numerous molecules with hepatokine functions have been described, and many of them have been associated with insulin resistance, obesity, and other diseases. Some of the more relevant ones are described in the next paragraphs.

19.8.1 Insulin-Like Growth Factor Hormone (IGF-1)

Insulin-like growth factor hormone (IGF-1) is synthesized in both the liver, where it functions as a systemic agent, and skeletal muscle, where it exerts autocrine and paracrine actions [24]. This dual role as a hepatokine and a myokine stimulates anabolic processes via the PI3K/Akt/mTOR pathway, thereby promoting muscle hypertrophy [50]. It is well-established that IGF-1 levels decline with age, consequently increasing the risk of developing sarcopenia [26]. Impairment of IGF-1 signaling is commonly observed in conditions associated with sarcopenia, leading to muscle atrophy [2]. It has also been hypothesized that intestinal microbiota may have role in sarcopenia, given that short-chain fatty acids produced by the gut microbiota are essential modulators of IGF-1 synthesis [49].

19.8.2 Fetuin-A

Fetuin-A, also referred to as α2-HS-glycoprotein, is a molecule synthesized by the liver and adipose tissue [44], functioning as a natural inhibitor of insulin receptor tyrosine kinase activity. This glycoprotein promotes a pro-inflammatory milieu through various mechanisms, including its interaction with toll-like receptor (TLR) 4, which mediates the induction of a pro-inflammatory state and insulin resistance by saturated fatty acids [30]. Implicated in the pathophysiology of several conditions, including sarcopenia, obesity, sarcopenic obesity, type 2 diabetes mellitus, and non-alcoholic fatty liver disease, fetuin-A underscores its multifaceted role in metabolic regulation [24].

19.8.3 Leukocyte-Derived Chemotaxin-2 (LECT2)

Leukocyte-derived chemotaxin-2 (LECT2), also recognized as chondromodulin-2, was initially characterized as a chemotactic factor for neutrophils. Despite its notable local anti-inflammatory and antitumor properties, LECT2 serves as a hepatokine capable of influencing skeletal muscle tissue [16]. LECT2 exerts detrimental effects on insulin action by activating c-Jun N-terminal kinase (JNK) in skeletal muscle and diminishes energy expenditure by modulating myogenesis [19]. Consequently, these actions culminate in a state of insulin resistance and sarcopenic obesity, a common manifestation observed in individuals with diabetes mellitus.

19.8.4 Fibroblast Growth Factor-21

Recent research indicates that fibroblast growth factor-21 (FGF21), functioning as both a myokine and hepatokine, exerts a significant influence on glucose and lipid metabolism. In animal models, it has demonstrated the ability to prevent diet-induced obesity and reduce levels of glucose, triglycerides, cholesterol, insulin, and glucagon in diabetes models [13]. In humans, FGF21 stimulates glucose uptake by enhancing GLUT1 expression in skeletal muscle [22]. Moreover, it activates the PI3K/AKT1 signaling pathway, promoting muscle hypertrophy and fat loss, thereby improving overall metabolism [14]. Both exercise and insulin administration have been shown to elevate muscular FGF21 secretion [13]. Low concentrations of FGF21 have been associated with sarcopenia and obesity due to its direct impact on muscle mass and its interaction with irisin [29].

19.9 Conclusions

This chapter elucidates the intricate interplay between skeletal muscle tissue and the liver, emphasizing the pivotal role of inter-organ communication in maintaining homeostatic equilibrium. Skeletal muscle, once perceived solely as a contractile apparatus, is now recognized as a multifaceted secretory organ, releasing myokines and exerkines that modulate various physiological processes in distal organs such as the liver and adipose tissue. Conversely, the liver, traditionally acknowledged for its metabolic functions, emerges as an endocrine entity capable of secreting hepatokines, thereby establishing bidirectional communication with skeletal muscle and other tissues. Perturbations in this communication network can precipitate adverse outcomes, including sarcopenia, insulin resistance, obesity, and other diseases. Understanding the molecular mechanisms underlying these interactions holds promise for the development of targeted therapeutic interventions aimed at ameliorating metabolic disorders and enhancing overall health outcomes.

References

1. Banzet S, Koulmann N, Simler N, et al. Control of gluconeogenic genes during intense/prolonged exercise: hormone-independent effect of muscle-derived IL-6 on hepatic tissue and PEPCK mRNA. J Appl Physiol. 2009;107:1830–9. https://doi.org/10.1152/JAPPLPHYSIOL.00739.2009.
2. Bilski J, Pierzchalski P, Szczepanik M, et al. Multifactorial mechanism of sarcopenia and sarcopenic obesity. Role of physical exercise, microbiota and myokines. Cells. 2022;11 https://doi.org/10.3390/CELLS11010160.
3. Bloch S, Polkey MI, Griffiths M, Kemp P. Molecular mechanisms of intensive care unit-acquired weakness. Eur Respir J. 2012;39:1000–11. https://doi.org/10.1183/09031936.00090011.
4. Boström P, Wu J, Jedrychowski MP, et al. A PGC1-α-dependent myokine that drives brown-fat-like development of white fat and thermogenesis. Nature. 2012;481:463–8. https://doi.org/10.1038/NATURE10777.
5. Braun TP, Marks DL. The regulation of muscle mass by endogenous glucocorticoids. Front Physiol. 2015;6 https://doi.org/10.3389/FPHYS.2015.00012.
6. Castillo-Quan JI. From white to brown fat through the PGC-1α-dependent myokine irisin: implications for diabetes and obesity. Dis Model Mech. 2012;5:293–5. https://doi.org/10.1242/DMM.009894.
7. Cruz-Jentoft AJ, Sayer AA. Sarcopenia. Lancet (London, England). 2019;393:2636–46. https://doi.org/10.1016/S0140-6736(19)31138-9.
8. Cruz-Jentoft AJ, Bahat G, Bauer J, et al. Sarcopenia: revised European consensus on definition and diagnosis. Age Ageing. 2019;48:16–31. https://doi.org/10.1093/AGEING/AFY169.
9. Fazzini B, Märkl T, Costas C, et al. The rate and assessment of muscle wasting during critical illness: a systematic review and meta-analysis. Crit Care. 2023;27 https://doi.org/10.1186/S13054-022-04253-0.
10. Han HQ, Zhou X, Mitch WE, Goldberg AL. Myostatin/activin pathway antagonism: molecular basis and therapeutic potential. Int J Biochem Cell Biol. 2013;45:2333–47. https://doi.org/10.1016/J.BIOCEL.2013.05.019.
11. Handschin C, Spiegelman BM. The role of exercise and PGC1alpha in inflammation and chronic disease. Nature. 2008;454:463–9. https://doi.org/10.1038/NATURE07206.

12. Hoene M, Runge H, Häring HU, et al. Interleukin-6 promotes myogenic differentiation of mouse skeletal muscle cells: role of the STAT3 pathway. Am J Physiol Cell Physiol. 2013;304 https://doi.org/10.1152/AJPCELL.00025.2012.
13. Hojman P, Pedersen M, Nielsen AR, et al. Fibroblast growth factor-21 is induced in human skeletal muscles by hyperinsulinemia. Diabetes. 2009;58:2797–801. https://doi.org/10.2337/DB09-0713.
14. Izumiya Y, Bina HA, Ouchi N, et al. FGF21 is an Akt-regulated myokine. FEBS Lett. 2008;582:3805–10. https://doi.org/10.1016/J.FEBSLET.2008.10.021.
15. Jensen-Cody SO, Potthoff MJ. Hepatokines and metabolism: deciphering communication from the liver. Mol Metab. 2021;44 https://doi.org/10.1016/J.MOLMET.2020.101138.
16. Kikuchi A, Takayama H, Tsugane H, et al. Plasma half-life and tissue distribution of leukocyte cell-derived chemotaxin 2 in mice. Sci Rep. 2020;10 https://doi.org/10.1038/S41598-020-70192-X.
17. Kim HJ, Higashimori T, Park SY, et al. Differential effects of interleukin-6 and -10 on skeletal muscle and liver insulin action in vivo. Diabetes. 2004;53:1060–7. https://doi.org/10.2337/DIABETES.53.4.1060.
18. Kitajima Y, Yoshioka K, Suzuki N. The ubiquitin-proteasome system in regulation of the skeletal muscle homeostasis and atrophy: from basic science to disorders. J Physiol Sci. 2020;70 https://doi.org/10.1186/S12576-020-00768-9.
19. Lan F, Misu H, Chikamoto K, et al. LECT2 functions as a hepatokine that links obesity to skeletal muscle insulin resistance. Diabetes. 2014;63:1649–64. https://doi.org/10.2337/DB13-0728.
20. Lim JY, Kim E. The role of Oorganokines in obesity and type 2 diabetes and their functions as molecular transducers of nutrition and exercise. Metabolites. 2023;13 https://doi.org/10.3390/METABO13090979.
21. MacDonald C, Wojtaszewski JFP, Pedersen BK, et al. Interleukin-6 release from human skeletal muscle during exercise: relation to AMPK activity. J Appl Physiol. 2003;95:2273–7. https://doi.org/10.1152/JAPPLPHYSIOL.00242.2003.
22. Mashili FL, Austin RL, Deshmukh AS, et al. Direct effects of FGF21 on glucose uptake in human skeletal muscle: implications for type 2 diabetes and obesity. Diabetes Metab Res Rev. 2011;27:286–97. https://doi.org/10.1002/DMRR.1177.
23. McElvaney OJ, Curley GF, Rose-John S, McElvaney NG. Interleukin-6: obstacles to targeting a complex cytokine in critical illness. Lancet Respir Med. 2021;9:643–54. https://doi.org/10.1016/S2213-2600(21)00103-X.
24. Minniti G, Pescinini-Salzedas LM, dos Minniti GAS, et al. Organokines, sarcopenia, and metabolic repercussions: the vicious cycle and the interplay with exercise. Int J Mol Sci. 2022;23 https://doi.org/10.3390/IJMS232113452.
25. Nadeau L, Aguer C. Interleukin-15 as a myokine: mechanistic insight into its effect on skeletal muscle metabolism. Appl Physiol Nutr Metab. 2019;44:229–38. https://doi.org/10.1139/APNM-2018-0022.
26. Naranjo JD, Dziki JL, Badylak SF. Regenerative medicine approaches for age-related muscle loss and sarcopenia: a mini-review. Gerontology. 2017;63:580–9. https://doi.org/10.1159/000479278.
27. Nie T, Zhu L, Yang Q. The classification and basic processes of autophagy. Adv Exp Med Biol. 2021;1208:3–16. https://doi.org/10.1007/978-981-16-2830-6_1.
28. Nielsen AR, Pedersen BK. The biological roles of exercise-induced cytokines: IL-6, IL-8, and IL-15. Appl Physiol Nutr Metab. 2007;32:833–9. https://doi.org/10.1139/H07-054.
29. Oflazoglu U, Caglar S, Yılmaz HE, et al. The relationship between sarcopenia detected in newly diagnosed colorectal cancer patients and FGF21, irisin and CRP levels. Eur Geriatr Med. 2022;13:795–803. https://doi.org/10.1007/S41999-022-00635-3.

30. Pal D, Dasgupta S, Kundu R, et al. Fetuin-A acts as an endogenous ligand of TLR4 to promote lipid-induced insulin resistance. Nat Med. 2012;18:1279–85. https://doi.org/10.1038/NM.2851.
31. Pankiv S, Clausen TH, Lamark T, et al. p62/SQSTM1 binds directly to Atg8/LC3 to facilitate degradation of ubiquitinated protein aggregates by autophagy. J Biol Chem. 2007;282:24131–45. https://doi.org/10.1074/JBC.M702824200.
32. Pedersen BK. IL-6 signalling in exercise and disease. Biochem Soc Trans. 2007;35:1295–7. https://doi.org/10.1042/BST0351295.
33. Pedersen BK, Febbraio M. Muscle-derived interleukin-6--a possible link between skeletal muscle, adipose tissue, liver, and brain. Brain Behav Immun. 2005;19:371–6. https://doi.org/10.1016/J.BBI.2005.04.008.
34. Pedersen BK, Febbraio MA. Muscles, exercise and obesity: skeletal muscle as a secretory organ. Nat Rev Endocrinol. 2012;8:457–65. https://doi.org/10.1038/NRENDO.2012.49.
35. Pedersen BK, Fischer CP. Physiological roles of muscle-derived interleukin-6 in response to exercise. Curr Opin Clin Nutr Metab Care. 2007;10:265–71. https://doi.org/10.1097/MCO.0B013E3280EBB5B3.
36. Pedersen BK, Steensberg A, Fischer C, et al. The metabolic role of IL-6 produced during exercise: is IL-6 an exercise factor? Proc Nutr Soc. 2004;63:263–7. https://doi.org/10.1079/PNS2004338.
37. Perakakis N, Triantafyllou GA, Fernández-Real JM, et al. Physiology and role of irisin in glucose homeostasis. Nat Rev Endocrinol. 2017;13:324–37. https://doi.org/10.1038/NRENDO.2016.221.
38. Quinn LBS, Strait-Bodey L, Anderson BG, et al. Interleukin-15 stimulates adiponectin secretion by 3T3-L1 adipocytes: evidence for a skeletal muscle-to-fat signaling pathway. Cell Biol Int. 2005;29:449–57. https://doi.org/10.1016/J.CELLBI.2005.02.005.
39. Ruderman NB, Keller C, Richard AM, et al. Interleukin-6 regulation of AMP-activated protein kinase. Potential role in the systemic response to exercise and prevention of the metabolic syndrome. Diabetes. 2006;55 Suppl 2 https://doi.org/10.2337/DB06-S007.
40. Sabio G, Das M, Mora A, et al. A stress signaling pathway in adipose tissue regulates hepatic insulin resistance. Science. 2008;322:1539–43. https://doi.org/10.1126/SCIENCE.1160794.
41. Sayer AA, Cruz-Jentoft A. Sarcopenia definition, diagnosis and treatment: consensus is growing. Age Ageing. 2022;51 https://doi.org/10.1093/AGEING/AFAC220.
42. Singer P, Blaser AR, Berger MM, et al. ESPEN guideline on clinical nutrition in the intensive care unit. Clin Nutr. 2019;38:48–79. https://doi.org/10.1016/J.CLNU.2018.08.037.
43. Singer P, Blaser AR, Berger MM, et al. ESPEN practical and partially revised guideline: clinical nutrition in the intensive care unit. Clin Nutr. 2023;42:1671–89. https://doi.org/10.1016/J.CLNU.2023.07.011.
44. Trepanowski JF, Mey J, Varady KA. Fetuin-A: a novel link between obesity and related complications. Int J Obes. 2015;39:734–41. https://doi.org/10.1038/IJO.2014.203.
45. Ueki K, Kondo T, Kahn CR. Suppressor of cytokine signaling 1 (SOCS-1) and SOCS-3 cause insulin resistance through inhibition of tyrosine phosphorylation of insulin receptor substrate proteins by discrete mechanisms. Mol Cell Biol. 2004;24:5434–46. https://doi.org/10.1128/MCB.24.12.5434-5446.2004.
46. Vanhorebeek I, Gunst J, Casaer MP, et al. Skeletal muscle myokine expression in critical illness, association with outcome and impact of therapeutic interventions. J Endocr Soc. 2023;7 https://doi.org/10.1210/JENDSO/BVAD001.
47. Vingren JL, Kraemer WJ, Ratamess NA, et al. Testosterone physiology in resistance exercise and training: the up-stream regulatory elements. Sports Med. 2010;40:1037–53. https://doi.org/10.2165/11536910-000000000-00000.
48. Xie G, Jin H, Mikhail H, et al. Autophagy in sarcopenia: possible mechanisms and novel therapies. Biomed Pharmacother. 2023;165 https://doi.org/10.1016/J.BIOPHA.2023.115147.

49. Yan J, Herzog JW, Tsang K, et al. Gut microbiota induce IGF-1 and promote bone formation and growth. Proc Natl Acad Sci USA. 2016;113:E7554–63. https://doi.org/10.1073/PNAS.1607235113.
50. Yoshida T, Delafontaine P. Mechanisms of IGF-1-mediated regulation of skeletal muscle hypertrophy and atrophy. Cells. 2020;9 https://doi.org/10.3390/CELLS9091970.
51. Zusman O, Theilla M, Cohen J, et al. Resting energy expenditure, calorie and protein consumption in critically ill patients: a retrospective cohort study. Crit Care. 2016;20 https://doi.org/10.1186/S13054-016-1538-4.

The Liver-Organs Axis in Gastrointestinal and Pancreatic Acute Injury

20

Katia Donadello, Marco Anderloni, Chiara Bruscagnin, and Leonardo Gottin

20.1 Introduction

In the last three decades, significant progress has been made in understanding how organs and tissues communicate in both physiological and pathological conditions. This communication occurs through the secretion of various substances including proteins, lipids, metabolites and small noncoding RNAs. It is now widely acknowledged that most tissues can communicate with nearby and distant organs through different mechanisms, such as autocrine, paracrine and endocrine signaling. Such interorgan communication is essential for maintaining balance within the body and for adapting to diseases [1].

The liver performs a wide range of essential functions related to detoxification, nutrient storage, digestion, metabolism and immunity. Thus, understanding the interorgan communication mechanisms, especially molecular mediators, is important for the development of targeted therapies [2].

K. Donadello (✉) · M. Anderloni
Department of Surgery, Dentistry, Gynaecology and Paediatrics, University of Verona, Verona, Italy

Anaesthesia and Intensive Care Unit B, Policlinico G.B. Rossi, University Hospital Integrated Trust of Verona, Verona, Italy
e-mail: katia.donadello@univr.it

C. Bruscagnin
Anaesthesia and Intensive Care Unit, Ospedale dell'Angelo di Mestre, Venezia, Italy

L. Gottin
Department of Surgery, Dentistry, Gynaecology and Paediatrics, University of Verona, Verona, Italy

Cardio-Thoracic Anaesthesia and Intensive Care Unit, Polo Chirurgico Confortini, University Hospital Integrated Trust of Verona, Verona, Italy
e-mail: leonardo.gottin@univr.it

D. Battaglini et al. (eds.), *Organ System Crosstalk in Critical Illness*,
https://doi.org/10.1007/978-3-032-01024-7_20

Despite initially being associated with metabolic diseases like nonalcoholic fatty liver disease (NAFLD) and type 2 diabetes, signaling proteins secreted specifically or predominantly by the liver, known as "hepatokines," have now been shown to play key roles in multiple disorders. Hepatocytes release over 560 different hepatokine types many of which play a regulatory role in metabolic and inflammatory disorders within the liver itself or in distant organs. For example, hepatokines have endocrine functions in tissues such as bones and heart, exerting their effects through the circulation. In situations of extreme challenge like prolonged starvation or overnutrition, the liver may secrete hepatokines to modulate energy balance and inflammation [3].

Nonetheless, normal liver function is crucial for resolving organ damage caused by infection. Liver performs indeed vital functions such as filtering systemic endotoxins, regulating the production and deactivation of inflammatory mediators and synthesizing acute-phase proteins [4]. In cases of endotoxin challenge, the uncontrolled release of biologically active substances from hepatic cells can initiate and sustain a systemic inflammatory response, potentially leading to multiple organ failure and ultimately to death [5].

Liver dysfunction is associated with impaired protein and carbohydrate metabolism, compromised detoxification system, coagulation system dysfunction, reduced urea synthesis, impaired bilirubin elimination and diminished fatty acid export [6]. Kupffer cells, constituting 80–90% of the body's resident macrophages, play a crucial role within the liver, and their number can significantly vary under specific conditions [7]. In response to endotoxin exposure or inflammation, Kupffer cell population increases dramatically due to both local proliferation and monocyte recruitment from the bloodstream [8]. Besides possessing macrophage functions, including phagocytosis and secretion of various biologically active molecules, Kupffer cells, due to their strategic location within the liver, play a critical role in clearing circulating endotoxin from the portal circulation, specifically originating from the gut [9].

20.2 Communications Between Liver, Gastrointestinal System, and Pancreas

- Liver and Gut

  The gastrointestinal tract, which is the largest mucosal surface in the human body, faces constant challenges from dietary antigens and microbes [10]. Recent research has provided compelling evidence that the entire gastrointestinal tract, spanning from the mouth to the anus, is inhabited by a diverse array of commensal microorganisms with various roles in both health and disease [11, 12]. This complex barrier comprises epithelial and endothelial cell types, together with innate and adaptive immune components and their mediators. Collectively, these elements enable the gastrointestinal system to function effectively [13]. The portal vein serves as a conduit for blood drainage from the small and large intestines, spleen, and pancreas, representing a significant anatomical point for gut and liver communication. Under normal circumstances, this blood drainage contains minimal amounts of potentially harmful or toxic substances, such as dietary components or commensal microorganisms and their metabolic byproducts. It is believed that a healthy liver, along with its immune system, can effectively handle such stressors [14]. Conversely, the liver secretes substances into the gut through the biliary tree, which are then taken up by the intestine, allowing for bidirectional communication along the liver-gut axis. For instance, bile facilitates the metabolism of bile acids by gut microbes and contains antimicrobial peptides that help control the commensal microbial population [15]. This communication between the gut and liver involves additional layers of complexity, such as lymphatic vessels connecting the gut and liver [16], intestine-derived lipid messengers [17] and liver vagal sensory afferent nerves [18].

- The liver gut vessel network: a guardian of volume status like no other
  The splanchnic circulation importance goes well beyond its basic anatomical and physiological aspects. Normovolemic healthy male adults have a blood volume of about 70 ml/kg body weight, with splanchnic organs containing 25% of this total blood volume, despite constituting only 10% of body weight [19]. The splanchnic vasculature acts as a significant reservoir for the circulatory system, capable of autotransfusing over 800 ml of blood into the systemic circulation rapidly if needed [20]. Under normal conditions, the volume of blood in splanchnic vessels is related to the transmural pressure so that a change in arterial flow leads to a proportional change in the pressure within these vessels [21]. When arterial flow decreases, venous blood volume and pressure decrease, and the veins recoil, a passive phenomenon that helps maintain transmural pressure sufficient to propel intravascular volume toward the systemic circulation. On the other hand, the release of catecholamines from sympathetic nerve terminals and the adrenal medulla is crucial in regulating arterial resistance and venous capacitance vessel tone. The net effect on splanchnic arteries, whether constriction or relaxion varies according to catecholamine type and concentration, and regional adrenoceptor density as shown in Table 20.1 and Fig. 20.1 [20].

Table 20.1 Distribution of adrenoceptor subtypes in the splanchnic vasculature [20]

Receptor subtype	Pre portal arterial	Hepatic arterial	Pre portal venous	Hepatic venous
α1	Vasoconstriction, high density	Vasoconstriction, high density	Vasoconstriction, high density	Vasoconstriction, moderate density
α2 peripheral	Vasoconstriction, moderate density	Vasoconstriction, low density	Vasoconstriction, low density	Vasoconstriction, low density
β2	Vasodilation, high density	Vasodilation, moderate density	Vasodilation, low density	Vasodilation, high density

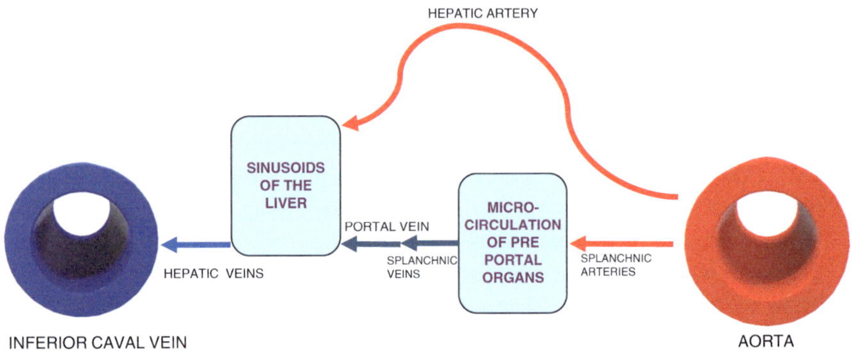

Fig. 20.1 Representation of the splanchnic vasculature [20]

Venoconstriction is a major effect of catecholamines on splanchnic vessels, thereby increasing capacitance vessel pressure and facilitating blood expulsion into the systemic circulation. Active (venoconstriction) and passive (elastic recoil) mechanisms work together to mobilize splanchnic blood volume toward the systemic circulation, thus providing a substantial contribution during sympathetic nervous system activation [22]. Through these mechanisms, splanchnic circulation plays a pivotal role in maintaining systemic hemodynamic stability, especially under varying physiological and pathophysiological conditions. Hemorrhage animal models have shown that considerable shifts in splanchnic blood compensate for systemic demands or blood loss. Hypovolemia, whether absolute or relative, triggers the activation of the sympathetic nervous system and elevates the levels of circulating catecholamines. This process results in the mobilization of blood from the body's reservoirs, notably the splanchnic capacitance vessels, into the systemic circulation, helping to offset reductions in circulating blood volume. A study in dogs demonstrated that a hemorrhage causing a 50% drop in mean aortic pressure coincided with a 50% decrease in cardiac output and an almost 90% decrease in intestinal blood volume [23]. Remarkably, while moderate changes in blood volume due to hypervolemia or hypovolemia did not significantly impact cardiac output, they did cause substantial changes in intestinal blood volume. When the intestinal blood volume was within 95–135% of baseline levels, cardiac output remained stable; however, volumes outside this range led to significant venous pressure and cardiac output fluctuations due to intestinal vessel constriction or dilation [23]. These findings highlight the critical role of splanchnic venous vasculature in moderating cardiac output fluctuations during acute fluid changes or blood loss, effectively keeping cardiac output stable across a broad spectrum of total vascular blood volumes [24]. Furthermore, the response to catecholamine administration during hypovolemia is influenced by the effective volume of blood within the splanchnic reservoir. In cases of severe hypovolemia, the splanchnic reservoir is likely depleted due to the body's intrinsic homeostatic responses to maintain blood pressure and cardiac output. Consequently, the effectiveness of exogenous catecholamines in augmenting systemic hemodynamics by acting on the splanchnic circulation diminishes as the sympathoadrenal response intensifies and the levels of endogenous catecholamines rise.

- Liver and pancreas
  Liver and pancreas play complementary roles, especially in glucose metabolism. In humans, interlobular and total pancreatic fat are both positively related to NAFLD, and total pancreatic fat is related to the presence of NAFLD [25]. It has been found in a retrospective study by Mikolasevic who analyzed 822 hospitalized patients with acute pancreatitis that NAFLD could have a prognostic role in acute pancreatitis, as it represents the hepatic manifestation of metabolic syndrome [26]. Of relevance, some hepatokines, like fetuin-A seems to play a role in pancreatic activity, especially in immunomodulation and metabolic regulation. Especially, it has been proposed that fetuin-A secreted by the fatty liver is able to augment pancreatic inflammation while impairing insulin secretion [27]. Other data suggest that the restoration of fibroblast growth factor 21 (FGF21) levels, a digestive secretagogue enzyme mainly secreted by liver and pancreas, involved in the maintenance of acinar cell proteostasis [28], may revert pancreatitis when induced by cerulein, alcohol, or endoscopic retrograde cholangiopancreatography [29]. However, whether the liver-secreted FGF21 participates in this process remains largely unknown. Moreover, damaged pancreas may secrete pro-inflammatory cytokines (e.g., TNF-α), which may directly attack the liver per se as explained forward.

20.3 Acute Pancreatitis and the Role of the Liver

Acute pancreatitis is a reversible inflammatory disorder that exhibits a wide spectrum of severity, ranging from focal edema and fat necrosis to extensive hemorrhagic necrosis. It is a relatively common and serious condition, with a global annual incidence of 33–74 cases per 100,000 individuals [30]. In the Western world, the incidence ranges from 5 to 35 cases per 100,000 individuals. The overall mortality rate is approximately 1–2% in cases without superimposed infection or organ failure [31]. Nowadays, its incidence is on the rise due to the escalating obesity epidemic and the associated increase in gallstone disease.

20.3.1 Etiology and Pathogenesis

In the United States, the most prevalent cause of acute pancreatitis is the obstruction of the common bile duct by gallstones, which impedes the passage of pancreatic secretions through the ampulla of Vater (referred to as “gallstone pancreatitis”). This is closely followed by pancreatitis due to excessive alcohol consumption. Together, gallstones and chronic alcohol use account for nearly 80% of acute pancreatitis cases, while the remaining cases are attributed to various factors:

- Unrelated to gallstone pancreatic duct obstruction, such as pancreatic cancer, periampullary neoplasms, pancreas divisum, bile precipitated solid particles ("biliary sludge") and parasitic infections (notably *Ascaris lumbricoides* and *Clonorchis sinensis*).
- Metabolic disorders, particularly hypertriglyceridemia, hyperparathyroidism and other hypercalcemic conditions. Hypertriglyceridemia (above 1000 mg/dL) has been reported to cause 5–10% of acute pancreatitis cases.
- Medications, including anticonvulsants, cancer chemotherapeutic agents, thiazide diuretics, estrogens, and many others.
- Infections with mumps virus or coxsackievirus, both of which can directly infect pancreatic exocrine cells [32].

Multiorgan dysfunction associated with acute pancreatitis is closely linked to the disease prognosis, and the liver is a critical extrapancreatic organ in this setting. Treating liver injury in patients with liver injury-associated acute pancreatitis (LIAAP) can improve the prognosis of acute pancreatitis. Therefore, it is crucial to investigate the potential mechanisms underlying LIAAP [30].

20.3.2 Cytokines and Inflammatory Cascade

Cytokines, classified into pro-inflammatory and anti-inflammatory cytokines, maintain a delicate balance in the body [33]. According to the theory of the inflammatory-anti-inflammatory factor balance, harmful stimuli trigger the activation of the inflammatory response as a protective mechanism, leading to the release of proinflammatory cytokines. Simultaneously, the anti-inflammatory system is engaged, releasing anti-inflammatory cytokines to regulate and inhibit the inflammatory response. This kind of balanced interaction is essential in order to guarantee both and adequate response to a harmful stimulus but at the same time to prevent an overactivation of the inflammatory response.

During acute pancreatitis, pancreatic acinar cells and hepatocytes are attacked by activated digestive enzymes. These stimulate neutrophils to release various inflammatory factors like interleukin-1 (IL-1) β, interleukin-6 (IL-6), and interleukin-8 (IL-8), leading to a systemic inflammatory response and subsequent organ damage. Pancreatic elastase activates the nuclear transcription factor-κB (NF-κB) pathway, inducing cytokine production in Kupffer cells (KCs). As a portion of pancreatic blood flows back through the portal vein, the liver is the first extrapancreatic organ to be exposed to high concentrations of activating enzymes and inflammatory mediators at the onset of acute pancreatitis.

20.3.3 Tumor Necrosis Factor-α (TNF-α)

Excessive TNF-α can activate neutrophils and stimulate the release of IL-1β, IL-6, IL-8, and other cytokines, leading to a wide range of pathological reactions. In severe acute pancreatitis, TNF-α serves as a significant trigger for complications, including liver damage. The mechanisms of TNF-α-induced liver injury include direct hepatotoxicity, excessive production of nitric oxide (NO) and oxygen free radicals (OFRs) by hepatic KCs and neutrophils and hepatocytes and KCs apoptosis. TNF-α alone can cause toxic shock symptoms and contribute to multiple organ dysfunction syndrome (MODS) [34, 35].

20.3.4 IL-6

In acute pancreatitis, IL-6 promotes B lymphocyte activation, leading to increased immunoglobulin synthesis, T lymphocyte activation and differentiation and acute phase reactions. These processes contribute to liver tissue injury, heightened neutrophil function and neutrophil recruitment factor-1. IL-6 activation also leads to leukocyte retention within the liver vascular system and their adhesion to endothelial cell surfaces. Leukocytes release toxic substances such as elastase and oxygen-free radicals (OFRs), directly damaging the liver vascular endothelium [36].

20.3.5 IL-8

IL-8 is primarily produced by neutrophils and acts as a neutrophil chemokine, mediating inflammation from the pancreas to extrapancreatic organs, including the liver. IL-8 intensifies tissue damage caused by neutrophils and enhances the phagocytosis and killing effect of natural killer (NK) cells on inflammatory tissues [30].

20.3.6 IL-18

IL-18 is a member of the IL-1 superfamily and is primarily produced by macrophages, although other cell types also contribute to its secretion. It has multiple effects on various cell types and acts as a proinflammatory cytokine that triggers a type 1 immune response. When exposed to microbial products like lipopolysaccharide (LPS), IL-18, along with IL-12, promotes cell-mediated immunity. In the context of liver damage, IL-18 induces hepatocyte apoptosis by increasing Fas ligand (FasL) expression and activates the Janus kinase/signal transducer and activator of transcription (JAK-STAT) signaling pathway [37].

20.3.7 High-Mobility Group Box-1

High mobility group protein B1 (HMGB1) is a highly conserved nuclear protein present in mammalian cells. When cells are damaged or undergo necrosis, HMGB1 can be released from the nucleus, triggering an inflammatory response. The presence of damaged cells that release HMGB1 and macrophages leads to the activation of NF-κB pathway, simulating an inflammatory response similar to tissue necrosis [38]. In this signaling pathway, ethyl pyruvate (EP) may have therapeutic effects in liver injury-associated acute pancreatitis (LIAAP) by modulating HMGB1 and other inflammatory cytokines in the high mobility group, suggesting a potential relationship between LIAAP and HMGB1 [39].

During severe acute pancreatitis (SAP), the liver is affected by pancreatic inflammation, resulting in reduced detoxification capacity and compromised barrier function against endotoxemia. This leads to the excessive release of endogenous inflammatory mediators, creating a vicious cycle. The systemic circulation becomes overwhelmed with these inflammatory mediators, leading to sustained systemic inflammatory response, tissue damage, and organ dysfunction. These chain reactions and amplification processes, known as cascade reactions, contribute to MODS [40].

20.3.8 Microcirculation Disturbances

Microcirculation disturbances are significant pathological features of AP [41]. In the early stages, microcirculatory disorders can occur mainly in the pancreas and liver [42]. In SAP, insufficient blood volume, due to the release of vasoactive substances, and impaired blood circulation within the liver contribute to liver injury. Decreased liver blood flow can result in mitochondrial ATP synthesis disorders and decreased cytochrome A and B phosphorylation rates [43]. Nonetheless blood flow dynamic alterations are caused also by imbalances in endothelin (ET), production, which promotes vasoconstriction, and nitric oxide (NO) synthesis, which, on the other hand, cause vasodilation. So, The imbalance of thromboxane A2/prostacyclin (TXA2/PGI2) and ET/NO ratios can lead to pathological changes, including vasomotor dysfunction, microthrombosis and vascular occlusion. In LIAAP, the balance of these regulatory factors is disrupted, impacting both liver injury and the secretion of ET, NO, TXA2, and PGI2 by vascular endothelial cells [36].

20.3.9 Tissue Factor

Tissue factor (TF), or CD142, is a protein produced by the F3 gene and present in various tissues, including subcutaneous tissue and white blood cells. It serves as a cellular coagulation initiator through its interaction with coagulation factor VII [44]. Both the coagulation and the fibrinolytic systems can be activated during SAP, but the fibrinolytic system function is relatively weak since TF and tissue factor-microparticle (TF-MP) levels are highly upregulated in both SAP patients and SAP mouse model [45]. In SAP, monocytes stimulated by LPS, TNF-α, or IL-1 express high levels of TF. This can be caught by platelets and contribute to pathological coagulation, leading to coagulation dysfunction and hypercoagulability. In SAP mouse models, TF expression is upregulated in KCs and the inhibition of this improves coagulation proper activity and reduces both serum TF levels and

TF-MP. In SAP, thus, imbalanced TF expression plays a crucial role in liver injury associated with microcirculation disturbances [45].

20.3.10 Oxidative Stress

Oxidative stress refers to an imbalance in the body that ultimately favors oxidation. This imbalance leads to the infiltration of inflammatory neutrophils, increased proteases secretion, and the generation of high levels of oxidative intermediates. Oxidative stress is thought to be a significant factor both in healthy aging and disease [46], and it can also contribute to liver injury through various mechanisms [47].

Reactive oxygen species (ROS), including oxygen ions, peroxides, and oxygen-containing free radicals, are byproducts of biological aerobic metabolism. Normally, there is a balance between ROS production and elimination through endogenous antioxidants. However, in AP, this balance is disrupted [48]. Animal experiments in rats have shown that an obstruction in the pancreatic duct leads to an excessive ROS production in the early stages of AP [48]. Highly active ROS directly attack lipids, proteins, and other components of cells, impairing their function; furthermore, increased ROS production by activated leukocytes causes cytoskeletal changes and damage to acinar cell membranes [49]. The disruption of the cytoskeleton interferes with the normal transport of digestive enzymes in cells, causing their activation [50]. Cell fragmentation and ROS-activated pancreatic enzymes promote damage to the capillary endothelium, increase the capillary permeability and result in tissue edema. Malondialdehyde (MDA), a product of oxidative damage, indicates the extent of oxidative stress-induced damage and could have a role as a biomarker of this process [51]. MDA reacts with DNA and proteins, leading to structural and functional changes, ultimately damaging cell membranes and hepatocytes. Accumulation of MDA alters mitochondrial membrane permeability, triggering the release of apoptosis-related cytokines and promoting apoptosis [30].

Experimental studies in mice have shown both decreased superoxide dismutase activity and increased MDA concentration in pancreatic tissue of caerulein-induced AP. This suggests that oxidative stress increases lipid peroxidation not only in pancreatic tissue but also in the liver, contributing thus to liver injury [52].

To mitigate liver injury induced by AP, various antioxidants, including melatonin, ascorbic acid, N-acetylcysteine, and L-cysteine, have shown potential in exerting antioxidant effects and ameliorating oxidative stress-related liver damage [52, 53].

20.3.11 The Clinical Management of Liver Injury Associated with Acute Pancreatitis

The clinical management of liver injury associated with acute pancreatitis (LIAAP) involves several aspects. It includes close monitoring of vital signs, fluid resuscitation, nutritional support, pain management, prevention of secondary infections, and local complication management [54]. The treatment of LIAAP is closely linked to the treatment of AP, since the extent of liver damage depends on the severity of pancreatitis. Based on the underlying mechanisms of LIAAP, treatment methods focus on anti-inflammatory and antioxidant therapies, improvement of microcirculation, inhibition of apoptosis, promotion of liver cell regeneration and supportive therapy.

In animal models, sodium butyrate has been shown to inhibit the activation of NF-κB in the liver, reduce the expression of the HMGB1 gene, decrease the level of HMGB1 protein and ultimately improve the outcomes of SAP in rats [38]. Antioxidants such as melatonin, ascorbic acid, and N-acetyl cysteine can mitigate pancreatic and liver damage in AP by restoring the activity of tissue antioxidant enzymes [52]. Recombinant human soluble thrombomodulin and prostaglandin E1 aid in maintaining microcirculation, reducing liver and pancreas damage, and improving the prognosis of SAP [52, 55]. Nilotinib, which inhibits the tyrosine kinase activity of the BCR-ABL protein, exhibits antioxidant and anti-inflammatory effects, reducing pancreatic and liver damage [56]. Heme oxygenase-1 can prevent pancreatic and liver damage through antioxidative, microcirculation maintenance, and anti-inflammatory mechanisms [57]. In cases where SAP is complicated by liver and kidney injuries, the administration of recombinant vascular endothelial growth factor (VEGF) can effectively improve liver and kidney function and inhibit cell apoptosis in these organs [58]. Somatostatin has the ability to inhibit the over-expression of serum TNF-α mRNA in AP rats' model, thereby reducing pancreatic and liver tissue damage [59]. In a SAP mouse model, ethyl pyruvate (EP) demonstrated anti-inflammatory and antioxidant effects, significantly reducing serum ALT levels and liver necrosis [60].

Given the multifactorial nature of AP, the combination of therapeutic agents may improve prognosis. Nonetheless, most of the molecules and drugs listed above have been studied either only in animal models or in humans in small numbers; moreover, the exploration of treatments targeting both the pancreas and extrapancreatic organs is promising, but further research remains necessary to prove efficacy and safety. Along with supportive therapy which nowadays remains of pivotal relevance, in the future we may see a paradigm shift with drugs that can affect the molecular processes underlying LIAAP.

20.4 Liver Role in Intestinal Failure

20.4.1 The Intestinal Barrier

The interaction between the gut mucosa and the liver, known as the gut-liver axis, is a consequence of a close anatomical and functional bidirectional interaction between the gastrointestinal tract and the liver, and it is mediated through the portal vein.

The gut-liver axis is fundamental in maintaining overall health and homeostasis because the interface between the liver and the microbiome is the gut barrier, consisting of an outer mucus layer, an inner epithelial layer, and the gut vascular barrier, where a network of metabolic, immune, and neuroendocrine interactions takes place. Otherwise, if the epithelium is breached by bacteria, the microorganisms are able to disseminate systemically [10].

The intestinal mucosa is responsible for the absorption of nutrients, and at the same time, it has a mucus barrier which physically separates the microbiota from the epithelial lining and is thicker in the terminal ileum and colon, where it consists of two layers: the outer one colonized by bacteria and the inner one, next to the epithelium, where very strict tight junctions and microbiota-excluding proteins work to preserve sterility [61, 62].

Below the mucus layer, the gut barrier is formed of epithelial cells that protect the gut from insults with a physical, electrical and chemical barrier. The gut-associated lymphoid tissue (GALT), which includes lymphoid cells and immune cells, constantly interacts with the intestinal microbiota. Antigens (coming from micro-organisms or from food) are recognized by dendritic cells or activate the immune system by modulating the T cell response. The lamina propria is indeed rich in plasma cells, capable of releasing IgA, and immune cells such as CD4+ T cells (T helper 17 that release IL-17A, IL-17F, and IL-22 and T regulatory cells), invariant NKT cells, mucosa-associated invariant T cells, innate lymphoid cells and mononuclear phagocytes [63].

However, some substances, including bacterial products and other metabolites, can cross the intestinal barrier and reach the liver through the portal vein.

Pathogen-associated molecular patterns (PAMPs), such as lipopolysaccharides (LPS), flagellin, and peptidoglycans, activate the nuclear factor kappa B (NF-κB) through toll-like receptors (TLRs) and nod-like receptors (NLRs), leading to the production of inflammatory cytokines and chemokines that enter portal circulation. PAMPs can also activate stellate cells and Kupffer cells, promoting liver fibrosis [64–67].

The exposure to gut-derived antigens and microbial products that are transported via the portal vein helps educate the immune system, maintaining a balance between immune tolerance and appropriate immune responses.

The liver acts as a gatekeeper and helps preventing the dissemination of potentially harmful substances, filtering the blood coming from the gut, and detoxifying various substances, such as drugs, alcohol, and metabolic waste products. Additionally, it produces the bile, which is essential for the digestion and absorption of dietary fats and which has direct antibacterial effects. Bile acids are primarily synthesized in the liver out of cholesterol and then converted to secondary bile acids by the gut microbiota and can enter enterohepatic circulation [10].

Bile acids activate the farnesoid-X receptor (FXR) in the enterocyte of the distal ileum and in the liver, during the enterohepatic cycle. In the enterocyte, FXR stimulates the secretion of fibroblast growth factor-19 (FGF19), which reaches the liver through the portal vein. In the hepatocyte, FGF19 downregulates cholesterol-7-alpha-hydroxylase-1, which inhibits the conversion of cholesterol into bile acids, thus providing negative feedback control of bile acids synthesis. In the liver, FXR further acts as a safeguard against bile acids toxicity by controlling the import and efflux of bile salts in the liver.

The FXR seems to play a role also in maintaining intestinal permeability and in repairing gut vascular barrier damage, thus protecting against bacterial and/or LPS translocation [68].

Disturbances in the gut-liver axis (such as in cholestasis and in critical illness) can contribute to the development of various liver diseases, such as non-alcoholic fatty liver disease (NAFLD), alcoholic liver disease (ALD), and liver fibrosis/cirrhosis or secondary sclerosing cholangitis [69]. Composition of gut microbiome, the gut barrier, bacterial translocation, and bile acid metabolism are the key features underlying these conditions and could represent a possible therapeutic target.

In critically ill patients, alterations in the gut-liver axis can also cause lung dysfunction (by cytokines, endotoxins, and pancreatic enzymes via lymphatics due to gut barrier dysfunction) and brain dysfunction (by an increased production of ammonia) that increase the overall clinical severity. For example, liver damage can contribute to the development of acute respiratory distress syndrome (ARDS), through production of acute-phase proteins (IL-1, IL-6), reduction in clearance of bacterial products (endotoxin) and the release of pro-coagulant and vasoactive mediators [70].

20.5 Intestinal Failure Associated Liver Disease

The intestinal failure associated liver disease (IFALD) is a common and potentially life-threatening condition for patients with short bowel syndrome, requiring long-term parenteral nutrition, more frequent in pediatric age [71].

The diagnosis is based on clinical, biochemical, radiological, and, at times, histologic elements. A persistent elevation of liver enzymes, alkaline phosphatase, and γ-glutamyl transferase 1.5 times above the upper limit reference range (for 6 months in adults or 6 weeks in children) are widely accepted criteria. By the way, no formally agreed criteria have been defined so far [72]. A typical sign of IFALD is the concomitant presence of cholestasis and steatosis, the former is more frequent in infants, the latter in older children and adults.

The absence of nutrients in the gut lumen can result in intestinal mucosal atrophy and increased permeability, with the risk of translocation of LPS into the portal circulation [71].

In IFALD, liver injury may arise from intrahepatic accumulation of bile acids and impaired FXR/FGF19-mediated liver repair. In patients with intestinal failure, serum FGF19 levels were found to be significantly lower than in healthy subjects and to correlate with portal inflammation or fibrosis, thus probably contributing to cellular apoptosis, fibrotic changes, and ultimately liver injury.

During parenteral nutrition, lipid emulsion and glucose overfeeding promote hepatic IFALD-steatosis, characterized by fat deposition in Kupffer cells and hepatic lysosomes, contributing to liver failure [73]. For the prevention of IFALD, ESPEN guideline recommends: prevention of infections (particularly the catheter related blood stream infections); preservation of small intestinal length as long as possible and retaining the colon in continuity during surgical procedures; maintenance of oral/enteral feeding; avoiding continuous PN infusion; avoiding PN overfeeding and limiting the dose of soybean-based (SO) intravenous fat emulsions (IVFEs) to less than 1 g/kg/d in adults [74].

20.6 Intestinal Ischemia-Reperfusion and the Role of the Liver

Intestinal ischemia-reperfusion (I/R) is a common pathophysiological process, which can occur in many conditions such as acute enteric ischemia, severe burns, small intestinal transplantation, etc. and it refers to the damage that occurs when blood flow is temporarily stopped (ischemia) and then restored (reperfusion). In the context of intestinal I/R injury, the correlation between the gut insult and the liver subsequent injury is due to the gut-liver axis [75].

The reduction in blood flow to the gut alters the gut barrier and results in increased membrane permeability, leading to bacteria, PAMPs, and DAMPs translocation into the portal circulation with consequent activation of the immune and inflammatory response [76]. In the liver, this stimulates Kupffer cells to release pro-inflammatory cytokines and mediators, inducing liver inflammation and injury. When blood flow is restored, the oxygen reintroduction generates reactive oxygen species (ROS) and oxidative stress, increasing tissue damage in the gut and the liver.

The pathways involved in I/R are many. The most commonly studied and identified are NF-κB signaling pathway, the P66shc signaling pathway, the HMGB1 signaling pathway, the Nrf2-ARE signaling pathway, and the AMPK-SIRT-1 signaling pathway [75].

20.6.1 NF-κB Pathway

During I/R context, ROS, DAMPs, and cytokines released from the injured tissue can activate the NF-κB pathway. The activation of NF-κB in Kupffer cells triggers a cascade of events that contribute to liver injury: NF-κB translocates to the nucleus [77], dissociates from IK-κB and acts as an enhancer or repressor to regulate transcription of genes, such as those encoding tumor necrosis factor-alpha (TNF-α), interleukin-1β (IL-1β), interleukin-6 (IL-6), intercellular adhesion molecule-1 (ICAM-1) and vascular cell adhesion molecule-1 (VCAM-1) [78]. This exacerbates inflammation and promotes the adhesion and infiltration of leukocytes into the liver tissue. NF-κB can also amplify the inflammation signaling, through the interaction with MAPK (mitogen-activated protein kinase) pathway [79] and the JAK-STAT (Janus kinase-signal transducer and activator of transcription) pathway [80].

20.6.2 HMGB1

High mobility group box 1 (HMGB1) plays an important role in liver injury after intestinal I/R. HMGB1 is a nuclear protein that can be released from damaged/necrotic cells or can be secreted by immune cells into the extracellular space and function as a DAMP molecule, contributing to inflammation and tissue damage also by increasing the polarization of Kupffer cells toward M1-type macrophages, which contribute to liver injury [81–83].

Indeed after intestinal I/R, RIP1 and RIP3 mediate the formation of a necrotic inducing protein complex, while causing mixed lineage kinase domain-like (MLKL) phosphorylation to greatly increase the release of intracellular damage-associated molecular patterns (DAMPs), of which HMGB1 is the predominant one [84].

HMGB1 acts as a pro-inflammatory cytokine: it activates immune cells stimulating the production of TNF-α, IL-1β, and IL-6, ROS species and it induces the expression of adhesion molecules, promoting leukocyte infiltration into the liver tissue. It also binds to several cell surface receptors [toll-like receptors TLR2, TLR4, and the receptor for advanced glycation end-products (RAGE)], activating NF-κB pathway (as discussed above) [85].

20.6.3 Ferroptosis and Intestinal Ischemia/Reperfusion (I/R) Injury

Intestinal I/R injury is associated with multiple types of regulated cell deaths, including apoptosis, necroptosis, autophagy, and ferroptosis.

Ferroptosis is a form of regulated cell death characterized by iron-dependent lipid peroxidation. Excessive iron produces ROS via the Fenton reaction, causing a depletion in reduced GSH and/or inhibition of glutathione peroxidase 4 (GPX4). At the same time, ROS attacks the polyunsaturated fatty acids (PUFAs) of lipid membranes, producing massive lipid peroxides and leading to membrane damage and cell death [86].

20.7 Clinical Management and Conclusions

The definition of gastrointestinal dysfunction or failure is not yet included in predictive scores to describe the severity of the critical patient, only the definition of liver dysfunction or failure is described via bilirubin value in SOFA score. Considering the relevant role played by gut inflammation, dysbiosis, and liver dysfunction in the immunological axis, targeting the interplay between microbiota, bile acids, and their signaling seems to be a possible treatment option. To date, there are still no approved treatments in clinical practice that can act on the pathophysiological mechanisms underlying I/R. Nevertheless, in the experimental setting, several molecules are being studied, such as curcumin, dexmedetomidine, N-acetylcysteine and carnosol, capable of interfering with Nf-kb signaling. Also, molecules capable of modifying macrophage polarization and plasticity are under study. While waiting for these molecules, old and new, to find application, supportive therapy remains to date the only real therapy in the clinical armamentarium.

In conclusion, we can say that from the clinical point of view, although therapeutic opportunities remain limited, it is central for the physician to take into account the existence of a deep interplay between liver, pancreas, and intestine, so that treating the pathology of an organ means, ultimately, taking care of a much more complex and articulated system.

References

1. Karsenty G, Olson EN. Bone and muscle endocrine functions: unexpected paradigms of inter-organ communication. Cell. 2016;164(6):1248–56.
2. Leitner LM, Wilson RJ, Yan Z, Gödecke A. Reactive oxygen species/nitric oxide mediated inter-organ communication in skeletal muscle wasting diseases. Antioxid Redox Signal. 2017;26(13):700–17.
3. Meex RCR, Watt MJ. Hepatokines: linking nonalcoholic fatty liver disease and insulin resistance. Nat Rev Endocrinol. 2017;13(9):509–20.
4. Matuschak GM, Rinaldo JE. Organ interactions in the adult respiratory distress syndrome during sepsis. Chest. 1988;94(2):400–6.
5. Gundersen Y, Saetre T, Scholz T, Carlsen H, Kjekshus H, Smiseth OA, et al. The NO donor sodium nitroprusside reverses the negative effects on hepatic arterial flow induced by endotoxin and the NO synthase inhibitor L-NAME. Eur Surg Res. 1996;28(5):323–32.
6. Cowley R, Trump B. Pathology and pathophysiology of the liver. In: Pathophysiology of shock, anoxia, and ischemia. Baltimore: Williams & Wilkins; 1982. p. 285–301.
7. Jones EA, Summerfield JA. Kupffer cells. In: The liver: biology and pathobiology. New York: Raven Press; 1982. p. 507–31.
8. Bouwens L, Knook DL, Wisse E. Local proliferation and extrahepatic recruitment of liver macrophages (Kupffer cells) in partial-body irradiated rats. J Leukoc Biol. 1986;39(6):687–97.
9. Ruiter DJ, van der Meulen J, Brouwer A, Hummel MJ, Mauw BJ, van der Ploeg JC, et al. Uptake by liver cells of endotoxin following its intravenous injection. Lab Investig J Tech Methods Pathol. 1981;45(1):38–45.
10. Tilg H, Adolph TE, Trauner M. Gut-liver axis: pathophysiological concepts and clinical implications. Cell Metab. 2022;34(11):1700–18.
11. De Vos WM, Tilg H, Van Hul M, Cani PD. Gut microbiome and health: mechanistic insights. Gut. 2022;71(5):1020–32.
12. Lee JY, Tsolis RM, Bäumler AJ. The microbiome and gut homeostasis. Science. 2022;377(6601):eabp9960.
13. Martel J, Chang SH, Ko YF, Hwang TL, Young JD, Ojcius DM. Gut barrier disruption and chronic disease. Trends Endocrinol Metab. 2022;33(4):247–65.
14. Guilliams M, Bonnardel J, Haest B, Vanderborght B, Wagner C, Remmerie A, et al. Spatial proteogenomics reveals distinct and evolutionarily conserved hepatic macrophage niches. Cell. 2022;185(2):379–396.e38.
15. Sarashina-Kida H, Negishi H, Nishio J, Suda W, Nakajima Y, Yasui-Kato M, et al. Gallbladder-derived surfactant protein D regulates gut commensal bacteria for maintaining intestinal homeostasis. Proc Natl Acad Sci. 2017;114(38):10178–83.
16. Juneja P, Tripathi DM, Kaur S. Revisiting the gut-liver axis: gut lymphatic system in liver cirrhosis and portal hypertension. Am J Physiol-Gastrointest Liver Physiol. 2022;322(5):G473–9.
17. Tellez LA, Medina S, Han W, Ferreira JG, Licona-Limón P, Ren X, et al. A gut lipid messenger links excess dietary fat to dopamine deficiency. Science. 2013;341(6147):800–2.
18. Teratani T, Mikami Y, Nakamoto N, Suzuki T, Harada Y, Okabayashi K, et al. The liver–brain–gut neural arc maintains the Treg cell niche in the gut. Nature. 2020;585(7826):591–6.
19. Greenway CV. Role of splanchnic venous system in overall cardiovascular homeostasis. Fed Proc. 1983;42(6):1678–84.
20. Gelman S, Mushlin PS, Weiskopf RB. Catecholamine-induced changes in the splanchnic circulation affecting systemic hemodynamics. Anesthesiology. 2004;100(2):434–9.

21. Greenway CV, Seaman KL, Innes IR. Norepinephrine on venous compliance and unstressed volume in cat liver. Am J Physiol-Heart Circ Physiol. 1985;248(4):H468–76.
22. Rothe CF. Venous system: physiology of the capacitance vessels. In: Terjung R, curatore. Comprehensive physiology [Internet]. 1a ed. Wiley; 1983 [citato 1 settembre 2024]. p. 397–452. Disponibile su: https://onlinelibrary.wiley.com/doi/10.1002/cphy.cp020313
23. Scott-Douglas NW, Robinson VJB, Smiseth OA, Wright CI, Manyari DE, Smith ER, et al. Effects of acute volume loading and hemorrhage on intestinal vascular capacitance: a mechanism whereby capacitance modulates cardiac output. Can J Cardiol. 2002;18(5):515–22.
24. Greenway CV, Lautt WW. Blood volume, the venous system, preload, and cardiac output. Can J Physiol Pharmacol. 1986;64(4):383–7.
25. Van Geenen EJM, Smits MM, Schreuder TCMA, Van Der Peet DL, Bloemena E, Mulder CJJ. Nonalcoholic fatty liver disease is related to nonalcoholic fatty pancreas disease. Pancreas. 2010;39(8):1185–90.
26. Mikolasevic I, Orlic L, Poropat G, Jakopcic I, Stimac D, Klanac A, et al. Nonalcoholic fatty liver and the severity of acute pancreatitis. Eur J Intern Med. 2017;38:73–8.
27. Gerst F, Wagner R, Kaiser G, Panse M, Heni M, Machann J, et al. Metabolic crosstalk between fatty pancreas and fatty liver: effects on local inflammation and insulin secretion. Diabetologia. 2017;60(11):2240–51.
28. Coate KC, Hernandez G, Thorne CA, Sun S, Le TDV, Vale K, et al. FGF21 is an exocrine pancreas secretagogue. Cell Metab. 2017;25(2):472–80.
29. Hernandez G, Luo T, Javed TA, Wen L, Kalwat MA, Vale K, et al. Pancreatitis is an FGF21-deficient state that is corrected by replacement therapy. Sci Transl Med. 2020;12(525):eaay5186.
30. Liu W, Du JJ, Li ZH, Zhang XY, Zuo HD. Liver injury associated with acute pancreatitis: the current status of clinical evaluation and involved mechanisms. World J Clin Cases. 2021;9(34):10418–29.
31. Lee PJ, Papachristou GI. New insights into acute pancreatitis. Nat Rev Gastroenterol Hepatol. 2019;16(8):479–96.
32. Forsmark CE, Swaroop Vege S, Wilcox CM. Acute pancreatitis. Campion EW, curatore. N Engl J Med. 2016;375(20):1972–81.
33. Neurath MF. Cytokines in inflammatory bowel disease. Nat Rev Immunol. 2014;14(5):329–42.
34. Suzuki M, Shimizu T, Kudo T, Shoji H, Ohtsuka Y, Yamashiro Y. Octreotide prevents l-asparaginase–induced pancreatic injury in rats. Exp Hematol. 2008;36(2):172–80.
35. Zhang XP, Zhang L, Yang P, Zhang RP, Cheng QH. Protective effects of Baicalin and octreotide on multiple organ injury in severe acute pancreatitis. Dig Dis Sci. 2008;53(2):581–91.
36. Zhang X, ping, Wang L, Zhang J. Study progress on mechanism of severe acute pancreatitis complicated with hepatic injury. J Zhejiang Univ Sci B. 2007;8(4):228–36.
37. Yuan BS, Zhu RM, Braddock M, Zhang XH, Shi W, Zheng MH. Interleukin-18: a pro-inflammatory cytokine that plays an important role in acute pancreatitis. Expert Opin Ther Targets. 2007;11(10):1261–71.
38. Zhang T, Xia M, Zhan Q, Zhou Q, Lu G, An F. Sodium butyrate reduces organ injuries in mice with severe acute pancreatitis through inhibiting HMGB1 expression. Dig Dis Sci. 2015;60(7):1991–9.
39. Luan ZG, Zhang H, Ma XC, Zhang C, Guo RX. Therapeutic treatment with ethyl pyruvate attenuates the severity of liver injury in rats with severe acute pancreatitis. Pancreas. 2012;41(5):729–37.
40. Mayer J. Inflammatory mediators in human acute pancreatitis: clinical and pathophysiological implications. Gut. 2000;47(4):546–52.
41. Cuthbertson CM, Christophi C. Disturbances of the microcirculation in acute pancreatitis. Br J Surg. 2006;93(5):518–30.
42. Lisman T, Porte R. Activation and regulation of hemostasis in acute liver failure and acute pancreatitis. Semin Thromb Hemost. 2010;36(04):437–43.
43. Trapnell JE. Pathophysiology of acute pancreatitis. World J Surg. 1981;5(3):319–23.
44. Carmeliet P, Collen D. Molecules in focus tissue factor. Int J Biochem Cell Biol. 1998;30(6):661–7.

45. Ou ZB, Miao CM, Ye MX, Xing DP, He K, Li PZ, et al. Investigation for role of tissue factor and blood coagulation system in severe acute pancreatitis and associated liver injury. Biomed Pharmacother. 2017;85:380–8.
46. Sies H, Berndt C, Jones DP. Oxidative stress. Annu Rev Biochem. 2017;86(1):715–48.
47. Sid B, Verrax J, Calderon PB. Role of oxidative stress in the pathogenesis of alcohol-induced liver disease. Free Radic Res. 2013;47(11):894–904.
48. Uruñuela A, Sevillano S, De La Mano AM, Manso MA, Orfao A, De Dios I. Time-course of oxygen free radical production in acinar cells during acute pancreatitis induced by pancreatic duct obstruction. Biochim Biophys Acta. 2002;1588(2):159–64.
49. Dąbrowski A, Konturek SJ, Konturek JW, Gabryelewicz A. Role of oxidative stress in the pathogenesis of caerulein-induced acute pancreatitis. Eur J Pharmacol. 1999;377(1):1–11.
50. Jungermann J, Lerch MM, Weidenbach H, Lutz MP, Kruger B, Adler G. Disassembly of rat pancreatic acinar cell cytoskeleton during supramaximal secretagogue stimulation. Am J Physiol-Gastrointest Liver Physiol. 1995;268(2):G328–38.
51. Wang G, Sun B, Gao Y, Meng QH, Jiang HC. The effect of Emodin-assisted early enteral nutrition on severe acute pancreatitis and secondary hepatic injury. Mediat Inflamm. 2007;2007:1–8.
52. Eşrefoğlu M, Gül M, Ateş B, Batçıoğlu K, Selimoğlu MA. Antioxidative effect of melatonin, ascorbic acid and *N*-acetylcysteine on caerulein-induced pancreatitis and associated liver injury in rats. World J Gastroenterol. 2006;12(2):259.
53. Chen F, Zhou YJ. Hepatic effect of NAC on sevear acute pancteatise of rats. Asian Pac J Trop Med. 2014;7(2):141–3.
54. Boxhoorn L, Voermans RP, Bouwense SA, Bruno MJ, Verdonk RC, Boermeester MA, et al. Acute pancreatitis. Lancet. 2020;396(10252):726–34.
55. Matsumoto M, Kamei K, Chikugo T, Matsumoto I, Kawaguchi K, Takeyama Y. Efficacy of recombinant human-soluble Thrombomodulin for severe acute pancreatitis in a rat experimental model. Pancreas. 2020;49(4):503–8.
56. Nader MA, Wagih HM. Nilotinib, a tyrosine kinase inhibitor exhibits protection against acute pancreatitis-induced lung and liver damage in rats. Naunyn Schmiedebergs Arch Pharmacol. 2017;390(3):291–300.
57. Zhang FH, Sun YH, Fan KL, Dong XB, Han N, Zhao H, et al. Protective effects of heme oxygenase-1 against severe acute pancreatitis via inhibition of tumor necrosis factor-α and augmentation of interleukin-10. BMC Gastroenterol. 2017;17(1):100.
58. Ueda T, Takeyama Y, Yasuda T, Matsumura N, Sawa H, Nakajima T, et al. Vascular endothelial growth factor increases in serum and protects against the organ injuries in severe acute pancreatitis. J Surg Res. 2006;134(2):223–30.
59. Zhang XP, Zhang J, Ren Z, Feng GH, Zhu W, Cai Y, et al. Study on protecting effects of Baicalin and octreotide on hepatic injury in rats with severe acute pancreatitis. World J Gastroenterol. 2008;14(42):6551.
60. Yang R, Shaufl AL, Killeen ME, Fink MP. Ethyl pyruvate ameliorates liver injury secondary to severe acute pancreatitis. J Surg Res. 2009;153(2):302–9.
61. Turner JR. Intestinal mucosal barrier function in health and disease. Nat Rev Immunol. 2009;9(11):799–809.
62. Abraham C, Abreu MT, Turner JR. Pattern recognition receptor signaling and cytokine networks in microbial defenses and regulation of intestinal barriers: implications for inflammatory bowel disease. Gastroenterology. 2022;162(6):1602–1616.e6.
63. Min YW, Rhee PL. The role of microbiota on the gut immunology. Clin Ther. 2015;37(5):968–75.
64. Abreu MT. Toll-like receptor signalling in the intestinal epithelium: how bacterial recognition shapes intestinal function. Nat Rev Immunol. 2010;10(2):131–44.
65. Artis D. Epithelial-cell recognition of commensal bacteria and maintenance of immune homeostasis in the gut. Nat Rev Immunol. 2008;8(6):411–20.
66. Gewirtz AT, Navas TA, Lyons S, Godowski PJ, Madara JL. Cutting edge: bacterial flagellin activates basolaterally expressed TLR5 to induce epithelial proinflammatory gene expression. J Immunol. 2001;167(4):1882–5.

67. Medzhitov R, Janeway Charle SJ. Innate immune recognition: mechanisms and pathways: innate immune recognition. Immunol Rev. 2000;173(1):89–97.
68. Chiang JYL, Ferrell JM. Discovery of farnesoid X receptor and its role in bile acid metabolism. Mol Cell Endocrinol. 2022;548:111618.
69. Blesl A, Stadlbauer V. The gut-liver axis in cholestatic liver diseases. Nutrients. 2021;13(3):1018.
70. Herrero R, Sánchez G, Asensio I, López E, Ferruelo A, Vaquero J, et al. Liver–lung interactions in acute respiratory distress syndrome. Intensive Care Med Exp. 2020;8(S1):48.
71. Zafirovska M, Zafirovski A, Rotovnik Kozjek N. Current insights regarding intestinal failure-associated liver disease (IFALD): a narrative review. Nutrients. 2023;15(14):3169.
72. Sasdelli AS, Agostini F, Pazzeschi C, Guidetti M, Lal S, Pironi L. Assessment of intestinal failure associated liver disease according to different diagnostic criteria. Clin Nutr. 2019;38(3):1198–205.
73. Pironi L, Sasdelli AS. Intestinal failure-associated liver disease. Clin Liver Dis. 2019;23(2):279–91.
74. Pironi L, Arends J, Bozzetti F, Cuerda C, Gillanders L, Jeppesen PB, et al. ESPEN guidelines on chronic intestinal failure in adults. Clin Nutr. 2016;35(2):247–307.
75. Jin B, Li G, Zhou L, Fan Z. Mechanism involved in acute liver injury induced by intestinal ischemia-reperfusion. Front Pharmacol. 2022;13:924695.
76. Grootjans J, Lenaerts K, Derikx JPM, Matthijsen RA, De Bruïne AP, Van Bijnen AA, et al. Human intestinal ischemia-reperfusion–induced inflammation characterized. Am J Pathol. 2010;176(5):2283–91.
77. Bellezza I, Giambanco I, Minelli A, Donato R. Nrf2-Keap1 signaling in oxidative and reductive stress. Biochim Biophys Acta. 2018;1865(5):721–33.
78. Xie M, Wang J, Gong W, Xu H, Pan X, Chen Y, et al. NF-κB-driven miR-34a impairs Treg/Th17 balance via targeting Foxp3. J Autoimmun. 2019;102:96–113.
79. Liu XM, Chen QH, Hu Q, Liu Z, Wu Q, Liang SS, et al. Dexmedetomidine protects intestinal ischemia-reperfusion injury via inhibiting p38 MAPK cascades. Exp Mol Pathol. 2020;115:104444.
80. Guo Q, Jin Y, Chen X, Ye X, Shen X, Lin M, et al. NF-κB in biology and targeted therapy: new insights and translational implications. Signal Transduct Target Ther. 2024;9(1):53.
81. Sica A, Mantovani A. Macrophage plasticity and polarization: in vivo veritas. J Clin Invest. 2012;122(3):787–95.
82. Linkermann A, Hackl MJ, Kunzendorf U, Walczak H, Krautwald S, Jevnikar AM. Necroptosis in immunity and ischemia-reperfusion injury. Am J Transplant. 2013;13(11):2797–804.
83. Andersson U, Yang H, Harris H. Extracellular HMGB1 as a therapeutic target in inflammatory diseases. Expert Opin Ther Targets. 2018;22(3):263–77.
84. Wen S, Li X, Ling Y, Chen S, Deng Q, Yang L, et al. HMGB1-associated necroptosis and Kupffer cells M1 polarization underlies remote liver injury induced by intestinal ischemia/reperfusion in rats. FASEB J. 2020;34(3):4384–402.
85. Tang SP, Mao XL, Chen YH, Yan LL, Ye LP, Li SW. Reactive oxygen species induce fatty liver and ischemia-reperfusion injury by promoting inflammation and cell death. Front Immunol. 2022;13:870239.
86. Zhou L, Han S, Guo J, Qiu T, Zhou J, Shen L. Ferroptosis—a new dawn in the treatment of organ Ischemia–reperfusion injury. Cells. 2022;11(22):3653.

Part V

The Heart

Brain-Heart Crosstalk: Mechanisms and Clinical Applications for Acute Brain Injury

21

Lavienraj Premraj, Denise Battaglini, and Pasquale Anania

21.1 Introduction

The interaction between the brain and heart (brain-heart crosstalk) during critical illness is poorly characterized. Patients with acute brain injury (ABI) in the intensive care unit (ICU) harbor a heterogeneous collection of pathology attributed to brain-heart crosstalk, including Takotsubo cardiomyopathy following subarachnoid hemorrhage (SAH), paroxysmal sympathetic hyperactivity post-TBI, and electrocardiographic anomalies following acute ischemic stroke (AIS). Non-specific cardiac injury in patients with ABI is well documented, manifesting as arrhythmia, cardiomyocyte injury (biomarker elevation), and/or echocardiographic changes.

Manifestations of brain-heart axis dysfunction are common across ABI subtypes. Electrocardiographic (ECG) changes in the acute phase of non-traumatic SAH (<72 hrs) are present in 25–75% [1–3] of patients with clinically significant arrhythmia occurring in around 4% [4]. Up to half of patients with TBI have arrhythmias [5]. Cardiac effects of acute ischemic stroke (AIS) are thought to depend on location [6–8]: broadly, in a cohort of AIS patients without primary heart disease, around half experienced arrhythmia and/or ischemic ECG changes [9]. Similarly injury to

L. Premraj
Australian and New Zealand Intensive Care Research Centre, Division of Acute and Critical Care, School of Public Health and Preventive Medicine, Faculty of Medicine, Nursing and Health Sciences, Monash University, Melbourne, VIC, Australia

D. Battaglini (✉)
Department of Surgical Sciences and Integrated Diagnostics, University of Genoa, Genoa, Italy
e-mail: denise.battaglini@unige.it

P. Anania
Division of Neurosurgery, IRCCS Ospedale Policlinico San Martino, Genoa, Italy

D. Battaglini et al. (eds.), *Organ System Crosstalk in Critical Illness*,
https://doi.org/10.1007/978-3-032-01024-7_21

cardiomyocytes, determined by cardiac enzyme elevation, is frequently reported in 29–36% of patients with SAH [10], around 60% in TBI [11, 12] and 5–34% with AIS [13, 14]. Elevation of these biomarkers in SAH patients is proportional to the severity of initial injury, independently predicts regional wall motion abnormalities [10], and is associated with increased risk of death and poor functional outcome [15, 16]. Similar relationships are demonstrated across a range of biomarkers and ABI types [10, 13, 14, 16]. While significant heterogeneity in the indicators of brain-heart crosstalk exists, cardiac dysfunction that develops in patients with ABI is associated with poor prognosis and morbidity, especially in those with severe injury. In fact, composite measures of brain-heart interaction derived from network modelling of longitudinal neuromonitoring data in TBI patients confirmed a negative relationship between mortality and brain-heart crosstalk indicators [17].

Despite evidence supporting the presence and prognostic significance of the brain-heart axis, its management remains largely conservative [2, 18, 19] though the rationale behind this approach is continually evaluated by neurointensivists [20]. A clinically oriented synthesis of literature may clarify hypotheses and inform pilot studies [12]. To this end, this chapter aims to (1) summarize the mechanisms of brain-heart crosstalk in critically ill patients and (2) evaluate their relevance in patients with AIS, SAH, and TBI admitted to ICU [7], accounting for the confounding effects of critical illness.

21.2 Mechanisms of Brain-Heart Crosstalk

Traditionally, brain-heart crosstalk implicates neurological pathways that directly modulate cardiac function (i.e., the autonomic nervous system and its reflexes). Autonomic outflow to the heart is regulated by the central autonomic network (CAN), which comprises interconnected areas of the telencephalon, diencephalon, and brain stem [7]. As per classical understanding, sympathetic outflow from the brain largely innervates the cardiac conduction system, ultimately shortening the RR-interval and increasing ventricular contractility, while parasympathetic preganglionic fibers located in the medulla project through into the cardiac conduction system and release acetylcholine, causing the opposite effect (prolons the RR interval and reduced atrial/ventricular contractility) [7].

Naturally, damage to CAN structures can result in autonomic hyperactivity. Ischemic damage to the right insular resulted in sympathetic hyperactivity (determined by reduced heart rate variability) and more complex arrythmias when compared to any other localization [21, 22]. Involvement of the insular cortex was also associated with higher troponin elevation [23, 24], Takotsubo syndrome [25], and post-stroke mortality [6, 26, 27] compared to other brain areas.

However, direct insult to the insular cortex or other CAN structures is not required to trigger the sympathetic hyperactivity responsible for cardiac injury. Through the Cushing reflex, the brain maintains cerebral perfusion pressure (CPP) despite large increases in intracranial pressure (ICP). When ICP exceeds (first demonstrated at ICP >40 mmHg) sympathetic overactivity is triggered, leading to tachycardia and hypertension [28]. More modest increases in ICP also cause sympathetic activation [29]. In ABI patients, neuroinflammation secondary to ischemia, trauma, and anatomical location may also amplify sympathetic hyperactivity [2, 30, 31]. In fact, a three-fold increase in total body norepinephrine was described within the first 48 h of SAH and persisted for up to 7 days. High circulating norepinephrine levels shift intracellular signaling in ventricular cardiomyocytes from G(s) to G(i) protein via the beta(2)-adrenoceptor. This protects against beta(1)-adrenoceptor-mediated proapoptotic effects but also reduces contractility in the apical myocardium (where beta-adrenoceptor density is greatest); a finding characteristic of Takotsubo syndrome [32, 33]. Severe sympathetic surges, as seen in brain death, are linked to myocardial contraction band necrosis [2, 34, 35]. Echocardiographic or ECG changes suggestive of ischemia reported post ABI may result from norepinephrine-driven increased oxygen demand [27] and impaired contractility due to uncoupling of myocardial beta-adrenergic receptors from mechanical response [36]. These mechanisms give rise to the characteristic features of "neurogenic stress cardiomyopathy" (NSC): contraction band necrosis, early calcification, perineural myofibrillary lesions, and reversible regional wall motion abnormalities inconsistent with a single vascular distribution [2, 35, 37].

Recent work has investigated the role of inflammation in the brain-heart axis. ABI often results in damage to the blood-brain barrier, which contributes to vasogenic oedema. The subsequent release of cytokines, if profound, may stimulate corticotropes in the hypothalamus, worsening the catecholamine surge [38, 39], which results in direct cardiac injury. Direct evidence linking neuroinflammation and cardiac injury is lacking: ischemic stroke was accompanied by cardiomyocyte death in a rat model though these results are not to be extrapolated to humans [2, 27, 40, 41]. Indirectly, Mashaly et al. posit that parasympathetic inhibition (due to sympathetic hyperactivity in SAH) may render cardiomyocytes more vulnerable to inflammatory injury as acetylcholine ordinarily inhibits the release of pro-inflammatory cytokines [42]. TBI patients with systemic inflammatory response syndrome (SIRS), observed in about one-fifth of moderate-to-severe TBI patients, had fourfold higher risk of systolic dysfunction than those without SIRS [43]. Other novel pathways may also contribute, gut pathogens contribute to the inflammatory response through platelet hyperactivation and thrombosis, mediated by conversion of choline and l-carnitine into trimethylamine-N-oxide (TMAO). TMAO also serves as an independent predictor for cardiac disease and, in addition to other biomarkers, can theoretically assist in predicting cardiac injury post-ABI [8, 38].

Even without direct injury structures responsible for autonomic control, ABI can cause cardiac dysfunction. Elevated ICP and neuroinflammation, common features of ABI, potentiate the catecholamine surge which may intensify cardiac injury.

21.3 Brain-Heart Axis Dysfunction in Acute Brain Injury

The main mechanisms involved in the bidirectional brain-heart and heart-brain pathways are presented in Fig. 21.1.

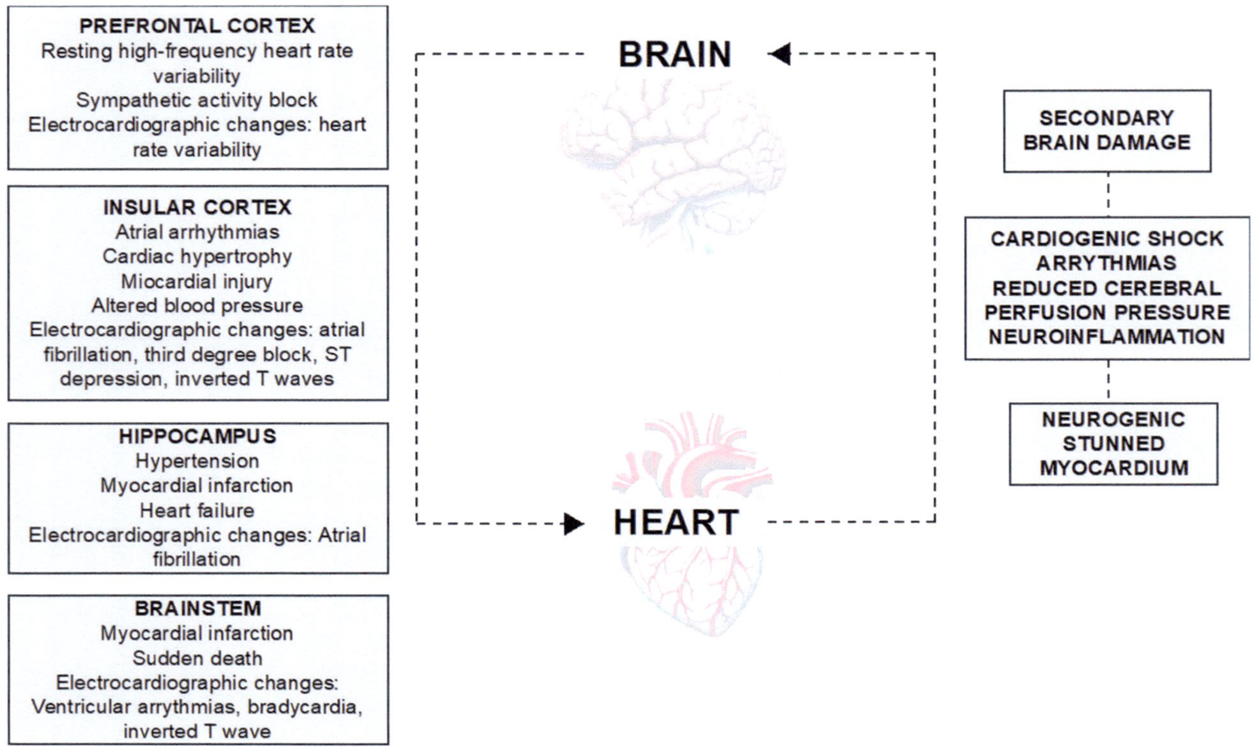

Fig. 21.1 The main mechanisms involved in the bidirectional brain-heart and heart-brain pathways. Acute brain injury can induce cardiac dysfunction through autonomic dysregulation, often without direct damage to autonomic centers like the insular cortex. Elevated intracranial pressure and neuroinflammation trigger a catecholamine surge, promoting myocardial injury via sympathetic overactivation, neurogenic stress cardiomyopathy, and inflammatory pathways. These mechanisms collectively contribute to cardiac complications such as arrhythmias, Takotsubo syndrome, and systolic dysfunction. Cardiac dysfunction can in turn cause secondary brain injury due to reduced cerebral perfusion pressure and neuroinflammatory markers release

21.4 Traumatic Brain Injury

The goal of TBI management is to prevent additional brain damage (secondary injury) and optimize conditions for brain recovery. Primary intracranial injury consists of parenchymal and/or vascular lesions which may occur as part of a larger polytrauma. Secondary injury develops during ICU stay due to the activation of various neuronal pathways [44]. In the acute phase ECG abnormalities, ventricular dysfunction, and direct cardiomyocyte injury are well documented, likely driven by the severity of initial insult. ECG changes include QTc prolongation, T-wave inversion, and ST segment changes indicative of ischemia in up to half of patients [5]. Ventricular dysfunction manifests in the acute phase of injury with hypertension and tachycardia followed by a drop in blood pressure in the subacute phase when circulating catecholamines and sympathetic activity have reduced [45, 46]. Though not routinely assessed, cohort studies report reduced left ventricular ejection fraction (LVEF) and regional wall motion abnormalities (RWMA) in 12% of TBI patients [47].

The prognostic value of cardiac dysfunction post-TBI is debated. While ECG alterations are common especially in the acute phase, they are largely transient and not associated with mortality. This is despite the long-standing association between raised ICP and ECG changes (especially in the context of SAH and ICH) [48, 49].

Clinical outcomes of ventricular dysfunction post-TBI are poorly described: takotsubo cardiomyopathy, known to occur in the acute phase, resolves within days [50]. Evidence examining the trajectory of patients with neurogenic stunned myocardium/stress cardiomyopathy is absent [2, 48]. Also, electrolyte derangements, thoracic trauma, and chronic cardiac disease confound measures of ABI-induced impairment of brain-heart crosstalk in TBI patients. Still, high-resolution longitudinal data from 226 patients were examined for interactions between heart rate and ICP at regular intervals. The algorithm detected the total number of brain-heart crosstalk events in patients with TBI and, through multilayer network modelling, determined an inverse relationship between these events and mortality [17]. Despite the variability among TBI patients and the complexity of their treatments, intact brain-heart crosstalk seems to play a crucial role in recovery and could eventually become a therapeutic target.

Paroxysmal sympathetic hyperactivity (PSH) syndrome is a serious complication of TBI (and other ABI) that is characterized by simultaneous, paroxysmal transient increases in sympathetic (elevated heart rate, blood pressure, respiratory rate, temperature, sweating), and motor (posturing) activity [51]. Prevalence of PSH syndrome ranges from 11% to 69% depending on the cohort and definition used: meta-analysis of studies from 2007 to 2021 estimates prevalence of 28.1% in TBI [52]. The PSH Assessment Measure incorporates heart rate and systolic blood pressure, which are sequalae of sympathetic hyperactivity [53, 54]. PSH syndrome resulted in longer hospital stay, higher proportion of tracheostomy, and worse functional outcome in adult and pediatric patients [51–53]. However, PSH syndrome is more likely to occur in severe brain injury [52, 55]. The prognostic value of the cardiac criteria (heart rate, systolic blood pressure) alone on the outcomes of TBI patients with PSH syndrome is unknown.

We conclude that the markers of brain-heart axis dysfunction (ECG echocardiographic and biomarker changes) are commonly observed post-TBI, (2) the value of these markers as prognostic tools nor their contribution to adverse outcome is not clear, (3) PSH post-TBI is not uncommon especially in severe TBI, results in cardiac dysfunction and is more clearly associated with poor neurological outcome and mortality. Dysregulation of the brain-heart axis may be most clinically relevant in the population with severe, diffuse brain injury with features of PSH syndrome.

21.5 Acute Ischemic Stroke

In addition to being a primary reason for ICU admission, acute ischemic stroke (AIS) can arise secondary to other critical illnesses (e.g., septic emboli), surgery (e.g., embolic complications), or medical interventions (e.g., post-thrombolysis blood pressure monitoring). Features of AIS requiring ICU admission include airway compromise, infarction complicated by seizure, large hemispheric infarction (LHI), and hemorrhagic transformation [56]. Brain-heart interaction in ICU patients with AIS is yet poorly characterized. Available evidence demonstrates that (1) patients with AIS are susceptible to cardiac injury, and stroke may lead to worse cardiac outcomes; and (2) AIS, particularly cases requiring ICU admission, can cause autonomic dysfunction that may further exacerbate brain injury.

The annual rate of myocardial infarction in post-AIS patients is 2.2% [57, 58] and long-term, 2–6% of all hospital-admitted stroke patients die from cardiac causes within 3 months of admission. Moreover, analysis of 14, 338 patients in metropolitan American centers between 2002 and 2018 showed that 5% of patients with AIS had left ventricular ejection fraction (LVEF) <40% [59] during hospitalization. The AIS population is vulnerable to cardiac injury at the outset and experiences a high rate of cardiac-related mortality post-stroke.

In non-ICU patients, 24% of patients with AIS developed autonomic dysfunction (as determined by a battery of autonomic reflex testing) [60]. In the acute phase of stroke and 7–10 days preceding, heart rate variability (HRV) parameters decreased significantly, indicating increased autonomic activity. While intravenous thrombolysis improved HRV measures, HRV in the acute phase was independently associated with unfavorable neurologic outcomes (mRS >2) [61]. Similarly, increased variability in blood pressure (BPV) in the acute phase is associated with poor long-term outcome [62, 63]. In a study of over half a million patients presenting to emergency with stroke, around 70% of AIS patients had initial BP >140mmHg [64]. Management of blood pressure in AIS balances risk of hypoperfusion with that of haemorrhage [8, 64]. Seizure or severe heart failure complicating AIS in the ICU may, in the context of impaired cardiac function secondary to autonomic hyperactivity, increase cerebral metabolic demand and restrict perfusion, preventing salvage of ischemic tissue.

The specific cardiovascular derangements secondary to AIS depend on the location and size of the lesion [7, 8, 41, 65]. Generally, involvement of the insular cortex is associated with greater likelihood of cardiovascular complications [41]. Lateralization is debated: left insular stroke is an independent predictor of serious cardiac events although troponins were increased in 6.7% of patients with infarction of the right insular cortex. Generally, studies demonstrate greater troponin elevation and incidence of Takotsubo syndrome in patients with insular/peri-insular (vs non-insular) stroke [41]. Strokes affecting the insula are generally larger than non-insular strokes. The insular is exclusively supplied by the middle cerebral artery (MCA), specifically by perforating arteries from the M2 segment, although some supply is drawn from M1 and M3 segments in 55% and 25% of hemispheres, respectively [66]. In patients with LHI, defined as stroke affecting the total or subtotal territory of the MCA involving the basal ganglia at least partially, the insular cortex is extremely likely to be involved [67]. In a study of consecutive patients admitted within 24 hours of LHI diagnosis, 54.5% had right hemispheric involvement, and these patients had a greater frequency of atrial fibrillation, malignant cerebral oedema, composite cardiovascular events during hospitalization, and one-month mortality [68, 69]. In such patients, with large infarcts warranting ICU admission, the prognostic relevance of brain-heart crosstalk requires more investigation. It is not clear if the numerous findings in the non-ICU population described previously are relevant in patients with AIS in the ICU.

21.6 Non-Traumatic Subarachnoid Hemorrhage

Unlike AIS and even mild TBI, the majority of SAH patients who survive the initial bleed are admitted to ICU. Cardiac complications in SAH patients are (1) common; (2) correlated with severity of SAH and (3) contribute to mortality and neurological recovery.

SAH may manifest the entire spectrum of cardiac dysfunction as discussed in the other forms of ABI. Of 11, 047 patients admitted to Australian and New Zealand ICUs with SAH, 3.9% had cardiac arrest 24 h preceding admission [70]. In US centers, SAH was the cause of out-of-hospital cardiac arrest in 4–8%; as a cause of in-hospital cardiac arrest prevalence was 0.5%. In both cases, the initial rhythms were asystole or pulseless electrical tachycardia [71]. At the onset of SAH, LV systolic dysfunction is commonly observed, though regresses over the first week coinciding with a decline in circulating catecholamine levels. Meta-analysis of studies comprising SAH patients who received echocardiographic evaluation of cardiac function from 2006 to 2014 concluded that one in five patients developed quantifiable ventricular dysfunction [72]. While cardiac dysfunction in SAH patients has long been documented and managed in the ICU, its prevalence should not be overestimated: older studies neglect the abandonment of triple H therapy (which carried significant risk of pulmonary oedema and myocardial ischemia) and advances in aneurysm securement.

Severity of SAH is related to markers of cardiac injury: on admission plasma catecholamines, BNP and troponin were higher in patients with higher WFNS score. Upon multivariate analysis of a cohort of 40 consecutive patients with acute SAH without known heart disease, only WFNS grade (and not age or plasma norepinephrine) was statistically associated with cardiac dysfunction on admission. In a separate study of 223 patients in 2004, Hunt-Hess score > 2 was among the independent predictors of troponin elevation. Recent studies have replicated these findings supporting the hypothesis that cardiac injury in SAH may be a neurally mediated process via the catecholamine-driven mechanisms discussed above [73–75].

Cardiac dysfunction in SAH patients is clearly associated with mortality and worse neurological outcomes. Meta-analysis of 25 studies (N = 2690) in SAH patients showed that mortality and poor neurological outcome were significantly associated with elevated troponin (relative risk; RR = 2.0) and ST-segment depression (RR = 2.4) [76]. Delayed cerebral ischemia (DCI), which occurs in roughly a third of SAH patients, undisputedly carries a dismal neurological prognosis. DCI was strongly associated with RWMAs (RR = 2.1) and biomarker elevation. Similarly, more recent meta-analyses reproduce the above findings, confirming that RWMAs (RR = 1.45) and troponin elevations (RR = 1.48) were consistently and significantly associated with DCI [10, 77].

Cardiac injury may be responsible, to some extent, for driving mortality in SAH. Equally, it may simply be that worse grades of SAH are associated with cardiac complications and, separately, mortality. Regardless of directionality, substantial evidence verifies that cardiac dysfunction in SAH patients is clinically important.

21.7 Conclusions

Brain-heart axis dysfunction is prevalent in ABI patients, with varying markers such as electrocardiographic changes, echocardiographic abnormalities, and cardiac biomarker elevation. The prognostic value of these markers in predicting outcomes remains uncertain, necessitating further investigation. Paroxysmal sympathetic hyperactivity in TBI patients is associated with significant cardiac dysfunction and poor neurological outcomes, underscoring the clinical importance of understanding brain-heart interactions in severe brain injuries.

References

1. Lanzino G, Kongable GL, Kassell NF. Electrocardiographic abnormalities after nontraumatic subarachnoid hemorrhage. J Neurosurg Anesthesiol. 1994;6(3):156–62.
2. Mazzeo AT, Micalizzi A, Mascia L, Scicolone A, Siracusano L. Brain-heart crosstalk: the many faces of stress-related cardiomyopathy syndromes in anaesthesia and intensive care. Br J Anaesth. 2014;112(5):803–15.
3. Togha M, Sharifpour A, Ashraf H, Moghadam M, Sahraian MA. Electrocardiographic abnormalities in acute cerebrovascular events in patients with/without cardiovascular disease. Ann Indian Acad Neurol. 2013;16(1):66–71.

4. Frontera JA, Parra A, Shimbo D, Fernandez A, Schmidt JM, Peter P, et al. Cardiac arrhythmias after subarachnoid hemorrhage: risk factors and impact on outcome. Cerebrovasc Dis Basel Switzerland. 2008;26(1):71–8.
5. Coppalini G, Salvagno M, Peluso L, Bogossian EG, Quispe Cornejo A, Labbé V, et al. Cardiac injury after traumatic brain injury: clinical consequences and management. Neurocrit Care. 2024;40(2):477–85.
6. Tokgözoglu SL, Batur MK, Topçuoglu MA, Saribas O, Kes S, Oto A. Effects of stroke localization on cardiac autonomic balance and sudden death. Stroke. 1999;30(7):1307–11.
7. Silvani A, Calandra-Buonaura G, Dampney RAL, Cortelli P. Brain–heart interactions: physiology and clinical implications. Philos Trans R Soc Math Phys Eng Sci. 2016;374(2067):20150181.
8. Battaglini D, Robba C, Lopes da Silva A, Dos Santos Samary C, Leme Silva P, Dal Pizzol F, et al. Brain-heart interaction after acute ischemic stroke. Crit Care Lond Engl. 2020;24(1):163.
9. Dogan A, Tunc E, Ozturk M, Kerman M, Akhan G. Electrocardiographic changes in patients with ischaemic stroke and their prognostic importance. Int J Clin Pract. 2004;58(5):436–40.
10. Zhang L, Zhang B, Qi S. Impact of echocardiographic wall motion abnormality and cardiac biomarker elevation on outcome after subarachnoid hemorrhage: a meta-analysis. Neurosurg Rev. 2020;43(1):59–68.
11. Salim A, Hadjizacharia P, Brown C, Inaba K, Teixeira PGR, Chan L, et al. Significance of troponin elevation after severe traumatic brain injury. J Trauma Acute Care Surg. 2008;64(1):46.
12. El-Menyar A, Asim M, Khan N, Rizoli S, Mahmood I, Al-Ani M, et al. Systemic and cerebro-cardiac biomarkers following traumatic brain injury: an interim analysis of randomized controlled clinical trial of early administration of beta blockers. Sci Rep. 2024;14(1):19574.
13. Kerr G, Ray G, Wu O, Stott DJ, Langhorne P. Elevated troponin after stroke: a systematic review. Cerebrovasc Dis. 2009;28(3):220–6.
14. Ahn S, Kim Y, Shin C, Lee J, Kim B, Kim Y, et al. Cardiac vulnerability to cerebrogenic stress as a possible cause of troponin elevation in stroke. J Am Heart Assoc. 2016;5(10):e004135.
15. Tung P, Kopelnik A, Banki N, Ong K, Ko N, Lawton MT, et al. Predictors of neurocardiogenic injury after subarachnoid hemorrhage. Stroke. 2004;35(2):548–51.
16. Tung PP, Olmsted E, Kopelnik A, Banki NM, Drew BJ, Ko N, et al. Plasma B-type natriuretic peptide levels are associated with early cardiac dysfunction after subarachnoid hemorrhage. Stroke. 2005;36(7):1567–9.
17. Dimitri GM, Beqiri E, Placek MM, Czosnyka M, Stocchetti N, Ercole A, et al. Modeling brain-heart crosstalk information in patients with traumatic brain injury. Neurocrit Care. 2022;36(3):738–50.
18. Jafari AA, Shah M, Mirmoeeni S, Hassani MS, Nazari S, Fielder T, et al. Paroxysmal sympathetic hyperactivity during traumatic brain injury. Clin Neurol Neurosurg. 2022;212:107081.
19. Battaglini D, De Rosa S, Godoy DA. Crosstalk between the nervous system and systemic organs in acute brain injury. Neurocrit Care. 2024;40(1):337–48.
20. Ripoll JG, Blackshear JL, Díaz-Gómez JL. Acute cardiac complications in critical brain disease. Neurol Clin. 2017;35(4):761–83.
21. Cheung RTF, Hachinski V. The insula and cerebrogenic sudden death. Arch Neurol. 2000;57(12):1685–8.
22. Colivicchi F, Bassi A, Santini M, Caltagirone C. Cardiac autonomic derangement and arrhythmias in right-sided stroke with insular involvement. Stroke. 2004;35(9):2094–8.
23. Krause T, Werner K, Fiebach JB, Villringer K, Piper SK, Haeusler KG, et al. Stroke in right dorsal anterior insular cortex is related to myocardial injury. Ann Neurol. 2017;81(4):502–11.
24. Ay H, Koroshetz WJ, Benner T, Vangel MG, Melinosky C, Arsava EM, et al. Neuroanatomic correlates of stroke-related myocardial injury. Neurology. 2006;66(9):1325–9.
25. Jung JM, Kim JG, Kim JB, Cho KH, Yu S, Oh K, et al. Takotsubo-like myocardial dysfunction in ischemic stroke: a hospital-based registry and systematic literature review. Stroke. 2016;47(11):2729–36.

26. Sposato LA, Cohen G, Wardlaw JM, Sandercock P, Lindley RI, Hachinski V, et al. Effect of right insular involvement on death and functional outcome after acute ischemic stroke in the IST-3 trial (Third international stroke trial). Stroke. 2016;47(12):2959–65.
27. Sposato LA, Hilz MJ, Aspberg S, Murthy SB, Bahit MC, Hsieh CY, et al. Post-stroke cardiovascular complications and neurogenic cardiac injury: JACC state-of-the-art review. J Am Coll Cardiol. 2020;76(23):2768–85.
28. Concerning a definite regulatory mechanism of the vaso-motor centre which controls blood pressure during cerebral compression - NLM Catalog - NCBI [Internet]. [cited 2024 Dec 28]. Available from: https://www.ncbi.nlm.nih.gov/nlmcatalog/101487551
29. Guild SJ, Saxena UA, McBryde FD, Malpas SC, Ramchandra R. Intracranial pressure influences the level of sympathetic tone. Am J Physiol-Regul Integr Comp Physiol. 2018;315(5):R1049–53.
30. Schmidt EA, Despas F, Pavy-Le Traon A, Czosnyka Z, Pickard JD, Rahmouni K, et al. Intracranial pressure is a determinant of sympathetic activity. Front Physiol. 2018;9:11.
31. Chen Z, Venkat P, Seyfried D, Chopp M, Yan T, Chen J. Brain-heart interaction: cardiac complications after stroke. Circ Res. 2017;121(4):451–68.
32. Lyon AR, Rees PSC, Prasad S, Poole-Wilson PA, Harding SE. Stress (Takotsubo) cardiomyopathy--a novel pathophysiological hypothesis to explain catecholamine-induced acute myocardial stunning. Nat Clin Pract Cardiovasc Med. 2008;5(1):22–9.
33. Paur H, Wright PT, Sikkel MB, Tranter MH, Mansfield C, O'Gara P, et al. High levels of circulating epinephrine trigger apical cardiodepression in a β2-adrenergic receptor/Gi-dependent manner: a new model of Takotsubo cardiomyopathy. Circulation. 2012;126(6):697–706.
34. Pérez López S, Otero Hernández J, Vázquez Moreno N, Escudero Augusto D, Alvarez Menéndez F, Astudillo González A. Brain death effects on catecholamine levels and subsequent cardiac damage assessed in organ donors. J Heart Lung Transplant. 2009;28(8):815–20.
35. Tavazzi G, Zanierato M, Via G, Iotti GA, Procaccio F. Are neurogenic stress cardiomyopathy and Takotsubo different syndromes with common pathways? JACC Heart Fail. 2017;5(12):940–2.
36. White M, Wiechmann RJ, Roden RL, Hagan MB, Wollmering MM, Port JD, et al. Cardiac beta-adrenergic neuroeffector systems in acute myocardial dysfunction related to brain injury. Evidence for catecholamine-mediated myocardial damage. Circulation. 1995;92(8):2183–9.
37. Gopinath R, Ayya SS. Neurogenic stress cardiomyopathy: what do we need to know. Ann Card Anaesth. 2018;21(3):228–34.
38. Fan X, Cao J, Li M, Zhang D, El-Battrawy I, Chen G, et al. Stroke related brain–heart crosstalk: pathophysiology, clinical implications, and underlying mechanisms. Adv Sci. 2024;11(14):2307698.
39. Santos Samary C, Pelosi P, Leme Silva P, Rieken Macedo Rocco P. Immunomodulation after ischemic stroke: potential mechanisms and implications for therapy. Crit Care. 2016;20(1):391.
40. Ishikawa H, Tajiri N, Vasconcellos J, Kaneko Y, Mimura O, Dezawa M, et al. Ischemic stroke brain sends indirect cell death signals to the heart. Stroke. 2013;44(11):3175–82.
41. Méloux A, Béjot Y, Rochette L, Cottin Y, Vergely C. Brain-heart interactions during ischemic processes: clinical and experimental evidences. Stroke. 2020;51(2):679–86.
42. Mashaly HA, Provencio JJ. Inflammation as a link between brain injury and heart damage: the model of subarachnoid hemorrhage. Cleve Clin J Med. 2008;75(Suppl 2):S26–30.
43. Chaikittisilpa N, Krishnamoorthy V, Lele AV, Qiu Q, Vavilala MS. Characterizing the relationship between systemic inflammatory response syndrome and early cardiac dysfunction in traumatic brain injury. J Neurosci Res. 2018;96(4):661–70.
44. Stocchetti N, Carbonara M, Citerio G, Ercole A, Skrifvars MB, Smielewski P, et al. Severe traumatic brain injury: targeted management in the intensive care unit. Lancet Neurol. 2017;16(6):452–64.
45. Krishnamoorthy V, Prathep S, Sharma D, Gibbons E, Vavilala MS. Association between electrocardiographic findings and cardiac dysfunction in adult isolated traumatic brain injury. Indian J Crit Care Med Peer-Rev. 2014;18(9):570–4.

46. Krishnamoorthy V, Chaikittisilpa N, Kiatchai T, Vavilala M. Hypertension after severe traumatic brain injury: friend or foe? J Neurosurg Anesthesiol. 2017;29(4):382–7.
47. Prathep S, Sharma D, Hallman M, Joffe A, Krishnamoorthy V, Mackensen GB, et al. Preliminary report on cardiac dysfunction after isolated traumatic brain injury. Crit Care Med. 2014;42(1):142–7.
48. Grunsfeld A, Fletcher JJ, Nathan BR. Cardiopulmonary complications of brain injury. Curr Neurol Neurosci Rep. 2005;5(6):488–93.
49. Jachuck SJ, Ramani PS, Clark F, Kalbag RM. Electrocardiographic abnormalities associated with raised intracranial pressure. Br Med J. 1975;1(5952):242–4.
50. Gruhl SL, Su J, Chua WC, Tay KV. Takotsubo cardiomyopathy in post-traumatic brain injury: a systematic review of diagnosis and management. Clin Neurol Neurosurg. 2022;213:107119.
51. Meyfroidt G, Baguley IJ, Menon DK. Paroxysmal sympathetic hyperactivity: the storm after acute brain injury. Lancet Neurol. 2017;16(9):721–9.
52. Qian J, Min X, Wang F, Xu Y, Fang W. Paroxysmal sympathetic hyperactivity in adult patients with brain injury: a systematic review and meta-analysis. World Neurosurg. 2022;166:212–9.
53. Rabinstein AA. Paroxysmal sympathetic hyperactivity in the neurological intensive care unit. Neurol Res. 2007;29(7):680–2.
54. Baguley IJ, Perkes IE, Fernandez-Ortega JF, Rabinstein AA, Dolce G, Hendricks HT, et al. Paroxysmal sympathetic hyperactivity after acquired brain injury: consensus on conceptual definition, nomenclature, and diagnostic criteria. J Neurotrauma. 2014;31(17):1515–20.
55. Fernandez-Ortega JF, Prieto-Palomino MA, Garcia-Caballero M, Galeas-Lopez JL, Quesada-Garcia G, Baguley IJ. Paroxysmal sympathetic hyperactivity after traumatic brain injury: clinical and prognostic implications. J Neurotrauma. 2012;29(7):1364–70.
56. McDermott M, Jacobs T, Morgenstern L. Chapter 10 - Critical care in acute ischemic stroke. In: Wijdicks EFM, Kramer AH, editors. Handbook of clinical neurology [Internet]. Elsevier; 2017 [cited 2025 Jan 12]. p. 153–176. (Critical Care Neurology Part I; vol. 140). Available from: https://www.sciencedirect.com/science/article/pii/B9780444636003000106
57. Touzé E, Varenne O, Chatellier G, Peyrard S, Rothwell PM, Mas JL. Risk of myocardial infarction and vascular death after transient ischemic attack and ischemic stroke: a systematic review and meta-analysis. Stroke. 2005;36(12):2748–55.
58. Prosser J, MacGregor L, Lees KR, Diener HC, Hacke W, Davis S, et al. Predictors of early cardiac morbidity and mortality after ischemic stroke. Stroke. 2007;38(8):2295–302.
59. Baker AD, Schwamm LH, Sanborn DY, Furie K, Stretz C, Mac Grory B, et al. Acute ischemic stroke, depressed left ventricular ejection fraction, and sinus rhythm: prevalence and practice patterns. Stroke. 2022;53(6):1883–91.
60. Xiong L, Tian G, Leung H, Soo YOY, Chen X, Ip VHL, et al. Autonomic dysfunction predicts clinical outcomes after acute ischemic stroke: a prospective observational study. Stroke. 2018;49(1):215–8.
61. Qu Y, Sun Y, Abuduxukuer R, Si X, Zhang P, Ren J, et al. Heart rate variability parameter changes in patients with acute ischemic stroke undergoing intravenous thrombolysis. J Am Heart Assoc. 2023;12(11):e028778.
62. Kang J, Hong JH, Jang MU, Choi NC, Lee JS, Kim BJ, et al. Change in blood pressure variability in patients with acute ischemic stroke and its effect on early neurologic outcome. PLoS One. 2017;12(12):e0189216.
63. Manning LS, Rothwell PM, Potter JF, Robinson TG. Prognostic significance of short-term blood pressure variability in acute stroke: systematic review. Stroke. 2015;46(9):2482–90.
64. Qureshi AI, Ezzeddine MA, Nasar A, Suri MFK, Kirmani JF, Hussein H, et al. Prevalence of elevated blood pressure in 563, 704 adult patients presenting to the emergency department with stroke in the United States. Am J Emerg Med. 2007;25(1):32–8.
65. Tahsili-Fahadan P, Geocadin RG. Heart-brain Axis: effects of neurologic injury on cardiovascular function. Circ Res. 2017;120(3):559–72.
66. Celik S, Bilge O, Yurttaş C, Turgut M. Anatomy of the insular arteries. In: Turgut M, Yurttaş C, Tubbs RS, editors. Island of Reil (insula) in the human brain: anatomical, functional, clinical

and surgical aspects [Internet]. Cham: Springer International Publishing; 2018 [cited 2025 Jan 12]. p. 39–53. Available from: https://doi.org/10.1007/978-3-319-75468-0_4.
67. Huttner HB, Schwab S. Malignant middle cerebral artery infarction: clinical characteristics, treatment strategies, and future perspectives. Lancet Neurol. 2009;8(10):949–58.
68. Laredo C, Zhao Y, Rudilosso S, Renú A, Pariente JC, Chamorro Á, et al. Prognostic significance of infarct size and location: the case of insular stroke. Sci Rep. 2018;8(1):9498.
69. Liebeskind DS, Jüttler E, Shapovalov Y, Yegin A, Landen J, Jauch EC. Cerebral edema associated with large hemispheric infarction. Stroke. 2019;50(9):2619–25.
70. Heaney J, Paul E, Pilcher D, Lin C, Udy A, Young PJ. Outcomes of patients with subarachnoid haemorrhage admitted to Australian and New Zealand intensive care units following a cardiac arrest. Crit Care Resusc. 2020;22(3):237–44.
71. Skrifvars MB, Parr MJ. Incidence, predisposing factors, management and survival following cardiac arrest due to subarachnoid haemorrhage: a review of the literature. Scand J Trauma Resusc Emerg Med. 2012;20(1):75.
72. Messina A, Longhitano Y, Zanza C, Calabrò L, Villa F, Cammarota G, et al. Cardiac dysfunction in patients affected by subarachnoid haemorrhage affects in-hospital mortality: a systematic review and metanalysis. Eur J Anaesthesiol. 2023;40(6):442–9.
73. Cammann VL, Scheitz JF, von Rennenberg R, Jäncke L, Nolte CH, Szawan KA, et al. Clinical correlates and prognostic impact of neurologic disorders in Takotsubo syndrome. Sci Rep. 2021;11:23555.
74. Catapano JS, Ducruet AF, Frisoli FA, Nguyen CL, Louie CE, Labib MA, et al. Predictors of the development of takotsubo cardiomyopathy in aneurysmal subarachnoid hemorrhage and outcomes in patients with intra-aortic balloon pumps. 2020 Sep 4 [cited 2025 Jan 29]; Available from: https://thejns.org/view/journals/j-neurosurg/135/1/article-p38.xml
75. Murthy SB, Shah S, Rao CPV, Bershad EM, Suarez JI. Neurogenic stunned myocardium following acute subarachnoid hemorrhage: pathophysiology and practical considerations. J Intensive Care Med. 2015;30(6):318–25.
76. van der Bilt IAC, Hasan D, Vandertop WP, Wilde AAM, Algra A, Visser FC, et al. Impact of cardiac complications on outcome after aneurysmal subarachnoid hemorrhage. Neurology. 2009;72(7):635–42.
77. Zhang L, Wang Z, Qi S. Cardiac troponin elevation and outcome after subarachnoid hemorrhage: a systematic review and meta-analysis. J Stroke Cerebrovasc Dis. 2015;24(10):2375–84.

Metabolic Crosstalk in Heart Failure

22

Simona Silvetti, Aaron Pagan, and Marina Pieri

22.1 Introduction

Heart failure (HF) is a complex clinical syndrome characterized by the inability of the heart to pump sufficient blood to meet the metabolic needs of tissues. It affects millions of individuals worldwide, playing a major contribution to morbidity and mortality. Recent research has shown that HF is not limited to a problem of impaired cardiac function; on the contrary, it is also closely tied to alterations in cellular metabolism. Understanding the metabolic changes that occur in HF has led to the recognition of "metabolic crosstalk," which plays a crucial role in the progression and pathophysiology of the disease [1, 2].

Metabolic crosstalk refers to the bidirectional communication between the heart and other organs, such as the liver, skeletal muscle, and adipose tissue. This interplay involves numerous signaling molecules, metabolic substrates, and enzymatic pathways that contribute to impact cardiac function. As HF progresses, disruptions in these pathways not only worsen cardiac dysfunction but also propagate systemic metabolic abnormalities [2, 3].

S. Silvetti (✉)
Department of Cardioanesthesia and Intensive Care, Policlinico San Martino IRCCS Hospital – IRCCS Cardiovascular Network, Genoa, Italy
e-mail: simona.silvetti@hsanmartino.it

A. Pagan
Department of Anesthesia and Intensive Care DISC, University of Genoa, Genoa, Italy

M. Pieri
Department of Anesthesia and Intensive Care, IRCCS San Raffaele Scientific Institute, Milan, Italy

School of Medicine, Vita-Salute San Raffaele, Milan, Italy
e-mail: Pieri.marina@hsr.it

D. Battaglini et al. (eds.), *Organ System Crosstalk in Critical Illness*,
https://doi.org/10.1007/978-3-032-01024-7_22

Metabolic crosstalk is a progressive, dynamic, and difficult to reverse phenomenon, whose impact is clear in chronic HF, but that can also impact acute decompensation episodes, affecting the response of the patients to treatment in the acute care scenario.

This chapter aims to explore the concept of metabolic crosstalk in heart failure, emphasizing the metabolic shifts that occur between various organs and cellular compartments. Additionally, we will discuss the potential therapeutic strategies targeting these metabolic pathways, providing insights into future treatment directions for HF [2, 4].

22.2 Metabolic Changes in Heart Failure

22.2.1 Energetic Dysregulation in the Failing Heart

Under normal physiological conditions, the heart primarily relies on fatty acid oxidation for its energy demands, with glucose and lactate serving as supplementary energy sources. However, in HF, a shift toward increased glucose and lactate utilization is observed. While this shift, known as metabolic remodeling, is thought to be an adaptive response to energy deficits, it often results in decreased efficiency in adenosine triphosphate (ATP) production [1, 2].

In HF, reduced fatty acid oxidation is linked to impaired mitochondrial function and decreased availability of oxygen. The reliance on glycolysis over oxidative phosphorylation leads to the accumulation of lactate and other intermediates, further contributing to metabolic inefficiency. Studies have shown that this energetic dysregulation correlates with worsening cardiac contractile function and adverse remodeling, thus exacerbating HF progression [3].

22.2.2 Mitochondrial Dysfunction

Mitochondria are essential for maintaining the energy demands of the heart, accounting for nearly 90% of its ATP production. In HF, mitochondrial dysfunction emerges as a central pathological feature. This dysfunction is characterized by reduced biogenesis, impaired electron transport chain activity, and increased production of reactive oxygen species (ROS) [2, 3].

ROS not only damages mitochondrial DNA but also disrupts membrane potential and compromise ATP production. Additionally, mitophagy, the process of clearing damaged mitochondria, is often dysregulated in HF, leading to the accumulation of defective organelles. These changes contribute to a vicious cycle where impaired mitochondrial function exacerbates energy deficits and promotes myocardial apoptosis, fibrosis, and inflammation.

22.3 Metabolic Crosstalk Between Organs

The pathophysiology of HF is not confined to the heart but involves complex interactions with peripheral organs, including the liver, skeletal muscle, adipose tissue, and kidneys. Understanding these inter-organ relationships is critical for developing comprehensive therapeutic strategies for HF patients [2, 4].

22.3.1 Heart-Liver Crosstalk

The liver plays a crucial role in maintaining metabolic homeostasis, including glucose and lipid metabolism. In heart failure, hepatic dysfunction, known also as "cardiohepatic syndrome," is frequently observed due to congestion and reduced perfusion. This results in impaired gluconeogenesis, dysregulated lipid metabolism, and increased systemic inflammation [3, 4].

The liver secretes hepatokines such as fetuin-A and fibroblast growth factor 21 (FGF21), which influence myocardial function. Conversely, pro-inflammatory cytokines and damage-associated molecular patterns (DAMPs) released by the failing heart exacerbate hepatic steatosis and fibrosis, creating a feedback loop that worsens systemic metabolic dysfunction [13].

22.3.2 Heart-Adipose Tissue Crosstalk

There is a well-documented association between obesity and HF. Multiple studies have established both pro- and anti-inflammatory effects of adipokines [7, 8].

Visceral fat is the most important depot of pro-inflammatory cytokines like IL-6, IL-8, and monocyte chemoattractant protein-1 (MCP-1), and there is a well-established positive correlation between visceral fat levels and HF [9–11]. Interestingly, peri and epicardial fat exhibit a similar phenotype to visceral fat with strong correlation to cardiac remodeling [12].

Adipose tissue is an active endocrine organ that secretes adipokines, such as adiponectin, leptin, and resistin, all of which influence cardiovascular health. In heart failure, altered adipokine profiles contribute to systemic inflammation and metabolic dysregulation. Epicardial adipose tissue (EAT), a specialized fat depot surrounding the myocardium, plays a particularly important role in local heart-adipose crosstalk [15, 17].

Increased EAT thickness is associated with adverse cardiac remodeling and impaired myocardial energetics. Conversely, signals from the failing heart, including natriuretic peptides and inflammatory cytokines, influence lipolysis and adipokine secretion, further disrupting metabolic homeostasis [2–4].

Proprotein convertase subtilisin/kexin type 9 (PCSK9) represents a novel therapeutic target in the management of dyslipidemias. PCSK9, secreted by liver, interacts with low-density lipoprotein receptor (LDL-R) and activates its degradation. In clinical trials involving patients with high LDL-C levels, anti-PCSK9 monoclonal antibodies, including evolocumab and alirocumab, reduced LDL-C levels by more than 60% and significantly reduced cardiovascular events [5].

22.3.3 Diabetic Cardiomyopathy

Extensive epidemiological and clinical data suggest that type 2 diabetes increases the risk for HF independently of other risk factors, such as hypertension [14]. One potential mechanism is that type 2 diabetes, often associated with obesity, leads to myocardial lipotoxicity that contributes to cell death, and thus, to HF [17].

Recent findings highlight the role of adipokines like adiponectin in mitigating these effects by enhancing fatty acid oxidation and reducing lipotoxicity [7].

Diabetic cardiomyopathy is also characterized by interstitial and perivascular fibrosis [16].

22.4 Molecular Mechanisms of Metabolic Crosstalk

The molecular mechanisms underpinning metabolic crosstalk in heart failure involve intricate signaling networks and molecular pathways. These include the activation of stress-response pathways, secretion of signaling molecules such as cytokines and hormones, and mitochondrial dysfunction. Understanding these mechanisms is critical for identifying therapeutic targets.

22.4.1 Cytokines and Inflammatory Pathways

Pro-inflammatory cytokines such as interleukin-1β (IL-1β), interleukin-6 (IL-6), and tumor necrosis factor-alpha (TNF-α) play a central role during heart failure. These cytokines are released by both cardiac and peripheral tissues in response to stress and contribute to systemic inflammation.

For example, the activation of the nucleotide-binding domain leucine-rich repeat-containing protein 3 (NLRP3) inflammasome in the myocardium triggers the release of IL-1β and IL-18, which can exacerbate cardiac dysfunction and promote adverse remodeling [6]. In addition, systemic inflammation driven by cytokines can impair glucose and lipid metabolism in the liver and skeletal muscle, further exacerbating metabolic dysregulation.

22.4.2 Role of Adipokines

Adipokines, including adiponectin, leptin, and resistin, mediate bidirectional communication between adipose tissue and the heart. In heart failure, altered adipokine profiles are observed, with decreased adiponectin levels contributing to increased inflammation and oxidative stress. Conversely, elevated leptin levels have been associated with cardiac hypertrophy and impaired myocardial function.

The interplay between adipokines and other signaling pathways highlights the complexity of metabolic crosstalk in heart failure. For instance, leptin resistance in adipose tissue can exacerbate lipolysis and release of free fatty acids, which may promote myocardial lipotoxicity and further compromise cardiac function.

Emerging Mechanisms

Novel pathways, including microRNA-mediated signaling and extracellular vesicles, are being explored for their role in metabolic crosstalk between adipose tissue and the heart. MicroRNAs, such as miR-223-3p, have been implicated in cardiac hypertrophy and inflammation, providing potential therapeutic targets for HF management [15, 17].

22.5 Clinical Implications of Metabolic Crosstalk in Heart Failure

The understanding of metabolic crosstalk in heart failure has significant clinical implications. By elucidating the interactions between the heart and peripheral organs, clinicians can better comprehend the systemic nature of heart failure, leading to more targeted therapeutic approaches.

Emerging biomarkers are expanding beyond traditional measures like B-type Natriuretic Peptide (BNP) and N-terminal pro-B-type Natriuretic Peptide (NT-proBNP). Recent evidence highlight the diagnostic potential of hepatokines and extracellular vesicles containing mitochondrial DNA. These markers indeed reflect systemic metabolic interference and organ-to-organ communication pathways, providing more nuanced insights into the pathophysiology of heart failure (HF) [18].

Exercise-induced hepatokines also demonstrate potential in modulating the liver-heart axis, with studies indicating improvements in myocardial and systemic metabolic homeostasis through enhanced glucose utilization and mitochondrial efficiency [19].

22.5.1 Diagnostic Biomarkers

Metabolic crosstalk offers potential biomarkers for the diagnosis and prognosis of heart failure. For instance, increased circulating levels of natriuretic peptides such as BNP and NT-proBNP reflect cardiac stress and volume overload. Similarly, alterations in adipokines, hepatokines, and other cytokines can provide insights into the systemic metabolic disturbances in HF patients.

Recently, a number of studies have used gene expression, array screening, cloning, and other techniques to identify new "cardiokines" to better understand the mechanism of how alterations in cell-cell communication contribute to heart disease and could identify new diagnostic and therapeutic targets.

22.6 Emerging Therapeutic Approaches

Advancements in our understanding of metabolic crosstalk have led to the development of innovative therapeutic strategies aimed at targeting the systemic nature of heart failure (HF). These approaches seek to address the underlying metabolic disturbances that contribute to HF progression. Although each of these approaches is supported by a strong rationale, it is essential to underscore the importance of comprehensive patient management, which encompasses both cardiac and extracardiac considerations (including the distinction between HF with preserved ejection fraction (EF) vs HF with reduced EF [26] and should be carried out in accordance with the most up-to-date guidelines and recommendations.

22.6.1 Pharmacological Interventions

The bidirectional communication between the heart and peripheral organs presents novel therapeutic targets. Modulating metabolic pathways through pharmacological or lifestyle interventions may disrupt the vicious cycle of heart failure progression.

Innovative therapies like Tirzepatide, a dual GLP-1/GIP receptor agonist, have shown efficacy in reducing HF-related hospitalizations and improving the quality of life in patients with HFpEF and obesity [27].

Vericiguat, a soluble guanylate cyclase stimulator, has the potential to reduce cardiovascular mortality and hospitalization rates in high-risk HF populations [23].

In patients with preexisting cardiovascular disease and overweight or obesity without diabetes, Semaglutide reduced the incidence of death from cardiovascular causes, nonfatal myocardial infarction, or nonfatal stroke [24].

Other strategies, such as anti-inflammatory agents targeting the NLRP3 inflammasome or therapies aimed at restoring mitochondrial function, are under active investigation.

Sodium-glucose cotransporter-2 (SGLT2) inhibitors, such as Empagliflozin and Dapagliflozin, originally developed for diabetes management, have demonstrated significant cardioprotective effects by improving cardiac energetics and reducing systemic inflammation. These agents are pivotal in disrupting the pathophysiological progression of HF [20].

Cardiac contractility modulation (CCM) therapy represents another breakthrough, particularly for patients with reduced ejection fraction. Studies reveal sustained improvements in functional capacity, left ventricular ejection fraction (LVEF), and quality of life, alongside marked reductions in HF hospitalizations over long-term follow-ups [21, 22].

Advanced pharmacological agents like sacubitril-valsartan have demonstrated significant reductions in NT-proBNP levels and improved outcomes in acute decompensated HF. These benefits underscore the necessity of early initiation of neprilysin inhibition in HF management [28].

Anti-inflammatory therapies, such as interleukin-1β monoclonal antibodies and NLRP3 inflammasome inhibitors, are under investigation for their potential to mitigate the systemic inflammatory response in HF. Additionally, agents that enhance mitochondrial biogenesis and reduce reactive oxygen species (ROS), such as PGC-1α agonists, are being explored as targeted treatments to restore energy balance in failing hearts.

Regular physical activity remains integral to managing HF, with its role in enhancing mitochondrial function and reducing systemic inflammation firmly established. Exercise-induced metabolic reprogramming not only optimizes glucose and lipid metabolism but also strengthens the heart-liver metabolic crosstalk [19].

22.6.2 Lifestyle and Non-pharmacological Interventions

In addition to pharmacological treatments, lifestyle interventions play a crucial role in managing heart failure. Regular physical activity has been shown to improve cardiac function and metabolic health by enhancing mitochondrial efficiency and reducing systemic inflammation. Structured exercise programs, such as cardiac rehabilitation, can positively influence inter-organ metabolic crosstalk and improve overall prognosis.

Dietary strategies, including ketogenic interventions and the incorporation of omega-3 fatty acids, have emerged as potent modifiers of oxidative stress and mitochondrial efficiency. Recent evidence also highlights the potential of intermittent fasting in promoting metabolic flexibility and reducing HF severity [25].

22.7 Conclusion

Metabolic crosstalk plays a pivotal role in the pathophysiology of heart failure, influencing not only the heart but also other organs involved in systemic metabolism. Disruptions in these metabolic pathways create a vicious cycle that exacerbates both cardiac and systemic dysfunction. Understanding the molecular mechanisms underlying these interactions has provided new insights into the complex nature of heart failure progression.

Recent advances in therapeutic strategies, including pharmacological and lifestyle interventions, highlight the potential to target metabolic crosstalk as a means of improving outcomes in HF patients. However, further research is needed to fully unravel all the aspects of these pathways and their contributions to disease progression. As our knowledge expands, it is likely that future treatment paradigms will incorporate both traditional heart failure management and metabolic-targeted therapies, emphasizing a holistic approach to care. Above all, indeed, robust data on the effects of pharmacological therapies that address the metabolic cross-talk in HF are needed to improve clinical management of HF patients. It is arguable that by addressing the intricate relationships between the heart, liver, skeletal muscle, adipose tissue, and other organs, clinicians will be able to develop and validate comprehensive strategies that improve both cardiac and systemic health, ultimately enhancing the quality of life for patients with heart failure.

References

1. Taegtmeyer H. Metabolic crosstalk in heart failure. J Am Coll Cardiol. 2011;58:1126.
2. Jahng JWS, Song E, Sweeney G. Crosstalk between the heart and peripheral organs in heart failure. Exp Mol Med. 2016;48:e217.
3. Ferrero KM, Koch WJ. Metabolic crosstalk between the heart and fat. Korean Circ J. 2020;50:379.
4. Mounesan A, Samadian Z. The effect of exercise on metabolic crosstalk between heart and liver. J Exerc Organ Crosstalk. 2023.
5. Zizhuo T, Yaozu X. Heart crosstalk with other organs and pharmacological strategies for Cardioprotection. J Holist Integr Pharm. 2022.
6. Abderrazak A, Syrovets T, Couchie D, El Hadri K, Friguet B, Simmet T, et al. NLRP3 inflammasome: from a danger signal sensor to a regulatory node of oxidative stress and inflammatory diseases. Redox Biol. 2015;4:296.
7. Park M, Sweeney G. Direct effects of adipokines on the heart: focus on adiponectin. Heart Fail Rev. 2013;18:631.
8. Turer AT, Hill JA, Elmquist JK, Scherer PE. Adipose tissue biology and cardiomyopathy: translational implications. Circ Res. 2012;111:1565.
9. Romacho T, Elsen M, Rohrborn D, Eckel J. Adipose tissue and its role in organ crosstalk. Acta Physiol (Oxf). 2014;210:733.
10. Sun K, Kusminski CM, Scherer PE. Adipose tissue remodeling and obesity. J Clin Invest. 2011;121:2094.
11. Amato MC, Giordano C. Visceral adiposity index: an indicator of adipose tissue dysfunction. Int. J Endocrinol. 2014;2014:1.
12. Britton KA, Fox CS. Ectopic fat depots and cardiovascular disease. Circulation. 2011;124.
13. Berezin AA. Cardiac hepatopathy: new perspectives on old problems through a prism of endogenous metabolic regulations by hepatokines. Antioxidants. 2023;12:516.
14. Wilson PW. Diabetes mellitus and coronary heart disease. Am J Kidney Dis. 1998;32:S89.
15. Lodewijks F, McKinsey TA, Robinson EL. Fat-to-heart crosstalk in health and disease. Front Genet. 2023;14:990155.
16. Boudina S, Abel ED. Diabetic cardiomyopathy, causes and effects. Rev Endocr Metab Disord. 2010;11:31.
17. Turera AT, et al. Adipose tissue biology and cardiomyopathy-translational implications. Circ Res. 2012;111:1565.
18. Tu Z, Xiang Y. Heart crosstalk with other organs and pharmacological strategies for cardioprotection. J Holist Integr Pharm. 2022;3:18.
19. Mounesan A, Samadian Z. The effect of exercise on metabolic crosstalk between heart and liver. J Exerc Organ Cross Talk. 2023;3:216–24.
20. Matsuura TR, et al. Ketones and the heart: metabolic principles and therapeutic implications. Circ Res. 2023;132:882.
21. Abraham WT, et al. A randomized controlled trial to evaluate the safety and efficacy of cardiac contractility modulation. Heart Fail. 2018;6:874–83.
22. Kuschyk J, et al. Long-term clinical experience with cardiac contractility modulation therapy delivered by the Optimizer Smart system. Eur J Heart Fail. 2021;23:1160.

23. Armstrong PW, et al. Vericiguat in patients with heart failure and reduced ejection fraction. N Engl J Med. 2020;382:1883.
24. Michael Lincoff A, et al. Semaglutide and cardiovascular outcomes in obesity without diabetes. N Engl J Med. 2023;389:2221.
25. Look AHEAD Research Group. Cardiovascular effects of intensive lifestyle intervention in type 2 diabetes. N Engl J Med. 2013.
26. Anker SD, et al. Patient phenotype profiling in heart failure with preserved ejection fraction to guide therapeutic decision making. A scientific statement of the Heart Failure Association, the European Heart Rhythm Association of the European Society of Cardiology, and the European Society of Hypertension. Eur J Heart Fail. 2023;25:936.
27. Packer M, et al. Tirzepatide for heart failure with preserved ejection fraction and obesity. N Engl J Med. 2024.
28. Velazquez EJ, et al. Angiotensin–neprilysin inhibition in acute decompensated heart failure. N Engl J Med. 2019;380:539.

Detrimental Role of Humoral Signaling in Cardiorenal Crosstalk

23

Shival Srivastav, Hemanshu Prabhakar, Indu Kapoor, and Charu Mahajan

23.1 Background

Cardiorenal syndrome (CRS) is a complex disorder observed in patients with kidney or heart diseases, wherein acute/chronic involvement of one organ induces disease in the other. The syndrome is important in the critical care context since co-involvement of the heart and kidney is commonly observed in many patients [1]. Its complex nature is underscored by the fact that the bidirectional crosstalk between these two organs is not well understood to date. Nevertheless, co-involvement markedly increases the morbidity and mortality of the patients, reduces lifespan and quality of life, and adds a significant burden to healthcare systems.

The syndrome is categorized into five subtypes based on the classification proposed by Acute Dialysis Quality Initiative Group in 2008 [2–5] (Table 23.1). As outlined in Chap. 16 ("Humoral Signaling in Cardiorenal Syndrome"), these clinical manifestations reflect the underlying neurohormonal and inflammatory crosstalk between the heart and kidneys. The classification clubs the subtypes into cardiorenal or renocardiac syndromes based on the primary organ which is involved. Further subdivision is based on the acute or chronic nature of the primary organ involvement. Type 5 is an independent entity, since it is secondary to a systemic disorder. Type 1 CRS refers to acute heart disease leading to injury to the kidney. Common causes include cardiogenic shock and heart failure. Type 2 CRS is kidney injury occurring secondary to chronic heart disease. This may be precipitated by heart failure and cardiomyopathies. Type 3 and 4 CRS are renocardiac syndromes, wherein acute or chronic injury to the kidney leads to heart failure. Type 5 CRS is

S. Srivastav
Department of Physiology, All India Institute of Medical Sciences, Jodhpur, India

H. Prabhakar (✉) · I. Kapoor · C. Mahajan
Department of Neuroanaesthesiology and Neurocritical Care, All India Institute of Medical Sciences, New Delhi, India

D. Battaglini et al. (eds.), *Organ System Crosstalk in Critical Illness*,
https://doi.org/10.1007/978-3-032-01024-7_23

Table 23.1 Classification of cardiorenal syndromes (CRS)

CRS type	Description	Also known as	Pathological event precipitating the CRS
I	Abrupt worsening of cardiac function leading to acute kidney injury	Acute cardiorenal syndrome	Acute decompensated heart failure (ADHF)
II	Chronic heart disease leading to kidney injury in the long run	Chronic cardiorenal syndrome	Congestive heart failure
III	Acute worsening of renal function leading to acute heart disease	Acute renocardiac syndrome	Acute kidney injury
IV	Chronic kidney disease leading to heart disease in the long term	Chronic renocardiac syndrome	Diabetic nephropathy
V	Systemic disease involving both the heart and the kidney	Secondary cardiorenal syndrome	Sepsis

Adapted from [2, 9, 10]

unique, since it occurs secondary to a systemic disease such as diabetes mellitus (DM), sepsis, hepatorenal syndrome, or other related disorders. This subtype is peculiar, since it does not satisfy the criteria for CRS, yet is included in the same [6]. Detailed classification with key precipitating causes is described elsewhere [7, 8].

The incidence of the syndrome varies according to the population under consideration. In the Indian context, incidence of cardiorenal syndrome varies from 27% to 34% in children and adults, respectively [11, 12]. In a systematic review, the pooled incidence of the syndrome was reported to be 33% [13].

23.2 Pathophysiology of CRS: The Detrimental Role of Humoral Signaling

The pathophysiology of different types of CRS depends on the primary organ involvement and the acute/chronic nature of the injury. The heart or the kidney may be the primary organ of injury depending on the subtype of CRS. This is followed by the involvement of the other organ via intricate signaling mechanisms. These mechanisms are a combination of neural and humoral signaling. Humoral signaling is specifically important since there are multiple bioactive molecules that can precipitate organ damage and lead to heart failure or renal shutdown. These mechanisms merit discussion, since understanding of these signaling mechanisms can help identify biomarkers and targets of therapy in the future.

23.2.1 CRS Type 1

The primary event precipitating cardiorenal syndrome 1 is acute decompensated heart failure (ADHF). ADHF leads to acute kidney injury leading to impairment of renal function and manifesting as elevated serum creatinine and/or reduction in estimated glomerular filtration rate, commonly referred to as acute kidney injury (AKI). The prevalence of patients with ADHF landing with AKI varies according to literature and is estimated to be 20–40% [14, 15]. Serum creatinine-based staging of AKI has been proposed as a part of the Kidney Disease: Improving Global Outcomes (KDIGO) criteria [16]. However, seemingly normal values may be seen in cases of volume overload observed in heart failure. Therefore, there is a need to exercise due caution when solely relying on creatinine values as the determinant of AKI [17]. The key pathophysiological mechanism attributed to this dysfunction is the reduction in cardiac output secondary to cardiac dysfunction. This leads to vascular underfilling, activating the sympathetic nervous system peripherally. This culminates in generalized vasoconstriction, including the renal bed, secondary to increased neurohumoral activity.

The role of humoral signaling in the process is mediated by a multitude of factors. Activation of the renin-angiotensin-aldosterone system (RAAS) plays an important role. Renin is released from macula densa cells of the juxtaglomerular apparatus in nephrons in response to alterations in tubular flow. It is released as a precursor form, which is activated and converts the protein angiotensinogen to angiotensin I (Ang-I), Ang-I is further processed in pulmonary vascular endothelium to form Angiotensin II (Ang-II), via angiotensin converting enzyme (ACE). Ang-II is an extremely potent vasoconstrictor, having renal as well as systemic effects. The intense vasoconstriction produced is aimed at correcting systemic blood pressure and tubular filtration simultaneously. In addition, adrenal synthesis and release of aldosterone are promoted by Ang-II. Aldosterone has sodium-converting effects in the body, mainly mediated by the insertion of epithelial sodium channels (ENaCs) in the renal tubules.

Unfortunately, the neuroendocrine activation produced has a detrimental effect on the cardiorenal axis. In the heart, this promotes ventricular hypertrophy and remodeling and leads to fibrotic changes as well as cell injury and death. In the kidney, this mechanism produces glomerulosclerosis and tubular fibrosis [18].

Another probable mechanism of humoral injury is through endothelial dysfunction. Elevated Ang-II levels promote endothelial injury, leading to a reduction in nitric oxide (NO) production. It is a well-known fact that NO, previously referred to as endothelium-derived relaxing factor (EDRF), is an important marker of endothelial integrity. During the normal state of affairs, NO is responsible for vasodilation and natriuresis. In addition, it has been shown to have beneficial roles in the inhibition of atherogenesis, reduction of smooth muscle hyperplasia, and facilitation of angiogenesis [19]. However, increased levels of Ang-II activate NAPH oxidase in the heart and the kidney, leading to impaired production of nitric oxide. Increased levels of reactive oxygen species (ROS) lead to the production of inflammatory mediators such as interleukin 6 and transforming growth factor–beta. Such a pro-oxidative milieu is responsible for fibrosis in the long term.

23.2.2 CRS Type 2

This subtype of CRS is kidney injury occurring secondary to chronic heart disease. Common causes of Type 2 CRS are myocardial infarction, hypertension, diabetes mellitus (DM), and metabolic syndrome. The key mechanisms bringing about renal insult are hypoperfusion of the kidney along with renal congestion. Increased right atrial pressure further complicates the situation. Chronic heart failure acts to put kidneys into a state of perpetual hypoxia, inflammation, and cellular damage [20]. The elevated levels of proinflammatory cytokines, such as tumor necrosis factor alpha, interleukins 1-beta, -6, and -18, are responsible for creating an inflammatory microenvironment that damages the endothelial glycocalyx coat in the renal and causes leakage of albumin in the urine [9]. These changes eventually culminate in glomerulosclerosis and interstitial fibrosis.

Renal fibrosis leading to end-stage renal disease (ESRD) in type 2 CRS is another example of pathological humoral signaling. Galectin-3 has been implicated as an important humoral mediator of fibrosis in this context. It is a beta-galactoside-binding lectin responsible for cell-to-cell and cell-to-matrix interactions in normal homeostasis by binding to glycans. It acts on myofibroblasts and leads to deposition of collagen in the renal tissue, leading to fibrosis in the long term. Its importance is being explored as a biomarker for ventricular remodeling and fibrosis [21]. In addition, multiple intricate signaling mechanisms have been described that lead to long-term renal injury. These include, but are not limited to, transforming growth factor-beta, Wnt/beta-catenin, trimethylamine-N-dioxide, and fibroblast growth factor 23-Klotho axis. A detailed description of these signaling mechanisms is described elsewhere [20].

23.2.3 CRS Type 3

Type 3 variant of CRS is also known as "renocardiac" syndrome, since the primary injury occurs at the level of the kidney. Acute kidney injury is the primary event leading to cardiac dysfunction. Causes that can precipitate AKI include glomerulonephritis, contrast/drug-induced kidney injury, rhabdomyolysis, and acute pyelonephritis [7]. This leads to cardiac dysfunction in the form of acute heart failure, acute coronary syndrome, and arrhythmias [22, 23]. Similar to previous subtypes, proinflammatory mediators such as TNF-alpha, IL-1, and IL-6 have been implicated as humoral markers leading to tissue injury. These mediators are shown to have direct depressant effects on the heart, probably by reducing calcium availability in the myocardium. This leads to negative ionotropic effects affecting cardiac output. In addition, these markers have been shown to cause left ventricular apoptosis and remodeling [24, 25].

Another detrimental effect of kidney injury on cardiac function occurs by means of dyselectrolytemia and reduced urine output. Oliguria has important consequences on sodium and water balance in the body, leading to cardiac overload and pulmonary congestion. Hyperkalemia occurring as a result of acute kidney injury predisposes the heart to the risk of arrhythmias. Impaired buffer action of the kidney causes an alteration in pH leading to additional myocardial injury [7]. Renal injury leading to uremia can additionally depress myocardial function, leading to the risk of injury and infarction [26].

23.2.4 CRS Type 4

Type 4 variant is cardiac injury occurring as a sequalae of chronic kidney disease (CKD). CKD acts as an independent risk factor for patients with chronic heart disease, since pre-existing kidney disease is considered an adverse prognostic factor. Chronic renal dysfunction causes a host of metabolic abnormalities such as uremia, dyselectrolytemia (especially calcium and phosphate imbalance), and acidosis in the blood. In addition, uremia also leads to anemia and endothelial dysfunction [27]. Hyperkalemia is another important factor that may lead to increased risk of arrhythmias and cardiotoxicity. Characteristic ECG changes may help in the early identification of this important and potentially fatal dyselectrolytemia. This disturbed humoral milieu creates a proinflammatory state that is responsible for cardiac interstitial fibrosis, hypertrophy, and systolic and diastolic dysfunction [28, 29]. Similar to previous CRS subtypes, deviant renin-angiotensin-aldosterone signaling is also implicated here as a culprit. Excess renin and Ang-II in the system signaling have a deleterious effect on the myocardium, further exacerbating the cardiac dysfunction.

23.2.5 CRS Type 5

This subtype of CRS is unique since it is secondary to a systemic disorder that affects both the heart and the kidney. Hence, this is also known as secondary cardiorenal syndrome. The prototype illness causing this disorder is an uncontrolled infection leading to sepsis. Other disorders such as can also precipitate Type 5 CRS. Uncontrolled hypertension observed during pre-eclampsia is another common entity in females that may lead to this condition [30].

This subtype is an important model of humoral dysregulation wherein circulating biomolecules can play havoc with cardiorenal axis. It is a well-established fact that systemic illness, especially after infection, can lead to a spillage of multiple humoral mediators in the bloodstream. These include pathogen- and damage-associated molecular patterns (PAMPs and DAMPs), such as bacterial lipopolysaccharides (LPS), peptidoglycans, bacterial DNA, heat shock proteins, and uric acid. These molecules lead to the activation of complement system, such as C5a and C3a, cell adhesion molecules like selectins and chemokines such as IL1, IL4, IL6, and IL10. Together, these mediators lead to widespread injury to the cardiovascular and renal systems. Long-term sequelae include chronic kidney disease and heart failure.

The key pathophysiological events that cause end-organ damage in CRS are summarized in Fig. 23.1. These events initiate a cascade of events that injure the heart and the kidney. Volume overload secondary to kidney injury can interfere with

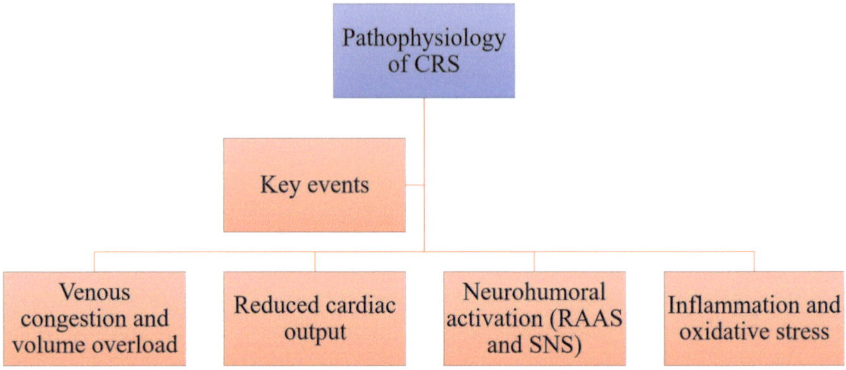

Fig. 23.1 Summary of key events that operate in CRS. (Adapted from [9, 17, 31])

cardiac function. Myocardial edema may develop, leading to injury and fibrosis. Neurohumoral dysregulation is an important consideration, especially with reference to RAAS activation. Contrary to the beneficial homeostatic roles of renin and angiotensin-II, their activation in CRS leads to cell injury, apoptosis, and fibrosis both in the heart and the kidney by multipronged mechanisms. The cardiotoxic effects of these two mediators are noteworthy. In addition, the creation of proinflammatory state in the body also worsens the situation. Inflammatory humoral mediators such as interleukins, cytokines, and TNF-alpha also act bidirectionally to aggravate cardiac and renal insult. In renocardiac syndromes (Type 3 and 4), elevated electrolytes and urea and pH imbalance act as agents of injury to the heart, leading to remodeling, cardiac fibrosis, and increasing the risk of arrhythmias. Acidemia resulting from kidney injury leads to generalized dilation of the vessels and may render vasopressors ineffective.

23.3 Summary

To summarize, dysregulated humoral signaling by a multitude of mediators has an extremely detrimental effect by causing cardiac and renal injury, irrespective of the primary origin of the CRS. Further understanding of these intricate signaling mechanisms is likely to usher us into an era of new biomarkers and therapies for this important clinical condition. As further explored in Chap. 24, advances in molecular imaging now allow the visualization of inflammatory crosstalk along the cardiorenal axis.

References

1. Cruz DN. Cardiorenal syndrome in critical care: the acute cardiorenal and renocardiac syndromes. Adv Chronic Kidney Dis. 2013;20:56–66.
2. Ronco C. Cardiorenal syndromes: definition and classification. Contrib Nephrol. 2010;164:33–8.

3. Ronco C, McCullough P, Anker SD, et al. Cardio-renal syndromes: report from the consensus conference of the Acute Dialysis Quality Initiative. Eur Heart J. 2010;31:703–11.
4. Di Lullo L, Ronco C. Cardio-renal axis: pathophysiological evidences and clinical implications. G Ital Nefrol. 2017;34:4–10.
5. Ronco C. Cardio-renal syndromes: from foggy bottoms to sunny hills. Heart Fail Rev. 2011;16:509–17.
6. Soni SS, Ronco C, Pophale R, et al. Cardio-renal syndrome type 5: epidemiology, pathophysiology, and treatment. Semin Nephrol. 2012;32:49–56.
7. Di Lullo L, Bellasi A, Russo D, et al. Cardiorenal acute kidney injury: epidemiology, presentation, causes, pathophysiology and treatment. Int J Cardiol. 2017;227:143–50.
8. Di Lullo L, Bellasi A, Barbera V, et al. Pathophysiology of the cardio-renal syndromes types 1–5: an uptodate. Indian Heart J. 2017;69:255–65.
9. McCullough PA, Kellum JA, Haase M, et al. Pathophysiology of the cardiorenal syndromes: executive summary from the Eleventh Consensus Conference of the Acute Dialysis Quality Initiative (ADQI). In: Kellum JA, McCullough PA, Mehta RL, et al. (eds) ADQI consensus on AKI biomarkers and cardiorenal syndromes. S. Karger AG.
10. Pathophysiology of the cardiorenal syndromes: executive summary from the Eleventh Consensus Conference of the Acute Dialysis Quality Initiative (ADQI). In: ADQI Consensus on AKI Biomarkers and Cardiorenal Syndromes. Karger.
11. Athwani V, Bhargava M, Chanchlani R, et al. Incidence and outcome of acute cardiorenal syndrome in hospitalized children. Indian J Pediatr. 2017;84:420–4.
12. Fernando K, Parthasarathy R, Mathew M, et al. Risk factors and outcomes of acute cardio-renal syndrome in a tertiary care setting in South India. J Assoc Physicians India. 2021;69:11–2.
13. Ru S-C, Lv S-B, Li Z-J. Incidence, mortality, and predictors of acute kidney injury in patients with heart failure: a systematic review. ESC Heart Fail. 2023;10:3237–49.
14. Heywood JT, Fonarow GC, Costanzo MR, et al. High prevalence of renal dysfunction and its impact on outcome in 118,465 patients hospitalized with acute decompensated heart failure: a report from the ADHERE database. J Card Fail. 2007;13:422–30.
15. Rewa O, Bagshaw SM. Acute kidney injury-epidemiology, outcomes and economics. Nat Rev Nephrol. 2014;10:193–207.
16. Khwaja A. KDIGO clinical practice guidelines for acute kidney injury. Nephron Clin Pract. 2012;120:c179–84.
17. Kumar U, Garimella PS, Wettersten N. Cardiorenal syndrome-pathophysiology. Cardiol Clin. 2019;37:251–65.
18. Palazzuoli A, Ruocco G. Heart-kidney interactions in cardiorenal syndrome type 1. Adv Chronic Kidney Dis. 2018;25:408–17.
19. Ronco C, Bellasi A, Di Lullo L. Cardiorenal syndrome: an overview. Adv Chronic Kidney Dis. 2018;25:382–90.
20. Xu X, Zhang B, Wang Y, et al. Renal fibrosis in type 2 cardiorenal syndrome: an update on mechanisms and therapeutic opportunities. Biomed Pharmacother. 2023;164:114901.
21. Hara A, Niwa M, Noguchi K, et al. Galectin-3 as a next-generation biomarker for detecting early stage of various diseases. Biomolecules. 2020;10:389.
22. Bagshaw SM, Cruz DN, Aspromonte N, et al. Epidemiology of cardio-renal syndromes: workgroup statements from the 7th ADQI Consensus Conference. Nephrol Dial Transplant. 2010;25:1406–16.
23. Bellomo R, Ronco C, Kellum JA, et al. Acute renal failure - definition, outcome measures, animal models, fluid therapy and information technology needs: the Second International Consensus Conference of the Acute Dialysis Quality Initiative (ADQI) Group. Crit Care Lond Engl. 2004;8:R204–12.
24. Edmunds NJ, Lal H, Woodward B. Effects of tumour necrosis factor-alpha on left ventricular function in the rat isolated perfused heart: possible mechanisms for a decline in cardiac function. Br J Pharmacol. 1999;126:189–96.
25. Rauchhaus M, Doehner W, Francis DP, et al. Plasma cytokine parameters and mortality in patients with chronic heart failure. Circulation. 2000;102:3060–7.

26. De Deyn PP, Vanholder R, D'Hooge R. Nitric oxide in uremia: effects of several potentially toxic guanidino compounds. Kidney Int Suppl. 2003;63:S25–8.
27. Goh CY, Vizzi G, De Cal M, et al. Cardiorenal syndrome: a complex series of combined heart/kidney disorders. Contrib Nephrol. 2011;174:33–45.
28. Gross M-L, Ritz E. Hypertrophy and fibrosis in the cardiomyopathy of uremia--beyond coronary heart disease. Semin Dial. 2008;21:308–18.
29. Remppis A, Ritz E. Cardiac problems in the dialysis patient: beyond coronary disease. Semin Dial. 2008;21:319–25.
30. Ilagan J, Sahani H, Saleh AB, et al. Type 5 cardiorenal syndrome: an underdiagnosed and underrecognized disease process of the American mother. J Clin Med Res. 2022;14:395–9.
31. Verma D, Firoz A, Garlapati SKP, et al. Emerging treatments of cardiorenal syndrome: an update on pathophysiology and management. Cureus. 2021;13:e17240.

24 Molecular Imaging of Inflammatory Crosstalk Across the Cardiorenal Axis Following Acute Heart Failure

Abdelrahman Elsebaie, Stephen H. Sams, Rakesh C. Arora, and Mohammad El-Diasty

Abbreviations

ADQI	Acute Dialysis Quality Initiative
AHF	Acute heart failure
AKI	Acute kidney injury
AMI	Acute myocardial infarction
Ang II	Angiotensin II
BNP	Brain-natriuretic peptide
CEUS	Contrast-enhanced ultrasound
CO	Cardiac Output
CRS	Cardiorenal syndrome
CT	Computed tomography (CT)
CVP	Central venous pressure

A. Elsebaie
Faculty of Health Sciences, Queen's University, Kingston, ON, Canada
e-mail: 19aoe@queensu.ca

S. H. Sams
Department of Anesthesiology, University of Utah Health, Salt Lake City, UT, USA
e-mail: stephen.sams@hsc.utah.edu

R. C. Arora (✉)
Harrington Heart and Vascular Institute, University Hospitals Cleveland Medical Center, Cleveland, OH, USA

M. El-Diasty
Harrington Heart and Vascular Institute, University Hospitals Cleveland Medical Center, Cleveland, OH, USA

Division of Cardiac Surgery, University Hospitals Cleveland Medical Center, Cleveland, OH, USA
e-mail: mohammad.eldiasty@uhhospitals.org

D. Battaglini et al. (eds.), *Organ System Crosstalk in Critical Illness*,
https://doi.org/10.1007/978-3-032-01024-7_24

CXCR4	C-X-C motif chemokine receptor 4
ET-1	Endothelin-1
GFR	Glomerular filtration rate
GMCSF	Granulocyte-macrophage colony-stimulating factor
IAP	Intra-abdominal pressure
IL	Interleukin 1 beta (β), 6, 18, etc.
MCP-1	Monocyte chemoattractant protein-1
MI	Molecular imaging
MNP	Magneto-fluorescent nanoparticle (MNP)
MPO	Myeloperoxidase
MRI	Magnetic resonance imaging
NF-κB	Nuclear factor kappa B
NIRF	Near-infrared fluorescence
NP	Natriuretic peptide
PAI	Photoacoustic imaging (PAI)
PET	Positron emission tomography
RANTES	Regulated on activation normal T-cell expressed and secreted
RASS	Renin-angiotensin-aldosterone system
RNS	Reactive nitrogen species
ROS	Reactive oxygen species
RS	Raman spectroscopy
sICAM	Soluble I form of cell adhesion molecule
SERS	Surface-enhanced-Raman spectroscopy
SNS	Sympathetic nervous system
SDF-1	Stromal-derived factor-1
SPECT	Single-photon emission tomography
TNF-α	Tumor necrosis factor-alpha
USPIO	Ultrasmall superparamagnetic iron oxide
WRF	Worsening renal failure

24.1 Introduction to Cardiorenal Syndrome

Crosstalk, along the cardiorenal axis, involves different bidirectional relationships, wherein each organ interacts synergistically to regulate critical physiological functions, including vascular tone, blood volume, and hemodynamic stability [1]. The heart and kidney are therefore interconnected in different pathological states, which result in a direct or indirect deleterious impact of one organ on the other via an intricate feedback system involving regulatory hormones, inflammatory molecules, and oxidative stress responses [1].

As early as 1836, Robert Bright articulated the nuanced and closely intertwined correlation between the kidney and heart after observing notable structural cardiac alterations in patients with advanced kidney disease [2]. Since then, various advances have been made in summarizing the cardiorenal crosstalk, including an initial attempt to arrive at a standardized definition by the Working Group of the National Heart, Lung, and Blood Institute in 2004 [3]. Specifically, they coined the term "cardiorenal syndrome" (CRS), the extreme result of cardiorenal dysregulation that manifests because of interactions between the kidneys and other circulatory compartments that increase circulating volume, exacerbating heart failure (HF) symptoms and disease progression [3]. While this cardio-centric definition remains the foundation of CRS in the context of acute HF (AHF), it is now recognized that cardiorenal dysregulation occurs on a broader, wider clinical spectrum [4].

In 2008, the Acute Dialysis Quality Initiative (ADQI) Group arrived at a consensus approach to describe and classify CRS that incorporates the bidirectional nature of organ interaction or "crosstalk." Specifically, this is defined as "disorders of the heart and kidneys whereby acute or chronic dysfunction in one organ may induce acute or chronic dysfunction of the other" [5]. They categorized CRS into two primary groups based on the syndrome's *primum movens* (cardiorenal and renocardiac) [5]. Further division of these groups involves factors like the acuity of onset (acute or chronic) and sequential organ involvement (Table 24.1) [5]. The nomenclature proposed by the ADQI's consensus aims to reduce confusion and ambiguity surrounding CRS with regards to its clinical management [4, 5]. This has enabled more reliable and precise characterization of cardiorenal dysregulation for diagnostics, management, and therapeutic endeavors [4, 5].

Epidemiological figures for CRS exhibit both variability across subtypes and disparities within each subtype when different definitions are used [5, 6]. The goal

Table 24.1 Classification and definitions of cardiorenal syndromes according to ADQI [5]

Syndrome	Denomination	Definition	Clinical examples
CRS type 1	Acute cardiorenal	Acute worsening of heart function leading to kidney injury and/or dysfunction	ACS or cardiogenic shock resulting in AHF followed by AKI
CRS type 2	Chronic cardiorenal	Chronic abnormalities in the heart function leading to kidney injury or dysfunction	CHF or CHD resulting in CKD
CRS type 3	Acute renocardiac	Acute worsening of kidney function leading to heart injury and/or dysfunction	AKI (due to volume overload, inflammatory surge and uremic metabolic disturbances) resulting AHF, ACS, or arrhythmias
CRS type 4	Chronic renocardiac	Chronic kidney disease leading to heart injury, disease, and/or dysfunction	CKD-associated cardiomyopathy resulting in LVH, CHF, and diastolic dysfunction
CRS type 5	Secondary cardiorenal	Systemic disease leading to simultaneous injury and/or dysfunction of the heart and kidney	CRS after sepsis, amyloidosis, cirrhosis, vasculitis, diabetes mellitus, noncardiogenic shock, COVID-19, or autoimmune diseases

Abbreviations: *ACS* acute coronary syndrome, *AHF* acute heart failure, *AKI* acute kidney injury, *CHD* chronic heart disease, *CHF* chronic heart failure, *CKD* chronic kidney disease, *COVID-19* coronavirus disease of 2019, *CRS* cardiorenal syndrome, *LVH* left ventricular hypertrophy of the ADQI's consensus definition on CRS is to reduce confusion and ambiguity when encountering multiple definitions for similar disease processes. For instance, nephrologists employ the term acute kidney injury (AKI), defined by criteria systems like RIFLE, KDIGO, and AKIN, while cardiologists use "worsening renal failure" (WRF) with its distinct definitions [5, 6]. This discrepancy may stem from complex pathophysiology and variations in studied patient populations and perfectly encapsulates the multifaceted nature of cardiorenal crosstalk, as explored in this chapter.

24.2 Pathophysiology of Acute CRS

The pathophysiological mechanisms driving acute kidney injury (AKI) and WRF after acute heart failure (AHF; whether acute decompensation of chronic HF or de novo) are intricate and not fully elucidated despite renal dysfunction being an independent mortality risk factor and most complication post-AHF, with a prevalence of 25–40% [7]. As introduced in Chap. 16 and further developed in Chap. 23, interorgan communication along the heart–kidney axis depends on tightly regulated neurohormonal and inflammatory pathways. Building upon this framework, the present chapter explores how cardiorenal crosstalk manifests in the setting of acute heart failure, focusing on its hemodynamic, neurohormonal, and immune-mediated mechanisms that can now be visualized through molecular imaging approaches. Proposed mechanisms for CRS type 1 include an imbalance in abnormal hemodynamics, neurohormonal activation, immune-mediated damage, overloading of counterregulatory systems, and varied responses to exogenous factors:

24.2.1 Hemodynamic Mechanisms

Numerous experimental and clinical findings suggest that the pathophysiology of CRS type 1 is predominantly triggered by hemodynamic mechanisms that culminate in renal function deterioration characterized by reduced renal arterial flow, oxygen consumption, and glomerular filtration rate (GFR) [6, 8]. Initially, WRF post-AHF was assumed to be linked to persistent renal dysfunction and ischemia resulting from hypoperfusion due to poor flow (i.e., low cardiac output (CO)) [9, 10]. More contemporary viewpoints, however, recognize the potential limitations of this perspective as it fails to capture the complexity of acute CRS [6, 9]. Moreover, in the acute setting, the impact of low CO appears to vary drastically, playing a more crucial role in patients with severe AHF, which comprises a small fraction of cases seen in daily clinical practice, thus making it less likely to be the primary determinant of WRF [6, 9].

An alternative hemodynamic mechanism proposes that the genesis of acute CRS in the setting of AHF is intricately linked to amplified volume overload, coupled with increased intra-abdominal (IAP) and central venous (CVP) pressures [9]. It is imperative to note that CVP as it pertains to pressure at the level of the renal veins is a product of a myriad of elements, such as right heart function, blood volume, and venous capacitance [11]. This proposed pathway arose from historical experimental data in which diuresis by an isolated canine kidney was markedly reduced at a renal venous pressure of 20 mmHg and improved above a threshold pressure > 25 mmHg [12]. Mechanistically, the kidneys demand continuous and ample perfusion, necessitating a favorable filtration pressure determined by the vast disparity between arterial pressure and venous outflow [9]. In the context of AHF, the significantly elevated CVP and IAP induce renal venous congestion, thereby reducing blood flow gradient through the glomerular capillary system, resulting in slow intravascular flow, glomerular functional impairment, and decreased GFR [6, 9, 13]. Furthermore, the simultaneous elevation of intrarenal interstitial pressure may induce tubular compression, parenchymal hypoxia, and a further reduction in GFR due to a decrease in net filtration pressure, finally marking the development of acute CRS [6]. These series of hemodynamic events and mechanisms are summarized in Fig. 24.1.

Recent investigations by Mullens et al. sought to validate the prevailing hypothesis that worsening renal function in patients with AHF is more dependent on IAP and CVP-induced systemic venous congestion than CO impairment [14, 15]. Findings from both studies confirmed that the correlation between elevated IAP and CVP and the manifestation of WRF surpasses the predictive value of arterial blood pressure, cardiac index, or pulmonary capillary wedge pressure in predicting the onset of CRS type 1 [14, 15]. To bridge these two hypothesized mechanisms, hemodynamic profiles have been developed to align with the clinical phenotype of individual patients [16, 17]. This classification is based on systemic

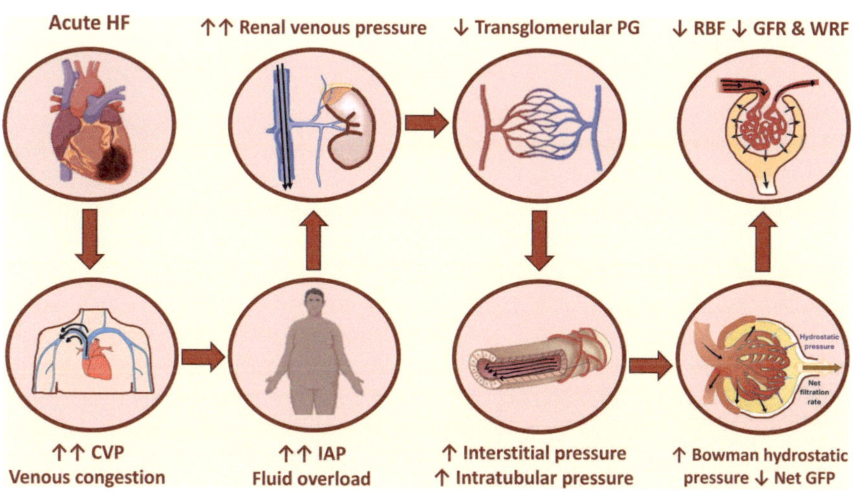

Fig. 24.1 Highlighting the hemodynamic mechanisms occurring down the cardiorenal axis that facilitate "worsening renal function" following acute heart failure. CVP central venous pressure, IAP intrabdominal pressure, RBF renal blood flow, GFR glomerular filtration rate, HF heart failure, WRF worsening renal function, GP gradient pressure, GFP glomerular filtration pressure

Table 24.2 Systemic hemodynamic profiles in acute CRS

Hemodynamic profiles	Characteristics
Wet and cold	↑ RVP, RIP, and CVP ↓ CO, ECFV, RBF, and RPP Impaired autoregulation (unable to preserve GFR) ↑ Pulmonary and/or systemic venous congestion Amplified systemic hypoperfusion
Wet and warm	↑ RVP, RIP, and CVP ↓ RPP and RBF Impaired autoregulation (unable to preserve GFR) Most common among AHF patients ↑ Pulmonary and/or systemic venous congestion Systemic perfusion is somewhat preserved
Dry and cold	↓ CO, ECFV, and RBF Impaired autoregulation (unable to preserve GFR) No signs of pulmonary and/or systemic venous congestion Amplified systemic hypoperfusion
Dry and warm	↓ RBF Intrarenal microvascular dysregulation No signs of pulmonary and/or systemic venous congestion Systemic perfusion is somewhat preserved

Abbreviations: *CO* cardiac output, *CVP* central venous pressure, *ECFV* effective circulation fluid volume, *GFR* glomerular filtration rate, *RBF* renal blood flow, *RIP* renal interstitial pressure, *RPP* renal perfusion pressure, *RVP* renal venous pressure

hemodynamics, considering perfusion adequacy (decreased CO and effective circulation fluid volume (ECFV)) and extent of congestion (elevated CVP or wedge pressure) [16, 17]. The outcome is four distinct AHF profiles (encapsulated in Table 24.2), each with a different pathogenesis contributing to the onset of acute CRS [16, 17].

24.2.2 Neurohormonal Activation

In addition to the hemodynamic pathway, numerous non-hemodynamic mechanisms that exacerbate cardiorenal injury are also operative in the pathogenesis of acute CRS [1–3]. At the core is the neurohormonal activation of the renin-angiotensin-aldosterone (RAAS) and sympathetic nervous (SNS) systems, facilitated by the baroreceptor reflex [17]. Activation enhances tissue perfusion and maintains GFR in response to renal hypoperfusion induced by reduced CO and ECFV along the renal arterial tree [1, 9]. The onset of biventricular failure is a likely trigger for the activation of these systems, which amplifies renin secretion and leads to an increased production of the neurohormone angiotensin II (Ang II). This culminates in an array of damaging effects that further exacerbate the complexities of the cardiorenal axis [11, 18].

From a cardiac perspective, the vasoconstrictive actions of Ang II result in a significantly augmented left ventricular afterload, potential myocardial ischemia, and endothelial dysfunction if the coronary arteries are severely constricted [19]. This potent neurohormone may also drive cardiac myocytes to undergo pathological hypertrophy and remodeling to compensate for hemodynamic impairment and overactive RAAS [20]. As for the propagation of kidney injury, Ang II is postulated to augment renal plasma flow filtered through the glomerulus and induce vasoconstriction of renal efferent arterioles [21]. This sequence results in diminished hydrostatic pressure, heightened salt reabsorption in the proximal tubule, and elevated peritubular oncotic pressure [21]. Moreover, Ang II amplifies the renal synthesis of endothelin-1 (ET-1), a potent vasoconstrictor with proinflammatory and profibrotic properties, instigating pathological renal alterations [21]. Concurrently, Ang II contributes to aldosterone-mediated salt retention in the distal tubules, culminating in heightened intra-abdominal pressure, edema, and venous congestion [1, 21].

Activation of the SNS induces a surge in catecholamines within the peripheral blood, leading to heightened systemic vascular tone, blood pressure, and heart rate [22]. This cascade results in increased cardiac workload and, ultimately, a reduction in CO and peripheral perfusion [22]. These orchestrated events, coupled with promoting apoptosis and fibrosis, collectively precipitate the deterioration of the cardiorenal axis within a vicious cycle [22]. Intriguingly, these neurohormonal pathways serve as proinflammatory agents and catalysts of oxidative stress, with discernible effects on renal fibroblasts, implicated as mechanisms responsible for renal damage arising from elevated Ang II levels [9]. This will be explored in the coming sections.

24.2.3 Immune-Mediated Damage and Humoral Signaling

Immune-mediated, humoral signaling and damage featuring inflammation and oxidative stress (induced by the imbalance of reactive oxygen species (ROS) to nitric oxide production) round out the remainder of non-hemodynamic pathways indicated CRS type 1's pathogenesis [3]. It has been previously established that disrupting redox homeostasis via oxidative processes involving ROS and reactive nitrogen species (RNS) activates the immune system, creating a proinflammatory and profibrotic milieu that culminates in cardiorenal structural and functional abnormalities [23, 24]. Specifically, after ischemic events (such as those that trigger AHF), oxygen depletion hinders mitochondrial function, producing ROS during reperfusion, further driving myocardial dysfunction and apoptosis as well as compensatory cardiac hypertrophy, remodeling, and fibrosis [25]. Furthermore, superoxide production mediates cellular proliferation, culminating in glomerular hypertrophy, scarring, and WRF [26].

The heightened presence of a dual oxidative stress pathway marked by the overproduction of RNS and ROS is likely responsible for CRS type 1-associated cardiorenal damage, as confirmed by Virzì et al.'s study [27]. After quantifying the levels of ROS, RSN, and a handful of other oxidative stress markers (i.e., myeloperoxidase (MPO)), in AKI-absent AHF, control, and acute CRS patients, the authors reported a significant elevation in circulating ROS and RNS levels for the latter [27].

Likewise, quantitative analysis of all markers revealed significantly lower oxidative stress levels in the non-acute CRS two groups [27]. It's evident that understanding the pervasive impact of oxidative stress in acute CRS is essential, as it holds the potential for reversibility in causing both heart and kidney injuries, serving as a critical pathway for tissue damage and organ failure [11]. The role of inflammatory mechanisms and ensuing apoptosis in acute CRS will be discussed in greater detail in the next section.

24.2.4 Failure of Counter-Regulatory Mechanisms

The natriuretic peptide (NP) system is vital to maintaining cardiorenal homeostasis alongside SNS and RAAS [1, 11]. Specifically, substantial crosstalk exists between these three regulatory systems, with the former being counterregulatory to the latter two, having the ability to reduce levels of catecholamines, Ang II, and aldosterone [1, 11]. By releasing NPs, such as brain-natriuretic peptide (BNP), that bind to NP receptors in the glomerulus and renal tubules, this system controls various cardiorenal processes, including vasodilation, natriuresis, diuresis, and inhibition of fibrosis and cardiomyocyte hypertrophy [1, 11]. However, during CRS type 1, these counterregulatory functions are severely overloaded as levels of NPs rise significantly, leading to WRF and oliguria [1, 11].

24.2.5 Exogenous/Iatrogenic Factors

Certain exogenous factors may affect the delicate cardiorenal balance, leading to progressive deterioration of both organs [11]. For example, the cornerstone of AHF treatment are oral and intravenous loop diuretics [28, 29]. However, these drugs create a double-edged-sword effect, as they are indicated to alleviate venous congestion, promote diuresis, and enhance GFR but can likewise contribute to WRF and reduced renal perfusion through arterial underfilling, renovascular reflexes, and increased activation of the SNS and RAAS, precipitating acute CRS [28, 29]. Additionally, during AHF hospitalization, the increased use of RAAS inhibitors (i.e., angiotensin-converting enzyme, Ang II-receptor, or aldosterone blockers) along with nephrotoxic drugs, such as iodized contrast media, non-steroidal anti-inflammatory medications, and some antibiotics, places these patients at a greater risk of cardiorenal impairment and thus acute CRS [11].

24.3 The Role of Inflammatory Processes and Markers in Acute CRS Pathogenesis

The dysregulation in immune system cell signaling pathways that promote or inhibit inflammation has been shown to be a contributing factor to the pathological interaction between the heart and kidneys in CRS type 1 [11]. This understanding stems from an initial analysis of sera from affected patients, revealing elevated levels of proinflammatory cytokines and pro-apoptotic factors [30]. Moreover, in initial preclinical studies, activated endothelial cells, acting as nonprofessional antigen-presenting cells, not only perpetuate acute CRS but also undergo apoptosis and necrosis in tandem with tubular epithelial cells [31, 32]. This response is triggered by stimulation of toll-like receptors and ischemic injury [31, 32].

A more recent study by Pastori et al. sought to understand how AHF inflammation can induce immune-mediated acute kidney damage by exploring the in vitro effect of plasma from CRS type 1 patients on a monocyte cell line and investigating the presence of typical cytokine plasma profiles in these patients [33]. This was achieved by incubating monocytes with plasma isolated from 15 controls and 40 patients with AHF, 11 labelled as having CRS type 1 (since they presented with AKI at admission for AHF or developed AKI during hospitalization) [33]. Consequently, cell apoptosis was assessed using DNA fragmentation, caspase activity, and cytofluorometric assay, while plasma cytokine quantification was attained using ELISA [33].

Their results indicated significantly higher apoptosis levels in monocytes treated with CRS type 1 plasma compared to the controls and the remaining 29 patients with AKI-absent AHF [33]. This was further corroborated by the considerably higher concentration of caspase-3 and -8 levels in cells incubated with plasma from these patients [33]. Lastly, a statistically significant upregulation of proinflammatory cytokines tumor necrosis factor-alpha (TNF-α) and interleukins-6 and -18 was observed in monocytes incubated with CRS type 1 plasma compared to the other groups [33]. Consequently, Pastori et al. verified the role of impaired regulation of monocyte apoptosis in CRS type 1 patients, indicating the participation of an inflammatory mechanism in the cardiorenal axis of those who develop AKI alongside AHF [33].

A later study by Virzì et al., aimed to delineate the putative role of inflammation and humoral markers in the pathogenesis of CRS type 1, resulted in comparable findings and conclusions [34]. Notably, the authors assessed the plasma levels of 53 AHF patients (17 of which were categorized as CRS type 1 using the same criteria used by Pastori et al.) to quantify levels of established proinflammatory cytokines [34]. These included IL-1β, TNF-α, IL-6, and IL-18, along with soluble I form of cell adhesion molecule (sICAM), regulated on activation normal T-cell expressed and secreted (RANTES) and granulocyte-macrophage colony-stimulating factor (GMCSF) [34]. Their findings unveiled a notable increase in the plasma levels of inflammatory markers IL-6 and -18 exclusively within the CRS type 1 group, as opposed to their AHF counterparts without AKI [34].

Intriguingly, the amplified increase in proinflammatory markers released during AHF has been hypothesized to obstruct the active process of reabsorption that tightly regulates the fluid quantity in the pulmonary interstitium and alveoli [35]. This, in turn, causes pulmonary fluid overload that unfolds without a reciprocal increase in total body fluid, thereby inducing a series of pathological events [36, 37]. These include insufficient renal perfusion pressures, peritubular edema, decreased glomerular filtration, and mixed inflammatory and ischemic tubular damage, culminating in the AKI seen in CRS type 1 [36, 37]. Alternative mechanisms for the contribution of inflammation in the pathogenesis of acute CRS suggest that augmented acute inflammatory responses, while attempting to lessen the main cardiac injury, further exacerbate damage throughout the cardiorenal axis [18]. Specific triggers of cardiac injury, such as hypertension and myocardial ischemia, can lower the ejection fraction and lead to increased central venous pressure, which ultimately decreases renal blood flow [18].

Subsequently, hyperactivity of the RAAS axis and amplified release of renin spearhead the Ang II-mediated overexpression of stromal-derived factor (SDF)-1 into circulation, inducing the infiltration of pro-fibrotic immune cells, namely monocytes, and fibroblasts into local inflammatory sites within the kidney and heart [38–40]. The infiltration occurs because of the interaction of SDF-1 with its cognate G protein-coupled chemokine receptor, C-X-C motif chemokine receptor 4 (CXCR4), which is commonly involved in the trafficking of immune cells to injured organs [38–40]. These immune cells, with the aid of angiotensin type-1 receptor-mediated nuclear factor kappa B (NF-κB) signaling, play a major role in propagating inflammation by regulating cytokines, chemokines, and adhesion molecule gene transcription and their subsequent release in the myocardium and renal tissue, thus promoting cardiorenal fibrosis [34, 38–40]. This proposed molecular mechanisms are pictured in Fig. 24.2.

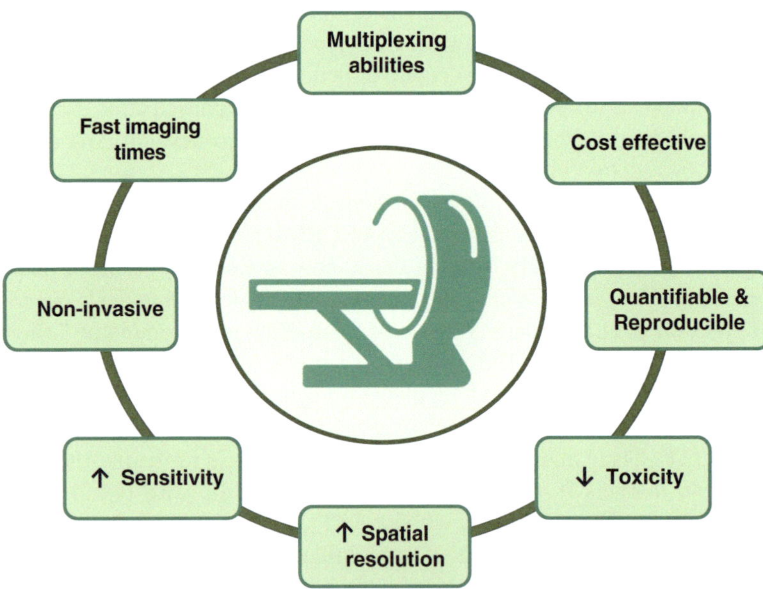

Fig. 24.2 Potential pathway of events highlighting the role of inflammation and inflammatory markers in the pathogenesis and physiological consequences of CRS type 1 post-acute heart failure. Ang II angiotensin II, BP blood pressure, HF heart failure, ICAM-1 intercellular adhesion molecule-1, IL-6 and -18 interleukin, MCP-1 monocyte chemoattractant protein-1, RBF renal blow flow, SDF-1 stromal cell-derived factor-1, TNF-α tumor necrosis factor alpha, VCAM-1 vascular cell adhesion protein-1

24.4 Modalities of Imaging of Inflammatory Markers and Processes

Introduced in the 1990s, molecular imaging (MI) is a growing biomedical research discipline that focuses on the visualization, detection, and quantification of the function of physiological and pathologic processes at the cellular or molecular level [41–43]. Its primary objective is to address questions related to the disease mechanism and characterize pathologies of diseased tissues in their physiologically authentic environment [41]. Additionally, it aims to identify cellular and molecular abnormalities causing the disease rather than focusing on the resulting anatomical and structural changes [41, 42]. By capturing the dynamics of biological processes in vivo over time through non-invasive methods, MI surpasses the constraints and demands of in vitro or ex vivo biopsy and cell culture laboratory techniques [42]. Achieving such intricate imaging necessitates using specialized instruments (modalities) in isolation or conjunction with imaging agents, namely endogenous biomolecules, or small molecule exogenous tracers, such as high-affinity pharmacological ligands or ligand-targeted nanomaterials [44].

Imaging at the molecular level provides functional data and anatomic information that can translate into significantly improved medical care, including earlier and more accurate diagnosis, grading, and staging, along with enhanced predicting and monitoring of responses to therapeutic methods [42–44]. This allows for personalized treatment planning based on a patient's disease state and a deeper understanding of complex biochemical pathways, streamlining the search for novel pharmaceutical discoveries [42–44]. Applying MI, in this regard, can potentially revolutionize the management of patients with conditions driven by inflammatory processes, such as CRS [42–44].

Molecular imaging modalities should have a set of optimal properties to provide clinically meaningful (i.e., actionable) information that justifies the use in routine diagnostic practices [44]. These include fast imaging times, heightened spatial resolution, and sensitivity, resulting in increased cost-effectiveness, lower motion artifacts, optimal patient comfort, improved molecular mapping of inflammatory sites, and detection of low-level imaging tracers or endogenous molecules [44]. Additionally, the MI modality should be quantifiable and reproducible for disease stratification and accurate monitoring across patients, lead to minimal toxicity, and be non-invasive such that it can image structures at depth within the body (except if exclusively used as an invasive catheter instrument) [44]. Lastly, it should have robust multiplexing capabilities to evaluate several targets and disease markers in a single scan, providing precise information for superior diagnostic accuracy [44]. These characteristics are encapsulated in Fig. 24.3.

Many of the established clinical imaging techniques have the potential to be employed in for the MI of inflammatory processes, including magnetic resonance imaging (MRI), contrast-enhanced ultrasound (CEUS), and computed tomography (CT), along with nuclear imaging modalities, such as positron emission tomography (PET) and single-photon emission tomography (SPECT) [42, 43]. A handful of other modalities in the pre-clinical stage have been shown to possess potentially

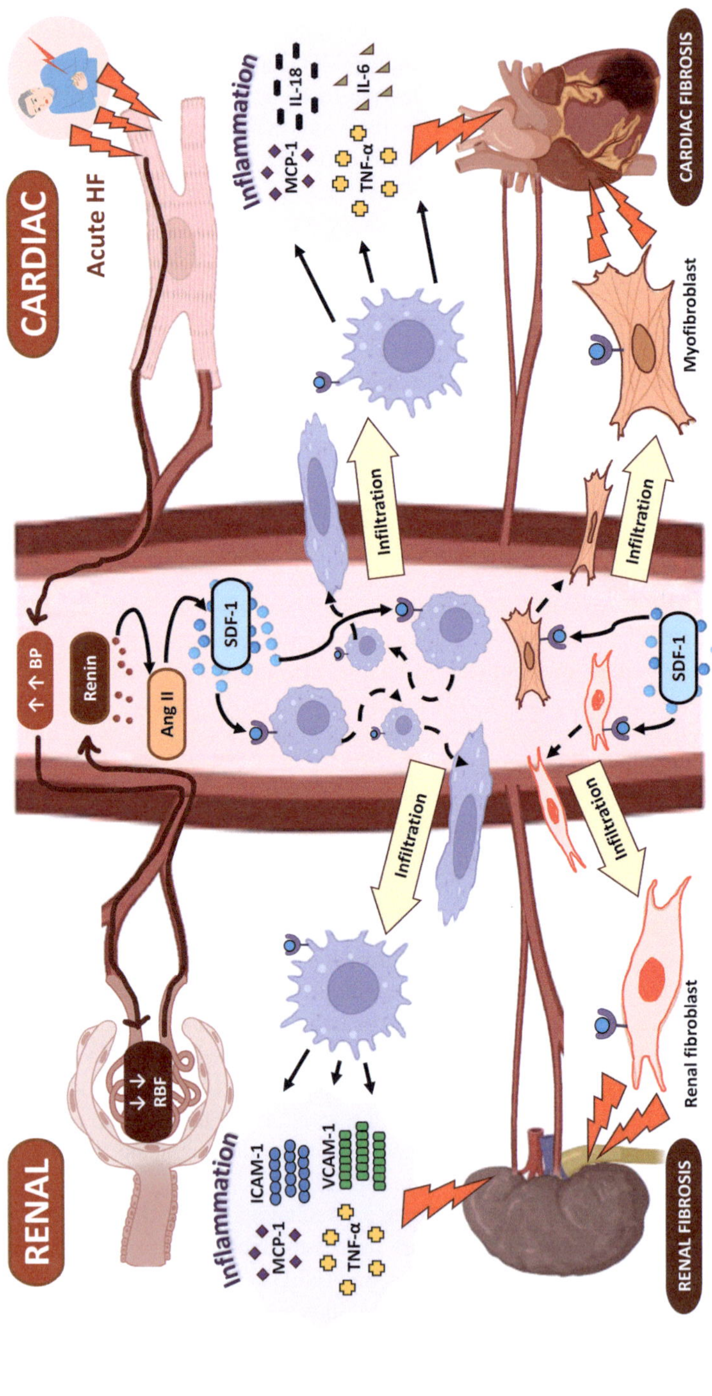

Fig. 24.3 Summarizing the key characteristics required for an ideal molecular imaging modality

beneficial MI abilities that fall under the umbrella of optical imaging and vibrational spectroscopy, comprising photoacoustic imaging (PAI) as well as Raman spectroscopy (RS) and surface-enhanced-Raman spectroscopy (SERS), respectively [42, 43]. Similarly, techniques such as near-infrared fluorescence (NIRF), where two or more photons are used to excite the fluorescent dye/nanoparticle, and spectral imaging using SERS for elevated multiplexing are not ready for common use in the clinic but exhibit great promise [42]. A more profound description of each prospective MI modality, their accompanying imaging/contrast agent, and the known strengths and drawbacks of each are detailed in Table 24.3 [42–44].

Existing modalities do not and may not simultaneously exhibit all these attributes at the ideal level, as a notable weakness typically offsets an adequate strength [44]. For instance, there is commonly an inverse correlation between sensitivity and spatial resolution, reducing the possibility of achieving intricate MI at a cellular level [44]. Nevertheless, these setbacks have led to the engineering of hybrid technologies, such as SPECT/CT and PET/CT, along with a strong push for multimodal MI, including the amalgamation of various optical imaging technologies onto a single probe [44].

Table 24.3 Summary of the characteristics associated with commonly used molecular imaging modalities

MI modality	Description	Imaging agent/radiotracers	Stage of development	Strengths	Weaknesses
CT	Constructs cross-sectional images based on measuring attenuation coefficients of X-ray beams passing through the object under study	Iodine Barium Krypton Xenon Bismuth and gold nanocrystals	Clinical	Fast imaging Non-invasive Good spatial resolution Unlimited depth penetration Provides whole-body imaging Inexpensive	Low sensitivity Poor soft tissue contrast Limited multiplexing Radiation exposure
PET	Involves the intravenous administration of a positron-emitting radiopharmaceutical into systemic distribution for detecting and quantification of bodily accumulation	Positron-emitting radioisotope bound to an organic ligand: Carbon-11 (i.e., ^{11}C acetate) Fluorine-18 (i.e., ^{18}F-FDG) Copper-64 (i.e., ^{64}Cu-BMV101) Gallium-68 (i.e., ^{68}Ga-pentixafor)	Clinical	Non-invasive Exquisitely high sensitivity Unlimited depth penetration Provides whole-body imaging Provides quantitative MI	Poor spatial resolution Radiation exposure Long imaging times Highly expensive No multiplexing abilities
SPECT	Integrates scintigraphy and CT for showcasing radionuclide distribution in a 3D manner for improved detail, contrast, and spatial information	Photon-emitting radioisotope bound to an organic ligand: Technetium-99m (i.e., ^{99m}Tc-teboroxime) Iodine-123 (i.e., ^{123}I) Indium-111 (i.e., ^{111}In-tilmanocept)	Clinical	Non-invasive High sensitivity Cheaper than PET Unlimited depth penetration Provides whole-body imaging Provides quantitative MI	Radiation exposure Poor spatial resolution Long imaging times Limited multiplexing capacity

MRI	Uses a radio wave antenna to transmit signals into the body that are then detected by a radiofrequency receiver, and converted into diagnostic images	Gadolinium chelates (Gd-DTPA) Iron and manganese oxide (i.e., SPIOs, USPIOs) Fluorine-19 (^{19}F)	Clinical	Lack of radiation exposure Non-invasive Excellent soft tissue contrast Good spatial resolution Unlimited depth penetration Provides whole-body imaging	Expensive Long imaging times Low sensitivity No multiplexing abilities Poor signal to noise ratio
CEUS	Utilizes transcutaneous contrast agents for elevated visualization and characterization of anatomical structures and lesions	Microbubbles in the form of gas bubbles stabilized by a shell	Clinical	Inexpensive Non-invasive High sensitivity No radiation exposure Fast, real-time imaging High spatial resolution Suitable for serial imaging across natural history of CRS	Cannot provide whole-body imaging as contrast agents are limited to vasculature Poor signal to noise ratio No multiplexing abilities
NIRF	Involves administering a fluorescence-imaging agent excitable at near-infrared wavelengths (650–1000 nm)	Fluorescent near-infrared organic dyes (i.e., ICG)	Pre-clinical	High-spatial resolution (but decreases as depth increases) No radiation exposure High sensitivity Relatively inexpensive Multiplexing abilities	Cannot provide whole-body imaging (restricted to superficial structures) Potential toxicity of pre-clinical imaging agents Invasive

(continued)

Table 24.3 (continued)

MI modality	Description	Imaging agent/radiotracers	Stage of development	Strengths	Weaknesses
PAI	Employs a hybrid method, combining optical illumination of endogenous materials or fluorescent tracers with the subsequent detection of ultrasound waves emitted due to thermoelastic expansion	Light absorbing organic or inorganic nanoparticles	Pre-clinical	High sensitivity Good spatial resolution Inexpensive No radiation exposure Good multiplexing capacity High speed, real-time imaging Superior penetration depths compared to other optical modalities	Poor penetration depths compared to clinical MI modalities Imaging agents not approved for human use
RS	Spectroscopic technique relying on inelastic scattering, where laser light interacts with a molecule, causing perturbations in its electron cloud and bonds	Nanoparticles	Pre-clinical	Inexpensive Portable Strong multiplexing capability Fast, real-time imaging High spatial resolution Can discriminate a wide set of molecular structures	Poor sensitivity Low imaging depths Requires complex chemometric analysis to separate analytes from spectra

SERS	Similar principles to RS, but also involves targeted nanoparticle functionalization for a specific marker, enabling indirect SERS signal production through the incorporation of a Raman nanoparticle	Silver or gold-based nanoparticles	Pre-clinical	Exquisitely high sensitivity Inexpensive Exquisitely high spatial resolution Portable Fast imaging times Deep-tissue imaging High multiplexing ability	Spectra can be sensitive to changes in nanoparticle orientation and interference from adjacent structures Requires complex statistical algorithms to quantify multiplexed spectra

Abbreviations—*CEUS* contrast-enhanced ultrasound, *CRS* cardiorenal syndrome, *CT* computed tomography, *DTPA* gadolinium diethylene triamine pentaacetic acid, *^{18}F-FDG* ^{18}F-fluorodeoxyglucose, *ICG* indocyanine green, *MI* molecular imaging, *MRI* magnetic resonance imaging, *NIRF* near-infrared fluorescence, *PAI* photoacoustic imaging, *PET* positron emission tomography, *RS* Raman spectroscopy, *SPECT* single photon emission tomography, *SERS* surface-enhanced Raman spectroscopy, *SPIOs* superparamagnetic iron oxides, *USPIOs* ultrasmall superparamagnetic iron oxides

24.5 Molecular Imaging of Inflammatory Crosstalk in CRS and Future Directions

Existing literature on using MI to understand further CRS type 1 heart-kidney crosstalk following AHF is notably insufficient and lacking. This is in part due to the limited progress in the preclinical development of several MI modalities and the underutilization of established techniques like PET, CT, and MRI in the context of CRS.

In pioneering studies relating to the use of MI in the milieu of CRS, Chang et al. gathered that, while cardiac inflammation is an excellent target for detection and therapy in CRS type 4 patients, the lack of effective detection techniques undermined their line of reasoning [45]. Nonetheless, the rapid improvements in nanotechnology-based MI prompted the authors to use, for the first time, a dual-modality magneto-fluorescent nanoparticle (MNP) containing an ultrasmall superparamagnetic iron oxide (USPIO) with Rhodamine B fluorescent dye, linked by poly-L-lysine and acrylic acid [45]. Through the conjugation of MRI, for improved diagnostic accuracy and optical imaging, for heightened sensitivity, Chang et al. sought to determine if this MNP can non-invasively diagnose myocardial inflammation in a CRS type 4 Sprague Dawley rat model and monitor the therapeutic efficacy of Ramipril-based anti-inflammatory therapy [45].

Their results revealed the dual-modality MNP's promising performance encapsulated through its high magnetization value and relaxation coefficient r2, indicative of a rapid and highly sensitive diagnostic tool [45]. Additionally, in vivo MRI demonstrated a significant negative contrast following MNP injection in the inflamed myocardium of type 4 CRS rats, closely relating to the percentage of infiltrated macrophages [45]. Further histopathological analysis verified MNP's ability to target monocyte/macrophages with high specificity [45]. These findings point to the dual-modality agent's potential to accurately identify inflammatory crosstalk, given the role infiltrated immune cells play in perpetuating inflammation throughout the cardiorenal axis post-AHF [45]. However, staining had to be utilized to confirm the increased expression of the previously established pro-inflammatory cytokines involved in CRS type 1 pathogenesis (i.e., TNF-a, IL-6, and monocyte chemoattractant protein-1 (MCP-1)), suggesting that MI is not yet sufficient as an individual technique to confirm inflammatory crosstalk after AHF [45].

Werner et al. launched an important study that included both animal and human subjects [46]. To date, it is one of the more robust studies focusing mainly on the potential use of MI to detect inflammatory crosstalk along the cardiorenal axis [46]. It is important to preface that these authors focused on inflammatory crosstalk in the context of acute myocardial infarction (AMI) rather than any subtype of CRS [46]. However, their findings should not be dismissed, as they offer valuable insights that can shape the future use of MI in the context of CRS type 1 and cardiorenal crosstalk post-AHF, given the strong association between AMI and AHF, with the former remaining the most common cause of the latter [47]. Nonetheless, Werner et al. used serial whole-body PET with the specific CXCR4-targeted radiotracer ^{68}Ga-Pentixafor to compare tracer retention in the heart and kidneys to other hematopoietic organs and access systemic inflammation in AMI-induced mice [46]. Furthermore, 96 patients underwent a 68Ga-Pentixafor PET probe within the first week after developing AMI for systems-based image analysis and to obtain a prognostic value for the adverse renal outcome [46].

Their primary finding was that AMI evoked a parallel temporal increase in cardiac and renal CXCR4 signal in the mouse model, suggesting an inflammatory link between the pair of organs [46]. Ex vivo autoradiography confirmed that the elevated CXCR4 signal corresponded to the amplified macrophage density in both the infarct territory of the myocardium and kidneys early post-AMI [46]. Additionally, distinguishing mice with severely impaired cardiac function in late follow-up was more accurate through renal CXCR4 radiotracer uptake 7 days post-MI than using the infarct PET signal [46]. This highlights the potential of the dual-organ targeting approach for outcome prediction. Not only did patients with renal functional decline (measured by blood based GFR) during follow-up have an elevated PET signal in the infarct early post-AMI, but CXCR4 signal intensity from renal parenchyma also correlated with the signal from infarct and remote myocardium [46]. This signifies a cardiorenal inflammatory link across species, emphasizing the translational potential of the animal model findings to humans [46].

This study establishes the groundwork for evaluating systemic inflammatory heart-kidney interactions through PET [46, 48]. Consequently, future investigations in the realm of CRS post-AHF should adopt the principles set forth by Werner et al., integrating whole-body MI for a comprehensive approach and exploring more novel contrast agents/tracers that target established key inflammatory molecules central to cardiorenal crosstalk.

24.6 Conclusion

In summary, this chapter explores cardiorenal syndrome, tracing its historical roots, evolution, and refined definitions by the ADQI. Examining the pathophysiology of acute CRS emphasizes the intricate interplay of hemodynamic, neurohormonal, and immune-mediated mechanisms. The role of inflammatory processes in CRS type 1 highlights the connection between immune responses and renal dysfunction. Additionally, the chapter probes into the promising realm of molecular imaging for inflammatory markers, offering new perspectives on diagnostics and treatment. This holistic overview enhances our understanding of crosstalk along the cardiorenal axis following acute heart failure, paving the way for future research and clinical applications.

Acknowledgments None

Declaration of Competing Interest None to declare.

Funding This research did not receive any specific grant from funding agencies in the public, commercial, or not-for-profit sectors.

References

1. Savira F, Magaye R, Liew D, et al. Cardiorenal syndrome: multi-organ dysfunction involving the heart, kidney and vasculature. Br J Pharmacol. 2020;177(13):2906–22. https://doi.org/10.1111/bph.15065.
2. Cases and Observations Illustrative of Renal Disease. Accompanied with the secretion of Albuminous urine. Med Chir Rev. 1836;25(49):23–35.
3. Cardio-Renal Connections in Heart Failure and Cardiovascular Disease | NHLBI, NIH. Accessed 17 Jan 2024. https://www.nhlbi.nih.gov/events/2004/cardio-renal-connections-heart-failure-and-cardiovascular-disease.
4. Rangaswami J, Bhalla V, Blair JEA, et al. Cardiorenal syndrome: classification, pathophysiology, diagnosis, and treatment strategies: a scientific statement from the American Heart Association. Circulation. 2019;139(16):e840–78. https://doi.org/10.1161/CIR.0000000000000664.
5. Ronco C, McCullough P, Anker SD, et al. Cardio-renal syndromes: report from the consensus conference of the acute dialysis quality initiative. Eur Heart J. 2010;31(6):703–11. https://doi.org/10.1093/eurheartj/ehp507.
6. Núñez J, Miñana G, Santas E, Bertomeu-González V. Cardiorenal syndrome in acute heart failure: revisiting paradigms. Rev Esp Cardiol (Engl Ed). 2015;68(5):426–35. https://doi.org/10.1016/j.rec.2014.10.016.
7. Harjola VP, Mullens W, Banaszewski M, et al. Organ dysfunction, injury and failure in acute heart failure: from pathophysiology to diagnosis and management. A review on behalf of the acute heart failure Committee of the Heart Failure Association (HFA) of the European Society of Cardiology (ESC). Eur J Heart Fail. 2017;19(7):821–36. https://doi.org/10.1002/ejhf.872.
8. Hanada S, Takewa Y, Mizuno T, Tsukiya T, Taenaka Y, Tatsumi E. Effect of the technique for assisting renal blood circulation on ischemic kidney in acute cardiorenal syndrome. J Artif Organs. 2012;15(2):140–5. https://doi.org/10.1007/s10047-011-0613-5.
9. Mitsas AC, Elzawawi M, Mavrogeni S, et al. Heart failure and Cardiorenal syndrome: a narrative review on pathophysiology, diagnostic and therapeutic regimens-from a cardiologist's view. J Clin Med. 2022;11(23):7041. https://doi.org/10.3390/jcm11237041.
10. Forman DE, Butler J, Wang Y, et al. Incidence, predictors at admission, and impact of worsening renal function among patients hospitalized with heart failure. J Am Coll Cardiol. 2004;43(1):61–7. https://doi.org/10.1016/j.jacc.2003.07.031.
11. Ronco C, Cicoira M, McCullough PA. Cardiorenal syndrome type 1: pathophysiological crosstalk leading to combined heart and kidney dysfunction in the setting of acutely decompensated heart failure. J Am Coll Cardiol. 2012;60(12):1031–42. https://doi.org/10.1016/j.jacc.2012.01.077.
12. Winton FR. The influence of venous pressure on the isolated mammalian kidney. J Physiol. 1931;72(1):49–61. https://doi.org/10.1113/jphysiol.1931.sp002761.
13. Ronco F, Mazzone P, Hosseinian L, Genovesi S. Recent advances in stroke prevention in patients with atrial fibrillation and end-stage renal disease. Cardiorenal Med. 2017;7(3):207–17. https://doi.org/10.1159/000470856.
14. Mullens W, Abrahams Z, Francis GS, et al. Importance of venous congestion for worsening of renal function in advanced decompensated heart failure. J Am Coll Cardiol. 2009;53(7):589–96. https://doi.org/10.1016/j.jacc.2008.05.068.
15. Mullens W, Abrahams Z, Skouri HN, et al. Elevated intra-abdominal pressure in acute decompensated heart failure: a potential contributor to worsening renal function? J Am Coll Cardiol. 2008;51(3):300–6. https://doi.org/10.1016/j.jacc.2007.09.043.
16. Nohria A, Tsang SW, Fang JC, et al. Clinical assessment identifies hemodynamic profiles that predict outcomes in patients admitted with heart failure. J Am Coll Cardiol. 2003;41(10):1797–804. https://doi.org/10.1016/S0735-1097(03)00309-7.
17. Haase M, Müller C, Damman K, et al. Pathogenesis of cardiorenal syndrome type 1 in acute decompensated heart failure: workgroup statements from the eleventh consensus conference

of the acute dialysis quality initiative (ADQI). Contrib Nephrol. 2013;182:99–116. https://doi.org/10.1159/000349969.
18. Dutta A, Saha S, Bahl A, Mittal A, Basak T. A comprehensive review of acute cardio-renal syndrome: need for novel biomarkers. Front Pharmacol. 2023:14. Accessed 12 Jan 2024. https://www.frontiersin.org/articles/10.3389/fphar.2023.1152055.
19. Bansal N, Keane M, Delafontaine P, et al. A longitudinal study of left ventricular function and structure from CKD to ESRD: the CRIC study. Clin J Am Soc Nephrol. 2013;8(3):355–62. https://doi.org/10.2215/CJN.06020612.
20. Buglioni A, Burnett JC. Pathophysiology and the cardiorenal connection in heart failure. Circulating hormones: biomarkers or mediators. Clin Chim Acta. 2015;443:3–8. https://doi.org/10.1016/j.cca.2014.10.027.
21. Prastaro M, Nardi E, Paolillo S, et al. Cardiorenal syndrome: pathophysiology as a key to the therapeutic approach in an under-diagnosed disease. J Clin Ultrasound. 2022;50(8):1110–24. https://doi.org/10.1002/jcu.23265.
22. Tarvasmäki T, Haapio M, Mebazaa A, et al. Acute kidney injury in cardiogenic shock: definitions, incidence, haemodynamic alterations, and mortality. Eur J Heart Fail. 2018;20(3):572–81. https://doi.org/10.1002/ejhf.958.
23. Gromadzka G, Tarnacka B, Flaga A, Adamczyk A. Copper dyshomeostasis in neurodegenerative diseases—therapeutic implications. Int J Mol Sci. 2020;21(23):9259. https://doi.org/10.3390/ijms21239259.
24. Virzì GM, Day S, de Cal M, Vescovo G, Ronco C. Heart–kidney crosstalk and role of humoral signaling in critical illness. Crit Care. 2014;18(1):201. https://doi.org/10.1186/cc13177.
25. Rubattu S, Mennuni S, Testa M, et al. Pathogenesis of chronic Cardiorenal syndrome: is there a role for oxidative stress? Int J Mol Sci. 2013;14(11):23011–32. https://doi.org/10.3390/ijms141123011.
26. Gelasco AK, Raymond JR. Indoxyl sulfate induces complex redox alterations in mesangial cells. Am J Physiol Renal Physiol. 2006;290(6):F1551–8. https://doi.org/10.1152/ajprenal.00281.2004.
27. Virzì GM, Clementi A, de Cal M, et al. Oxidative stress: dual pathway induction in cardiorenal syndrome type 1 pathogenesis. Oxidative Med Cell Longev. 2015;2015:391790. https://doi.org/10.1155/2015/391790.
28. Damman K, Ng Kam Chuen MJ, MacFadyen RJ, et al. Volume status and diuretic therapy in systolic heart failure and the detection of early abnormalities in renal and tubular function. J Am Coll Cardiol. 2011;57(22):2233–41. https://doi.org/10.1016/j.jacc.2010.10.065.
29. Chiong JR, Cheung RJ. Loop diuretic therapy in heart failure: the need for solid evidence on a fluid issue. Clin Cardiol. 2010;33(6):345–52. https://doi.org/10.1002/clc.20771.
30. Elmore S. Apoptosis: a review of programmed cell death. Toxicol Pathol. 2007;35(4):495–516. https://doi.org/10.1080/01926230701320337.
31. Jentzer JC, Chawla LS. A clinical approach to the acute Cardiorenal syndrome. Crit Care Clin. 2015;31(4):685–703. https://doi.org/10.1016/j.ccc.2015.06.006.
32. Akcay A, Nguyen Q, Edelstein CL. Mediators of inflammation in acute kidney injury. Mediat Inflamm. 2010;2009:e137072. https://doi.org/10.1155/2009/137072.
33. Pastori S, Virzì GM, Brocca A, et al. Cardiorenal syndrome type 1: a defective regulation of monocyte apoptosis induced by proinflammatory and proapoptotic factors. Cardiorenal Med. 2015;5(2):105–15. https://doi.org/10.1159/000371898.
34. Virzì GM, Breglia A, Brocca A, et al. Levels of Proinflammatory cytokines, oxidative stress, and tissue damage markers in patients with acute heart failure with and without Cardiorenal syndrome type 1. Cardiorenal Med. 2018;8(4):321–31. https://doi.org/10.1159/000492602.
35. Colombo PC, Banchs JE, Celaj S, et al. Endothelial cell activation in patients with decompensated heart failure. Circulation. 2005;111(1):58–62. https://doi.org/10.1161/01.CIR.0000151611.89232.3B.
36. Mutlu GM, Sznajder JI. Mechanisms of pulmonary edema clearance. Am J Physiol Lung Cell Mol Physiol. 2005;289(5):L685–95. https://doi.org/10.1152/ajplung.00247.2005.

37. Cotter G, Metra M, Milo-Cotter O, Dittrich HC, Gheorghiade M. Fluid overload in acute heart failure--re-distribution and other mechanisms beyond fluid accumulation. Eur J Heart Fail. 2008;10(2):165–9. https://doi.org/10.1016/j.ejheart.2008.01.007.
38. Chu PY, Zatta A, Kiriazis H, et al. CXCR4 antagonism attenuates the cardiorenal consequences of mineralocorticoid excess. Circ Heart Fail. 2011;4(5):651–8. https://doi.org/10.1161/CIRCHEARTFAILURE.110.960831.
39. Chu PY, Mariani J, Finch S, et al. Bone marrow-derived cells contribute to fibrosis in the chronically failing heart. Am J Pathol. 2010;176(4):1735–42. https://doi.org/10.2353/ajpath.2010.090574.
40. Jin L, Li Q, Li J, et al. Apela inhibits systemic and renal inflammatory reactions in mice with type I cardiorenal syndrome. FASEB J. 2021;35(10):e21907. https://doi.org/10.1096/fj.202101030R.
41. James ML, Gambhir SS. A molecular imaging primer: modalities, imaging agents, and applications. Physiol Rev. 2012;92(2):897–965. https://doi.org/10.1152/physrev.00049.2010.
42. MacRitchie N, Frleta-Gilchrist M, Sugiyama A, Lawton T, McInnes IB, Maffia P. Molecular imaging of inflammation - current and emerging technologies for diagnosis and treatment. Pharmacol Ther. 2020;211:107550. https://doi.org/10.1016/j.pharmthera.2020.107550.
43. Pysz MA, Gambhir SS, Willmann JK. Molecular imaging: current status and emerging strategies. Clin Radiol. 2010;65(7):500–16. https://doi.org/10.1016/j.crad.2010.03.011.
44. MacRitchie N, Noonan J, Guzik TJ, Maffia P. Molecular imaging of cardiovascular inflammation. Br J Pharmacol. 2021;178(21):4216–45. https://doi.org/10.1111/bph.15654.
45. Chang D, Wang YC, Zhang SJ, et al. Visualizing myocardial inflammation in a rat model of type 4 cardiorenal syndrome by dual-modality molecular imaging. Biomaterials. 2015;68:67–76. https://doi.org/10.1016/j.biomaterials.2015.07.050.
46. Werner RA, Hess A, Koenig T, et al. Molecular imaging of inflammation crosstalk along the cardio-renal axis following acute myocardial infarction. Theranostics. 2021;11(16):7984–94. https://doi.org/10.7150/thno.61423.
47. Jenča D, Melenovský V, Stehlik J, et al. Heart failure after myocardial infarction: incidence and predictors. ESC Heart Fail. 2020;8(1):222–37. https://doi.org/10.1002/ehf2.13144.
48. Werner RA, Pomper MG, Buck AK, Rowe SP, Higuchi T. SPECT and PET radiotracers in renal imaging. Semin Nucl Med. 2022;52(4):406–18. https://doi.org/10.1053/j.semnuclmed.2021.12.003.

Effects of Atrial Natriuretic Peptide on Interorgan Crosstalk

25

Gian Marco Rosa, Paolo Costa, and Vered Gil Ad

Data from literature show a crosstalk between various organs such as heart, kidney, adipose tissue, and metabolism. This crosstalk is particularly evident in the presence of heart failure, which is characterized by impaired muscular and oxidative function and by insulin resistance [voce 1, 2]. It has been previously shown that natriuretic peptides, and in particular ANP, which are commonly considered cardiovascular and renal hormones may interact with lipid and glucose metabolism [3]. The aim of this chapter is to explore the effects of natriuretic peptides on interorgan crosstalk, which is peculiar to cardiovascular and metabolic diseases.

25.1 Natriuretic Peptides (General Features)

In 1984, the discovery of atrial natriuretic peptide (ANP) represented a significant breakthrough. ANP, along with its counterparts like brain natriuretic peptides (BNP) and C-type natriuretic peptide (CNP), forms a common family of biochemically similar 17-amino acids-ring-structured molecules.

The genes for ANP and BNP are located in tandem on Chromosome 1.

ANP and BNP are circulating hormones secreted by the cardiac atria and ventricles, respectively. Both peptides are synthesized as preprohormones and stored as prohormones in intracellular granules. Stretching of atrial or ventricular

G. M. Rosa (✉)
Cardiology Clinic, Department of Internal Medicine and Medical Specialties, University of Genoa, Genoa, Italy

IRCCS Ospedale Policlinico San Martino, Genoa, Italy

P. Costa
Cardiology Clinic, Department of Internal Medicine and Medical Specialties, University of Genoa, Genoa, Italy

V. G. Ad
IRCCS Ospedale Policlinico San Martino, Genoa, Italy

D. Battaglini et al. (eds.), *Organ System Crosstalk in Critical Illness*,
https://doi.org/10.1007/978-3-032-01024-7_25

cardiomyocytes, whether due to physical exercise, increased sodium intake, or diseases associated with volume overload, can trigger their release. The primary effect of ANP and BNP is to promote sodium excretion by the kidneys, thereby influencing the filtration fraction. In contrast, CNP is not produced by the heart and does not exert the natriuretic effects observed for ANP and BNP.

ANP and BNP responses are primarily mediated by the GCA (guanylyl cyclase-coupled natriuretic peptide) receptor, also known as NPR-A (natriuretic peptide receptor A).

In addition, natriuretic peptides are enzymatically cleaved by neprilysin, which additionally degrades other peptides involved in cardiovascular and metabolic regulation, such as bradykinin, endothelin-1, and glucagon-like peptide [3].

25.2 Renal and Cardiovascular Effects of ANP

Natriuretic peptides play a pivotal role in hemodynamic regulation; their global hemodynamic effects are complex and interconnected. ANP primarily induces increased natriuresis and diuresis, and elicits vasodilation by antagonizing the renin-angiotensin system. In this regard, genetic variants associated with increased natriuretic peptide concentrations present lower blood pressure and reduced odds of arterial hypertension.

Furthermore, natriuretic peptides also attenuate sympathetic nervous system activity at least in part through interaction with central vasopressin pathways [4].

From a nephrological perspective, ANP has direct effects on nephron collecting ducts and presents inhibitory action on angiotensin II effects. It increases the glomerular filtration rate (GFR) by dilating afferent arterioles and constricting efferent arterioles to increase the glomerular capillary hydraulic pressure [5].

Particularly, ANP has also been shown to enhance recovery from renal ischemia reperfusion injury (IRI) by increasing renal medullary blood flow in rats [6].

IRI is a common cause of acute kidney injury and has a frequent occurrence in critically ill patients. Renal IRI releases proinflammatory cytokines within the kidney that induce crosstalk between the kidney and other organ systems.

In his interesting study, Mitaka showed that ANP infusion, in a rat model of unilateral renal IRI, presented both direct tissue protective effects and anti-inflammatory effects, which may potentially inhibit interorgan crosstalk [7].

In a clinical setting, ANP infusion improves pulmonary capillary wedge pressure and cardiac index in patients with acute heart failure [8] and preserves renal function after cardiovascular surgery [9].

Beyond its role as circulating endocrine factors, inside the heart ANP and BNP act as local antihypertrophic (ANP) and antifibrotic (BNP) cardiac factors, thus acting on cardiac remodeling [10].

Due to these important hemodynamic effects, recombinant ANP (carperitide) and BNP (nesiritide) have been developed for intravenous treatment of acutely decompensated heart failure. Their short plasma half-life and the need for intravenous or subcutaneous infusion preclude their chronic use [3].

Therefore, newer natriuretic peptides that differ from the native peptides in terms of efficacy, specificity, and resistance to enzymatic degradation have been developed [11].

25.3 Metabolic Effects and Effects on Adipose Tissue

ANP presents various effects on lipidic metabolism; indeed, it has been shown to increase of lipid oxidation concomitantly with a decrease of blood pressure after short-term ANP infusion.

In this regard, a recent study has established robust associations between plasma NT-proBNP and NT-proANP levels and various components of metabolic syndrome [3]. Notably, an inverse relationship between natriuretic peptide levels and insulin resistance is identified.

In the early 2000, a potent lipolytic effect was demonstrated of natriuretic peptides in human isolated adipocytes [12]. Furthermore, it has been demonstrated that treatment with atrial natriuretic peptide induces adipose tissue browning and exerts thermogenic actions in vivo.

Furthermore, it has been shown that, after intravenous ANP infusion, adipose tissue lipolysis may occur in a dose-dependent manner. This phenomenon is observed only in adipose tissue but not in skeletal muscle.

Kimura et al., in an interesting study, demonstrated that exogenous ANP administration significantly improved the high-fat diet (HFD)-induced insulin resistance by attenuating hepatic steatosis and inducing morphological changes of adipose tissue. These changes consisted in browning of adipose tissue in association with the activation of the brown fat thermogenic program.

Accordingly, the mice treated with ANP developed tolerance to cold exposure, indicating the adaptive heat-retaining property of NPs when body temperature falls via interorgan metabolic crosstalk with adipose tissues [13].

In the context of heart failure, certain obesity-related parameters are associated with reduced NT-pro-BNP levels. Moreover, evidences suggest that sex-specific differences exist, indicating that younger age and male sex may play a role [14].

These results contribute significantly to understanding the complex interrelationships between cardiac, sex endocrine systems, and obesity-related parameters.

Furthermore, the link between obesity and hypertension may be considered a conundrum; undoubtedly, sodium retention and excessive sympathetic tone are key contributors Owing to the fact that NP are important regulators of sodium hemostasis and neurohormonal activation, it may be hypothesized that obese individuals have an impaired natriuretic peptides response. In this regard, the interesting study conducted by Mitaka has demonstrated that in HFD-mice, ANP treatment decreased body weight and blood pressure [7].

Finally, it has been demonstrated that also diabetes was associated with low plasma natriuretic peptide levels, and the negative effects of obesity and diabetes on natriuretic peptide levels were additive [15].

25.4 Effects on Inflammatory Pathways

ANP presents intricate links also with inflammatory pathways.

Recent evidence suggests that during chronic inflammation, the mRNA expression of TNF-α, IL-6, and IL-1β increases significantly, whereas ANP and BNP may help prevent or reduce the elevation of these proinflammatory cytokines [16].

Particularly, in induced AKI rats, ANP treatment decreased TNF-α, IL-6, and NF-κB expression scores of the lung [7].

25.5 Conclusions

In summary, this chapter provides a comprehensive overview of the multifaceted roles of ANP and its counterparts, shedding light on their physiological and pathophysiological implications. The intricate network of interactions with various systems, including cardiovascular, renal, and endocrine systems, underscores the role of natriuretic peptides in maintaining homeostasis and responding to critical clinical conditions.

References

1. Holditch SJ, Schreiber CA, Nini R, Tonne JM, Peng KW, Geurts A, Jacob HJ, Burnett JC, Cataliotti A, Ikeda Y. B-type natriuretic peptide deletion leads to progressive hypertension, associated organ damage, and reduced survival: novel model for human hypertension. Hypertension. 2015;66:199–210. https://doi.org/10.1161/HYPERTENSIONAHA.115.05610. Crossref. PubMed.
2. Kemppainen J, Tsuchida H, Stolen K, Karlsson H, Björnholm M, Heinonen OJ, Nuutila P, Krook A, Knuuti J, Zierath JR. Insulin signalling and resistance in patients with chronic heart failure. J Physiol. 2003;550(pt 1):305–15.
3. Jordan J, Birkenfeld AL, Melander O. Natriuretic peptides in cardiovascular and metabolic crosstalk implications for hypertension management. Hypertension. 2018;72(2):270–6.
4. Yusof AP, Yusoff NH, Suhaimi FW, Coote JH. Role of supraspinal vasopressin neurones in the effects of atrial natriuretic peptide on sympathetic nerve activity. Auton Neurosci. 2009;148:50–4.
5. Marin Grez M, Fleming JT, Steinhausen M. Atrial natriuretic peptide causes pre-glomerular vasodilation and post-glomerular vasoconstriction in rat kidney. Nature. 1986;324:473–6.
6. Chujo K, Ueno M, Asaga T, Sakamoto H, Shirakami G, Ueki M. Atrial natriuretic peptide enhances recovery from ischemia/reperfusion-induced renal injury in rats. J Biosci Bioeng. 2010;109:526–30.
7. Mitaka C, et al. Effects of atrial natriuretic peptide on inter-organ crosstalk among the kidney, lung, and heart in a rat model of renal ischemia-reperfusion injury. Intensive Care Med Exp. 2014;2(1):1–17.
8. Kobayashi D, Yamaguchi N, Takahashi O, Deshpande G, Fukui T. Human atrial natriuretic peptide treatment for acute heart failure: a systematic review of efficacy and mortality. Can J Cardiol. 2012;28:102–9.
9. Sezai A, Hata M, Niino T, et al. Results of low dose human atrial natriuretic peptide infusion in non dialysis patients with chronic kidney disease undergoing coronary artery bypass grafting. J Am Coll Cardiol. 2011;58:897–903.

10. Sarzani R, Allevi M, Di Pentima C, et al. Role of cardiac natriuretic peptides in heart structure and function. Int J Mol Sci. 2022;23(22):14415.
11. Meems LMG, Burnett JC. Innovative therapeutics: designer natriuretic peptides. JACC Basic Transl Sci. 2016;1:557–67.
12. Sengenes C, Berlan M, De Glisezinski I, et al. Natriuretic peptides: a new lipolytic pathway in human adipocytes. FASEB J. 2000;14(10):1345–51.
13. Kimura H, Nagoshi T, Oi Y, et al. Treatment with atrial natriuretic peptide induces adipose tissue browning and exerts thermogenic actions in vivo. Sci Rep. 2021;11(1):17466.
14. Madamanchi C, Alhosaini H, Sumida A, et al. Obesity and natriuretic peptides, BNP and NT-proBNP: mechanisms and diagnostic implications for heart failure. Int J Cardiol. 2014;176(3):611–7.
15. Wang TJ, Larson MG, Levy D, et al. Impact of obesity on natriuretic peptide levels. Circulation. 2004;109(5):594–600.
16. Ramakrishnan V, Burnett JC, Sumida A, et al. Natriuretic peptides, inflammation, and sounding the alarm. Circ Heart Fail. 2020;13(7):e007208.

Part VI

The Lungs

Brain-Lung Crosstalk and Mechanical Ventilation

26

Renata Mendes, Gloria Martins, Denise Battaglini, Chiara Robba, Pedro L. Silva, and Patricia R. M. Rocco

26.1 Introduction

Crosstalk between organs is a biological process which includes cellular, soluble, immune, and neurohormonal pathways [1]. It is a two-way communication responsible for coordinating and maintaining physiological homeostasis; however, during pathological processes, crosstalk can trigger or exacerbate injury to one or multiple organs [2] (Fig. 26.1).

Acute brain injuries, including traumatic brain injury (TBI), intracerebral hemorrhage, subarachnoid hemorrhage, and acute ischemic stroke, may damage not only the central nervous system but also distal organs [3]. The local inflammatory process plays a crucial role in brain recovery and neurogenesis, but it can also be responsible for distal organ injury. Extensive research on the crosstalk between brain and distal organs is underway seeking to better understand the associated

R. Mendes
Department of Nephrology, State University of Rio de Janeiro, Rio de Janeiro, Brazil

Department of Nephrology, Federal University of Rio de Janeiro, Rio de Janeiro, Brazil

G. Martins
Neurointensive Care, Barra D'Or Hospital, Rio de Janeiro, Brazil

D. Battaglini
Department of Surgical Sciences and Integrated Diagnostics, University of Genoa, Genoa, Italy

C. Robba
Anesthesia and Intensive Care, IRCCS Ospedale Policlinico San Martino, Genoa, Italy

Department of Surgical Sciences and Integrated Diagnostics (DISC), University of Genoa, Genoa, Italy

P. L. Silva · P. R. M. Rocco (✉)
Laboratory of Pulmonary Investigation, Carlos Chagas Filho Institute of Biophysics, Federal University of Rio de Janeiro, Rio de Janeiro, Brazil
e-mail: pedroleme@biof.ufrj.br

D. Battaglini et al. (eds.), *Organ System Crosstalk in Critical Illness*,
https://doi.org/10.1007/978-3-032-01024-7_26

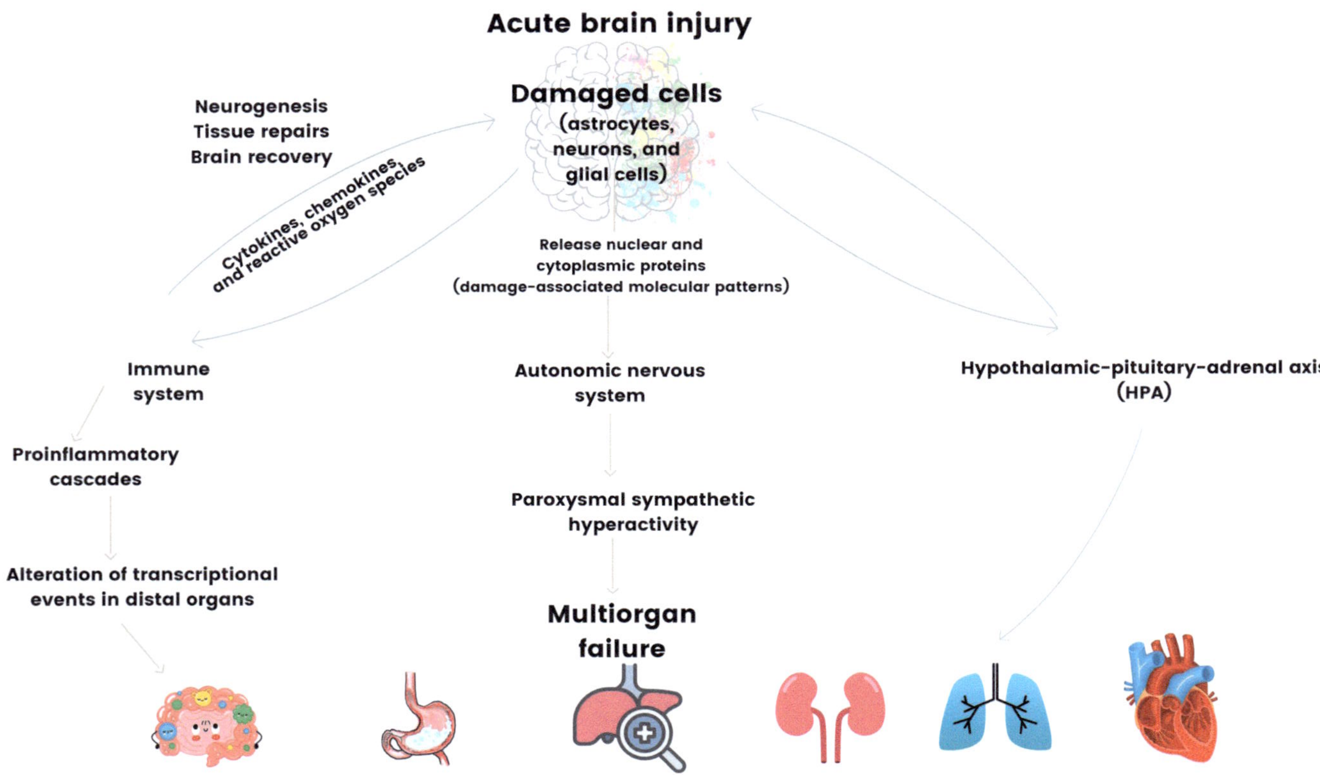

Fig. 26.1 Pathophysiological mechanisms of multiorgan failure following acute brain injury

pathways, which may serve as targets for future therapies and thus improve outcomes of critically ill neurological patients [4, 5].

Lungs seem to be the distal organ most vulnerable to damage after brain injury, which often leads to systemic and pulmonary inflammation, as well as increased endothelial cell permeability and edema [6], thus impairing respiratory system mechanics [7]. This may result in the need for ventilatory and hemodynamic support [8–10], which, in turn, can have deleterious effects of its own on brain and lungs alike.

This chapter aims to investigate crosstalk between the brain and lungs and address the impact of mechanical ventilation in neurocritical patients, as well as to evaluate the lung-brain crosstalk.

26.2 Pathophysiology of Crosstalk Between Organs After Brain Injury

Acute brain injury, regardless of its cause, triggers metabolic, hormonal, and humoral responses following activation of the immune system, the autonomic nervous system (both sympathetic and parasympathetic), and the hypothalamic-pituitary-adrenal axis [11]. After a brain insult, damaged cells in the central nervous system (astrocytes, neurons, and glial cells) release their cytoplasmic and nuclear contents, which act as damage-associated molecular patterns (DAMPs) [5, 12] (Fig. 26.1). This mechanism triggers the innate and adaptive immune responses, with local and then systemic effects. Once the inflammatory process is activated, an increase in biomarkers (cytokines, chemokines, and free radicals) is observed [3] in the central nervous system, leading to multiorgan dysfunction. On the other hand, this inflammatory response is also important for repair, neurogenesis, and neuronal recovery [13]. In this line, neuronal survival appears to be controlled by regulatory T cells, which have a neuroprotective effect [5].

Another pathway that can affect the lungs indirectly following acute brain injury is paroxysmal sympathetic hyperactivity (PSH) [14], which may occur in up to 80% of these patients. PSH is characterized by a transient increase in sympathetic and motor activities that may be mediated by direct disruption between brainstem centers and cortical inhibitory centers or by a two-stage process involving loss of descending inhibition, thus allowing the development of excitatory spinal circuits. PSH activates the release of central neurotransmitters (catecholamines and corticosteroids), which can enhance the peripheral response to acute brain injury [5] (Fig. 26.1). It has been demonstrated that direct myocardial injury, such as Takotsubo cardiomyopathy, can contribute to neurogenic pulmonary edema and cardiac failure with hemodynamic instability. Indeed, following brain injury, there is a massive sympathetic discharge that can lead to direct myocardial damage and heart wall motion abnormalities, which correspond to the pattern of sympathetic nerve innervation. The neuro-hemodynamic theory suggests that this indirect impairment of ventricular compliance occurs due to rapid increases in systemic and pulmonary pressures. This results in a translocation of blood flow from the highly resistant systemic circulation to the low-resistance pulmonary circulation, ultimately causing hydrostatic pulmonary edema [14].

26.3 Brain-Lung Crosstalk: The Brain-to-Lung Pathway

A communication pathway between the brain and the lungs (known as the brain-lung axis) has been described, as well as a strict communication between the lungs and the brain. This communication becomes evident as patients with brain injuries often exhibit pulmonary complications, which may worsen both brain and lung damage. Patients with brain injury often require mechanical ventilation due to the risk of aspiration and deteriorated neurological status [15, 16].

Pulmonary complications such as ventilator-associated pneumonia (VAP) and the acute respiratory distress syndrome (ARDS) are in fact more common in brain-injured patients than in the general ICU population [17, 18] (Fig. 26.2). This is likely due not only to the initial local inflammatory cascade but also to use of non-protective mechanical ventilation strategies, which is more common in brain-injured patients [17]. Moreover, the hypoxemia and systemic inflammatory responses encountered in ARDS can further precipitate secondary brain injury [16].

Timely diagnosis and treatment of VAP and ARDS are imperative, as they worsen the outcomes of patients with acute brain injury [17]. The use of mechanical ventilation in this population has been associated with higher need for tracheostomy, increased incidence of VAP, unfavorable neurological outcomes, extended intensive care unit and hospital stays, and increased mortality [17]. The pathophysiological mechanisms of the most frequent pulmonary complications in acute brain injury patients are described below.

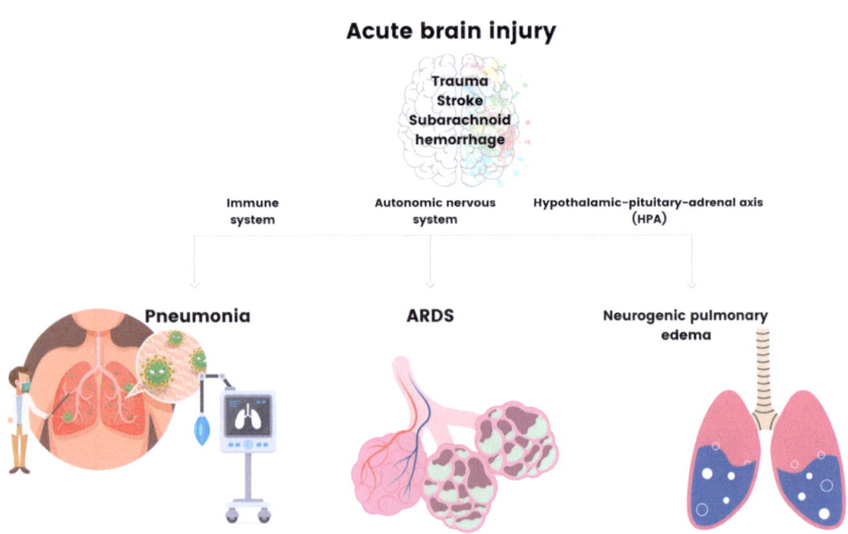

Fig. 26.2 Lung damage following acute brain injury. ARDS acute respiratory distress syndrome

26.3.1 Neurogenic Pulmonary Edema

Neurogenic pulmonary edema (NPE) is a condition that has been known for over 100 years and consists of pulmonary edema that develops following a severe neurological injury (such as traumatic brain injury, subarachnoid hemorrhage, stroke, status epilepticus, meningitis, or subdural hemorrhage) once other causes have been ruled out. In a review exploring cases of NPE, the primary etiology was subarachnoid hemorrhage (43%), and symptoms typically manifested approximately 4 hours after brain injury [19]. The most widely accepted theory proposes that a sudden rise in intracranial pressure (ICP) triggers excessive sympathetic stimulation and a significant release of catecholamines into the systemic circulation, which bind to adrenergic receptors in the pulmonary vasculature, causing vasoconstriction and an increase in pulmonary vascular resistance [20, 21]. This vasoconstriction impairs blood flow through the pulmonary capillaries, leading to increased hydrostatic pressure and fluid leakage into the alveolar spaces [20, 21].

In addition to sympathetic activation, disruption of the blood-brain barrier (BBB) plays an important role in NPE development. CNS insults can result in an inflammatory response and the release of inflammatory mediators, which can compromise the integrity of the BBB [22]. This allows the entry of plasma proteins, such as albumin and fibrinogen, into the brain parenchyma. The presence of these proteins in the CNS triggers an inflammatory cascade, which further contributes to increased vascular permeability and pulmonary edema [22]. Another contributing factor in NPE is an imbalance between the sympathetic and parasympathetic systems. CNS insults can disrupt the normal autonomic regulation, leading to sympathetic overactivity and parasympathetic withdrawal. This imbalance can result in uncontrolled release of vasoconstrictive substances, such as endothelin-1, and a decrease in vasodilatory substances, such as nitric oxide [23]. This dysregulation of vascular tone promotes pulmonary vasoconstriction, further exacerbating pulmonary hypertension and edema formation [23].

Patients with NPE may present with symptoms such as dyspnea, tachypnea, hypoxemia, pink-colored frothy sputum, and signs of pulmonary congestion on chest imaging. Clinical evaluation, assessment of the underlying CNS pathology, and exclusion of other causes of pulmonary edema, such as cardiogenic causes.

Treatment of NPE focuses on managing the underlying CNS insult while providing supportive care for the pulmonary edema [21].

26.3.2 Ventilator-Associated Pneumonia (VAP)

The incidence of VAP in neurological patients ranges from 21% to 61% [24–26] and has been associated with reduced level of consciousness, need for prolonged mechanical ventilation, and the occurrence of aspiration [27]. The most common pathogens in this population are *Staphylococcus aureus*, *Klebsiella pneumoniae*, *Acinetobacter baumannii*, *Pseudomonas aeruginosa*, *Streptococcus pneumoniae*, and *Enterobacter aerogenes* [28]. VAP increases length of hospital stay and mortality in stroke and TBI patients [29]. Early feeding and proper oral hygiene may reduce the risk of VAP.

An analysis of secondary data from the "Extubation strategies in Neuro-Intensive care unit (ICU) patients and associations with Outcomes" (ENIO) cohort study revealed a VAP prevalence of 39.5%. Several factors were found to be associated with VAP, including male gender, invasive procedures such as intracranial pressure (IP) monitoring and external ventricular drain (EVD) placement, tracheobronchitis, and the use of therapeutic hypothermia. While VAP did not impact mortality, it was found to prolong ICU stay [18].

Invasive mechanical ventilation can also induce lung injury, leading to pulmonary inflammation (especially if non-protective ventilation strategies are used) and infection (Fig. 26.3). Tracheal intubation and prolonged mechanical ventilation impair local immune defenses and pulmonary hostprotection mechanisms, facilitating the colonization of the lower respiratory tract by pathogenic microorganisms and predisposing to the development of pneumonia. The use of VAP prevention bundles effectively decreases the occurrence of VAP. These bundles encompass several components, including education and appropriate airway management, hand hygiene prior to airway handling, maintenance and regulation of cuff pressure, oral hygiene with chlorhexidine, semi-recumbent positioning, reduction in mechanical ventilation duration, and avoidance of elective modifications to the ventilator circuit and its components [30].

26.3.3 Acute Respiratory Distress Syndrome

ARDS is common in patients with severe acute brain injury: it is reported in up to 30% of patients with TBI [31], 38% of patients with non-traumatic subarachnoid

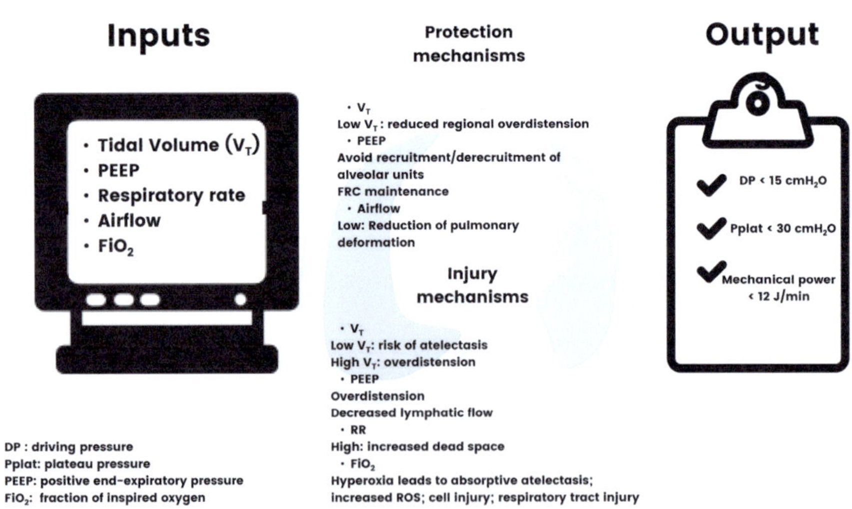

Fig. 26.3 Ventilatory variables able to protect or induce lung injury. ROS reactive oxygen species

hemorrhage [32], 28% of patients with spontaneous intracranial hemorrhage [2, 6], and 4% of patients with acute ischemic stroke [33].

Regardless of the neurological insult, the presence of ARDS impacts morbidity and mortality in these patients, yielding a threefold increase in hospital mortality [31, 34]. ARDS is associated with worse neurological outcomes and longer ICU and hospital stays [34].

The risk factors associated with ARDS in this population include the severity of brain injury, as represented by a low Glasgow Coma Score (GCS 3–4); abnormalities observed on computed tomography scan, such as midline shift; the presence of hypertension; the need for vasopressor administration; a history of drug abuse; young age; male gender; and comorbidities such as diabetes, hypertension, and chronic obstructive pulmonary disease [35].

A lung-protective mechanical ventilation strategy, consisting of low tidal volume (6 ml/kg), plateau pressure < 30 cmH_2O, driving pressure < 15 cmH_2O, and mechanical power < 12 J/min [34], minimizes the risk of ARDS in acutely brain-injured patients (Fig. 26.3). The ventilator management of patients with severe neurologic injury appears to be a crucial aspect in the development of ARDS and aligns with the "double hit" model. The distribution of ARDS exhibits a bimodal pattern, characterized by an early peak on days 2–3 following the initiation of mechanical ventilation and a later peak on days 7–8, at which time it is often associated with pneumonia (Fig. 26.3).

26.4 Lung-Brain Crosstalk: The Other Side of the Pathway

ARDS-associated brain dysfunction is a prevalent complication observed in critically ill patients with ARDS, representing one of the most common organ dysfunctions in this population. It can persist for several months beyond hospital discharge [36]. The exact mechanism behind this interaction is not yet fully understood; however, multiple factors have been identified as contributors to ARDS-associated brain injury. These include inflammation, hypoxemia, neurologic adverse events related to lung-protective ventilation (such as hypercapnia and vasoconstriction), hypotension, disruption of the BBB, and altered neurotransmission [20] (Fig. 26.4).

26.4.1 Role of Inflammation and Mechanical Ventilation

ARDS is characterized by acute inflammation, resulting in the release of proinflammatory mediators into the systemic circulation. Key mediators involved in this process include interleukin (IL)-6, IL-1 beta, IL-8, and tumor necrosis factor (TNF)-alpha. These mediators have the potential to cause dysfunction in distant organs and systems [37, 38].

Mechanical ventilation, which is often necessary in ARDS patients, can further exacerbate the inflammatory process by triggering the release of inflammatory mediators into the circulation. This process, known as biotrauma, worsens the primary pulmonary injury and can lead to dysfunction of distant organs if left unchecked [37, 38].

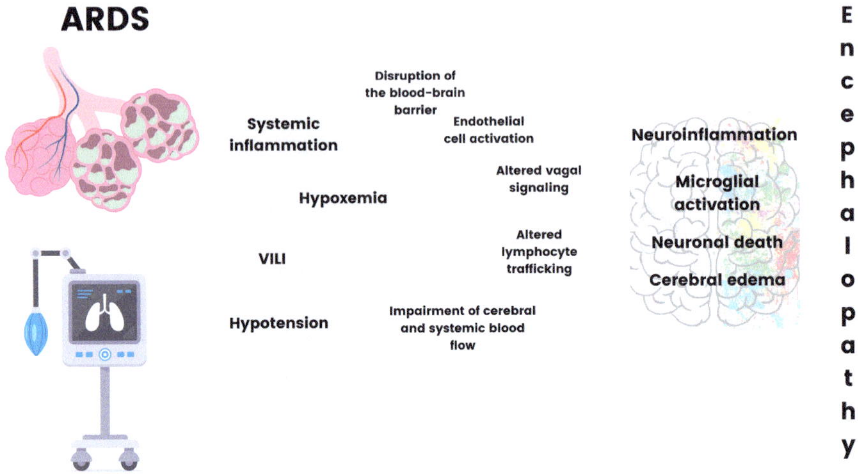

Fig. 26.4 Lung-brain crosstalk: The other side of the pathway. VILI ventilator-induced lung injury

In ARDS, the pulmonary circulation receives the entire cardiac output and contains a significant number of neutrophils. Consequently, the damage to the pulmonary microvasculature caused by ARDS allows inflammatory mediators to enter the systemic circulation [39]. Moreover, most causes of ARDS result in systemic inflammation, endothelial dysfunction, BBB disruption, neuroinflammation, and death of neuroglial cells [40]. Cytokines such as IL-1 beta and TNF-alpha play a central role in neuroregeneration, indicating a potential link between lung injury and the development of cerebral dysfunction. Additionally, cytokines can induce direct neuronal apoptosis, leading to various neurological symptoms [41].

In addition to potentially enhancing the inflammatory process, as noted above, mechanical ventilation can induce changes in vagal signaling, leading to neuroinflammation and neural death. The type of mechanical ventilation employed also influences this inflammatory process. The use of high tidal volumes can increase the release of mediators such as IL-1 beta, IL-6, and TNF-alpha, which can have distant impacts, including augmentation of cerebral inflammation [42]. Pathogenic mechanisms involve overstretching, recurrent alveolar collapse, and re-expansion during each respiratory cycle.

To minimize the risk of ventilation-induced lung injury (VILI), it is crucial to minimize the duration of mechanical ventilation. Patients should be regularly reassessed to determine if mechanical ventilation is still necessary. While positive pressure is required, ventilator variables such as tidal volume (V_T), positive end-expiratory pressure (PEEP), respiratory rate (RR), flow rate, and fraction of inspired oxygen (FiO_2) should be individualized and constantly monitored. Ventilator readouts, including plateau pressure (Pplat), driving pressure, and mechanical power, are essential for monitoring the effects of predefined parameters and reducing the risk of VILI (Fig. 26.3).

26.4.2 The Role of Blood Gases

The brain has a high metabolic rate and consumes approximately 20% of the body's oxygen despite accounting for only 2% of body weight. Therefore, it is extraordinarily susceptible to hypoxemic conditions. In the presence of hypoxemia, compensatory cerebral blood flow increases; however, hypoxemia stimulates chemoreceptors, leading to hyperventilation and a subsequent decrease in $PaCO_2$ [43].

Brain hemorrhagic complications are observed in 25% of patients with ARDS [44]. Although the pathophysiology is not fully understood, it is hypothesized that hypoxemia and inflammation contribute to epithelial dysfunction and BBB disruption, resulting in extravasation of erythrocytes and diffuse cerebral microbleeding [45]. Cerebral ischemic injury is also commonly observed in patients with lung injury. The pathophysiological mechanisms include endothelial activation, systemic inflammation, coagulation system activation, and thrombus formation. Factors such as hypoxemia can also lead to mitochondrial dysfunction, neuronal apoptosis, necrosis, and cytotoxic edema [44]. The ideal partial pressures of oxygen (PaO_2) and carbon dioxide ($PaCO_2$) in patients with brain injury are still unclear. $PaCO_2$ is a critical parameter in controlling cerebral blood flow: hypercapnia can contribute to cerebral vasodilation and increase ICP, while hypocapnia can lead to vasoconstriction and reduction in ICP but cause ischemic injury [46]. $PaCO_2$ titration should have maintenance of normocapnia as its overarching goal.

However, the ideal $PaCO_2$ is controversial, especially in patients with increased intracranial pressure. There has been extensive discussion regarding $PaCO_2$ targets in ABI, with consideration given to existing guidelines that recommend short-term mild hyperventilation for managing TBI patients with increased intracranial pressure. Profound hyperventilation should be reserved to life-threatening situations such as risk of brain herniation [46]. A state of normoxia (PaO_2 80–120 mmHg) should be the target. Hypoxemia is a well-known cause of secondary damage. However, recent evidence also suggests that hyperoxemia can have detrimental effects on patient outcomes [47].

When concomitant brain injury and refractory hypoxemia occur, e.g., in cases of ARDS, some rescue therapies can be considered, such as prone positioning if ICP is stable [46].

26.4.3 Role of Hemodynamic Impairment

Hemodynamic instability is common in patients with ARDS and is associated with increased mortality. It may arise from *cor pulmonale*, the deleterious effect of mechanical ventilation on the right ventricle, alterations in pulmonary vasculature, and sepsis [48]. Additionally, mechanical ventilation leads to changes in lung volume, which subsequently affect pulmonary vascular tone and resistance. Particularly, when high tidal volumes are used, ventilation can lead to cardiac tamponade by compressing the heart within its pericardial space. Furthermore, transpulmonary pressure influences the afterload of the right ventricle as pleural pressure reduces venous return, contributing to hemodynamic instability [49].

As the brain has a high metabolic demand, its autoregulation is efficient within mean arterial pressures of 60–150 mmHg. However, in septic patients, this autoregulatory capacity may be disrupted [50]. The hemodynamic instability commonly observed in patients with ARDS disrupts cerebral homeostasis, playing a significant role in cognitive impairment in these patients [50]. Clinical and experimental data have shown that hypoperfusion is associated with metabolic and energetic dysregulation, capillary degeneration, loss of cholinergic receptors, altered protein synthesis, and neuronal damage, particularly in regions highly sensitive to hypoperfusion (predominantly the hippocampus) [51]. In addition, disruption of the BBB, activation of the coagulation cascade, and subsequent ischemic injury may occur, further contributing to brain damage [52].

26.5 Conclusion

In this chapter, we have explored the pathophysiology of brain-lung crosstalk. Therapeutic strategies should protect both the brain and the lungs. Understanding the bidirectional interactions between these organs is crucial for optimizing patient management strategies and developing targeted therapeutic interventions. The need for a multidisciplinary approach to ensure comprehensive care for patients with brain and lung injuries cannot be overstated.

Further investigations are warranted to elucidate the underlying molecular mechanisms and identify potential therapeutic targets. Future studies should also focus on the development of advanced imaging techniques and biomarkers to enhance early detection and monitoring of brain-lung crosstalk.

In short, the interplay between the brain and the lungs is a complex phenomenon with profound implications for patient outcomes. The brain's high metabolic demands and susceptibility to hypoxemia, as well as the high prevalence of cerebral ischemic injury in patients with lung injury, underscore the importance of recognizing and addressing brain-lung crosstalk in clinical practice. By unraveling the intricacies of this relationship, we can pave the way for improved diagnostic and therapeutic strategies, ultimately enhancing the care and outcomes of patients with brain and lung disorders.

References

1. Mrozek S, Constantin JM, Geeraerts T. Brain-lung crosstalk: implications for neurocritical care patients. World J Crit Care Med. 2015;4(3):163–78.
2. Battaglini D, De Rosa S, Godoy DA. Crosstalk between the nervous system and systemic organs in acute brain injury. Neurocrit Care. 2023;40:337.
3. Anthony DC, Couch Y. The systemic response to CNS injury. Exp Neurol. 2014;258:105–11.

4. Battaglini D, da Silva AL, Felix NS, Rodrigues G, Antunes MA, Rocha NN, et al. Mild hypothermia combined with dexmedetomidine reduced brain, lung, and kidney damage in experimental acute focal ischemic stroke. Intensive Care Med Exp. 2022;10(1):53.
5. Smith M, Meyfroidt G. Focus on the brain and systemic organ systems: when essential interactions become toxic relationships. Intensive Care Med. 2018;44(12):2263–6.
6. Elmer J, Hou P, Wilcox SR, Chang Y, Schreiber H, Okechukwu I, et al. Acute respiratory distress syndrome after spontaneous intracerebral hemorrhage. Crit Care Med. 2013;41(8):1992–2001.
7. Bruni A, Garofalo E, Pelaia C, Longhini F, Navalesi P. Mechanical ventilation in brain injured patients: seeing the forest for the trees. J Thorac Dis. 2017;9(10):3483–7.
8. National Heart L, Blood Institute Acute Respiratory Distress Syndrome Clinical Trials N, Wiedemann HP, Wheeler AP, Bernard GR, Thompson BT, et al. Comparison of two fluid-management strategies in acute lung injury. N Engl J Med. 2006;354(24):2564–75.
9. Mendes RS, Oliveira MV, Padilha GA, Rocha NN, Santos CL, Maia LA, et al. Effects of crystalloid, hyper-oncotic albumin, and iso-oncotic albumin on lung and kidney damage in experimental acute lung injury. Respir Res. 2019;20(1):155.
10. Mendes RS, Martins G, Oliveira MV, Rocha NN, Cruz FF, Antunes MA, et al. Iso-oncotic albumin mitigates brain and kidney injury in experimental focal ischemic stroke. Front Neurol. 2020;11:1001.
11. Battaglini D, Pimentel-Coelho PM, Robba C, Dos Santos CC, Cruz FF, Pelosi P, et al. Gut microbiota in acute ischemic stroke: from pathophysiology to therapeutic implications. Front Neurol. 2020;11:598.
12. Blanch L, Quintel M. Lung-brain cross talk in the critically ill. Intensive Care Med. 2017;43(4):557–9.
13. Eppensteiner J, Kwun J, Scheuermann U, Barbas A, Limkakeng AT, Kuchibhatla M, et al. Damage- and pathogen-associated molecular patterns play differential roles in late mortality after critical illness. JCI Insight. 2019;4(16):e127925.
14. Meyfroidt G, Baguley IJ, Menon DK. Paroxysmal sympathetic hyperactivity: the storm after acute brain injury. Lancet Neurol. 2017;16(9):721–9.
15. Pelosi P, Rocco PR. The lung and the brain: a dangerous cross-talk. Crit Care. 2011;15(3):168.
16. Mrozek S, Gobin J, Constantin JM, Fourcade O, Geeraerts T. Crosstalk between brain, lung and heart in critical care. Anaesth Crit Care Pain Med. 2020;39(4):519–30.
17. Robba C, Rebora P, Banzato E, Wiegers EJA, Stocchetti N, Menon DK, et al. Incidence, risk factors, and effects on outcome of ventilator-associated pneumonia in patients with traumatic brain injury: analysis of a large, multicenter, prospective, Observational Longitudinal Study. Chest. 2020;158(6):2292–303.
18. Battaglini D, Parodi L, Cinotti R, Asehnoune K, Taccone FS, Orengo G, et al. Ventilator-associated pneumonia in neurocritically ill patients: insights from the ENIO international prospective observational study. Respir Res. 2023;24(1):146.
19. Fontes RB, Aguiar PH, Zanetti MV, Andrade F, Mandel M, Teixeira MJ. Acute neurogenic pulmonary edema: case reports and literature review. J Neurosurg Anesthesiol. 2003;15(2):144–50.
20. Busl KM, Bleck TP. Neurogenic pulmonary edema. Crit Care Med. 2015;43(8):1710–5.
21. Davison DL, Terek M, Chawla LS. Neurogenic pulmonary edema. Crit Care. 2012;16(2):212.
22. Galea I. The blood-brain barrier in systemic infection and inflammation. Cell Mol Immunol. 2021;18(11):2489–501.
23. Duan GX, Zhou KS, Zhao CX, Jing YL, Hu YQ. Function of endothelin-1 in neurogenic pulmonary edema. Zhongguo Ying Yong Sheng Li Xue Za Zhi. 2004;20(3):268–71.
24. Bronchard R, Albaladejo P, Brezac G, Geffroy A, Seince PF, Morris W, et al. Early onset pneumonia: risk factors and consequences in head trauma patients. Anesthesiology. 2004;100(2):234–9.
25. Woratyla SP, Morgan AS, Mackay L, Bernstein B, Barba C. Factors associated with early onset pneumonia in the severely brain-injured patient. Conn Med. 1995;59(11):643–7.
26. Lepelletier D, Roquilly A, Demeure Dit Latte D, Mahe PJ, Loutrel O, Champin P, et al. Retrospective analysis of the risk factors and pathogens associated with early-onset venti-

lator-associated pneumonia in surgical-ICU head-trauma patients. J Neurosurg Anesthesiol. 2010;22(1):32–7.
27. Kollef MH, Morrow LE, Niederman MS, Leeper KV, Anzueto A, Benz-Scott L, et al. Clinical characteristics and treatment patterns among patients with ventilator-associated pneumonia. Chest. 2006;129(5):1210–8.
28. Lee HS, Moon J, Shin HR, Ahn SJ, Kim TJ, Jun JS, et al. Pneumonia in hospitalized neurologic patients: trends in pathogen distribution and antibiotic susceptibility. Antimicrob Resist Infect Control. 2019;8:25.
29. Kasuya Y, Hargett JL, Lenhardt R, Heine MF, Doufas AG, Remmel KS, et al. Ventilator-associated pneumonia in critically ill stroke patients: frequency, risk factors, and outcomes. J Crit Care. 2011;26(3):273–9.
30. Alvarez-Lerma F, Palomar-Martinez M, Sanchez-Garcia M, Martinez-Alonso M, Alvarez-Rodriguez J, Lorente L, et al. Prevention of ventilator-associated pneumonia: the multimodal approach of the Spanish ICU "pneumonia zero" program. Crit Care Med. 2018;46(2):181–8.
31. Rincon F, Ghosh S, Dey S, Maltenfort M, Vibbert M, Urtecho J, et al. Impact of acute lung injury and acute respiratory distress syndrome after traumatic brain injury in the United States. Neurosurgery. 2012;71(4):795–803.
32. Kahn JM, Caldwell EC, Deem S, Newell DW, Heckbert SR, Rubenfeld GD. Acute lung injury in patients with subarachnoid hemorrhage: incidence, risk factors, and outcome. Crit Care Med. 2006;34(1):196–202.
33. Rincon F, Maltenfort M, Dey S, Ghosh S, Vibbert M, Urtecho J, et al. The prevalence and impact of mortality of the acute respiratory distress syndrome on admissions of patients with ischemic stroke in the United States. J Intensive Care Med. 2014;29(6):357–64.
34. Mascia L, Zavala E, Bosma K, Pasero D, Decaroli D, Andrews P, et al. High tidal volume is associated with the development of acute lung injury after severe brain injury: an international observational study. Crit Care Med. 2007;35(8):1815–20.
35. Contant CF, Valadka AB, Gopinath SP, Hannay HJ, Robertson CS. Adult respiratory distress syndrome: a complication of induced hypertension after severe head injury. J Neurosurg. 2001;95(4):560–8.
36. Sasannejad C, Ely EW, Lahiri S. Long-term cognitive impairment after acute respiratory distress syndrome: a review of clinical impact and pathophysiological mechanisms. Crit Care. 2019;23(1):352.
37. Hegeman MA, Hennus MP, Heijnen CJ, Specht PA, Lachmann B, Jansen NJ, et al. Ventilator-induced endothelial activation and inflammation in the lung and distal organs. Crit Care. 2009;13(6):R182.
38. Khadaroo RG, Marshall JC. ARDS and the multiple organ dysfunction syndrome. Common mechanisms of a common systemic process. Crit Care Clin. 2002;18(1):127–41.
39. Huppert LA, Matthay MA, Ware LB. Pathogenesis of acute respiratory distress syndrome. Semin Respir Crit Care Med. 2019;40(1):31–9.
40. Simard AR, Rivest S. Do pathogen exposure and innate immunity cause brain diseases? Neurol Res. 2005;27(7):717–25.
41. Dantzer R. Cytokine-induced sickness behaviour: a neuroimmune response to activation of innate immunity. Eur J Pharmacol. 2004;500(1–3):399–411.
42. Crimi E, Slutsky AS. Inflammation and the acute respiratory distress syndrome. Best Pract Res Clin Anaesthesiol. 2004;18(3):477–92.
43. Hoiland RL, Bain AR, Rieger MG, Bailey DM, Ainslie PN. Hypoxemia, oxygen content, and the regulation of cerebral blood flow. Am J Physiol Regul Integr Comp Physiol. 2016;310(5):R398–413.
44. Huang M, Gedansky A, Hassett CE, Price C, Fan TH, Stephens RS, et al. Pathophysiology of brain injury and neurological outcome in acute respiratory distress syndrome: a scoping review of preclinical to clinical studies. Neurocrit Care. 2021;35(2):518–27.
45. Fanou EM, Coutinho JM, Shannon P, Kiehl TR, Levi MM, Wilcox ME, et al. Critical illness-associated cerebral microbleeds. Stroke. 2017;48(4):1085–7.

46. Robba C, Poole D, McNett M, Asehnoune K, Bosel J, Bruder N, et al. Mechanical ventilation in patients with acute brain injury: recommendations of the European Society of Intensive Care Medicine consensus. Intensive Care Med. 2020;46(12):2397–410.
47. Robba C, Battaglini D, Cinotti R, Asehnoune K, Stevens R, Taccone FS, et al. Individualized thresholds of hypoxemia and hyperoxemia and their effect on outcome in acute brain injured patients: a secondary analysis of the ENIO study. Neurocrit Care. 2023;40(2):515–28.
48. Vieillard-Baron A, Matthay M, Teboul JL, Bein T, Schultz M, Magder S, et al. Experts' opinion on management of hemodynamics in ARDS patients: focus on the effects of mechanical ventilation. Intensive Care Med. 2016;42(5):739–49.
49. Mahmood SS, Pinsky MR. Heart-lung interactions during mechanical ventilation: the basics. Ann Transl Med. 2018;6(18):349.
50. Taccone FS, Castanares-Zapatero D, Peres-Bota D, Vincent JL, Berre J, Melot C. Cerebral autoregulation is influenced by carbon dioxide levels in patients with septic shock. Neurocrit Care. 2010;12(1):35–42.
51. Wang X, Cui L, Ji X. Cognitive impairment caused by hypoxia: from clinical evidences to molecular mechanisms. Metab Brain Dis. 2022;37(1):51–66.
52. Sharshar T, Annane D, de la Grandmaison GL, Brouland JP, Hopkinson NS, Francoise G. The neuropathology of septic shock. Brain Pathol. 2004;14(1):21–33.

Host-Microbe Crosstalk in the Lung Microenvironment

27

Corrado Carpanelli, Francesca Gualdi, and Denise Battaglini

27.1 Introduction

The microbiota represents the set of microorganisms (bacteria, fungi, viruses, archaea) that live in a given environment, establishing a symbiotic relationship with a host organism including mutualism, commensalism, and parasitism [1]. In the human body, the microbiota is present in multiple regions; a significant example is the intestinal microbiota, a complex population of microorganism that plays an important role in maintaining metabolic and immune homeostasis [2].

The human respiratory tract, which extends from the pulmonary alveoli to the nostrils, is inhabited by niche-specific bacterial communities that play distinct roles in maintaining respiratory homeostasis [3]. For example, in the upper respiratory tract (i.e., nostrils, nasal cavity, oral cavity, pharynx, larynx), the microbiota presumably prevents potential pathogens from spreading to the lungs, thus acting as a guardian of the respiratory system. Similarly, in the lower respiratory tract (i.e., trachea, bronchi, bronchioles, alveoli), the microbiota plays a role in host immune homeostasis [3].

While the respiratory microbiota plays a fundamental role in maintaining local homeostasis by protecting the body from pathogens and contributing to the balance of immune responses in the respiratory tract [4], its interactions with other microbiota in the human body extend its impact far beyond the pulmonary boundaries.

C. Carpanelli · F. Gualdi
Department of Surgical Sciences and Integrated Diagnostics, University of Genoa, Genoa, Italy

Anesthesia and Intensive Care, IRCCS Ospedale Policlinico San Martino, Genoa, Italy

D. Battaglini (✉)
Department of Surgical Sciences and Integrated Diagnostics, University of Genoa, Genoa, Italy
e-mail: denise.battaglini@unige.it

D. Battaglini et al. (eds.), *Organ System Crosstalk in Critical Illness*, https://doi.org/10.1007/978-3-032-01024-7_27

A growing understanding of how the microbial communities of extrapulmonary organs, such as the gut, interact with the lung microbiota is revealing a complex network of biochemical and cellular signals that mediate this communication [5]. The gut and lungs are anatomically distinct, but potential anatomic communications and complex pathways involving their respective microbiota have reinforced the existence of a gut–lung axis (GLA). Compared to the better-studied gut microbiota, the lung microbiota, only considered in recent years, represents a more discreet part of the whole microbiota associated with human hosts. While the vast majority of studies focused on the bacterial component of the microbiota in healthy and pathological conditions, recent works have highlighted the contribution of fungal and viral kingdoms at both digestive and respiratory levels. Moreover, growing evidence indicates the key role of inter-kingdom crosstalks in maintaining host homeostasis and in disease evolution. In fact, the recently emerged GLA concept involves host–microbe as well as microbe–microbe interactions, based both on localized and long-reaching effects. GLA can shape immune responses and interfere with the course of respiratory diseases. In this review, we aim to analyze how the lung and gut microbiota influence each other and may impact on respiratory diseases. Due to the limited knowledge on the human virobiota, we focused on gut and lung bacteriobiota and mycobiota, with a specific attention on inter-kingdom microbial crosstalks which are able to shape local or long-reached host responses within the GLA [6]. Especially, the gut-lung crosstalk is a complex communication system that works bidirectionally, so the two systems influence each other [7]. Several studies investigate the association between dysbiosis and diseases in the lung and intestine, although a clear link is yet to be identified.

The purpose of this chapter is to explore the dialogue that exists between the lung microbiota and other microbiota, the potential clinical implications of this interaction, and the possible therapeutic options available.

27.2 The Lung Microbiota

According to culture-based results, the lung has been considered for decades as "bacteria-free" environment under physiological conditions [8]. Nowadays, thanks to the use of culture-independent molecular techniques, it is now clear that the lower airways host diverse bacterial communities composed of various microorganisms [9].

The composition of the lung microbiota likely occurs during the first weeks of life, and it is influenced by several elements such as the mode of delivery (vaginal vs. cesarean), nutrition (breast vs. formula feeding), environment exposure (siblings, daycare attendance at nursery school), as well as the specific characteristics of the lung niche. It is possible that an early respiratory microbiota can predict subsequent susceptibility to respiratory tract infections [10].

In healthy individuals, the upper respiratory tract is the main source of the lung microbiome, which is determined by the balance between microbial immigration and elimination [3]. Three key ecological factors are believed to shape. Microbial immigration occurs due to phenomena such as microaspiration, inhalation of bacteria, mucosal dispersion. In contrast, microbial elimination in the airways is achieved through coughing, mucociliary clearance, and both innate and adaptive host defenses. Regional growth conditions include factors such as temperature, pH, humidity, local microbial competition, partial pressure of oxygen, nutrient availability [9], as summarized in Fig. 27.1.

Regarding the composition of the lung microbiota, it seems to vary according to the environment, disease, and therapy. Regarding the phylum (taxonomic group), the most frequently identified in a healthy microbiota of the lungs are *Bacteroidetes, Proteobacteria, Firmicutes*. As regards the genus, the most frequently identified are *Streptococcus, Pseudomonas, Fusobacteria, Veillonella, Prevotella,* and to a lesser extent *Haemophilus* and *Neisseria* [8]. Another study observed the presence of five main bacterial phyla in the healthy lungs: *Firmicutes* (51.8%), *Proteobacteria* (30.1%), *Bacteroidetes* (14.2%), *Actinobacteria* (2.4%), and *Fusobacteria* (1.2%). In this study, at least 16 phyla in total and over 179 bacterial species were identified, among which the most abundant were *Streptococcus* (26.1%), *Haemophilus* (4.1%), *Moraxella* (5.6%), *Pseudomonas* (4.4%), *Prevotella* (8.15%), Neisseria (7.75%), Gemella (6.12%), and *Veillonella* (5.5%). In addition, pathogenic bacteria were also detected, including *Acinetobacter* (4.3%) and *Klebsiella* (3.2%) [11]. It seems reasonable to believe that the microorganisms present vary based on climate, environmental microbiota, and exposure to animals, other individuals, and other variables. This is plausible considering how much the microbiota of the human gastrointestinal tract varies based on geographical exposure [12]. Several studies consider the geographic influence on bacterial communities in the airways. In this particular study [13], 38 patients with cystic fibrosis were considered, 19 from the UK and 19 from the USA, matched on the basis of clinical parameters. Two culture-independent methods were used to study the lung microbiota, one with 16S rRNA clone

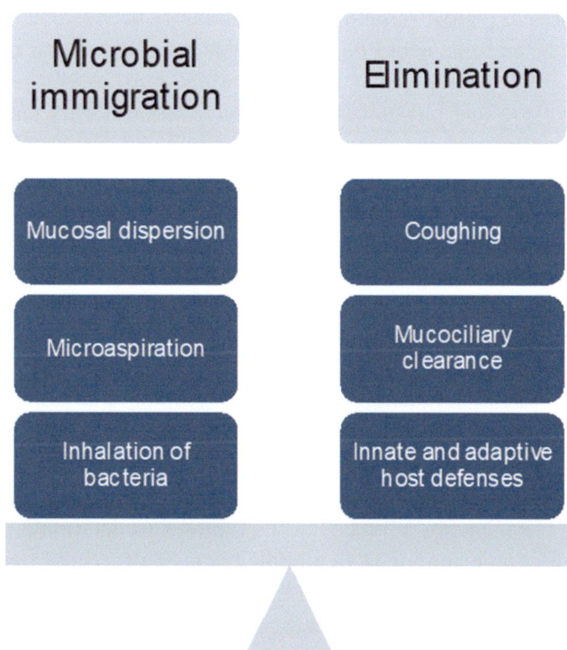

Fig. 27.1 Origin and dynamics of the lung microbiome in healthy individuals. The balance between microbial immigration from the upper respiratory tract and elimination determines the composition of the lung microbiome

sequencing and the other using terminal restriction fragment length polymorphism (T-RFLP) profiling. Overall, substantial similarities in bacterial communities were detected. Among the main common species detected in this analysis we find *Pseudomonas aeruginosa*, *Staphylococcus aureus*, *Stenotrophomonas maltophilia*, *S. aureus*, *Prevotella*, *Achromobacter*, *Bordetella*, *Actinomyces*, *Parvimonas*, *Neisseria*, and *Veillonella*. Small geographical differences between the sample groups are represented, for example, by the presence of *Phenylobacterium koreense* and *S. maltophilia*, detected only in the group of patients from the UK [13]. Another large study [14] examines, through 16S rRNA sequencing, the composition of the lower respiratory tract microbiota in 64 healthy individuals, divided between smokers and non-smokers. In this study, the oral microbiota differed significantly between smokers and non-smokers in species such as *Porphyromonas*, *Neisseria,* and *Gemella*, with less variation in other species. Other studies have shown that the oropharynx of smokers has a more diverse population than non-smokers, with a reduction in organisms typical of the normal microbiota, sometimes with harmful effects [15, 16].

Interestingly, most of the bacteria which were found in the lung were also identified in the oral cavity, while at the lung level, some bacteria were much more represented than in the oral cavity, among these we recognize *Haemophilus, Methylobacterium,* Enterobacteriaceae, *Ralstonia*. These bacteria have probably adapted to the lung environment. Furthermore, the size of the study allowed us to also find rare bacteria such as *Tropheryma whipplei*, which was found in the lung but not in the mouth. In addition to describing some components of the lung microbiota, this study demonstrates that it does not derive solely from the oral cavity, but it is necessary to consider other sources including the outside, the nasal cavities, throat, gastrointestinal tract [14]. We can therefore suppose that in healthy subjects, there is a great variability in the similarity between the lung and oral microbiota [17, 18], and this could be linked to factors such as oral hygiene, possible respiratory system pathologies, laryngeal dysfunctions, esophageal reflux. It is reasonable to believe that physiological micro-aspiration occurs mainly during sleep, in supine position, where the protective cough and laryngeal reflexes are reduced [19]. Therefore, the similarity between oral and pulmonary microbiota could be circadian, high during the night and reduced during the day, when immigration is reduced and elimination is increased [20].

Considering the evidence, the healthy lung is not "sterile" but presents a complex community of microorganisms. This has been clarified over the last decades, and can be summarized as follows:

1. Identification of lung-specific microbiota was possible, thanks to molecular biology techniques independent of culture. Molecular biology techniques allow the analysis of nucleic acids, proteins and metabolites of a biological sample [21]. Among the most commonly used techniques, deoxyribonucleic acid (DNA) sequencing, a procedure that allows to determine the order of the nucleotides composing the DNA sample being analyzed [22], is the most known. However, the most commonly used for the research of bacterial communities is the

sequencing of the 16S ribosomal ribonucleic acid (rRNA) gene [20]. The 16S rRNA gene is a typical locus in the bacterial genome, small and highly conserved. Once the DNA is isolated from the sample, it is classified according to taxonomic databases. Conventionally, sequences that are at least 97% homologous are grouped into operational taxonomic units (OTUs), which allow microorganisms to be organized by species and provide a population census for each sample, obtaining a population census for each sample. These sequencing-based techniques overcome the limitations of conventional culture techniques which often fail to identify most human-associated microbes [20].

2. The lung microbiota derives mainly from the exchange with nasopharynx, oropharynx, ambient air [23], and is determined by the balance between immigration and elimination of microbes, according to the ecological factors described above.
3. Evidence suggests a variability between subjects, geographic variability, and a temporal variability. According to evidence, the most common bacterial genera found in the healthy respiratory tract include *Pseudomonas, Streptococcus, Prevotella, Fusobacterium, Haemophilus, Veillonella, Porphyromonas, Haemophilus,* and Enterobacteriaceae [14, 24, 4, 20].

27.3 Dysbiosis of the Lung Microbiota in Critical Illnesses

The lung microbiota plays an important role in maintaining the body's homeostasis. There are several conditions that can cause dysbiosis, a condition of alteration of the microbiota, contributing to the development of major lung diseases [25]. Among these conditions, mechanical ventilation, hospitalization in intensive care, ongoing pathological conditions, and the use of some drugs may substantially contribute to the changes occurred in the lung microenvironment. In patients undergoing mechanical ventilation, dysbiosis quickly occurs with a gradual decline in the macrobiotic variety and the progressive predominance of a pathogenic bacterium. This condition favors the onset of a lung infection [26].

Several studies hypothesize that intubation and mechanical ventilation reduce the variety of respiratory microbiota, and it seems that this reduction is predominant in patients who develop ventilator-associated pneumonia (VAP). This suggests an association between dysbiosis and the onset of respiratory diseases. Alagna et al. [27] found that the dysbiosis of the respiratory microbiota was more profound in patients who developed VAP (11 patients) than those without VAP (18 patients), by analyzing samples using the 16S rRNA gene sequencing [27].

Another study confirmed the differences in lung microbiota according to different lung diseases. Bronchoalveolar lavage (BAL) was collected from patients with different types of pneumonia: (VAP) ventilator-associated pneumonia, (CAP) community-acquired pneumonia, aspiration pneumonia, and non-ventilator-associated ICU pneumonia. Samples were analyzed using 16s rDNA and 18s rDNA gene sequencing, as well as cultures and detection of urinary antibodies and antigens. Based on these tests, approximately 160 bacterial species were identified, of which

73 were not previously detected in pneumonia. In addition, 24 fungal species were identified (mycobiota), of which 6 were never previously reported in pneumonia, and 7 were viruses. A considerable difference in the microbiota of patients with pneumonia acquired or not in the ICU setting was found [28].

Drugs play another important role in the composition of lung microbiota, especially antacids. Rosen et al. found [29] an association between the use of antacids and changes in gastric and lung flora. The use of antacid drugs was associated with a higher prevalence and abundance of potential pathogens including *Staphylococcus*, *Streptococcus*, *Veillonella*, *Dermabacter*, and *Rothia*. Among these, *Staphylococcus* and *Streptococcus* can act as potential pathogens at the respiratory tract level, suggesting that there may be a link between the use of antacids and lung infections. This theory was explored through a study founding an overlap between gastric and pulmonary microflora. In a study involving 50 patients, an association was found between gastric microbiota present in non-acid reflux and pulmonary microbiota. Overlapping bacteria identified included *Corynebacterium*, *Propionibacterium*, *Bacillus*, *Dermabacter*, *Lactobacillus*, *Peptostreptococcus*, and *Capnocytophaga*. In patients treated with antacids, primary pulmonary bacterial growth was not observed, suggesting that gastroesophageal reflux may influence pulmonary bacterial growth, leading to microbiotic overlap between the two environments [29].

Further experiments involved administering antibiotics, such as streptomycin, to deplete the intestinal microbiota before PR8 infection. These treated mice exhibited lung damage from PR8 but showed protection in the intestine. Additionally, fecal transplantation from PR8-infected mice to healthy controls resulted in increased enterobacteria and intestinal damage due to dysbiosis, even without viral infection. Direct infection of control mice with *E. coli* also caused intestinal immune damage [30]. Factors affecting lung microbiota in critical Illness are presented in Fig. 27.2.

27.4 Host-Microbe Crosstalk in the Lung Microenvironment

According to current evidence, the pulmonary microbiota can be influenced by other microbiota present in the body. All external surfaces—such as the skin, intestines, reproductive system, excretory system, and respiratory tract—are colonized by distinct microbiota [31]. These microbiotas can vary based on local factors, including carbon dioxide levels, pH, oxygen availability, nutrient composition, immune responses, and environmental pollutants. For instance, the skin is characterized by nutrient scarcity and high oxygen levels, leading to the predominance of aerobic organisms. In contrast, the lower gastrointestinal tract has low oxygen availability and abundant nutrients, favoring anaerobic microorganisms [10]. There are several communication pathways between the various microbiota in the body, which are the focus of intensive research. Some pathways are discussed in the following sections.

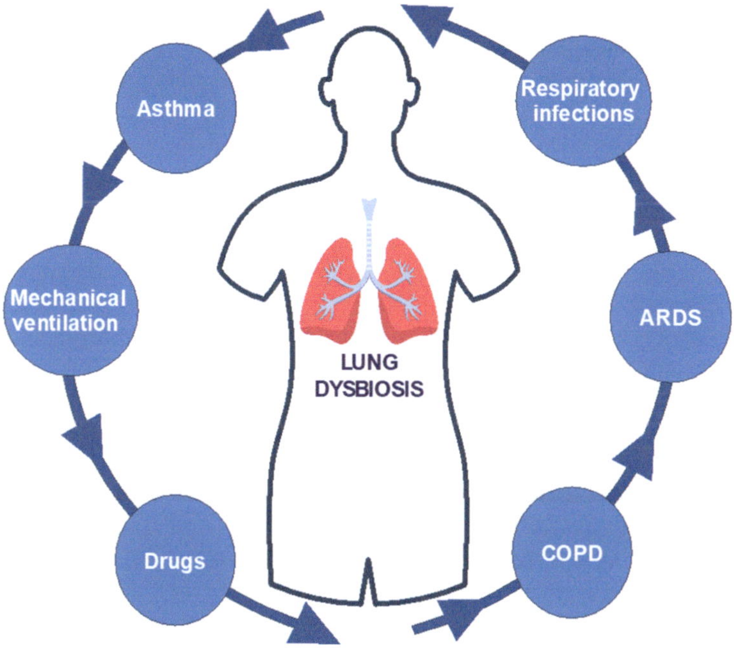

Fig. 27.2 Factors affecting lung microbiota in critical illness

27.4.1 Gut-Lung Crosstalk

A particularly fascinating aspect is the discovery that the reciprocal modulation between the lung and intestinal microbiota can influence not only respiratory health but also other vital functions, including overall immune system function [32, 33]. This crosstalk between the lung and extrapulmonary organ microbiota is defined by a complex interaction mediated by neurohormones, soluble mediators, and cellular signals [34]. Specifically, the connection between the intestinal and lung microbiota—known as the "gut-lung axis"—is emerging as a critical area of research [6, 35]. Alterations in the composition of the intestinal microbiota appear to have significant effects on the host's immune status and may be involved in the development of lung diseases. In fact, many studies have shown that the intestinal microbiota in the early stages of life plays a fundamental role in the development and function of the immune system and at the same time the immune system regulates the composition of the microbiota [36]. Numerous microbiota components influence the immune system, as evidenced by reliable studies. For instance, *Bacteroides fragilis* helps modulate the balance of Th1 and Th2 cells [37], segmented filamentous bacteria promote Th17 cell differentiation [38], and *Clostridium* species stimulate the production of regulatory T cells (Treg) [39].

Although the investigation into how these microbial alterations may either promote or respond to pulmonary diseases remains an ongoing debate, these interactions could have fundamental clinical implications [6, 35]. The respiratory microbiota communicates with the host immune system, providing signals that appear to play roles in immune training, the maintenance of immune tolerance, and the overall health of the respiratory system and the body as a whole [3]. Multiple studies have examined the bidirectional dialogue between the intestinal and pulmonary microbiota—the 'gut–lung axis'—although causality remains uncertain [6, 35]. Recently, researchers have investigated how alterations in intestinal microbial species may be linked to changes in immune responses as well as the development of lung diseases. However, it remains uncler whether microbial alteration is the cause or the effect of lung diseases [40].

Respiratory diseases frequently encountered in critical care setting, such as ARDS, asthma, COPD, and respiratory infections, can lead to dysbiosis and gastrointestinal symptoms; similarly intestinal alterations or diseases could participate in the onset of respiratory diseases [41].

27.4.1.1 Acute Respiratory Distress Syndrome

Several studies supported the influence of gut bacteria on the lung microbiota of experimental models or patients with ARDS. Wakisaka et al. [42] developed an experimental model of abdominal sepsis, through the ligation and puncture of the cecum of murine guinea pigs. This technique causes a transient systemic inflammation that is similar to the septic response in humans [43]. Sequencing was then performed on murine BAL and a significant variation was found between the lung microbiota of mice with and without sepsis. The microbiota of sepsic mice was significantly enriched with bacteria, which are normally present in the murine intestine, including *Bacteroidales* sp., *Enterococcus* sp., and *Lachnospiraceae* sp. The intestinal and pulmonary microbiota were more similar in septic mice than non-septic ones. From this study derives the possibility that the pulmonary microbiota in case of sepsis is enriched by intestinal bacteria also in other species, as demonstrated in the murine species. In the same study [42], the lung microbiota of patients with ARDS was also compared to that of healthy volunteers. In BAL samples from ARDS patients, atypical bacteria were common and abundant, including intestinal bacteria such as *Bacteroides* sp. and other bacteria such as *B. thetaiotaomicron*, *B. faecichinchillae*, and *B. salyersiae*, while these were not found in BAL samples from healthy volunteers. In addition, a significant association was observed between the abundance of *Bacteroides* spp., and the presence of *Proteobacteria* and serum tumor necrosis factor (TNF-α) and alveolar concentration, respectively. Indeed, TNF-α is an important mediator of inflammation in ARDS. This study suggests that gut-lung bacterial translocation, when present, is related to the degree of inflammation and consequently the inflammation affects the lung microbiota [42]. Dysbiosis of lung microbiota has been observed in other cohorts of patients with ARDS. An increase of microorganisms of intestinal origin, especially Enterobacteriaceae, was found in the lung microbiota, suggesting again a possible interaction between gut and lung [26].

27.4.1.2 Asthma

In a study by Settembre et al., researchers investigated the relationship between variations in intestinal microbiota and allergic asthma using murine models sensitized with ovalbumin (OVA). The mice were divided into groups treated with vancomycin and an untreated control group [44]. Vancomycin treatment led to increased inflammatory cell infiltrates, including eosinophils and elevated immunoglobulin E levels, in BAL compared to the controls. Additionally, airway hyperreactivity to methacholine (MCh) was significantly greater in the vancomycin-treated mice, and histopathological analysis confirmed a stronger presence of allergic disease in these animals. Furthermore, the study noted changes in intestinal flora, particularly a reduction in *Clostridium* and *Bacteroides* species, which are known to induce regulatory T cells (Treg). There was also a marked decrease in Treg cells and Th17 cells in the intestines of the vancomycin-treated mice. Overall, these findings suggest that early vancomycin treatment disrupts intestinal flora and immune regulatory cells, correlating with heightened inflammatory responses and asthma-related symptoms. The observed decrease in colonic $CD4^{+}CD25^{+}FOXP3^{+}$ Treg cells and in small-intestinal Th17 cells in vancomycintreated mice has been previously demonstrated by other studies [39, 45]. In summary, subjects treated early with vancomycin present alterations of the intestinal flora and of the regulatory cells of the immune system, in conjunction with increased levels of inflammatory cells, eosinophils, immunoglobulin-E, hyperreactivity of the airways, and histopathological confirmation as compared to control subjects.

Treatment of adult mice with the antibiotics did not induce asthma, indicating that early administration of vancomycin may associate with the onset or exacerbation of asthma in the studied subjects. The precise mechanisms remain unclear, but it is likely that vancomycin-induced alterations in microbiota lead to different microbial signals compared to healthy controls. This dysbiosis may disrupt the signaling pathways of intestinal epithelial cells and modify both innate and adaptive immune responses. In summary, the early depletion of specific microbiota species and immune cell phenotypes due to vancomycin can dysregulate the immune system, contributing to increased susceptibility to experimental allergic asthma [44].

27.4.1.3 Chronic Obstructive Pulmonary Disease

In the context of COPD, alterations in gut microbiota have been linked to tobacco smoke and other inhalable particles, which can affect gut composition via the circulatory system. COPD patients exhibit an increase in *Enterocloster clostridioformis* and *Escherichia coli*, along with a decrease in *Lactobacillus* sp. and *Ruminococcus albus*. This dysbiosis appears to damage the intestinal barrier by activating MAPK/ERK pathways, although the exact mechanisms are still being investigated. The rise of harmful intestinal bacteria in COPD patients likely contributes significantly to the prevalence of intestinal disorders in this population [46, 11].

27.4.1.4 Respiratory Infections

Respiratory infections can disrupt respiratory microbiota and have indirect effects on other systems. For instance, influenza is often associated with gastrointestinal symptoms, highlighting an association between these conditions.

A study by Wang et al. [30] examined how influenza virus infection can lead to intestinal immune damage through microbiota alterations, resulting in intestinal inflammation via Th17 cell dysregulation. Mice infected with the influenza virus strain A/PR/8/34 (PR8) showed a gradual decrease in body weight compared to saline-treated controls, along with shortened intestinal length and diarrhea. Notably, the liver and kidneys appeared normal, and the presence of the influenza virus in the intestine was ruled out, indicating that the damage was not directly caused by the virus. To explore the involvement of microbiota alterations in this intestinal damage, the composition of the microbiota post-PR8 infection was analyzed. The study found an increase in Enterobacteriaceae, including *E. coli*, and a decrease in segmented filamentous bacteria (SFB) and *Lactobacillus/Lactococcus*. These findings suggest that intestinal dysbiosis, particularly the increase of *E. coli*, plays a significant role in intestinal immune damage during influenza infection [30].

To explore the mechanisms underlying immune damage during PR8 infection, the study revealed notable changes in respiratory mucosal lymphocytes, particularly a significant increase in CCR9 + CD4 + T cells [10]. These cells likely migrate to the intestinal mucosa via the CCL25-CCR9 chemokine axis, impacting intestinal flora and elevating IFN-γ levels. CCL25 is consistently expressed on the intestinal epithelium [47], which may explain why PR8 infection specifically induces immune damage in the intestine without affecting the liver or kidneys. Dysbiosis contributed to an increase in certain microorganisms, including those that produce cytokines like IL-6, IL-15, and IL-23, which promote Th17 cell polarization. Another critical factor is interleukin 17A (IL-17A), a cytokine produced by various cells, including Th17 lymphocytes, that regulates immune responses. Notably, no intestinal damage was observed in IL-17A-deficient mice. PR8 infection heightened the expression of the Th17 transcription factor RORγt and IL-17A. Following infection, Th17 cell numbers and percentages increased in the intestine, while no such increase occurred in the liver or kidneys. Treatment with an anti-IL-17A antibody significantly reduced intestinal damage, suggesting that Th17 cells play a vital role in the immune damage induced by influenza.

Although the complete mechanism remains unclear, ongoing studies continue to investigate this topic [30]. In summary, alterations in intestinal microbiota may contribute to respiratory diseases, while changes in lung microbiota could similarly impact gastrointestinal health, as demonstrated in various studies [10].

27.4.2 Brain-Lung Crosstalk

Recently it has been demonstrated how the lung microbiota can intervene in the regulation of the immune system, and through this it can influence autoimmune inflammation also at the brain level, in the context of an interaction that we could call the brain-lung axis.

In an animal model of multiple sclerosis with experimental autoimmune encephalomyelitis (EAE) [48], inflammation was induced to affect the myelin of the central nervous system, resulting in demyelination and neurodegeneration. The rats were treated with intratracheal neomycin which resulted in an alteration of microbial community structure mainly characterized by a significant increase in *Bacteriodetes*. Subsequently, these treated rats were immunized with T cells specific for myelin basic protein (MBP) to develop the model of EAE. The study showed that the alteration of the airway microbiota with neomycin protected the rats from EAE. To further test this hypothesis, EAE rats that had not received neomycin were given a transfer of bronchoalveolar lavage (BAL)–derived microbiota collected from neomycin-treated donor rats; this BAL-microbiota transfer reproduced the protection against EAE. Neomycin therapy seems to alter the composition of the microbiota by increasing the presence of bacteria producing lipopolysaccharide, which pushes microglia to produce interferon type 1, which has a neuroprotective capacity limiting the progression in MS disease with EAE [49, 48].

Furthermore, there are further connections between lung and brain; in fact several studies demonstrate how variations in the lung microbiota can influence the polarization of autoreactive T cells. These autoreactive T cells, including Th1, Th17, and CD8 + T cells, are key players in the initiation and progression of some central nervous system diseases [50]. They reside transiently in pulmonary lymph nodes and then reach the central nervous system through the blood circulation [51].

27.5 Therapeutic Options

Considering the alteration of microbiota as one of the possible causes of the onset of some diseases, it is natural to believe that a therapy capable of restoring the microbiota can contribute to the healing of the subject. There are several therapeutic hypotheses that are the subject of various studies.

27.5.1 Probiotics and Synbiotics

Probiotics are defined as "live microorganisms" and many of them have demonstrated beneficial properties; of these, we can mention *Lactobacillus* spp., *Bifidobacterium* spp., *Enterococcus* spp., *Propionibacterium* spp., *Streptococcus* spp., *Bacillus cereus, Saccharomyces boulardii*, and some strains of *Escherichia coli*. Probiotics play a crucial role in maintaining the integrity of the intestinal barrier, inhibiting pathogen proliferation, decreasing bacterial translocation, and elevating anti-inflammatory cytokine levels, all of which contribute to immunomodulation and infection prevention. A systematic review revealed that groups consuming prebiotics had higher energy intake, but only one out of four randomized controlled trials (RCTs) showed that those taking probiotics reached caloric goals more quickly. Regarding diarrhea, seven of the twelve RCTs noted beneficial effects from probiotics; however, changes in gut microbiota generally did not lead to better clinical outcomes, such as shorter hospital or ICU stays [52].

Lactobacillus is one of the most used probiotics, with over 200 known species of bacteria belonging to this genus. They are gram-positive anaerobic bacteria that produce lactic acid through the fermentation of carbohydrates. They are widely used in biotechnology to produce food or in medical applications. In the human body, *Lactobacillus* spp. can be found in the gastrointestinal tract where they represent about 6% of the total bacteria. Furthermore, they can also be found in the vagina, oral cavity, respiratory tract, and on the skin. The immunobiotic and immunomodulatory capacity of these probiotics, related to gastrointestinal and vaginal disorders, is already well described, while there are ongoing studies and emerging evidence about their function with respect to the respiratory system, for which they could represent a new therapeutic strategy. Although the mechanisms by which *Lactobacillus enteric* influences pulmonary immunity through the gut-lung axis are not yet fully understood, several assumptions and evidence already exist [53]. The mechanism of action of probiotics on the microbiota is shown in Fig. 27.3.

The most known etiological aspects of COPD are cigarettes and air pollutants. Some studies have shown that *Lactobacillus rhamnosus* NutRes1 can reduce inflammatory mediators produced by human macrophages activated by cigarettes. Furthermore, oral feeding of *Lactobacillus rhamnosus* increases the levels of IL-10, SOCS3, and TIMP1/2 reducing lung damage in C57BL/6 mice with cigarette-induced COPD [54]. Finally, the development of COPD is associated with the reduction of *Lactobacillus* spp. in the lungs. This suggests an association between lung microbiota and the pathological condition, therefore possible therapies. Based

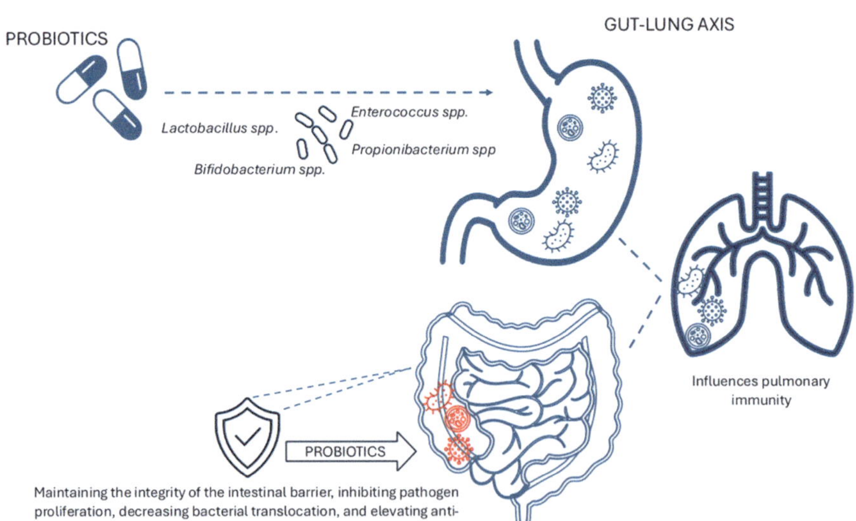

Fig. 27.3 The mechanism of action of probiotics on the microbiota

on the "hygiene hypothesis," exposure to some microbial components at an early age can reduce the predisposition to asthma and allergic conditions. Therefore, oral administration of the probiotic *Lactobacillus* at an early age could also play a role in the prevention of asthma [53, 55].

Some studies indicate that a reduction of intestinal *Lactobacillus* may contribute to the development of pulmonary arterial hypertension, while its intestinal integration with *Lacticaseibacillus paracasei* strain Shirota may reduce the incidence of VAP in hospitalized patients [56, 57].

Some current research does not endorse the use of probiotics for microbiota modulation. For instance, Johnstone et al. reported no significant differences in the development of VAP when comparing L-rhamnosus GG to a placebo. Additionally, the PROPATRIA trial demonstrated that in patients with a predicted severe acute pancreatitis, the use of mixed probiotic strains for prophylaxis was linked to an increased risk of mortality and did not reduce the incidence of infectious complications [58].

A meta-analysis found that probiotics and synbiotics may help decrease the incidence of VAP, sepsis, length of hospital stay, duration of mechanical ventilation, and ICU mortality. However, they did not demonstrate a significant impact on diarrhea, hospital-acquired infections, or overall mortality rates [59].

27.5.2 Selective Decontamination of the Digestive Tract

Selective digestive decontamination (SDD) aims to minimize infections acquired in the ICU by preventing the colonization of Gram-negative bacteria, *Staphylococcus aureus*, and yeasts in the digestive system, ultimately enhancing patient outcomes [60]. SDD significantly alters the composition of the intestinal microbiota compared to standard care and selective oral decontamination, particularly influencing *Enterobacteriales* [61]. The gut microbiome of ICU patients undergoing SDD often differs markedly from that of healthy individuals, and there is a risk of antibiotic-resistant bacteria recolonizing the gut after patients leave the ICU and SDD treatment ends [62].

In a recent RCT, patients receiving SDD exhibited unique gut microbial profiles compared to controls, including phyla that are not specifically targeted by SDD. This suggests that while SDD effectively reduces the colonization of harmful Gram-negative bacteria in the gastrointestinal tract, it also diminishes the levels of beneficial gut flora, altering the overall microbiome composition [63]. In the ARCTIC trial, SDD demonstrated a greater effect on alpha and beta diversity, except for the oral microbiome, among critically ill children when compared to standard treatment. However, the implementation of SDD did not significantly alter the burden of antibiotic resistance genes compared to usual care [64]. Additionally, a recent meta-analysis indicated that SDD was associated with a reduced risk of VAP, ICU-acquired bacteremia, and hospital mortality compared to conventional treatment [65].

27.5.3 Fecal Microbiota Transplantation

One of the most promising approaches seems to be the transfer of entire microbiota through fecal microbiota transplantation (FMT). In some studies, the introduction of physiological microbiota in pathological hosts has restored immunity, demonstrating that the intestinal microbiota can modulate host immunity [32]. For example, FMT has had significant success in the treatment of antibiotic-resistant *Clostridium difficile* colitis [66]. Despite the encouraging data, it is still necessary to study whether FMT can influence lung health, whether lung microbiota transplantation is feasible, whether it can last over time as a therapy for chronic lung diseases, whether it does not involve complications related to the transfer of antibiotic-resistant bacteria.

27.5.4 Other Treatments for Specific Diseases

In addition to the use of live bacteria, specific molecules of microbial origin are being studied. Several studies have already used bacterial metabolites to treat allergic airway disease (AAD) in mouse models. Among these metabolites, D-tryptophan, bacterial polysaccharide A, oligodeoxynucleotides with bacterial CpG motifs, LPS from *Escherichia coli* O111, flagellin B, short-chain fatty acids, and neutrophil activation protein from *Helicobacter pylori* have been investigated. All of these reduced airway eosinophilia and T helper 2-mediated immune response, in AAD mouse models [10].

In addition to bacterial metabolites, some molecules derived from helminth parasites have also been identified, including the TGF-β mimetic (TGM) and the *Heligmosomoides polygyrus* alarm release inhibitor (HpARI) from *H. polygyrus*, Cystatin (AvCystatin) and excretory-secretory (ES)-62 from *Acanthocheilonema viteae*, and the IL-4 inducing principle from schistosome eggs (IPSE). These molecules appear to have an effect on mouse models of allergic asthma [10]. Another therapeutic example can be found in this study [53], which studies the beneficial effects of probiotics on respiratory health.

27.6 Conclusions

The lung microbiota plays a fundamental role in maintaining homeostasis and regulating immune responses. Once considered sterile, the lung harbors a diverse microbial community influenced by environmental, geographical, and host factors. The balance between microbial immigration and elimination determines its composition, which can be disrupted by factors such as mechanical ventilation, antibiotic use, and critical illnesses.

Dysbiosis of the lung microbiota has been linked to various respiratory diseases, including asthma, COPD, ARDS, and respiratory infections. The gut-lung axis highlights the bidirectional communication between intestinal and pulmonary microbiota, where gut dysbiosis can contribute to respiratory inflammation and vice versa. Additionally, emerging evidence supports a brain-lung connection, where lung microbiota alterations may influence neuroimmune responses, potentially affecting neurological conditions such as multiple sclerosis.

Therapeutic strategies targeting the microbiota, such as probiotics, SDD, FMT, and microbial metabolites, are promising but require further research. Probiotics, particularly *Lactobacillus* spp., have shown potential in modulating immune responses and reducing inflammation in respiratory diseases. However, challenges remain regarding the long-term efficacy, safety, and mechanisms of microbiota-based interventions.

Future research should aim to elucidate the full spectrum of microbial interactions within the lung, exploring viral and fungal components, and developing targeted therapies to restore microbiota balance in disease states. Integrating microbiota modulation with conventional treatments could open new avenues for managing respiratory and systemic diseases.

References

1. Berg G, Rybakova D, Fischer D, Cernava T, Vergès MC, Charles T, et al. Microbiome definition re-visited: old concepts and new challenges. Microbiome [Internet]. 2020 [citato 8 febbraio 2025];8(1). Disponibile su: https://pubmed.ncbi.nlm.nih.gov/32605663/.
2. Thursby E, Juge N. Introduction to the human gut microbiota. Biochem J. 2017;474(11):1823–36.
3. Wu CH, Chien YC, Chou MT, Huang YM. Integrating computational thinking, game design, and design thinking: a scoping review on trends, applications, and implications for education. Humanit Soc Sci Commun. 2025;12(1):1–12.
4. Hilty M, Burke C, Pedro H, Cardenas P, Bush A, Bossley C, et al. Disordered microbial communities in asthmatic airways. PLoS One. 2010;5(1):e8578.
5. Ullah H, Arbab S, Tian Y, Chen Y, Qing LC, Li Q, et al. Crosstalk between gut microbiota and host immune system and its response to traumatic injury. Front Immunol [Internet]. 2024 [citato 8 febbraio 2025];15. Disponibile su: https://www.frontiersin.org/journals/immunology/articles/10.3389/fimmu.2024.1413485/full.
6. Enaud R, Prevel R, Ciarlo E, Beaufils F, Wieërs G, Guery B, et al. The gut-lung axis in health and respiratory diseases: a place for inter-organ and inter-kingdom crosstalks. Front Cell Infect Microbiol. 2020;10:9.
7. Schuijt TJ, Lankelma JM, Scicluna BP, de Sousa e Melo F, Roelofs JJTH, de Boer JD, et al. The gut microbiota plays a protective role in the host defence against pneumococcal pneumonia. Gut. 2016;65(4):575–83.
8. Beck JM, Young VB, Huffnagle GB. The microbiome of the lung. Transl Res J Lab Clin Med. 2012;160(4):258–66.
9. Yagi K, Huffnagle GB, Lukacs NW, Asai N. The lung microbiome during health and disease. Int J Mol Sci. 2021;22(19):10872.
10. Gosens R, Hiemstra PS, Adcock IM, Bracke KR, Dickson RP, Hansbro PM, et al. Host-microbe cross-talk in the lung microenvironment: implications for understanding and treating chronic lung disease. Eur Respir J. 2020;56(2):1902320.
11. Sun Z, Zhu QL, Shen Y, Yan T, Zhou X. Dynamic changes of gut and lung microorganisms during chronic obstructive pulmonary disease exacerbations. Kaohsiung J Med Sci. 2020;36(2):107–13.

12. Yatsunenko T, Rey FE, Manary MJ, Trehan I, Dominguez-Bello MG, Contreras M, et al. Human gut microbiome viewed across age and geography. Nature. 2012;486(7402):222–7.
13. Blanchard LS, Armstrong TP, Kresken M, Emery CL, Ying YX, Sauvonnet V, et al. Multicenter clinical evaluation of ETEST eravacycline for susceptibility testing of enterobacteriaceae and enterococci. J Clin Microbiol. 2023;61(3):e0165022.
14. Morris A, Beck JM, Schloss PD, Campbell TB, Crothers K, Curtis JL, et al. Comparison of the respiratory microbiome in healthy nonsmokers and smokers. Am J Respir Crit Care Med. 2013;187(10):1067–75.
15. Charlson ES, Chen J, Custers-Allen R, Bittinger K, Li H, Sinha R, et al. Disordered microbial communities in the upper respiratory tract of cigarette smokers. PLoS One. 2010;5(12):e15216.
16. Shchipkova AY, Nagaraja HN, Kumar PS. Subgingival microbial profiles of smokers with periodontitis. J Dent Res. 2010;89(11):1247–53.
17. Bassis CM, Erb-Downward JR, Dickson RP, Freeman CM, Schmidt TM, Young VB, et al. Analysis of the upper respiratory tract microbiotas as the source of the lung and gastric microbiotas in healthy individuals. mBio. 2015;6(2):e00037.
18. Segal LN, Alekseyenko AV, Clemente JC, Kulkarni R, Wu B, Chen H, et al. Enrichment of lung microbiome with supraglottic taxa is associated with increased pulmonary inflammation. Microbiome. 2013;1(1):19.
19. Sullivan CE, Murphy E, Kozar LF, Phillipson EA. Waking and ventilatory responses to laryngeal stimulation in sleeping dogs. J Appl Physiol. 1978;45(5):681–9.
20. Dickson RP, Erb-Downward JR, Martinez FJ, Huffnagle GB. The microbiome and the respiratory tract. Annu Rev Physiol. 2016;78:481–504.
21. Rapley R. Basic molecular biology techniques. 2021 [citato 12 febbraio 2025]; Disponibile su: https://books.rsc.org/books/edited-volume/866/chapter/633461/Basic-Molecular-Biology-Techniques.
22. Treccani [Internet]. [citato 12 febbraio 2025]. Sequenziamento del dna - Enciclopedia. Disponibile su: https://www.treccani.it/enciclopedia/sequenziamento-del-dna_res-bcb7d282-9b5e-11e1-9b2f-d5ce3506d72e_%28Dizionario-di-Medicina%29/.
23. Tsay JCJ, Wu BG, Sulaiman I, Gershner K, Schluger R, Li Y, et al. Lower airway dysbiosis affects lung cancer progression. Cancer Discov. 2021;11(2):293–307.
24. Erb-Downward JR, Thompson DL, Han MK, Freeman CM, McCloskey L, Schmidt LA, et al. Analysis of the lung microbiome in the "healthy" smoker and in COPD. PLoS One. 2011;6(2):e16384.
25. Zhou J, Hou W, Zhong H, Liu D. Lung microbiota: implications and interactions in chronic pulmonary diseases. Front Cell Infect Microbiol. 2024;14:1401448.
26. Dickson RP, Schultz MJ, van der Poll T, Schouten LR, Falkowski NR, Luth JE, et al. Lung microbiota predict clinical outcomes in critically ill patients. Am J Respir Crit Care Med. 201(5):555–63.
27. Alagna L, Mancabelli L, Magni F, Chatenoud L, Bassi G, Del Bianco S, et al. Changes in upper airways microbiota in ventilator-associated pneumonia. Intensive Care Med Exp. 2023;11:17.
28. Bousbia S, Papazian L, Saux P, Forel JM, Auffray JP, Martin C, et al. Repertoire of intensive care unit pneumonia microbiota. PLoS One. 2012;7(2):e32486.
29. Rosen R, Amirault J, Liu H, Mitchell P, Hu L, Khatwa U, et al. Changes in gastric and lung microflora with acid suppression: acid suppression and bacterial growth. JAMA Pediatr. 2014;168(10):932–7.
30. Wang J, Li F, Wei H, Lian ZX, Sun R, Tian Z. Respiratory influenza virus infection induces intestinal immune injury via microbiota-mediated Th17 cell-dependent inflammation. J Exp Med. 2014;211(12):2397–410.
31. Marsland BJ, Gollwitzer ES. Host-microorganism interactions in lung diseases. Nat Rev Immunol. 2014;14(12):827–35.
32. Round JL, Mazmanian SK. The gut microbiota shapes intestinal immune responses during health and disease. Nat Rev Immunol. 2009;9(5):313–23.

33. Tuganbaev T, Mor U, Bashiardes S, Liwinski T, Nobs SP, Leshem A, et al. Diet diurnally regulates small intestinal microbiome-epithelial-immune homeostasis and enteritis. Cell. 2020;182(6):1441–1459.e21.
34. Battaglini D, Rocco PRM. Editorial: crosstalk between lung and brain, heart, kidney and vascular system in critical illness. Front Physiol. 2024;15:1516682.
35. Khoruts A, Staley C, Sadowsky MJ. Faecal microbiota transplantation for Clostridioides difficile: mechanisms and pharmacology. Nat Rev Gastroenterol Hepatol. 2021;18(1):67–80.
36. Kamada N, Núñez G. Regulation of the immune system by the resident intestinal bacteria. Gastroenterol. 2014;146(6):1477–88.
37. Mazmanian SK, Liu CH, Tzianabos AO, Kasper DL. An immunomodulatory molecule of symbiotic bacteria directs maturation of the host immune system. Cell. 2005;122(1):107–18.
38. Ivanov II, Atarashi K, Manel N, Brodie EL, Shima T, Karaoz U, et al. Induction of intestinal Th17 cells by segmented filamentous bacteria. Cell. 2009;139(3):485–98.
39. Atarashi K, Tanoue T, Shima T, Imaoka A, Kuwahara T, Momose Y, et al. Induction of colonic regulatory T cells by indigenous clostridium species. Science. 2011;331(6015):337–41.
40. Zhang D, Li S, Wang N, Tan HY, Zhang Z, Feng Y. The cross-talk between gut microbiota and lungs in common lung diseases. Front Microbiol [Internet]. 2020;11. Disponibile su: https://www.frontiersin.org/journals/microbiology/articles/10.3389/fmicb.2020.00301/full.
41. Sencio V, Machado MG, Trottein F. The lung-gut axis during viral respiratory infections: the impact of gut dysbiosis on secondary disease outcomes. Mucosal Immunol. 2021;14(2):296–304.
42. Wakisaka Y, Suzuki Y, Iwata O, Nakashima A, Ito T, Hirose M, et al. Probing the metabolic heterogeneity of live Euglena gracilis with stimulated Raman scattering microscopy. Nat Microbiol. 2016;1(10):16124.
43. Walley KR, Lukacs NW, Standiford TJ, Strieter RM, Kunkel SL. Balance of inflammatory cytokines related to severity and mortality of murine sepsis. Infect Immun. 1996;64(11):4733–8.
44. Settembre C, Zoncu R, Medina DL, Vetrini F, Erdin S, Erdin S, et al. A lysosome-to-nucleus signalling mechanism senses and regulates the lysosome via mTOR and TFEB. EMBO J. 2012;31(5):1095–108.
45. Ivanov II, de Frutos RL, Manel N, Yoshinaga K, Rifkin DB, Sartor RB, et al. Specific microbiota direct the differentiation of IL-17-producing T-helper cells in the mucosa of the small intestine. Cell Host Microbe. 2008;4(4):337–49.
46. Du B, Fu Y, Han Y, Sun Q, Xu J, Yang Y, et al. The lung-gut crosstalk in respiratory and inflammatory bowel disease. Front Cell Infect Microbiol. 2023;13:1218565.
47. Papadakis KA, Prehn J, Nelson V, Cheng L, Binder SW, Ponath PD, et al. The role of thymus-expressed chemokine and its receptor ccr9 on lymphocytes in the regional specialization of the mucosal immune system. J Immunol. 2000;165(9):5069–76.
48. Azzoni R, Marsland BJ. The lung-brain axis: a new frontier in host-microbe interactions. Immunity. 2022;55(4):589–91.
49. Akkasheh G, Kashani-Poor Z, Tajabadi-Ebrahimi M, Jafari P, Akbari H, Taghizadeh M, et al. Clinical and metabolic response to probiotic administration in patients with major depressive disorder: a randomized, double-blind, placebo-controlled trial. Nutr Burbank Los Angel Cty Calif. 2016;32(3):315–20.
50. Baecher-Allan C, Kaskow BJ, Weiner HL. Multiple sclerosis: mechanisms and immunotherapy. Neuron. 2018;97(4):742–68.
51. Odoardi F, Sie C, Streyl K, Ulaganathan VK, Schläger C, Lodygin D, et al. T cells become licensed in the lung to enter the central nervous system. Nature. 2012;488(7413):675–9.
52. Seifi N, Jafarzadeh Esfahani A, Sedaghat A, Rezvani R, Khadem-Rezaiyan M, Nematy M, et al. Effect of gut microbiota modulation on feeding tolerance of enterally fed critically ill adult patients: a systematic review. Syst Rev. 2021;10(1):95.
53. Du T, Lei A, Zhang N, Zhu C. The beneficial role of probiotic lactobacillus in respiratory diseases. Front Immunol. 2022;13:908010.

54. Mortaz E, Adcock IM, Ricciardolo FLM, Varahram M, Jamaati H, Velayati AA, et al. Anti-inflammatory effects of Lactobacillus Rahmnosus and Bifidobacterium breve on cigarette smoke activated human macrophages. PLoS One. 2015;10(8):e0136455.
55. Drago L, Rodighiero V. Probiotici: possibilità di regolazione della risposta allergica. Riv Immunol Allergol Pediatr. 2011;3:25–33. [Italian]. Available from: https://old.riaponline.it/article/probiotici-possibilita-regolazione-dellarisposta-allergica/ (accessed 4 Sep 2025).
56. Randomized controlled study of probiotics containing Lactobacillus casei (Shirota strain) for prevention of ventilator-associated pneumonia. J Med Assoc Thail Chotmaihet Thangphaet. 2015;98(3):253–9.
57. Dong W, Ma L, Huang Q, Yang X, Mei Z, Kong M, et al. Gut microbiome alterations in pulmonary hypertension in highlanders and lowlanders. ERJ Open Res [Internet]. 2023;9(3). Disponibile su: https://publications.ersnet.org/content/erjor/9/3/00617-2022.
58. Johnstone J, Meade M, Lauzier F, Marshall J, Duan E, Dionne J, et al. Effect of probiotics on incident ventilator-associated pneumonia in critically ill patients: a randomized clinical trial. JAMA. 2021;326(11):1024–33.
59. Lou J, Cui S, Huang N, Jin G, Chen C, Fan Y, et al. Efficacy of probiotics or synbiotics in critically ill patients: a systematic review and meta-analysis. Clin Nutr ESPEN. 2024;59:48–62.
60. Bonten M. Selective decontamination of the digestive tract: an answer at last? JAMA. 2022;328(23):2310–1.
61. Benus RF, Harmsen HJ, Welling GW, Spanjersberg R, Zijlstra JG, Degener JE, et al. Impact of digestive and oropharyngeal decontamination on the intestinal microbiota in ICU patients. Intensive Care Med. 2010;36(8):1394–402.
62. Buelow E, Bello González TDJ, Fuentes S, de Steenhuijsen Piters WAA, Lahti L, Bayjanov JR, et al. Comparative gut microbiota and resistome profiling of intensive care patients receiving selective digestive tract decontamination and healthy subjects. Microbiome. 2017;5(1):88.
63. van Doorn-Schepens MLM, Abis GSA, Oosterling SJ, van Egmond M, Poort L, Stockmann HBAC, et al. The effect of selective decontamination on the intestinal microbiota as measured with IS-pro: a taxonomic classification tool applicable for direct evaluation of intestinal microbiota in clinical routine. Eur J Clin Microbiol Infect Dis. 2022;41(11):1337–45.
64. Kean IRL, Clark JA, Zhang Z, Daubney E, White D, Ferrando-Vivas P, et al. Short-duration selective decontamination of the digestive tract infection control does not contribute to increased antimicrobial resistance burden in a pilot cluster randomised trial (the ARCTIC Study). Gut. 2024;73(6):910–21.
65. Hammond NE, Myburgh J, Seppelt I, Garside T, Vlok R, Mahendran S, et al. Association between selective decontamination of the digestive tract and in-hospital mortality in intensive care unit patients receiving mechanical ventilation: a systematic review and meta-analysis. JAMA. 2022;328(19):1922–34.
66. Britton RA, Young VB. Role of the intestinal microbiota in resistance to colonization by Clostridium difficile. Gastroenterology. 2014;146(6):1547–53.

Lung Cell Crosstalk in Obese Patients with ARDS

28

Eleonora Balzani and Lorenzo Ball

28.1 Introduction

Since 1975, the prevalence of obesity has tripled globally, and by 2030, it is predicted that over 51% of people would be obese, underscoring the expanding public health concern [1]. It appears that genetic, environmental, and behavioral factors are the main causes of this epidemic. According to the World Health Organization (WHO), urbanization and technology have led to sedentary lifestyles and a rise in the consumption of foods high in calories but low in nutrients, which is why obesity rates are on the rise [2]. This "*nutrition transition,*" as defined by Popkin et al., underscores how, no longer limited to high-income countries, a shift toward high-energy, processed foods rich in fats and sugars, is exacerbating the problem also in mid- and low-income countries [3].

In fact, social environment is only a part of the main determinants of obesity: genetic predispositions also play a significant role. Advances in genome-wide association studies have identified a number of loci influencing appetite regulation, energy expenditure, and fat distribution [4].

From a biological standpoint, chronic low-grade inflammation, metabolic syndrome, and coexisting conditions like diabetes, hypertension, and dyslipidemia are hallmarks of obesity making this clinical condition, in fact, a syndrome [5, 6]. This pro-inflammatory condition characterized by cytokine overproduction—primarily TNF-α, IL-6, and IL-1β—impairs at multiple levels the function of several organs, including but not limited to the lungs, skeletal muscle, and liver [7–9].

E. Balzani
Centre for Medical Sciences-CISMed, University of Trento, Trento, Italy

L. Ball (✉)
Department of Surgical Sciences and Integrated Diagnostics, University of Genoa, Genoa, Italy

Anesthesia and Intensive Care, San Martino Policlinico Hospital, Genoa, Italy

D. Battaglini et al. (eds.), *Organ System Crosstalk in Critical Illness*,
https://doi.org/10.1007/978-3-032-01024-7_28

Acute respiratory distress syndrome (ARDS) is a life-threatening condition characterized by severe hypoxemia, increased pulmonary vascular permeability, and loss of alveolar tissue integrity [10]. Despite advancements in supportive therapies, ARDS continues to have a high mortality rate, estimated to be over 34% in intensive care unit patients [11].

Obesity adds complexity to ARDS through both macroscopic and microscopic mechanisms. Macroscopically, obesity leads to increased intra-abdominal pressure, reduced functional residual capacity (FRC) and total lung capacity (TLC), impaired lung compliance, and increased work of breathing [12, 13]. Microscopically, it is characterized by chronic inflammation and systemic immune dysregulation [14, 15]. Elevated levels of pro-inflammatory cytokines, such as IL-6 and TNF-α, further exacerbate lung damage, increasing susceptibility to ARDS of patients admitted to the ICU for other reasons and complicating ventilation management [16].

28.2 Obesity and ARDS Outcomes: A Complex Relationship

The finding that people who are fat may have better clinical outcomes than non-obese patients is referred to as the "obesity paradox" [17], and it is confirmed by several epidemiological studies in acute conditions including ARDS. Obese people appear to have increased survival rates when admitted to the ICU for critical illness than their non-obese counterparts [18]. This phenomenon has been described in sepsis, ARDS, and the general ICU population; however, the mechanisms underlying this association between obesity and improved survival are matter of debate [18–20]. Several authors questioned the interpretation of the "obesity paradox" in ARDS, highlighting the heterogeneity of patient populations and study designs, which may contribute to the diverse conclusions regarding the paradox. In particular, critically ill obese patients seem to be admitted more promptly to the ICU, possibly resulting in less severe obese patients being identified as "critically ill" as compared to non-obese [13].

Potential biological explanations have been investigated, hypothesizing that adipose tissue in obese people may contribute to systemic inflammation through several mechanisms. Adipose tissue is a major source of pro-inflammatory cytokines such as TNF-α and IL-6, which are implicated in systemic inflammation and obesity-associated comorbidities like atherosclerosis, hypertension, and insulin resistance [21]. These elevated cytokine levels contribute to the chronic low-grade inflammatory state characterizing obesity [21]. On the other hand, adipose tissue generates anti-inflammatory adipokines, such as adiponectin, which inhibit inflammatory pathways and aid in tissue repair [18].

This dual role—amplifying inflammation through cytokines while mitigating it through adipokines—may influence outcomes in acute inflammatory conditions such as ARDS [18]: increased levels of anti-inflammatory factors in obese individuals may help modulating the hyperinflammatory state observed in the hyperinflammatory phenotype of ARDS, possibly explaining to the "obesity paradox."

In addition to these mechanistic explanations, it has been proposed that the "obesity paradox" may, at least in part, be explained by the different clinical management of obese critically ill patients as compared to non-obese. Clinician may tend to prefer higher positive end-expiratory pressure (PEEP) levels in obese patients [22]. While higher PEEP showed conflicting results when used routinely in unselected ARDS patients [23, 24], trials on PEEP focusing on obese patients with ARDS are lacking. Observational studies suggested that higher PEEP in obese patients with ARDS is associated with improved oxygenation and reduced mortality [25].

However, not all findings consistently support the "obesity paradox" concept. In fact, obesity is associated with impaired respiratory mechanics, including reduced lung compliance and increased chest wall elastance, which exacerbate hypoxemia and increases the risk of complications related to mechanical ventilation [26]. In a large observational study on extremely obese patients (BMI >40 kg/m^2) admitted to the ICU, while unadjusted analyses suggested an improved mortality, this finding was not confirmed when adjusting for confounding factors; moreover, extremely obese patients had longer ICU stay and mechanical ventilation duration [27].

Nonetheless, moderate obesity (BMI 30–35 kg/m^2) appears to confer protective benefits in ARDS, while extreme obesity remains a significant risk factor [18]. The interplay between adipose tissue, inflammation, and clinical management highlights the necessity of individualized approaches to ARDS treatment, focusing on patient-specific factors such as fat distribution and metabolic profiles.

Biases in ICU admission practices may further complicate interpretations of the "obesity paradox." Obese patients admitted to ICUs are often younger and have fewer preexisting comorbidities compared to their non-obese counterparts, which may distort statistics focused on mortality in their favor [18]. Additionally, BMI, the most commonly used metric of obesity, fails to differentiate between subcutaneous and visceral fat compartments [28]. While subcutaneous fat may confer protective effects, visceral fat is associated with adverse outcomes, further emphasizing the limitations of BMI-based analyses.

All these factors contribute to the complexity of interpreting findings in the literature, potentially generating further confusion within the so-called "obesity paradox."

28.3 Molecular Mechanisms in Obesity-ARDS Crosstalk

The interaction between obesity and ARDS is driven by complex molecular mechanisms involving endothelial dysfunction, epithelial dysregulation, and immune cell modulation. These pathways highlight how adipose tissue actively modulates the response to pathophysiological alterations in ARDS, particularly in obese individuals.

28.3.1 Endothelial Dysfunction

Obesity is linked to a chronic inflammatory state driven by an imbalance between pro- and anti-inflammatory adipokines, which alter endothelial function [29]. Pro-inflammatory adipokines such as leptin, resistin, and TNF-α play a key role in this process by activating TLR4 receptors and the NF-κB pathway, leading to sustained inflammation [29, 30]. On the other hand, anti-inflammatory adipokines, including adiponectin, omentin, IL-10, and SFRP5, which usually help control inflammation and maintain endothelial health, are significantly reduced in individuals with obesity [29].

This inflammatory state is characterized by a shift in immune cell activity. Macrophages transition from an M2 phenotype, associated with anti-inflammatory and tissue-repair functions, to an M1 phenotype that promotes inflammation [31]. Similarly, there is a shift in T-cell populations, with an increase in pro-inflammatory Th1 and Th17 cells and a decline in the protective Th2 and Treg subsets [29]. Together, these changes drive the release of pro-inflammatory cytokines such as TNF-α, IL-6, and IFN-γ, as well as reactive oxygen species (ROS), which directly damage endothelial cells [29]. This damage triggers endothelial activation, marked by increased production of adhesion molecules like ICAM-1 and VCAM-1, enhancing leukocyte recruitment and disrupting vascular integrity [32].

In the context of COVID-19-related ARDS, these mechanisms are further aggravated by the direct viral effect on endothelial cells exerted by SARS-CoV-2. This infection induces endothelitis, intensifies vascular injury, and accelerates microvascular thrombosis and capillary leak [33].

28.3.2 Immune Cell Modulation in Obesity and ARDS

Obesity profoundly alters immune cell function, creating a complex interplay between systemic inflammation, immune dysregulation, and pulmonary homeostasis. A hallmark change in obesity is the polarization of macrophages toward the M1 (pro-inflammatory) from the M2 anti-inflammatory phenotype [31]. While M2 macrophages are normally involved in tissue repair and resolution of inflammation, in obesity a paradoxical shift toward M1 phenotype has been described [31].

This maladaptive polarization from M2 to M1 macrophage phenotypes in obesity is determined by the combined effect of various factors, which also sustains the altered balance between these macrophage populations. Among the key actors of this switch, adipose tissue expansion and hypoxia induce the expression of hypoxia-inducible factors (HIFs) that promote the recruitment and activation of M1 macrophages [34]. Additionally, adipocyte stress promotes the production of danger-associated molecular patterns (DAMPs) and the release of pro-inflammatory cytokines [35]. Additional contributors, such as monocyte chemoattractant protein 1 (MCP-1) and free fatty acid secretion, further enhance the pro-inflammatory milieu [29]. Together, these factors sustain chronic inflammation, creating a molecular environment that perpetuates and reinforces this pathological macrophage polarization.

Adding another layer of complexity, it is important to note that the lung is highly susceptible to the presence of M1 macrophages. Alveolar M1 macrophages are critically important in pulmonary infections due to their strong pro-inflammatory and microbicidal properties [36]. They play a crucial role in various pulmonary inflammatory conditions, including streptococcal pneumonia, *Mycobacterium tuberculosis* infections, viral infections, and asthma [36]. However, their presence increases the lung susceptibility to inflammation and injury [36]. This imbalance also disrupts the resolution of inflammation—a process normally mediated by M2 macrophages—which is essential for preventing chronic damage and fibrosis. Neutrophil dysfunction contributes to inflammation in the lung tissue of obese patients [37]. In obese mice, neutrophils exhibit impaired chemotaxis, particularly to the alveolar spaces, due to reduced CXCR2 expression, indicating a decreased neutrophil response [37]. These findings were corroborated by a reduced presence of neutrophils in the bronchoalveolar lavage fluid of the same animals [37].

28.3.3 Cytokine Storm in Obese ARDS Patients

In both ARDS and COVID-19, there is extensive literature discussing the cytokine storm. This could result in complex interactions with the pro-inflammatory state seen in obesity.

COVID-19 has strongly reinforced the concept of cytokine storm in the context of critical illness: a massive release of cytokines in a short time period, driving multisystemic effects on host cells. However, cytokine storm has been defined heterogeneously across the medical literature [38].

The term "cytokine storm" refers to a hyper-inflammatory response characterized by an excessive release of cytokines such as IL-6, TNF-α, IL-1β, and other inflammatory mediators [38–40]. This phenomenon is triggered by pathogen-associated molecular patterns (PAMPs) or damage-associated molecular patterns (DAMPs), activating immune pathways including the Janus kinase/signal transducer and activator of transcription (JAK/STAT) signaling pathway for IL-6, NF-κB signaling for TNF-α, and the NLRP3 inflammasome for IL-1β. These signaling cascades amplify inflammation, creating a positive feedback loop that overwhelms the body's ability to regulate the immune response.

The cytokine storm in obese ARDS patients acts as a pathological crosstalk between adipose tissue, endothelial cells, and immune mediators, potentially exacerbating pulmonary damage.

In the lungs, this can promote diffuse alveolar damage (DAD), characterized by endothelial dysfunction, increased vascular permeability, fluid leakage, and impaired gas exchange [41, 42].

In obese patients, the cytokine storm is often more severe due to underlying metabolic and immune dysregulation [29, 36, 43]. Adipose tissue acts as an endocrine organ, secreting pro-inflammatory mediators such as leptin, resistin, and visfatin, while producing lower levels of anti-inflammatory adipokines like adiponectin [39]. In murine models and in clinical studies, elevated leptin levels promote macrophage polarization toward the M1 phenotype, driving the release of IL-6 and TNF-α [39, 44, 45]. Simultaneously, reduced adiponectin fails to counteract inflammation, exacerbating cytokine release [46].

Given this adipose-driven pro-inflammatory environment, the immune system of obese patients is primed for an exaggerated response, which delays inflammation resolution and predisposes to worse pulmonary outcomes. From a molecular point of view, the storm involves a series of intra- and extracellular mechanisms that exacerbate lung injury. IL-6 is a key player, activating the JAK-STAT pathway, sustaining neutrophilic inflammation and delaying resolution, as seen in COVID-19 ARDS [38, 40]. On the other hand, TNF-α, through NF-κB signaling, enhances vascular leakage and endothelial dysfunction, facilitating immune cell extravasation and alveolar injury, as shown in murine models of acute lung injury [29, 37, 40].

IL-1β activates the inflammasome complex, driving neutrophil recruitment and amplifying cytokine production, as observed in experimental and clinical studies of inflammatory lung diseases [37, 38, 40].

These mechanisms were corroborated by studies across different contexts, including COVID-19 obese patients, where cytokine levels correlate with disease severity, and rodent models, which revealed the molecular mechanisms of cytokine activation [38–40].

In other words, the cytokine storm in obese patients represents a complex interplay of metabolic and immune dysregulation. Elevated levels of IL-6, TNF-α, and IL-1β, combined with adipose-driven inflammation, exacerbate pulmonary damage, as supported by both human and murine studies [38–40]. Cytokine modulation could be crucial for ARDS and lung injury treatment, especially in obese patients. New therapies targeting the regulation of cytokine release may offer promising options for improving outcomes in this population.

28.4 Mechanical Ventilation Strategies in Obesity and ARDS Patients

This section will look at how mechanical ventilation techniques differ between obese and non-obese individuals, with a focus on the particular problems and physiological changes associated with obesity.

Obese patients differ from the non-obese from a physiological point of view due to their increased body mass which leads to altered respiratory mechanics [13].

From a practical perspective, obesity significantly reduces functional residual capacity (FRC) and total lung capacity due to their increased intra-abdominal pressure and chest wall resistance. These changes compress the lungs promoting atelectasis, particularly in dependent lung regions [12, 13].

The reduction in FRC is coupled with increased pleural pressure due to the weight of the chest wall and elevated intra-abdominal pressure exerting force on the lungs. This is more commonly observed when patients are in the supine position.

The consequences of an elevated pleural pressure are a reduction of end-expiratory transpulmonary pressure—the pressure keeping alveoli open—making them prone to collapse at end-expiration, especially in dorsal, dependent, lung zones [47]. This pressure may reach low to negative values, translating into an increased risk of development of atelectasis [47].

For this reason, end-expiratory transpulmonary pressure is crucial parameter to consider in obese patients because it indicates alveolar stability at the end of expiration, a critical moment when alveoli are prone to collapse due to high pleural pressures [48].These factors contribute to ventilation-perfusion mismatch and hypoxemia, conditions that worsen during mechanical ventilation [47].

Individualized PEEP levels through decremental PEEP trial, based on the lowest respiratory system elastance, could improve oxygenation in obese patients [47]. This intervention achieved in a population of critically ill obese patients a balance between alveolar recruitment and avoidance of overdistension, reducing intratidal recruitment/derecruitment and enhancing oxygenation [47].

On the other hand, reduced FRC leads to diminished lung volumes, increasing the likelihood of airway closure, particularly in dependent lung regions. This phenomenon exacerbates the risk of airway closure during mechanical ventilation, resulting in an elevated airway opening pressure (AOP). Up to 60% of obese patients without lung injury undergoing robotic surgery in the anti-Trendelenburg position exhibited complete airway closure during pneumoperitoneum, with a median AOP of 17 cm H_2O [49].

RMs play a critical role in reopening collapsed lung regions, improving oxygenation and pulmonary compliance. Stepwise pressure increases during RMs, often combined with higher PEEP, are termed gradual RMs, facilitating a controlled and progressive increase in transpulmonary pressure [49, 50].

In this context, it is essential to fine-tune ventilator settings to ensure that inspiratory pressure exceeds the AOP, thereby maintaining effective ventilation while minimizing the risk of ventilator-induced lung injury.

Ventilatory management of obese patients remains controversial due to unresolved challenges and limited evidence. Higher PEEP is crucial to counteract elevated pleural pressures and prevent alveolar collapse; however, higher PEEP also increases intrathoracic pressure, which can reduce venous return to the heart, lower cardiac output, and compromise hemodynamics [12]. Despite the frequent call for individualized PEEP titration strategies in obese patients, the lack of standardized protocols for PEEP titration and RMs highlights a critical gap in clinical practice [47, 51]. Similarly, RMs are essential for reopening collapsed alveoli, improving oxygenation, and enhancing lung compliance, particularly in obese patients prone to atelectasis due to reduced functional residual capacity and increased pleural pressure [49, 51]. However, they must be used with caution, as excessive airway pressures can lead to alveolar overdistension and barotrauma. This risk is especially significant in patients with heterogeneous lung parenchyma, where varying responses of lung regions to increased pressures may exacerbate ventilation-induced lung injury.

Q&A Section

1. **Q:** The "obesity paradox" in ARDS remains a debated phenomenon. Which of the following factors is most likely to contribute to the paradoxical observation of improved survival in moderately obese patients?

   (a) The anti-inflammatory effects of adipokines such as adiponectin.
   (b) Biases in ICU admission criteria, favoring younger and less comorbid obese patients.
   (c) Uniformly better respiratory mechanics in obese individuals due to higher chest wall compliance.
   (d) Neutrophil recruitment to alveolar spaces, reducing the risk of infection but increasing inflammation.
   (e) A combination of the above.

   A: (e) Several molecular and epidemiological factors could explain the "obesity paradox."
2. **Q:** Obesity modulates immune responses in ARDS through complex molecular pathways. Which of the following best describes the interplay between immune cells and adipokines in obese ARDS patients?

   (a) M1 macrophages predominate due to the upregulation of hypoxia-inducible factors (HIFs) and the release of pro-inflammatory cytokines such as TNF-α and IL-6.
   (b) Neutrophil recruitment to the lungs is enhanced by increased CXCR2 expression, counteracting alveolar collapse.
   (c) Anti-inflammatory adipokines such as leptin reduce endothelial dysfunction and promote lung repair mechanisms.
   (d) Elevated adiponectin levels exacerbate cytokine storm development through activation of the NF-κB pathway.

   A: (a) M1 macrophages predominate due to the upregulation of hypoxia-inducible factors (HIFs) and the release of pro-inflammatory cytokines such as TNF-α and IL-6.
3. **Q**: What is the primary physiological reason for using higher PEEP levels in mechanically ventilated obese patients with ARDS?

   (a) To enhance cardiac output by reducing intrathoracic pressure.
   (b) To maintain alveolar stability by counteracting elevated pleural pressures.
   (c) To avoid the need for recruitment maneuvers.
   (d) To increase functional residual capacity and decrease respiratory compliance.

   A: (b) To maintain alveolar stability by counteracting elevated pleural pressures.

References

1. World Obesity Federation. World obesity atlas 2023 [Internet]. London: World Obesity Federation; 2023 [cited 2025 Apr 27]. Available from: https://data.worldobesity.org/publications/WOF-Obesity-Atlas-V5.pdf.
2. World Health Organization. Obesity and overweight [Internet]. Geneva: World Health Organization; 2021 Jun 9 [cited 2025 Apr 27]. Available from: https://www.who.int/news-room/fact-sheets/detail/obesity-and-overweight.
3. Popkin BM, Gordon-Larsen P. The nutrition transition: worldwide obesity dynamics and their determinants. Int J Obes Relat Metab Disord. 2004;28(Suppl 3):S2–9.
4. Loos RJF, Yeo GSH. The genetics of obesity: from discovery to biology. Nat Rev Genet. 2022;23(2):120–33.
5. Powell-Wiley TM, Poirier P, Burke LE, Després JP, Gordon-Larsen P, Lavie CJ, et al. Obesity and cardiovascular disease: a scientific statement from the American Heart Association. Circulation. 2021;143(21):e984–e1010.
6. Khanna D, Khanna S, Khanna P, Kahar P, Patel BM. Obesity: a chronic low-grade inflammation and its markers. Cureus. 2022;14(2):e22711.
7. Milano W, Carizzone F, Foia M, Marchese M, Milano M, Saetta B, et al. Obesity and its multiple clinical implications between inflammatory states and gut microbiotic alterations. Diseases. 2022;11(1)
8. Kern PA, Di Gregorio GB, Lu T, Rassouli N, Ranganathan G. Adiponectin expression from human adipose tissue: relation to obesity, insulin resistance, and tumor necrosis factor-alpha expression. Diabetes. 2003;52(7):1779–85.
9. Esposito K, Pontillo A, Ciotola M, Di Palo C, Grella E, Nicoletti G, et al. Weight loss reduces interleukin-18 levels in obese women. J Clin Endocrinol Metab. 2002;87(8):3864–6.
10. Matthay MA, Zemans RL, Zimmerman GA, Arabi YM, Beitler JR, Mercat A, et al. Acute respiratory distress syndrome. Nat Rev Dis Prim. 2018;5(1)
11. Bellani G, Laffey JG, Pham T, Fan E, Brochard L, Esteban A, et al. Epidemiology, patterns of care, and mortality for patients with acute respiratory distress syndrome in intensive care units in 50 countries. JAMA. 2016;315(8):788–800.
12. Bonatti G, Robba C, Ball L, Silva PL, Rocco PRM, Pelosi P. Controversies when using mechanical ventilation in obese patients with and without acute distress respiratory syndrome. Expert Rev Respir Med. 2019;13(5):471–9.
13. Ball L, Serpa Neto A, Pelosi P. Obesity and survival in critically ill patients with acute respiratory distress syndrome: a paradox within the paradox. Crit Care. 2017;21(1):114.
14. Hornung F, Rogal J, Loskill P, Löffler B, Deinhardt-Emmer S. The inflammatory profile of obesity and the role on pulmonary bacterial and viral infections. Int J Mol Sci. 2021;22(7)
15. Dixon AE, Peters U. The effect of obesity on lung function. Expert Rev Respir Med. 2018;12(9):755–67.
16. Dreyfuss D, Ricard JD, Saumon G. On the physiologic and clinical relevance of lung-borne cytokines during ventilator-induced lung injury. Am J Respir Crit Care Med. 2003;167(11):1467–71.
17. Di Angelantonio E, Bhupathiraju SN, Wormser D, Gao P, Kaptoge S, De Gonzalez AB, et al. Body-mass index and all-cause mortality: individual-participant-data meta-analysis of 239 prospective studies in four continents. Lancet. 2016;388(10046):776–86.
18. Schetz M, De Jong A, Deane AM, Druml W, Hemelaar P, Pelosi P, et al. Obesity in the critically ill: a narrative review. Intensive Care Med. 2019;45(6):757–69.
19. De Jong A, Verzilli D, Jaber S. ARDS in obese patients: specificities and management. Crit Care. 2019;23(1):74.
20. Gong MN, Bajwa EK, Thompson BT, Christiani DC. Body mass index is associated with the development of acute respiratory distress syndrome. Thorax. 2010;65(1):44–50.
21. Stapleton RD, Dixon AE, Parsons PE, Ware LB, Suratt BT. The association between BMI and plasma cytokine levels in patients with acute lung injury. Chest. 2010;138(3):568–77.

22. Gattinoni L, Caironi P, Cressoni M, Chiumello D, Ranieri VM, Quintel M, et al. Lung recruitment in patients with the acute respiratory distress syndrome. N Engl J Med. 2006;354(17):1775–86.
23. Dianti J, Tisminetzky M, Ferreyro BL, Englesakis M, Del Sorbo L, Sud S, et al. Association of positive end-expiratory pressure and lung recruitment selection strategies with mortality in acute respiratory distress syndrome: a systematic review and network meta-analysis. Am J Respir Crit Care Med. 2022;205(11):1300–10.
24. Ball L, Serpa Neto A, Trifiletti V, Mandelli M, Firpo I, Robba C, et al. Effects of higher PEEP and recruitment manoeuvres on mortality in patients with ARDS: a systematic review, meta-analysis, meta-regression and trial sequential analysis of randomized controlled trials. Intensive Care Med Exp. 2020;8(Suppl 1):39.
25. Bime C, Fiero M, Lu Z, Oren E, Berry CE, Parthasarathy S, et al. High positive end-expiratory pressure is associated with improved survival in obese patients with acute respiratory distress syndrome. Am J Med. 2017;130(2):207–13.
26. Syed MKH, Selickman J, Evans MD, Dries D, Marini JJ. Elastic power of mechanical ventilation in morbid obesity and severe hypoxemia. Respir Care. 2021;66(4):626–34.
27. Martino JL, Stapleton RD, Wang M, Day AG, Cahill NE, Dixon AE, et al. Extreme obesity and outcomes in critically ill patients. Chest. 2011;140(5):1198–206.
28. Buckley E, Mullen MM, Nizamuddin RA, Stein JH, Kuroki LM, Fuh KC, et al. High visceral fat to subcutaneous fat ratios portend a poor prognosis in patients with advanced endometrial cancer. Gynecol Oncol. 2022;167(3):496–501.
29. Wang C. Obesity, inflammation, and lung injury (OILI): the good. Mediat Inflamm. 2014;2014:978463.
30. Adya R, Tan BK, Randeva HS. Differential effects of leptin and adiponectin in endothelial angiogenesis. J Diabetes Res. 2015;2015:648239.
31. Jung HN, Jung CH. The role of anti-inflammatory adipokines in cardiometabolic disorders: moving beyond adiponectin. Int J Mol Sci. 2021;22(24)
32. Singh V, Kaur R, Kumari P, Pasricha C, Singh R. ICAM-1 and VCAM-1: gatekeepers in various inflammatory and cardiovascular disorders. Clin Chim Acta. 2023;548:117487.
33. Mosleh W, Chen K, Pfau SE, Vashist A. Endotheliitis and endothelial dysfunction in patients with COVID-19: its role in thrombosis and adverse outcomes. J Clin Med. 2020;9(6)
34. Norouzirad R, González-Muniesa P, Ghasemi A. Hypoxia in obesity and diabetes: potential therapeutic effects of hyperoxia and nitrate. Oxidative Med Cell Longev. 2017;2017:5350267.
35. Grant RW, Dixit VD. Adipose tissue as an immunological organ. Obesity (Silver Spring). 2015;23(3):512–8.
36. Arora S, Dev K, Agarwal B, Das P, Syed MA. Macrophages: their role, activation and polarization in pulmonary diseases. Immunobiology. 2018;223(4–5):383–96.
37. Kordonowy LL, Burg E, Lenox CC, Gauthier LM, Petty JM, Antkowiak M, et al. Obesity is associated with neutrophil dysfunction and attenuation of murine acute lung injury. Am J Respir Cell Mol Biol. 2012;47(1):120–7.
38. Sinha P, Matthay MA, Calfee CS. Is a "cytokine storm" relevant to COVID-19? JAMA Intern Med. 2020;180(9):1152–4.
39. Post A, Bakker SJL, Dullaart RPF. Obesity, adipokines and COVID-19. Eur J Clin Investig. 2020;50(8):e13313.
40. Maurya R, Sebastian P, Namdeo M, Devender M, Gertler A. COVID-19 severity in obesity: leptin and inflammatory cytokine interplay in the link between high morbidity and mortality. Front Immunol. 2021;12:649359.
41. Swenson KE, Swenson ER. Pathophysiology of acute respiratory distress syndrome and COVID-19 lung injury. Crit Care Clin. 2021;37(4):749–76.
42. Ranieri VM, Suter PM, Tortorella C, De Tullio R, Dayer JM, Brienza A, et al. Effect of mechanical ventilation on inflammatory mediators in patients with acute respiratory distress syndrome: a randomized controlled trial. JAMA. 1999;282(1):54–61.
43. Ray A, Bonorden MJL, Pandit R, Nkhata KJ, Bishayee A. Infections and immunity: associations with obesity and related metabolic disorders. J Pathol Transl Med. 2023;57(1):28–42.

44. Han Y, Huang Y, Gao P, Yang Q, Jia L, Zheng Y, et al. Leptin aggravates periodontitis by promoting M1 polarization via NLRP3. J Dent Res. 2022;101(6):675–85.
45. Luo M, Zhao F, Cheng H, Su M, Wang Y. Macrophage polarization: an important role in inflammatory diseases. Front Immunol. 2024;15:1352946.
46. Choi HM, Doss HM, Kim KS. Multifaceted physiological roles of adiponectin in inflammation and diseases. Int J Mol Sci. 2020;21(4)
47. Fumagalli J, Berra L, Zhang C, Pirrone M, Santiago RRS, Gomes S, et al. Transpulmonary pressure describes lung morphology during decremental positive end-expiratory pressure trials in obesity. Crit Care Med. 2017;45(8):1374–81.
48. Grieco DL, Chen L, Brochard L. Transpulmonary pressure: importance and limits. Ann Transl Med. 2017;5(14):285.
49. Grieco DL, Russo A, Anzellotti GM, Romanò B, Bongiovanni F, Dell'Anna AM, et al. Lung-protective ventilation during Trendelenburg pneumoperitoneum surgery: a randomized clinical trial. J Clin Anesth. 2023;85:111037.
50. Scharffenberg M, Mandelli M, Bluth T, Simonassi F, Wittenstein J, Teichmann R, et al. Respiratory mechanics and mechanical power during low vs. high positive end-expiratory pressure in obese surgical patients – a sub-study of the PROBESE randomized controlled trial. J Clin Anesth. 2024;92:111242.
51. Pirrone M, Fisher D, Chipman D, Imber DA, Corona J, Mietto C, et al. Recruitment maneuvers and positive end-expiratory pressure titration in morbidly obese ICU patients. Crit Care Med. 2016;44(2):300–7.

Organ Crosstalk in Pulmonary Hypertension

29

Giovanni Barbati and Claudio Picariello

29.1 Introduction

Pulmonary hypertension (PH) is a pathophysiological disorder that affects about 1% of the global population and up to 10% of individuals over 65 years old [1]. PH is mainly suspected by echocardiography and confirmed by right heart catheterization, defined by a mean pulmonary arterial pressure (mPAP) > 20 mmHg at rest. Measurements of pulmonary arterial wedge pressure (PAWP) and of pulmonary vascular resistance (PVR) allow subclassification PH in pre-capillary, post-capillary, and combined pre- and post-capillary PH [2] (Table 29.1).

PH is a consequence of multiple underlying diseases and can be clinically classified in five groups (Table 29.2): (1) pulmonary arterial hypertension, (2) PH associated with left heart disease, (3) PH associated with lung disease and/or hypoxia, (4) PH associated with pulmonary artery obstructions, (5) PH with unclear and/or multifactorial mechanisms [2]. Among these conditions, PH is most commonly associated with left-sided heart disease and chronic lung disease, especially in elderly people [3, 4].

These different diseases may all cause severe PH with increased right ventricle (RV) afterload, which can lead to RV dilation and dysfunction, and finally to right-sided heart failure (RHF). Transthoracic echocardiography is a simple noninvasive and valuable tool to detect right ventricle pressure overload and dysfunction and to noninvasively estimate the systolic pulmonary arterial pressure (sPAP) with different grades of PH probability (low, intermediate, high) [2, 5] (Figs. 29.1 and 29.2).

G. Barbati (✉)
Cardiology Unit, San Bortolo Hospital, Vicenza, Italy
e-mail: giovanni.barbati@aulss8.veneto.it

C. Picariello
Cardiology Unit, Santa Maria della Misericordia Hospital, Rovigo, Italy
e-mail: claudio.picariello@aulss5.veneto.it

D. Battaglini et al. (eds.), *Organ System Crosstalk in Critical Illness*,
https://doi.org/10.1007/978-3-032-01024-7_29

Table 29.1 Definitions of pulmonary hypertension [2]

Pre-capillary PH	mPAP >20 mmHg PAWP ≤15 mmHg PVR >2 Wood Units (WU)
Post-capillary PH	mPAP >20 mmHg PAWP >15 mmHg PVR ≤2 WU
Combined pre- and post-capillary PH	mPAP >20 mmHg PAWP >15 mmHg PVR >2 WU

RHF can in turn involve multiple organ systems including left heart, brain, kidneys, liver, gastrointestinal tract, skeletal muscle, and the endocrine, immune, and autonomic systems, determining a complex clinical syndrome [4].

29.2 Organ Crosstalk

The concept of organ crosstalk (OC) in PH refers to a set of multiple biological mechanisms and feedback secondary to RHF, which can increase morbidity and mortality inducing functional and structural changes in multiple organs [3, 6]. Among the OC mechanisms, there are the hemodynamic consequences of RHF, such as systemic venous congestion, impaired peripheral perfusion, and reduced systemic output, as well as maladaptive neurohormonal activation, oxidative stress, hormonal imbalance, and abnormal immune cell signaling [4]. OC involves circulating pro-inflammatory cytokines and may occur in acute, chronic, or acute-on-chronic settings [4]. Organ targets and systemic consequences of PH and RHF can be numerous and relevant (Table 29.3).

29.2.1 Left Ventricle

RV structural and functional changes related to RHF directly affect the left ventricle (LV), producing impairment of its geometry, structure, and function. These effects are consequences of the RV/LV interdependency, determined by shared septal myocardium, pericardial restraint, and the anatomy of circulatory system [4]. Therefore, a volume and pressure right ventricle overload causes mechanical septal leftward shift leading to paradoxical septal movement and a "D-shaped" and compressed LV, determining an increased left ventricular eccentricity index [7]. The reduced stroke volume and cardiac output (CO) of right ventricle, contribute to underfill LV, especially during exercise [8]. LV diastolic filling pressures may be elevated even when LV preload is reduced and LV is underfilled due to mechanisms of interdependency [9]. Reduced workload and chronic underutilization of the LV both lead to reductions of LV end-diastolic volume and LV mass by about 10–20% and 5–15%, respectively, and reductions in LV systolic strain, stroke volume, and ejection

Table 29.2 Clinical classification of pulmonary hypertension [2]

GROUP 1: *Pulmonary arterial hypertension (PAH)*
1. Idiopathic
1.1. Nonresponders at vasoreactivity testing
1.2. Responders at vasoreactivity testing
2. Heritable
3. Associated with drugs and toxins
4. Associated with:
4.1. Connective tissue disease
4.2. HIV
4.3. Portal hypertension
4.4. Congenital heart disease
4.5. Schistosomiasis
5. PAH with venous/capillary involvement
6. Persistent PH of the newborn
GROUP 2: *PH associated with left heart disease*
1. Heart failure with:
1.1. Preserved ejection fraction
1.2. Reduced ejection fraction
2. Valvular heart disease
3. Congenital/acquired cardiovascular conditions leading to post-capillary PH
GROUP 3: *PH associated with lung diseases and/or hypoxia*
1. Obstructive lung disease or emphysema
2. Restrictive lung disease
3. Lung disease with mixed restrictive/obstructive pattern
4. Hypoventilation syndromes
5. Hypoxia without lung disease
6. Developmental lung disorders
GROUP 4: *PH associated with pulmonary artery obstructions*
1. Chronic thrombo-embolic PH (CTEPH)
2. Other pulmonary artery obstructions
GROUP 5: *PH with unclear and/or multifactorial mechanisms*
1. Hematological disorders
2. Systemic disorders
3. Metabolic disorders
4. Chronic renal failure with or without hemodialysis
5. Pulmonary tumor thrombotic microangiopathy
6. Fibrosing mediastinitis

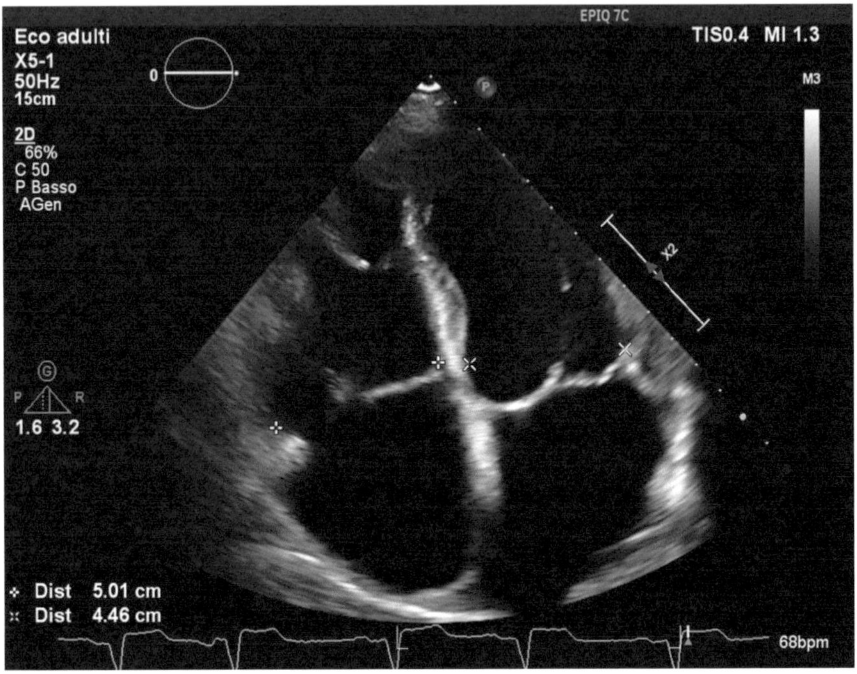

Fig. 29.1 Right ventricular dilation in a patient with chronic thromboembolic PH (CTEPH)

fraction [10]. Furthermore, pulmonary artery (PA) dilation may occasionally cause compression of the left main coronary artery triggering myocardial ischemia and fatal/nonfatal arrhythmias [11]. Indeed, a significant number of PAH patients die from sudden death, and a PA diameter 48 mm was associated with a 7.5-fold increased risk of sudden unexplained death in patients with severe PAH or CTEPH [12]. At cellular and molecular point of view, LV myocardium of patients with severe PH displays cardiomyocyte atrophy and contractile dysfunction, as well as lower cellular content of myosin, impaired phosphorylation of sarcomeric proteins, reduced number of available myosin-based cross-bridges, and a leftward shift in the force relationship, which may explain the impairment of the LV diastolic function [9, 13]. All this explains post-lung transplantation failure: there is an increased post-operative LV filling and inability to manage a normalized preload. In this context, it is important to use veno-arterial extracorporeal membrane oxygenation (V-A ECMO) as a bridge to recovery [14].

29.2.2 Kidneys

Elevated serum creatinine values and/or a reduced estimated glomerular filtration rate (eGFR) are present in 12–29% of PAH patients, and even slight abnormalities are clinically relevant [15]. The REVEAL registry (Registry to Evaluate the Early

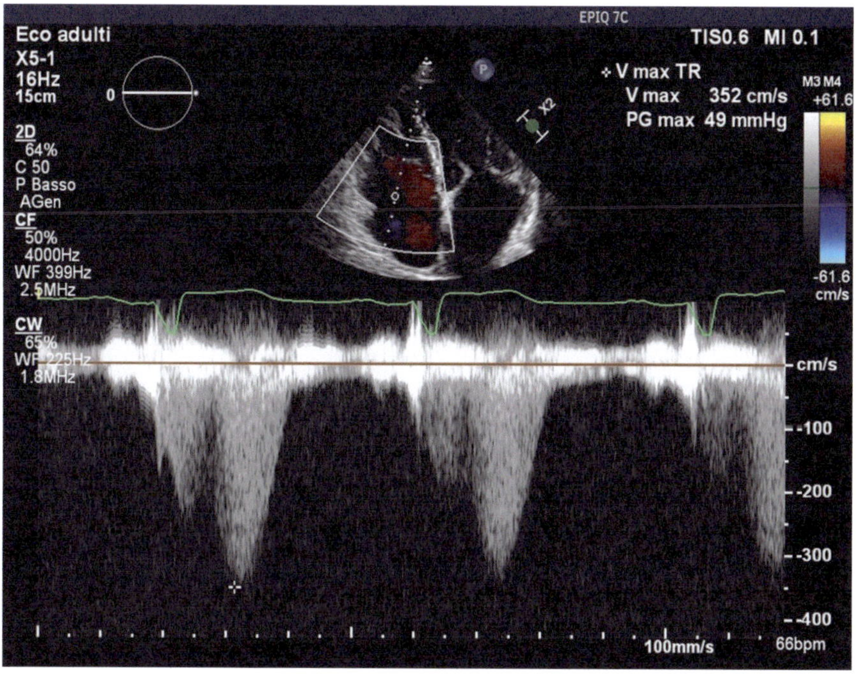

Fig. 29.2 Elevated sPAP/high probability PH: estimation based on peak tricuspid regurgitation velocity

Table 29.3 Systemic consequences of PH and RHF

1. *Left heart*: Mechanical compression, underfilling/deconditioning, functional (systolic/diastolic dysfunction), cardiomyocyte dysfunction
2. *Kidneys*: Low perfusion renal injury, congestive nephropathy, renal fibrosis/sclerosis, acute-on-chronic renal injury
3. *Liver*: Congestive hepatopathy, hepatic fibrosis, cardiac cirrhosis, ischemic hepatitis
4. *Gut/bowel*: Leaky bowel syndrome, malabsorption, appetite loss/cachexia, gut microbiota
5. *Iron homeostasis*: Iron deficiency, impaired adsorption, anemia
6. *Thyroid*: Hypothyroidism, hyperthyroidism, graves's disease
7. *Endocrine system*: Metabolic syndrome, diabetes, estrogen/testosterone
8. *Skeletal muscle*: Deconditioning, impaired function of skeletal and respiratory muscles, reduced aerobic capacity
9. *Immune system*: Systemic inflammation, innate/adaptive immunity, autoimmunity
10. *Autonomic system*: Sympathetic hyperactivity, increased susceptibility for syncope and arrhythmias, endothelial dysfunction
11. *Eyes*: Open-angle glaucoma, retinal detachment, venous stasis retinopathy, central retinal vein occlusion
12. *Brain*: Cognitive function, depression, anxiety, sleep
13. *Skin*: Subacute prurigo simplex

and Long-term Pulmonary Arterial Hypertension Disease Management), a large US registry of PAH patients, has shown a strong association between renal failure and death and that both the absolute value and a 10% decline in eGFR from baseline over 1 year are associated with an increased risk of death [16, 17]. In PH, neurohormonal activation, secondary to increased PVR, leads to water and salt retention, venous congestion, and reduced CO [4]. In RHF, renal dysfunction occurs secondary to renal hypoperfusion, but chronic venous congestion also plays a central role in acute and chronic kidney injury [6, 18]. In PAH, central venous pressure is one of the most important hemodynamic determinants of worsening renal function, and both a decreased cardiac index and an increased right atrial pressure are independent determinants of reduced eGFR over time [18]. Renal congestion, as a consequence of elevated central venous pressure present in patients with RHF, is characterized by renal edema, increased interstitial pressure, tubular compression, and intracapsular tamponade, which may further decrease renal perfusion pressure and eGFR [4]. Furthermore, activation of venous endothelium acts as a stimulus for release of inflammatory mediators, which causes structural glomerular and interstitial damage, sclerosis/fibrosis as well as functional abnormalities, such as diminished tubular reabsorption, proteinuria, and retention of salt and water [6]. During the progression of PH, repetitive episodes of subclinical acute kidney injury occur in a slow progressive degenerative process that predispose to the development of subsequent chronic kidney disease [19]. Sensitive markers of early kidney injury include L-type fatty acid-binding protein (L-FABP), neutrophil gelatinase-associated lipocalin (NGAL), and kidney injury molecule-1 (KIM-1) [20, 21]. In patients with RHF patients and acute kidney injury, deterioration of either organ function may conduce to a vicious circle leading to refractory congestive RHF [4]. Patients with acute-on-chronic renal injury have a narrow window for fluid management of venous congestion and are at high risk of worsening cardiorenal function and death, but the benefits of intensive decongestion may outweigh over time transient increase in serum creatinine or in tubular injury markers [22]. It is important to underline the OC between the pulmonary vasculature, the RV, and kidneys [6]. Kidneys are dependent on blood flow and perfusion pressure provided by the heart, and this one is dependent on the regulation of fluid homeostasis and of salt and water content by the kidneys. Furthermore, renal dysfunction may aggravate PH, because circulatory factors can be involved in pulmonary inflammation after renal injury [6]. To date, few data are available on the impact of targeted PAH therapies on renal function and only the phosphodiesterase type 5 inhibitor (sildenafil) demonstrated an improvement of kidney function [23].

29.2.3 Liver

The liver of patients with PH and RHF may be exposed to decreased arterial perfusion, hypoxemia, and venous congestion [4, 24]. Hepatic hypoperfusion may cause ischemic hepatitis, histologically characterized by centri-lobular necrosis. Laboratory findings are a rapid increase in serum amino-transferases (>20 times the upper level of normal) and lactate dehydrogenase. Serum bilirubin is only mildly elevated, but it can be significantly increased in cases of liver failure or secondary ischemic cholangiopathy. The majority of cases are reversible when the underlying cause is resolved, but a progressive liver dysfunction or an acute liver failure are also possible [24]. The risk of acute ischemic hepatitis is increased in case of chronic hepatic venous congestion due to preexisting RHF [25]. Chronic congestive hepatopathy, related to elevated right-sided filling pressures, may result in fibrosis or, rarely, in cardiac cirrhosis. The extent of hepatic fibrosis is associated with right atrial (RA) pressure and dilation, and RV dilation, thus correlating with the degree and severity of RHF [26]. In patients with precapillary PH, elevated level of a liver fibrosis marker, P4NP7S (7S domain of collagen type IV) is associated with higher central venous pressure, right-sided volume overload, and mortality [27]. Clinical features are enlarged and pulsating jugular veins, edema, jaundice, and ascites. Larger amounts of ascites in the absence of edema may indicate cardiac cirrhosis. Laboratory findings include elevated levels of γ-glutamyltransferase (GGT), alkaline phosphatase (ALP) and bilirubin, and normal or mildly elevated serum aminotransferases. Reduced serum albumin and impaired hepatic drug metabolism may be found in advanced cases [24]. Liver stiffness, evaluated by FibroScan technique, and elevated serum bilirubin levels are associated with RHF clinical severity and with an increased mortality risk [28, 29].

29.2.4 Gut and Bowel

Gut mucosa of PH and RHF patients may lose its barrier function, due to impaired arterial perfusion and venous congestion. Altered gut permeability results in bacterial translocation and endotoxinemia [30]. Venous congestion is probably the main determinant of leaky gut, and so diuretics can reduce endotoxin levels [31]. A gut–lung crosstalk has also been proposed. Bacterial translocation and endotoxinemia are consequences of RHF-related gut congestion, but at the same time, they exacerbate inflammation and pulmonary vascular remodeling. Lipopolysaccharide translocation from gut lumen to bloodstream activate pulmonary and systemic TLR4 (Toll-like receptor 4), which is associated with increased levels of soluble CD14, a marker of macrophage activation. Blood levels of lipopolysaccharide, TLR4, and soluble CD14 are elevated in patients with PAH [32]. Lastly, bowel congestion, due to elevated right-sided filling pressure, together with systemic inflammation contributes to gut dysfunction and then to development of cachexia [33].

29.2.5 Iron Homeostasis

Iron deficiency is common in patients with PAH, with prevalence ranging from 30% to 63%, independently of anticoagulation status [34]. Iron deficiency is associated with lower exercise capacity, worse hemodynamics, higher NT-proBNP levels, and increased mortality [34]. Enteric iron absorption is negatively regulated by hepcidin, a hormone released from liver in presence of an iron loading. Hepcidin levels were inappropriately elevated in patients with PAH, contributing so to iron deficiency [34]. Iron is a significant regulator of pulmonary vascular tone, and it has been demonstrated that in healthy individuals, an exaggerated hypoxic vasoconstrictive response related to iron deficiency can be corrected with intravenous iron supplementation [35]. Iron deficiency is also associated with reduced myoglobin, impaired mitochondrial oxidative capacity, and anemia, thereby limiting the aerobic capacity of muscle tissue and affecting myocardial metabolic substrates use through mitochondrial dysfunction [36]. Intravenous iron replacement in patients with iron deficiency and PAH improves exercise capacity and delays the time to the anaerobic threshold [37].

29.2.6 Thyroid Disease

Thyroid disease has a prevalence of about 20% in PAH patients. It is a predictor of poor prognosis, and subclinical hyper- or hypothyroidism is associated with an increased risk of incident atrial fibrillation [38, 39]. The prevalence of hypothyroidism in PAH is 10–24%, but data on the direct link between hypothyroidism and pulmonary circulation are limited [40]. Conversely, hyperthyroidism can lead to arrhythmias and can worsen RHF, increasing myocardial inotropism and so exacerbating RV dysfunction. In addition, hyperthyroidism may also exert direct remodeling or functional effects on pulmonary vasculature through enhanced catecholamine sensitivity, increased metabolism of intrinsic pulmonary vasodilators, and decreased metabolism of vasoconstrictors [41]. In patients with hyperthyroidism, Graves's disease antibody levels directly correlate with PAP [41].

29.2.7 Metabolic Syndrome and Diabetes

Metabolic syndrome is associated with loss of myocardial compliance and increased LV mass, leading to increased afterload and postcapillary PH. Patients with PAH and metabolic syndrome present reduced exercise capacity, higher functional class, and increased risk of mortality [42]. There is also a higher prevalence of diabetes in PAH patients and their association leads to higher mortality [43]. Insulin resistance and hyperglycemia, acting on pulmonary microcirculation, may modify the course of PH [44]. Insulin resistance is related to deficiency of the nuclear receptor PPARγ (peroxisome proliferator-activated receptor gamma), that are also reduced in patients with PH, and that are involved in regulation of endothelial cells and smooth muscle cells [45]. Hyperglycemia inhibits endothelial NO synthase and, promoting the liberation of reactive oxygen species and the activation of protein kinase C, leads to vasoconstriction and inflammation [44]. In addition, hyperglycemia induces RV fibrosis and ischemia through the expression of endothelin-1, platelet-derived growth factor, and TGF-β [44]. Similarly, insulin resistance induces cardiac fibroblasts to increase collagen production and myocardial fibrosis, promoting ischemia [46]. All these mechanisms eventually alter the RV/PA coupling.

29.2.8 Skeletal Muscles and Diaphragm

In PAH patients, the function of skeletal (including respiratory) muscles may be altered during exercise by reduced oxygen delivery related to RHF, but the strength of skeletal muscles may be impaired too, because of decreased maximal force generation [47]. Mechanisms of muscle dysfunction may be both systemic and local. Circulatory proinflammatory cytokines can lead to muscle fiber atrophy and impaired contractile function through proteolysis [48]. Reduced physical activity in PH, in the presence of elevated ventilatory demand, increases protein turnover and makes skeletal muscles susceptible to systemic factors, such as iron deficiency and reduced CO/oxygen delivery that contribute to impair aerobic muscle capacity [47].

29.2.9 Inflammation and Immune System

Inflammation may be involved in PAH pathophysiology or may be its consequence. Soluble inflammatory mediators and regulators of innate and adaptive immunity, secreted in response to PH-associated RV hypertrophy/dilation and kidney injury, may act locally or affect distant organs [6]. Elevated circulating levels of inflammatory mediators are predictive for survival [49]. PAH lesions contain pulmonary perivascular inflammatory infiltrates composed of T and B lymphocytes, mast cells, dendritic cells, and macrophages: both B and T cells contribute to a proinflammatory environment [50]. Activation, proliferation, and differentiation of B lymphocytes are promoted by the increased production of interleukin-1 and interleukin-6, while regulatory T-cells are dysfunctional in various forms of PAH [49, 51]. To date, it is still not clear if immune dysregulation may represent the cause or the effect of PAH.

29.2.10 Coagulation System and Thrombocytopenia

Increased plasma concentrations of pro-coagulative factors such as fibrinogen, von Willebrand factor, and plasminogen-activator inhibitor-1 have been described in patients with PAH and CTEPH [52]. Thrombi are commonly detected in the small pulmonary arteries in idiopathic PAH (iPAH) [53]. Current European guidelines don't recommend routine anticoagulation in PH, except for CTEPH, for which lifelong anticoagulation is strongly recommended [2]. Thrombocytopenia (platelet count $<150 \times 10^9/l$) has been reported in up to 20% of idiopathic PAH patients, commonly found in patients with portopulmonary hypertension as consequence of hypersplenism, and it seems to be related to disease severity [54]. Thrombocytopenia in IPAH may be related to pulmonary thrombotic microangiopathy. It is present in patients with PAH and hematological conditions or Eisenmenger syndrome, who have higher risk of thrombosis and bleeding due to thrombocytopenia and platelet dysfunction [55].

29.2.11 Autonomic Function and Peripheral Endothelial Function

Sympathetic and parasympathetic abnormalities and autonomic dysfunction may be disease modifiers in PAH patients. They can also occur in early stages of RHF and represent independent predictors of clinical deterioration [56]. Impairment of autonomous control reduces heart rate variability in RHF, which correlates with PAP in iPAH patients [57]. Lower adrenergic baroreflex sensitivity is associated with greater susceptibility to orthostatic hypotension, cerebral hypoperfusion, and syncope [58]. Sympathetic hyperactivity and electrophysiological cellular remodeling were associated with an increased incidence of atrial fibrillation and atrial flutter, both determinants of poor outcome in PAH [59]. Furthermore, in several studies, PAH patients display impaired peripheral endothelial function, assessed by measurement of brachial artery flow-mediated dilation or the peripheral arterial tone ratio [60].

29.2.12 Eyes

Open-angle glaucoma, retinal detachment, venous stasis retinopathy, ciliary detachment, and central retinal vein occlusion are reported in patients with PAH and RHF. It is possible that systemic venous congestion affecting eyes can cause choroidal and retinal venous stasis. The frequency and clinical relevance of such findings are unknown [61].

29.2.13 Cognitive Function, Depression, and Anxiety

Moderate-to-severe depression and anxiety are common in patients with PH and are associated with the severity of disease [62]. Impairment of cognitive function is also present, although there are no clear differences in disease severity [63]. It has been suggested that cognitive impairment may be related to reduced cerebral tissue oxygenation, but an interventional study has demonstrated that PAH therapies may improve cognitive function without change in cerebral tissue oxygenation [62]. In patients with CTEPH undergoing pulmonary endoarterectomy, a randomized trial showed no difference between deep hypothermic circulatory arrest and antegrade cerebral perfusion in terms of impact on cognitive function [64].

29.2.14 Sleep Apnea and Hypoxemia

In patients with PH, poor sleep quality is associated with worse functional status, reduced exercise capacity, poor quality of life and psychological disorders [65]. Sleep-disordered breathing is common and rates of obstructive sleep apnea vary from 10% to 50% [65]. Furthermore, hypoxemia may occur or worsen during the night, and it can be due to ventilation-perfusion mismatch, obstructive sleep apnea, or both [65]. The degree of nocturnal hypoxemia correlates with worse daytime PaO_2 and distal airways narrowing. There are insufficient data to evaluate prognostic effect of sleep-disordered breathing or nocturnal hypoxemia, but nocturnal oxygen therapy over 1 week may improve 6-min walking distance, nocturnal heart rate, and corrected QT interval [66].

29.3 Conclusion

RHF is the main consequence of PH, regardless of its etiology. Systemic venous congestion, impaired peripheral perfusion, and reduced systemic output, all related to RHF, can contribute together to alter multiple organ systems by mechanisms of organ crosstalk and a systemic pro-inflammatory state. The final result is an increasing morbidity and mortality in PH. It is crucial to recognize the systemic consequences of PH, often neglected and underestimated, because they represent other targets of treatment that can strongly impact the course and severity of the disease and provide an example of precision medicine in PH [4]. Therefore, the best management of PH requires a holistic, multidisciplinary approach with a strong collaboration between cardiologists and other specialists [2].

References

1. Hoeper MM, Humbert M, Souza R, Idrees M, Kawut SM, Sliwa-Hahnle K, et al. A global view of pulmonary hypertension. Lancet Respir Med. 2016;4(4):306–22.
2. Humbert M, Kovacs G, Hoeper MM, Badagliacca R, Berger RMF, Brida M, et al. 2022 ESC/ERS guidelines for the diagnosis and treatment of pulmonary hypertension. Eur Heart J. 2022;43(38):3618–731.
3. Rosenkranz S, Gibbs JS, Wachter R, De Marco T, Vonk-Noordegraaf A, Vachiéry JL. Left ventricular heart failure and pulmonary hypertension. Eur Heart J. 2016;37(12):942–54.
4. Rosenkranz S, Howard LS, Gomberg-Maitland M, Hoeper MM. Systemic consequences of pulmonary hypertension and right-sided heart failure. Circulation. 2020;141(8):678–93.
5. Lang RM, Badano LP, Mor-Avi V, Afilalo J, Armstrong A, Ernande L, et al. Recommendations for cardiac chamber quantification by echocardiography in adults: an update from the American Society of Echocardiography and the European Association of Cardiovascular Imaging. Eut Heart J Cardiovasc Imaging. 2015;16(3):233–70.
6. Husain-Syed F, McCullough PA, Birk HW, Renker M, Brocca A, Seeger W, Ronco C. Cardio-pulmonary-renal interaction – a multidisciplinary approach. J Am Coll Cardiol. 2015;65(22):2433–48.
7. Gan C, Lankhaar JW, Marcus JT, Westerhof N, Marques KM, Bronzwaer JG, et al. Impaired left ventricular filling due to right-to-left ventricular interaction in patients with pulmonary arterial hypertension. Am J Physiol Heart Circ Physiol. 2006;290(4):H1528–33.
8. Gorter TM, Obokata M, Reddy YNV, Melenovsky V, Borlaug BA. Exercise unmasks distinct pathophysiologic features in heart failure with preserved ejection fraction and pulmonary vascular disease. Eur Heart J. 2018;39(30):2825–35.
9. Tonelli AR, Plana JC, Heresi GA, Dweik RA. Prevalence and prognostic value of left ventricular diastolic dysfunction in idiopathic and heritable pulmonary arterial hypertension. Chest. 2012;141(6):1457–65.

10. Kishiki K, Singh A, Narang A, Gomberg-Maitland M, Goyal N, Maffessanti F, et al. Impact of severe pulmonary arterial hypertension on the left heart and prognostic implications. J Am Soc Echocardiogr. 2019;32(9):1128–37.
11. Galiè N, Saia F, Palazzini M, Manes A, Russo V, Bacchi Reggiani ML, et al. Left main coronary artery compression in patients with pulmonary arterial hypertension and angina. J Am Coll Cardiol. 2017;69(23):2808–17.
12. Zyłkowska J, Kurzyna M, Florczyk M, Burakowska B, Grzegorczyk F, Burakowski J, et al. Pulmonary artery dilatation correlates with the risk of unexpected death in chronic arterial or thromboembolic pulmonary hypertension. Chest. 2012;142(6):1406–16.
13. Manders E, Bogaard HJ, Handoko ML, van de Veerdonk MC, Keogh A, Westerhof N, et al. Contractile dysfunction of left ventricular cardiomyocytes in patients with pulmonary arterial hypertension. J Am Coll Cardiol. 2014;64(1):28–37.
14. Tudorache I, Sommer W, Kühn C, Wiesner O, Hadem J, Fühner T, et al. Lung transplantation for severe pulmonary hypertension awake extracorporeal membrane oxygenation for postoperative left ventricular remodelling. Transplantation. 2015;99:451–8.
15. Shah SJ, Thenappan T, Rich S, Tian L, Archer SL, Gomberg-Maitland M. Association of serum creatinine with abnormal hemodynamics and mortality in pulmonary arterial hypertension. Circulation. 2008;117:2475–83.
16. Benza RL, Miller DP, Gomberg-Maitland M, Frantz RP, Foreman AJ, Coffey CS, et al. Predicting survival in pulmonary arterial hypertension: insights from the registry to evaluate early and long-term pulmonary arterial hypertension disease management (REVEAL). Circulation. 2010;122(2):164–72.
17. Chakinala MM, Coyne DW, Benza RL, Frost AE, McGoon MD, Hartline BK, et al. Impact of declining renal function on outcomes in pulmonary arterial hypertension: a REVEAL registry analysis. J Heart Lung Transplant. 2018;37(6):696–705.
18. Bitker L, Sens F, Payet C, Turquier S, Duclos A, Cottin V, Juillard L. Presence of kidney disease as an outcome predictor in patients with pulmonary arterial hypetension. Am J Nephrol. 2018;47(2):134–43.
19. Haase M, Kellum JA, Ronco C. Subclinical AKI – an emerging syndrome with important consequences. Nat Rev Nephrol. 2012;8(12):735–9.
20. Torregrosa I, Montoliu C, Urios A, Andrés-Costa MJ, Giménez-Garzó C, Juan I, et al. Urinary KIM-1, NGAL and L-FABP for the diagnosis of AKI in patients with acute coronary syndrome or heart failure undergoing coronary angiography. Heart Vessel. 2015;30(6):703–11.
21. Ko GJ, Grigoryev DN, Linfert D, Jang HR, Watkins T, Cheadle C, et al. Transcriptional analysis of kidneys during repair from AKI reveals possible roles for NGAL and KIM-1 as biomarkers of AKI-to- CKD transition. Am J Physiol Renal Physiol. 2010;298(6):F1472–83.
22. Rao VS, Ahmad T, Brisco-Bacik MA, Bonventre JV, Wilson FP, Siew ED, et al. Renal effects of intensive volume removal in heart failure patients with preexisting worsening renal function. Circ Heart Fail. 2019;12(6):e005552.
23. Webb DJ, Vachiery JL, Hwang LJ, Maurey JO. Sildenafil improves renal function in patients with pulmonary arterial hypertension. Br J Clin Pharmacol. 2015;80(2):235–41.
24. Samsky MD, Patel CB, DeWald TA, Smith AD, Felker GM, Rogers JG, Hernandez AF. Cardiohepatic interactions in heart failure: an overview and clinical implications. J Am Coll Cardiol. 2013;61(24):2397–405.
25. Fuhrmann V, Kneidinger N, Herkner H, Heinz G, Nikfardjam M, Bojic A, et al. Hypoxic hepatitis: underlying conditions and risk factors for mortality in critically ill patients. Intensive Care Med. 2009;35(8):1397–405.
26. Dai DF, Swanson PE, Krieger EV, Liou IW, Carithers RL, Yeh MM. Congestive hepatic fibrosis score: a novel histologic assessment of clinical severity. Mod Pathol. 2014;27(12):1552–8.
27. Yoshihisa A, Kimishima Y, Kiko T, Sato Y, Watanabe S, Kanno Y, et al. Liver fibrosis marker, 7S domain of collagen type IV, in patients with pre-capillary pulmonary hypertension. Int J Cardiol. 2018;258:269–74.

28. Taniguchi T, Ohtani T, Kioka H, Tsukamoto Y, Onishi T, Nakamoto K, et al. Liver stiffness reflecting right-sided filling pressure can predict adverse outcomes in patients with heart failure. JACC Cardiovasc Imaging. 2019;12(6):955–64.
29. Takeda Y, Takeda Y, Tomimoto S, Tani T, Narita H, Kimura G. Bilirubin as a prognostic marker in patients with pulmonary arterial hypertension. BMC Pulm Med. 2010;10:22.
30. Sundaram V, Fang JC. Gastrointestinal and liver issues in heart failure. Circulation. 2016;133(17):1696–703.
31. Niebauer J, Volk HD, Kemp M, Dominguez M, Schumann RR, Rauchhaus M, et al. Endotoxin and immune activation in chronic heart failure: a prospective cohortstudy. Lancet. 1999;353(9167):1838–42.
32. Ranchoux B, Bigorgne A, Hautefort A, Girerd B, Sitbon O, Montani D, et al. Gut-lung connection in pulmonary arterial hypertension. Am J Respir Cell Mol Biol. 2017;56(3):402–5.
33. Valentova M, von Haehling S, Bauditz J, Doehner W, Ebner N, Bekfani T, et al. Intestinal congestion and right ventricular dysfunction: a link with appetite loss, inflammation, and cachexia in chronic heart failure. Eur Heart J. 2016;37(21):1684–91.
34. Rhodes CJ, Howard LS, Busbridge M, Ashby D, Kondili E, Gibbs JS, et al. Iron deficiency and raised hepcidin in idiopathic pulmonary arterial hypertension: clinical prevalence, outcomes, and mechanistic insights. J Am Coll Cardiol. 2011;58(3):300–9.
35. Frise MC, Cheng HY, Nickol AH, Curtis MK, Pollard KA, Roberts DJ, et al. Clinical iron deficiency disturbs normal human responses to hypoxia. J Clin Invest. 2016;126(6):2139–50.
36. Melenovsky V, Petrak J, Mracek T, Benes J, Borlaug BA, Nuskova H, et al. Myocardial iron content and mitochondrial function in human heart failure: a direct tissue analysis. Eur J Heart Fail. 2017;19(4):522–30.
37. Viethen T, Gerhardt F, Dumitrescu D, Knoop-Busch S, ten Freyhaus H, Rudolph TK, et al. Ferric carboxymaltose improves exercise capacity and quality of life in patients with pulmonary arterial hypertension and iron deficiency: a pilot study. Int J Cardiol. 2014;175(2):233–9.
38. Chu JW, Kao PN, Faul JL, Doyle RL. High prevalence of autoimmune thyroid disease in pulmonary arterial hypertension. Chest. 2002;122(5):1668–73.
39. Baumgartner C, da Costa BR, Collet TH, Feller M, Floriani C, Bauer DC, et al. Thyroid studies collaboration. Thyroid function within the normal range, subclinical hypothyroidism, and the risk of atrial fibrillation. Circulation. 2017;136(22):2100–16.
40. Curnock AL, Dweik RA, Higgins BH, Saadi HF, Arroliga AC. High prevalence of hypothyroidism in patients with primary pulmonary hypertension. Am J Med Sci. 1999;318(5):289–92.
41. Osmak-Tizon L, Poussier M, Cottin Y, Rochette L. Non-genomic actions of thyroid hormones: molecular aspects. Arch Cardiovasc Dis. 2014;107(4):207–11.
42. Poms AD, Turner M, Farber HW, Meltzer LA, McGoon MD. Comorbid conditions and outcomes in patients with pulmonary arterial hypertension: a REVEAL registry analysis. Chest. 2013;144(1):169–76.
43. Pugh ME, Robbins IM, Rice TW, West J, Newman JH, Hemnes AR. Unrecognized glucose intolerance is common in pulmonary arterial hypertension. J Heart Lung Transplant. 2011;30(8):904–11.
44. Grinnan D, Farr G, Fox A, Sweeney L. The role of hyperglycemia and insulin resistance in the development and progression of pulmonary arterial hypertension. J Diabetes Res. 2016;2016:2481659.
45. Ameshima S, Golpon H, Cool CD, Chan D, Vandivier RW, Gardai SJ, et al. Peroxisome proliferator-activated receptor gamma (PPARgamma) expression is decreased in pulmonary hypertension and affects endothelial cell growth. Circ Res. 2003;92(10):1162–9.
46. Arnold N, Koppula PR, Gul R, Luck C, Pulakat L. Regulation of cardiac expression of the diabetic marker microRNA miR-29. PLoS One. 2014;9(7):e103284.
47. Manders E, Rain S, Bogaard HJ, Handoko ML, Stienen GJ, Vonk- Noordegraaf A, et al. The striated muscles in pulmonary arterial hypertension: adaptations beyond the right ventricle. Eur Respir J. 2015;46(3):832–42.

48. de Man FS, van Hees HW, Handoko ML, Niessen HW, Schalij I, Humbert M, et al. Diaphragm muscle fiber weakness in pulmonary hypertension. Am J Respir Crit Care Med. 2011;183(10):1411–8.
49. Soon E, Holmes AM, Treacy CM, Doughty NJ, Southgate L, Machado RD, et al. Elevated levels of inflammatory cytokines predict survival in idiopathic and familial pulmonary arterial hypertension. Circulation. 2010;122(9):920–7.
50. Huertas A, Perros F, Tu L, Cohen-Kaminsky S, Montani D, Dorfmüller P, et al. Immune dysregulation and endothelial dysfunction in pulmonary arterial hypertension: a complex interplay. Circulation. 2014;129(12):1332–40.
51. Huertas A, Phan C, Bordenave J, Tu L, Thuillet R, Le Hiress M, et al. Regulatory T cell dysfunction in idiopathic, heritable and connective tissue-associated pulmnary arterial hypertension. Chest. 2016;149(6):1482–93.
52. Huber K, Beckmann R, Frank H, Kneussl M, Mlczoch J, Binder BR. Fibrinogen, t-PA, and PAI-1 plasma levels in patients with pulmonary hypertension. Am J Respir Crit Care Med. 1994;150(4):929–33.
53. Stacher E, Graham BB, Hunt JM, Gandjeva A, Groshong SD, McLaughlin VV, et al. Modern age pathology of pulmonary arterial hypertension. Am J Respir Crit Care Med. 2012;186:261–72.
54. Mojadidi MK, Goodman-Meza D, Eshtehardi P, Pamerla M, Msaouel P, Roberts SC, et al. Thrombocytopenia is an independent predictor of mortality in pulmonary hypertension. Heart Lung. 2014;43(6):569–73.
55. Remková A, Šimková I, ValkoviÊová T, Kaldarárová M. Platelet abnormalities in adults with severe pulmonary arterial hypertension related to congenital heart defects (Eisenmenger syndrome). Blood Coagul Fibrinolysis. 2016;27(8):925–9.
56. Maron BA, Leopold JA. Emerging concepts in the molecular basis of pulmonary arterial hypertension: part II: neurohormonal signaling contributes to the pulmonary vascular and right ventricular pathophenotype of pulmonary arterial hypertension. Circulation. 2015;131(23):2079–91.
57. Yi HT, Hsieh YC, Wu TJ, Huang JL, Lin WW, Liang KW, et al. Heart rate variability parameters and ventricular arrhythmia correlate with pulmonary arterial pressure in adult patients with idiopathic pulmonary arterial hypertension. Heart Lung. 2014;43(6):534–40.
58. Mar PL, Nwazue V, Black BK, Biaggioni I, Diedrich A, Paranjape SY, et al. Valsalva maneuver in pulmonary arterial hypertension: susceptibility to syncope and autonomic dysfunction. Chest. 2016;149(5):1252–60.
59. Zhao Q, Deng H, Jiang X, Dai Z, Wang X, Wang X, et al. Effects of intrinsic and extrinsic cardiac nerves on atrial arrhythmia in experimental pulmonary artery hypertension. Hypertension. 2015;66(5):1042–9.
60. Perros F, Ranchoux B, Izikki M, Bentebbal S, Happé C, Antigny F, et al. Nebivolol for improving endothelial dysfunction, pulmonary vascular remodeling, and right heart function in pulmonary hypertension. J Am Coll Cardiol. 2015;65(7):668–80.
61. Yang S, Jeong J, Kim JG, Yoon YH. Progressive venous stasis retinopathy and open-angle glaucoma associated with primary pulmonary hypertension. Ophthalmic Surg Lasers Imaging. 2006;37(3):230–3.
62. Somaini G, Stamm A, Müller-Mottet S, Hasler E, Keusch S, Hildenbrand FF, et al. Disease-targeted treatment improves cognitive function in patients with precapillary pulmonary hypertension. Respiration. 2015;90(5):376–83.
63. White J, Hopkins RO, Glissmeyer EW, Kitterman N, Elliott CG. Cognitive, emotional, and quality of life outcomes in patients with pulmonary arterial hypertension. Respir Res. 2006;7(1):55.

64. Vuylsteke A, Sharples L, Charman G, Kneeshaw J, Tsui S, Dunning J, et al. Circulatory arrest versus cerebral perfusion during pulmonary endarterectomy surgery (PEACOG): a randomised controlled trial. Lancet. 2011;378:1379–87.
65. Jilwan FN, Escourrou P, Garcia G, Jaïs X, Humbert M, Roisman G. High occurrence of hypoxemic sleep respiratory disorders in precapillary pulmonary hypertension and mechanisms. Chest. 2013;143(1):47–55.
66. Ulrich S, Keusch S, Hildenbrand FF, Lo Cascio C, Huber LC, Tanner FC, et al. Effect of nocturnal oxygen and acetazolamide on exercise performance in patients with pre-capillary pulmonary hypertension and sleep-disturbed breathing: randomized, double-blind, cross-over trial. Eur Heart J. 2015;36(10):615–23.

The Role of Osteopontin in Kidneys and Respiratory Failure

30

Francesco Cundari, Marco Monfroni, Pietro Dallapiccola, and Silvia De Rosa

30.1 Introduction

Osteopontin (OPN) is a versatile glycoprotein involved in numerous physiological and pathological processes within the human body. First identified for its role in bone metabolism, OPN has since been recognized as a key regulator of immune responses, wound healing, and tissue remodeling across various organ systems, including the kidneys and lungs. Its importance stems from its ability to interact with cellular receptors such as integrins and CD44, mediating inflammatory processes and promoting cellular survival under stress conditions [1] (Fig. 30.1).

The kidneys play a critical role in maintaining homeostasis by filtering waste products from the blood and regulating fluid balance [2]. They are also crucial in controlling electrolyte levels, blood pressure, and red blood cell production [3]. However, in pathological states such as acute kidney injury (AKI) or chronic kidney disease (CKD), these functions can be impaired, leading to significant morbidity [2, 3]. The respiratory system, similarly, ensures gas exchange to supply oxygen and remove carbon dioxide. It is particularly vulnerable to secondary damage from other organ failures, such as the kidneys, due to the interconnectedness of systemic inflammation and fluid overload, which can lead to acute respiratory distress or failure [4].

F. Cundari · M. Monfroni
Department of Surgical, Medical, Molecular Pathology and Critical Care Medicine, University of Pisa, Pisa, Italy
e-mail: f.cundari@studenti.unipi.it; m.monfroni@studenti.unipi.it

P. Dallapiccola
Centre for Medical Sciences – CISMed, University of Trento, Trento, Italy
e-mail: pietro.dallapiccola@studenti.unitn.it

S. De Rosa (✉)
Centre for Medical Sciences-CISMed, University of Trento, Trento, Italy
e-mail: silvia.derosa@unitn.it

D. Battaglini et al. (eds.), *Organ System Crosstalk in Critical Illness*,
https://doi.org/10.1007/978-3-032-01024-7_30

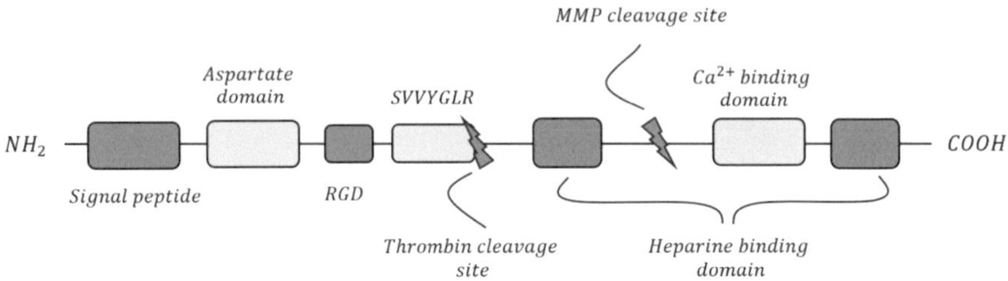

Fig. 30.1 Schematic representation of osteopontin (OPN) structure with functional domains and cleavage sites. This diagram illustrates the structural domains and cleavage sites of OPN, showing the arrangement from the N-terminus (NH_2) to the C-terminus (COOH). Key functional regions include the signal peptide, aspartate domain, RGD sequence, thrombin and MMP cleavage sites, Ca^{2+} binding domain, and heparin binding domain

Table 30.1 Functions of osteopontin (OPN) in various biological processes

Biological process	Role of OPN	Key interactions
Bone metabolism	Links bone cells to the extracellular matrix	Integrins, CD44
Immune response	Modulates immune cell migration and survival	CD44, integrins
Wound healing	Promotes tissue repair	–
Tissue remodeling	Aids in matrix formation and cell adhesion	Integrins, RGD domain
Inflammatory regulation	Modulates cytokine release and immune cell activity	CD44, IL-1β, TNF-α, IL-17A, etc.

Notes: OPN, Osteopontin; CD44, Cluster of Differentiation 44; RGD, Arginine-Glycine-Aspartic acid sequence IL, Interleukin; IL-1β, Interleukin-1 beta; IL-17A, Interleukin-17A; TNF-α, Tumor Necrosis Factor alpha.

This interdependence between the kidneys and lungs highlights the relevance of OPN as it plays a central role in mediating the inflammation and damage that can occur in both organs during such failures [1]. Understanding the role of OPN in these contexts can provide insight into potential therapeutic interventions (Table 30.1).

30.2 Osteopontin and Its Biological Role

OPN is a multifunctional protein that plays crucial roles in various biological processes, influencing both physiological and pathological conditions. As a pleiotropic protein, it exerts multiple effects and is produced by diverse cell types, including endothelial cells, epithelial cells, osteoclasts, and activated immune cells such as macrophages and T cells. The protein's name, derived from "osteo" (bone) and "pontin" (bridge), reflects its role in linking bone cells to the bone extracellular matrix [5–7]. The OPN gene, also known as the secreted phosphoprotein 1 (SPP1) gene, encodes a protein comprising approximately 314 amino acids, structured into seven highly conserved exons [8]. The functional complexity of OPN is enhanced by multiple interacting domains and protease cleavage sites. These include an arginine-glycine-aspartic (RGD) domain, a

Table 30.2 Regulatory mechanisms and modifications of osteopontin (OPN)

Regulatory factor	Effect on OPN expression	Post-translational modification	Functional implications
Protein kinase C (PKC)	Suppresses OPN release	Phosphorylation	Affects protein stability and function
Glucose, glucocorticoids, vitamin D	Increases transcription and release	Glycosylation, transglutamination	Alters binding interactions and stability
Cytokines (IL-1β, IL-6, TGF-β)	Upregulates OPN transcription	Sulfation	Modulates immune response
Alternative splicing	Produces five isoforms	–	Isoform diversity in immune response
Translation variation	Produces sOPN and iOPN forms	–	sOPN for extracellular signaling, iOPN in immune regulation

Notes: PKC, Protein kinase C; OPN, Osteopontin; IL, Interleukin; IL-1β, Interleukin-1 beta; IL-6, Interleukin-6; TGF-β, Transforming Growth Factor beta; sOPN, secreted Osteopontin; iOPN, intracellular Osteopontin.

serine-valine-valine-tyrosine-glutamate-leucine-arginine (SVVYGLR) domain, binding sites for heparin and thrombin, a calcium-binding site, and specific sequences that interact with CD44 variants and integrin receptors [5, 6] (Fig. 30.1; Table 30.2).

OPN synthesis is regulated by several factors. Protein kinase C (PKC), for example, suppresses OPN release, while factors such as glucose, glucocorticoids, vitamin D, and certain cytokines—including interleukin-1β, IL-6, TGF-β, IL-17A, TNF-α, and interferon-stimulating elements—increase its transcription and release [5, 9, 10]. These regulatory mechanisms underscore OPN's complexity in cellular signaling and function. Following transcription, OPN undergoes several post-translational modifications, including sulfation, glycosylation, transglutamination, and, most prominently, phosphorylation [11]. These modifications add further complexity, contributing to the protein's functional diversity and its presence in different molecular weights, ranging from 44 to 75 kDa [5, 12]. Alternative splicing of the SPP1 gene produces five isoforms of varying lengths (including a full-length and other shorter variant missing certain exons), while alternative translation of the full gene generates two primary isoforms: a secreted form (sOPN) and an intracellular form (iOPN). While research has largely focused on sOPN, evidence increasingly suggests that iOPN plays vital roles, especially in regulating immune responses to infections. However, additional research is needed to fully elucidate iOPN's functions and implications [12]. In summary, osteopontin is a critical protein with wide-ranging roles in bone biology, immune responses, and beyond, highlighting its potential as both a biomarker and a therapeutic target in various diseases.

30.3 Role of OPN in Kidney Structure and Function

OPN is a multifunctional glycoprotein that takes part in both physiological and pathological processes in the kidney. It is synthesized in the thick ascending limb of the loops of Henle and in the collecting duct epithelium [13]. One of the main roles of osteopontin in the kidney is to modulate the inflammatory response. By binding to integrins, particularly with CD44, OPN triggers a sequence of intracellular signals that promote the migration and activation of immune cells such as T, B, natural killer (NK), macrophages, and Kupffer cells [14]. It has been observed that during kidney injury, OPN levels increase in both blood and urine, indicating its role in the local inflammatory response [15]. Moreover, OPN in kidney structure and function reduces cellular apoptosis (via AQP1), and its ability to attract macrophages, as well as to stimulate TGF-β activity and collagen I and IV deposition, suggests that OPN has profibrotic properties apoptosis, and its ability to attract macrophages, as well as stimulating TGF-β activity and collagen I and IV deposition, suggests that OPN has profibrotic properties [16].

30.4 OPN in Acute Kidney Injury (AKI) and Chronic Kidney Disease (CKD)

AKI is a common condition in critically ill patients, often lately diagnosed due to difficulties in early identification with common renal function markers such as creatinine or urine output [17]. OPN has been proposed as a biomarker to help identify these patients early. A study by Lorenzen's group [18] observed that plasma concentrations of OPN in critically ill patients were higher in those with more advanced renal injury, both acute and chronic, and that these values remained elevated in patients that had become dependent on renal replacement therapy (RRT). Interestingly, an association was found between OPN levels and 28-day mortality, but its usefulness as a surrogate for GFR has not been demonstrated in AKI conditions, unlike in CKD patients [19]. More recently, the measurements of OPN in patients at risk of developing sepsis did not show a significant difference in this marker's concentration between those patients with renal injury and those without [20], More recently, measurements of OPN in patients at risk of developing sepsis, AKI, and CKD did not show a significant difference in OPN concentrations between patients with renal injury and those without, leaving open the question of whether the increase in OPN levels is a consequence of AKI or a causative factor. However, another study on a population with advanced AKI observed significantly higher osteopontin concentrations in AKI patients ± 13.64 ng/mL, p 0.001), particularly in non-survivors the increase in OPN levels a consequence of AKI or a causative factor is. However, another study on a population with advanced acute renal injury observed higher osteopontin concentrations in AKI patients (395 ± 197.49 ng/mL vs. 48.74 ± 13.64 ng/mL, $p < 0.001$), and in non-survivors [16, 21].

While the role of OPN in intensive care settings remains unclear, its role in inflammatory processes, regardless of etiology, is certain [21, 22]. One of the most common mechanisms of renal injury in hospitalized patients is related to hypoperfusion, particularly through ischemia/reperfusion damage. Preclinical studies in this context are also conflicting: some have shown that in OPN-knockout mice, ischemia-reperfusion injury is reduced due to decreased NK cells infiltration in the kidney, which are important mediators of renal tubular cell apoptosis [23, 24]. Indeed, Persy et al. demonstrated the profibrotic role of OPN in renal pathophysiology, showing reduced collagen production 12 weeks after ischemia-reperfusion injury induction in OPN-knockout mice compared to wild-type controls [24].

Conversely, another study observed a negative role of OPN in protecting the kidney against ischemia, demonstrating that mice with targeted deletion of the osteopontin gene have an enhanced sensitivity to acute renal ischemia (evaluated by the retention of BUN and creatinine) [25]. These differences could be explained by different ischemia models and/or different methods of OPN gene knockout [24].

In the case of AKI, data are still conflicting and further studies are certainly needed, but in the context of chronic kidney disease, the role of OPN is more established. In CKD, persistent expression of OPN supports the inflammatory process and provokes fibrosis development, the central drivers in disease progression. OPN promotes fibroblast proliferation and their transformation into myofibroblasts, responsible for extracellular matrix production. This fibrotic response leads to a gradual reduction of functional renal tissue, contributing to the gradual decline in renal function. Moreover, serum OPN levels in CKD patients inversely correlate with GFR values and directly with the albumin/creatinine ratio [19, 26]. This makes OPN a marker of disease progression in CKD and opens the door to therapeutic strategies aimed at reducing its levels to mitigate renal fibrosis [26]. OPN levels are elevated in various chronic kidney diseases; among these, diabetic nephropathy, being a common outcome, is an important condition to investigate. Due to the fact that albuminuria, traditionally used to assess renal involvement, has limitations in recognizing early renal damage [27], osteopontin could bridge this gap, serving as an effective marker for disease progression [14].

30.5 Pathophysiology of OPN in Kidney Diseases

OPN is a protein that exerts several functions in the kidney. Firstly, it seems to have a role in the embryogenesis of renal tubules, while in developed kidneys, it participates in tissue inflammatory response and kidney stone formation. In fact, one of OPN's main roles in renal physiology is its involvement in nephrolithiasis. OPN can inhibit the formation, growth, and aggregation of calcium oxalate crystals. However, there are contrasting data since some studies show that OPN might promote kidney stone formation too. This dual role is supported by observations that urinary OPN levels are often lower in patients with kidney stones compared to healthy individuals, which could suggest that the reduction in urinary OPN might be due to its incorporation into stone matrices [12].

OPN is also implicated in renal damage and inflammation. OPN expression recruits not only macrophages but also T and B cells, triggering the local inflammatory response [12]. In this context, OPN seems to have a dual role: on the one hand, it appears to protect host cells by activating intracellular signals that reduce apoptosis and protect them from reactive species by inhibiting iNOS [28], allowing cells to repair damage caused by toxic or ischemic insults. On the other hand, it has been observed that OPN can support macrophage activity and the inflammatory response in renal tissue, perpetuating chronic inflammation and fibrosis, particularly in chronic kidney disease [29].

30.6 Therapeutic Implications

Given the role of OPN in various pathological conditions, from inflammatory states to tumors, the possibility of blocking the biological signals triggered by this protein is attractive in a therapeutic context. Although many data still derive from preclinical studies, this strategy appears promising. Inhibiting its expression using silencing RNA or molecules capable of preventing the binding between OPN and integrins has shown reduced neoplastic proliferation and migration in melanoma and prostate cancer models [30, 31].

In the context of renal diseases, blocking OPN could prevent ischemia-reperfusion injury: for example, in mice in which OPN-mediated signaling was blocked through genetic knockout techniques or anti-OPN antibodies, results showed reduced local NK cell infiltration, less local cytotoxic damage, and faster functional recovery following this type of injury [15, 25]. Further studies found out a reduction in renal damage related to the effects of angiotensin II in knockout mice compared to wild-type controls [32]. Although studies are still far from clinical practice, diabetic nephropathy could be an interesting field of application since individuals with high OPN levels develop diabetic nephropathy more frequently [26]. Given that OPN also contributes to healing processes, blocking it may pose challenges, but in patients with rheumatoid arthritis, although not effective, OPN inhibition appeared safe [33].

30.7 Interaction Between Kidney Disease and Respiratory Failure Mediated by OPN

Different organs, anatomically separated, can communicate with each other through neurohormonal and cellular signals. This mechanism is called organ crosstalk and is essential in maintaining the physiological activities of organs, but it has significant repercussions in the case of mono−/multiorgan pathologies [34]. Chronic or acute kidney damage thus affects the functions of various organs, including the lungs. Kidney damage results in reduced clearance of soluble substances present in the plasma, which particularly causes damage in the lungs due to its extensive capillary network and the high susceptibility of this organ to fluid overload [35, 36].The main mediators of this interaction are IL6, TNFa, IL 8, and T lymphocytes [36]. OPN also seems to play a role in this interaction. To evaluate the role of OPN in the organ crosstalk between the kidney and lungs, a recent study [37] used murine models in which acute lung injury (ALI) was induced because of ischemic damage. This study concluded that OPN released from kidney tubules damaged by ischemic insult, interacting with CD44 receptors at the lung level, induces the inflammatory damage typical of ALI as observed in the bronchoalveolar lavage (BAL) performed days after the induction of AKI. The use of OPN-neutralizing antibodies was associated with a reduced concentration of neutrophils and interstitial macrophages in the lung, while ALI did not develop in OPN-knockout mice. Even endothelial vascular permeability, a paradigmatic sign of ALI, does not occur in the absence of the OPN gene, given the maintenance of tight junctions in these mice [37]. Additionally, the same study observed that the transplantation of kidneys with ischemia-reperfusion injury into healthy mice resulted in increased OPN in the transplanted animals, leading to the development of ALI; the damage did not develop if the ischemia–/reperfusion-injured kidney came from OPN-knockout mice [37].Transplantation of a wild-type kidney into OPN-knockout mice led to an increase in OPN levels in the knockout mice, indicating that OPN was synthesized by the transplanted kidney. Another interesting finding from this experiment was the evaluation of OPN as a sufficient mediator for the development of AKI-ALI. Investigators induced moderate AKI by reducing the ischemia time [37]. BUN levels were lower compared to mice with severe AKI, as were circulating OPN levels. It was observed that exogenous OPN injection resulted in the development of AKI-ALI, which otherwise did not develop. Infusion of OPN in healthy mice did not produce any organ changes. Thus, OPN is a key factor in the development of AKI-ALI, although it is not the only actor, as an underlying functional alteration of AKI is required [37].

In vivo studies in intensive care patients showed that serum OPN levels were associated with increased mortality and longer days of ventilation [21]. Although promising, studies remain at a preclinical level but open up interesting opportunities for modulating lung damage or damage to other organs following primary renal damage, within the context of organ crosstalk.

30.8 Conclusion

In conclusion, OPN emerges as a pivotal factor in the complex interplay between kidney function and respiratory health, particularly in conditions such as AKI and CKD. Through its ability to modulate immune responses, reduce apoptosis, and influence fibrosis, OPN contributes significantly to the progression of kidney diseases. Its potential role as a biomarker in early diagnosis and disease progression monitoring further underscores its clinical relevance. Moreover, the phenomenon of organ crosstalk, where kidney damage influences lung function, highlights the broader systemic implications of OPN's activity. Research into OPN's role in acute lung injury following renal damage opens promising avenues for therapeutic interventions that target this protein. Although much of the data is still preclinical, inhibiting OPN could offer new strategies for mitigating both renal and respiratory failures. However, further studies are essential to fully understand its dual role in both protecting and perpetuating tissue damage and inflammation.

References

1. Lund SA, Giachelli CM, Scatena M. The role of osteopontin in inflammatory processes. J Cell Commun Signal. 2009;3(3–4):311–22.
2. Devarajan P. The current state of the art in acute kidney injury. Front Pediatr. 2020;8:70.
3. Basile DP, Anderson MD, Sutton TA. Pathophysiology of acute kidney injury. In: Prakash YS, editor. Comprehensive physiology [internet]. 1st ed. Wiley; 2012. [citato 3 maggio 2024]. p. 1303–53. Disponibile su: https://onlinelibrary.wiley.com/doi/10.1002/cphy.c110041.
4. Doi K, Ishizu T, Fujita T, Noiri E. Lung injury following acute kidney injury: kidney-lung crosstalk. Clin Exp Nephrol. 2011;15(4):464–70.

5. Icer MA, Gezmen-Karadag M. The multiple functions and mechanisms of osteopontin. Clin Biochem. 2018;59:17–24.
6. Kumari A, Kashyap D, Garg VK. Osteopontin in cancer. In: Advances in clinical chemistry [internet]. Elsevier; 2024. [citato 27 ottobre 2024]. p. 87–110. Disponibile su: https://linkinghub.elsevier.com/retrieve/pii/S0065242323001105.
7. Franzén A, Heinegård D. Isolation and characterization of two sialoproteins present only in bone calcified matrix. Biochem J. 1985;232(3):715–24.
8. Cao DX. Osteopontin as potential biomarker and therapeutic target in gastric and liver cancers. WJG. 2012;18(30):3923.
9. Liu W-L, Zhang H, Zheng Y, Wang H-T, Chen F-H, Xu L, et al. Expression and regulation of osteopontin in chronic rhinosinusitis with nasal polyps. Clin Exp Allergy. 2015;45(2):414–22.
10. Cai M, Bompada P, Atac D, Laakso M, Groop L, De Marinis Y. Epigenetic regulation of glucose-stimulated osteopontin (OPN) expression in diabetic kidney. Biochem Biophys Res Commun. 2016;469(1):108–13.
11. Jono S, Peinado C, Giachelli CM. Phosphorylation of Osteopontin is required for inhibition of vascular smooth muscle cell calcification. J Biol Chem. 2000;275(26):20197–203.
12. Jia Q, Huang Z, Wang G, Sun X, Wu Y, Yang B, et al. Osteopontin: an important protein in the formation of kidney stones. Front Pharmacol. 2022;13:1036423.
13. Imig JD. Osteopontin regulates phosphate solubility to prevent mineral aggregates in CKD. Kidney360. 2022;3(9):1477–9.
14. Sinha SK, Mellody M, Carpio MB, Damoiseaux R, Nicholas SB. Osteopontin as a biomarker in chronic kidney disease. Biomedicine. 2023;11(5):1356.
15. de Borst MH, Carrero JJ. Will osteopontin bridge the gap towards clinical application in chronic kidney disease? Nephrol Dial Transplant. 2023;38(6):1352–4.
16. Varalakshmi B, Kiranmyai VS, Aparna B, Ram R, Rao PVLNS, Kumar VS. Plasma osteopontin levels in patients with acute kidney injury requiring dialysis: a study in a tertiary care institute in South India. Int Urol Nephrol. 2020;52(5):917–21.
17. Ostermann M, Chang RWS. Acute kidney injury in the intensive care unit according to RIFLE. Crit Care Med. 2007;35(8):1837–43; quiz 1852.
18. Lorenzen JM, Hafer C, Faulhaber-Walter R, Kümpers P, Kielstein JT, Haller H, et al. Osteopontin predicts survival in critically ill patients with acute kidney injury. Nephrol Dial Transplant. 2011;26(2):531–7.
19. Lorenzen J, Krämer R, Kliem V, Bode-Boeger SM, Veldink H, Haller H, et al. Circulating levels of osteopontin are closely related to glomerular filtration rate and cardiovascular risk markers in patients with chronic kidney disease. Eur J Clin Invest. 2010;40(4):294–300.
20. Kul'skiĭ LA, Potapchenko NG, Savluk OS. Adaptation of Escherichia coli to silver. Mikrobiol Zh (1978). 1986;48(6):21–4.
21. Roderburg C, Benz F, Cardenas DV, Lutz M, Hippe HJ, Luedde T, et al. Persistently elevated osteopontin serum levels predict mortality in critically ill patients. Crit Care. 2015;19(1):271.
22. Vaschetto R, Nicola S, Olivieri C, Boggio E, Piccolella F, Mesturini R, et al. Serum levels of osteopontin are increased in SIRS and sepsis. Intensive Care Med. 2008;34(12):2176–84.
23. Zhang D. Correlation analysis of early renal injury in elderly patients with acute exacerbations of chronic obstructive pulmonary disease. COPD. 2022;17:2109–15.
24. Persy VP, Verhulst A, Ysebaert DK, De Greef KE, De Broe ME. Reduced postischemic macrophage infiltration and interstitial fibrosis in osteopontin knockout mice. Kidney Int. 2003;63(2):543–53.
25. Noiri E, Dickman K, Miller F, Romanov G, Romanov VI, Shaw R, et al. Reduced tolerance to acute renal ischemia in mice with a targeted disruption of the osteopontin gene. Kidney Int. 1999;56(1):74–82.
26. Steinbrenner I, Sekula P, Kotsis F, von Cube M, Cheng Y, Nadal J, et al. Association of osteopontin with kidney function and kidney failure in chronic kidney disease patients: the GCKD study. Nephrol Dial Transplant. 2023;38(6):1430–8.
27. Colhoun HM, Marcovecchio ML. Biomarkers of diabetic kidney disease. Diabetologia. 2018;61(5):996–1011.

28. Guo H, Cai CQ, Schroeder RA, Kuo PC. Osteopontin is a negative feedback regulator of nitric oxide synthesis in murine macrophages. J Immunol. 2001;166(2):1079–86.
29. Domagala W, Woźniak L, Lasota J, Weber K, Osborn M. Vimentin is preferentially expressed in high-grade ductal and medullary, but not in lobular breast carcinomas. Am J Pathol. 1990;137(5):1059–64.
30. Desai B, Rogers MJ, Chellaiah MA. Mechanisms of osteopontin and CD44 as metastatic principles in prostate cancer cells. Mol Cancer. 2007;6:18.
31. Kiss T, Jámbor K, Koroknai V, Szász I, Bárdos H, Mokánszki A, et al. Silencing Osteopontin expression inhibits proliferation, invasion and induce altered protein expression in melanoma cells. Pathol Oncol Res. 2021;27:581395.
32. Wolak T, Kim H, Ren Y, Kim J, Vaziri ND, Nicholas SB. Osteopontin modulates angiotensin II-induced inflammation, oxidative stress, and fibrosis of the kidney. Kidney Int. 2009;76(1):32–43.
33. Boumans MJH, Houbiers JGA, Verschueren P, Ishikura H, Westhovens R, Brouwer E, et al. Safety, tolerability, pharmacokinetics, pharmacodynamics and efficacy of the monoclonal antibody ASK8007 blocking osteopontin in patients with rheumatoid arthritis: a randomised, placebo controlled, proof-of-concept study. Ann Rheum Dis. 2012;71(2):180–5.
34. Armutcu F. Organ crosstalk: the potent roles of inflammation and fibrotic changes in the course of organ interactions. Inflamm Res. 2019;68(10):825–39.
35. Husain-Syed F, Birk HW, Ronco C, Schörmann T, Tello K, Richter MJ, et al. Doppler-derived renal venous stasis index in the prognosis of right heart failure. J Am Heart Assoc. 2019;8(21):e013584.
36. Domenech P, Perez T, Saldarini A, Uad P, Musso CG. Kidney-lung pathophysiological crosstalk: its characteristics and importance. Int Urol Nephrol. 2017;49(7):1211–5.
37. Khamissi FZ, Ning L, Kefaloyianni E, Dun H, Arthanarisami A, Keller A, et al. Identification of kidney injury released circulating osteopontin as causal agent of respiratory failure. Sci Adv. 2022;8(8):eabm5900.

Index

D. Battaglini et al. (eds.), *Organ System Crosstalk in Critical Illness*,
https://doi.org/10.1007/978-3-032-01024-7

J

K

M

FSC
www.fsc.org
MIX
Papier aus verantwortungsvollen Quellen
Paper from responsible sources
FSC® C105338

If you have any concerns about our products,
you can contact us on
ProductSafety@springernature.com

In case Publisher is established outside the EU,
the EU authorized representative is:
Springer Nature Customer Service Center GmbH
Europaplatz 3, 69115 Heidelberg, Germany

Printed by Libri Plureos GmbH
in Hamburg, Germany